Wound Closure Biomaterials and Devices

Wound Closure Biomaterials and Devices

Edited by

Chih-Chang Chu, Ph.D.
Fiber Science Program
Department of Textiles and Apparel
College of Human Ecology
and
Bioengineering Program
Cornell University
Ithaca, New York

J. Anthony von Fraunhofer, Ph.D., F.A.S.M., F.R.S.C.
Department of Restorative Dentistry
School of Dentistry University of Maryland at Baltimore
Baltimore, Maryland

Howard P. Greisler, M.D.
Department of Surgery
Department of Cell Biology, Neurobiology, and Anatomy
Stritch School of Medicine
Loyola University
and
Department of Surgery Hines V.A. Hospital
Maywood, Illinois

CRC Press
Boca Raton   Boston   London   New York   Washington, D.C.

Acquiring Editor:	Marsha Baker
Editorial Assistant	Jean Jarboe
Project Editor:	Gail Renard
Marketing Manager:	Susie Carlisle
Direct Marketing Manager:	Becky McEldowney
Cover Designer:	Dawn Boyd
PrePress:	Kevin Luong
Manufacturing:	Sheri Schwartz

Library of Congress Cataloging-in-Publication Data

Wound closure biomaterials and devices / edited by Chih-Chang Chu, J. Anthony
    von Fraunhofer, Howard P. Greisler.
            p.   cm.
        Includes bibliographical references and index.
        ISBN 0-8493-4964-8
        1. Ligature (Surgery). 2. Sutures. 3. Adhesives in surgery. I. Chu, Chih-Chang.
    II. Von Fraunhofer, J. A. (Joseph Anthony). III. Greisler, Howard P.
    RD73.L5W68   1996
    617′.9178—dc20
                                                                                96-8975
                                                                                    CIP

CONTRIBUTORS

Chih-Chang Chu, Ph.D.
Professor, Fiber Science Program
Department of Textiles & Apparel
College of Human Ecology and
  Bioengineering Program
Cornell University
Ithaca, New York
cc62@cornell.edu

J. Anthony von Fraunhofer, Ph.D., F.A.S.M., F.R.S.C.
Professor, Department of Restorative Dentistry
School of Dentistry
University of Maryland at Baltimore
Baltimore, Maryland
avf001@dental3.ab.umd.edu

Howard P. Greisler, M.D.
Professor, Department of Surgery
Department of Cell Biology,
  Neurobiology and Anatomy
Stritch School of Medicine
Loyola University
and
Department of Surgery
Hines V.A. Hospital
Maywood, Illinois
hgreisl@wpo.it.luc.edu

Mark K. Hirko, M.D.
Department of Surgery
North Side Medical Center
Youngstown, Ohio

Yoshito Ikada, D.Eng., D.Med.Sc.
Professor
Research Center for Biomedical Engineering
Kyoto University
Kyoto, Japan
yyikada@medeng.kyoto-u.ac.jp

William Irvin, M.D.
1030 S. Jefferson
Suite 110
Roanoke, Virginia

Steven S. Kang, M.D.
Assistant Professor of Surgery
Department of Surgery
Loyola University Medical Center
Maywood, Illinois
skang@wpo.it.luc.edu

Peter H. Lin, M.D.
Department of Surgery
Finch University of Health Science
The Chicago Medical School
Chicago, Illinois
LIN1906@aol.com

J. R. Perez-Sanz, M.D.
College of Medicine
University of Illinois–Chicago
Chicago, Illinois
and
Christ Hospital and Medical Center
Oak Lawn, Illinois
and
Little Company of Mary Hospital
Evergreen Park, Illinois

PREFACE

Wound closure biomaterials and devices have played a critical role in human survival since the dawn of history. It is not an overstatement to say that human lives have been saved by tiny threads of silk or linen almost since the beginning of time. Wound closure biomaterials have the longest history among all biomaterials. These biomaterials and devices concern every surgeon because every surgery or wound requires the use of biomaterials to close them for successful healing. The proper closing of wounds can influence the success of surgery. Many complications, such as infection, wound dehiscence, and sinus formation can occur in the wound closure line.

There are three types of wound closure biomaterials and devices: sutures, clips/staples, and tissue adhesives. Sutures are the most frequently used and have the longest history. As early as 4000 years ago, linen was used as a suture material. Since then, numerous materials like iron wire, gold, silver, dried gut, horse hair, strips of hide, bark fibers, silk, linen, and tendon have been used as suture materials. Among them, catgut and silk dominated the suture market until 1930. The introduction of synthetic polymers during and after World War II revolutionized the chemical origin of suture materials. The use of ligating clip/stapler systems in wound closure is relatively new and allows accurate apposition with minimal tension, reduced operating time, and easy removal. Further, these devices achieve good cosmetic results. Although metallic clips/staples have the longest history in this group, their use is limited to skin closure, and synthetic absorbable clips/staples have recently become the dominant player, particularly for tissues and organs beneath skin. Coover discovered tissue adhesives in the mid-1950s. Although they are not as popular as suture materials and clips/staples, particularly in the United States, they have a unique role among wound closure biomaterials. The significant advances in materials science and engineering over the past decades provide surgeons with a wide range of choices of wound closure biomaterials with vast differences in chemical, mechanical, biological and often biodegradable properties, and clinical performance. As a result of this continuous advance in materials, the art of wound closure has become far more complex and demanding. Although there has been fragmented review literature describing suture materials in the past two decades, to date there has been virtually no single English-language volume that systematically and comprehensively describes all required properties of available wound closure biomaterials and devices. We believe such a comprehensive and timely reference source for surgeons in the modern health care environment is long overdue.

Meeting the needs of surgeons is half of the goal of this book. Biomaterials scientists have played a crucial role in the research and development of wound closure biomaterials for the past several decades. Because of the multidisciplinary nature of wound closure biomaterials and devices, a book that will also satisfy biomaterials scientists and engineers must have ample information about structures and basic material properties, such as molecular weight, synthesis, and tensile properties, so that they can use the book as a major reference for future research and development of improved wound closure biomaterials and devices.

With these goals in mind, we are introducing this book to both the medical and biomaterials science/engineering communities. The book has five basic parts: wound healing, suture materials, clips/staples, tissue adhesives, and emerging new wound closure biomaterials. It has 12 chapters with a distinct emphasis on suture materials because of their preeminence in wound closure use. Coherence within this book has been maintained by linking and cross-referencing the contents of the 12 chapters. In doing this, we feel we have avoided the common failing of many monographs that resemble a series of unrelated reviews by different authors.

After the first chapter, *Introduction*, a review of the basics of wound healing, particularly relating to wound closure biomaterials, is given in Chapter 2. This chapter should provide readers with a reasonable background in the basic phenomena and some recent findings of wound healing that wound closure biomaterials experience all the time. Chapter 3, *Surgical Needles*, describes an integral part of sutures, particularly their biomechanical properties, that are frequently ignored in the published literature. Chapter 4, *Classification and General Characteristics of Suture Materials*, provides comprehensive classifications of suture materials in terms of size, biodegradability, physical form, and coating materials and an overview of four general characteristics that every suture material should have, namely physical/mechanical, handling, biocompatibility, and biodegradation, if applicable. Following an overview of suture materials in Chapter 4, Chapter 5, *Chemical Structure and Manufacturing Processes*, provides far more detailed information about the basic chemical properties of suture materials and how they are made. This chapter is written mainly for chemists, material scientists, and engineers rather than surgeons.

However, surgeons may use this chapter to acquire additional in-depth material information about the suture materials that they use every day.

Chapters 6 through 8 cover the three most important properties of suture materials in great detail, i.e., mechanical, biodegradable, and biological properties. These three chapters provide the core information for both the medical profession and materials scientists/engineers for their comprehensive understanding of the vast differences in the three most essential properties of suture materials. Several properties of suture materials that are often unfamiliar to the medical profession, such as viscoelasticity, carcinogenicity, and many new findings in biodegradation properties like computational chemical modeling of the biodegradation property of absorbable suture materials and plasma surface modification of absorbable sutures to alter their biodegradation properties, are also explained in these three chapters.

Chapter 9, *Suture Techniques and Selection*, is written primarily for surgeons and has practical information about the actual use of sutures in a variety of fields of surgery.

Chapters 10, *Ligating Clips and Staples*, and 11, *Tissue Adhesives*, provide detailed technical information about the other two types of wound closure biomaterials and devices. Because they are less frequently used than sutures, there are relatively few reported studies of these two alternative wound closure biomaterials and devices. However, the landscape of wound closure biomaterials and devices may change in the next century when new materials and technology emerge.

Chapter 12, *New Emerging Materials for Wound Closure*, provides a preview of some new inventions and developments that could have major impact on wound closure biomaterials and devices in the next century. Those wound closure biomaterials that are currently used outside the United States but have not been approved by the FDA are also mentioned in this chapter. This chapter also suggests the direction of new research and development efforts in wound closure biomaterials by addressing some of the challenging problems, such as efficient control of wound infection, the promotion of wound healing via the incorporation of growth factors into wound closure biomaterials/devices, control of their biodegradation behavior for better and more predictable wound healing in demanding clinical cases, and improved handling properties of sutures.

We have done our best to provide readers with the most up-to-date and core information that we could find in the published literature. We primarily limited our database to English journals to ensure timely publication and wider appeal. A lot of the information used in this book is from the authors' own research activities over the past several decades. Some of the information provided in this book is not yet in the public domain, such as pending patents. We have also tried our best to balance the content of this book between the needs of clinicians and basic biomaterials scientists/engineers. We wrote this book with two basic goals in mind: clinicians would be provided with a book that has much practical information for their daily practice while researchers of either biomaterials science/engineering or with a medical background would find that this book has a wealth of research information for their research and development work on wound closure biomaterials and devices.

Finally, we would particularly like to thank Dennis D. Jamiolkowski of Ethicon, Drs. Griffin Lewis and Walter Sabisiak of Davis & Geck, and Drs. C.K. Liu and Y. Jiang of US Surgical for their continuous support with samples, some illustrations, and information. We would also like to acknowledge the graduate students, postdoctoral fellows, and interns of the editors for their research work, upon which this book is largely based.

Chih-Chang Chu
Cornell University

Howard P. Greisler
Loyola University

J. Anthony von Fraunhofer
University of Maryland at Baltimore

DEDICATION

We would like to dedicate this book to

Martha A. Mutschler-Chu, Chen-Wei and Hope Ho-Hui Chu, and Shirley C. Chu, for their encouragement, patience, sacrifice, and understanding during those many evenings, weekends, and holidays that were consumed for the past two decades of R/D of wound closure biomaterials that led to the publication of this book.

C. C. Chu

Elizabeth, whose unswerving support, understanding, and social conscience have enabled me to not become my own enemy.

Howard P. Greisler

Nancy, for her patience and support, and to my friends for not letting me lose my sense of humor during the writing of this book.

J. Anthony von Fraunhofer

CONTENTS

Chapter 1

Introduction

C.C. Chu

Wound closure biomaterials and devices concern every surgeon. Every operation requires the use of biomaterials to close the wound for subsequent successful healing. The proper closing of wounds can influence the success of surgery. Many complications such as infection, wound dehiscence, and sinus formation occur in the wound closure line. The wound closure biomaterials required depend, to some extent, on the type of wound to be closed; however, all wound closure biomaterials must retain adequate tensile strength during the critical period of healing. They should also induce minimal tissue reaction that might interfere with the healing process.

The complexity involved in wound healing, such as the involvement of more than one type of tissue in a wound, the various degrees of wound strength during the process of healing, the exposure of the biomaterials to body fluids, or the variety of surgical wounds, each with its own healing problems, call for different types of wound closure materials. The choice of these biomaterials is based largely on the type of wound and surgeons' preferences.

In general, wound closure biomaterials are divided into three major categories: suture materials, staplers/ligating clips, and tissue adhesives. Sutures have received the most attention and are the most widely used in wound closure. Ligating clips and staplers facilitate anastomosis with minimal trauma, necrosis, or interruption of tissue function, and their use has steadily increased in specific clinical conditions, particularly the availability of synthetic absorbable ligating clips and staplers. Tissue adhesives are the least frequently used for wound closure at the present time, even though they received considerable attention in the 1960s.

A suture, by definition, is a strand of material, either natural or synthetic, used to ligate blood vessels and to approximate tissue together. Suture materials are the earliest and most frequent application of textile materials for surgical wound closure. As early as 4000 years ago, linen was used as a suture material. Since then, numerous materials have been used as ligatures and sutures: iron wire, gold, silver, dried gut, horse hair, strips of hide, bark fibers, silk, linen, and tendon. Among them, catgut and silk dominated the suture market until 1930. The introduction of steel wire and synthetic nonabsorbable fibers like nylon, polyester, and polypropylene during and after World War II greatly expanded the chemical composition of suture materials. During the early 1970s, the successful introduction of two synthetic absorbable suture materials, Dexon® (Davis & Geck Corp., Wayne, NJ) and Vicryl® (Ethicon, Inc., Somerville, NJ), opened a new chapter for suture materials. Owing to their precisely controlled manufacturing processes and uniform and reproducible properties, these absorbable biomaterials have received a great deal of attention from both surgeons and researchers. Recently several new synthetic absorbable suture materials like PDSII® (Ethicon), Maxon® (Davis & Geck), Monocryl® (Ethicon), and Biosyn® (US Surgical, Norwalk, CT) have been commercially available. The most important advantage of synthetic absorbable sutures is their reproducible degradability inside a biological environment. This property will enable the sutures to minimize chronic undesirable tissue reactions after the sutures have lost their function. Due to the development of these synthetic fibers, they have gradually replaced some natural fibers like cotton, linen, and catgut for wound closure purposes. Today, surgeons can choose among a large number of suture materials with various chemical, physical, mechanical, and biological properties.

The use of a ligating clip/stapler system in wound closure is relatively new. It allows accurate apposition with minimal tension and time and can be removed easily. It also has good cosmetic results. The earliest record of using ligating clips was found in early 1900 with metallic (i.e., silver) ligating clips. Subsequently, other metals like stainless steel and titanium have become available as ligating clip materials. Although these metallic wound closure devices have become acceptable for securing anastomosis, particularly in the regions difficult to access, the handling property, radiolucency, and tissue reactions of these metallic clips were the major concerns until the introduction in the 1980s of synthetic biodegradable clips/staplers based on glycolide-lactide copolymers and polydioxanone. These biodegradable clips/staplers have largely replaced nonbiodegradable metallic ones for internal use, but metallic clips/staplers still dominate external use (e.g., skin closure).

H.W. Coover discovered tissue adhesives in the mid-1950s. Although they are not as popular as suture materials, particularly in the United States, they have a unique role among wound closure biomaterials. Unlike sutures, which hold the wound together mechanically, tissue adhesives chemically bond to the wounded tissues. Some surgeons prefer tissue adhesives over suture materials in certain types of surgery, such as joining blood vessels and closing lacerated solid organs. The special environment of tissues, their regenerative capacity, biodegradability, and tissue reactions to biodegradable products, however, make tissue adhesives more difficult to develop. The most representative tissue adhesives come from either the homologs of alkyl-α-cyanoacrylates or fibrin glues. They are used most frequently in the anastomosis of blood vessels and the small and large intestine. Other applications, such as the treatment of fragile tissues in liver, spleen, and kidney wounds, and in repairing ophthalmological, genitourinary, and cardiovascular systems, have also been reported. Even though tissue adhesives have certain advantages over suture materials, such as hemostatic capability and the lesser degree of tissue deformation that is important in plastic surgery, better properties like biodegradability and biocompatibility are required for satisfactory sutureless closure of wounds with these tissue adhesives. Several recent advances in biomaterials have addressed these critical concerns.

One of the greatest concerns surrounding all wound closure biomaterials is the degree of tissue response. These responses range from an inflammatory reaction due to the trauma of insertion and foreign body reaction due to the chemical, physical, and mechanical properties of the wound closure biomaterials. For optimal wound healing, it is critical to minimize these reactions because the healing process, its rate, and complications are greatly influenced by the tissue reactions elicited by wound closure biomaterials. The degree of tissue reaction depends not only on the chemical and physical nature of the wound closure biomaterials and the type of tissues, but also on the mass of the biomaterials and the duration of their presence in the tissue, i.e., the biodegradation rate. It is thus ideal to have wound closure biomaterials like sutures that would serve their function satisfactorily during the critical wound healing period and then quickly disappear once they are not needed. The longer a wound closure biomaterial stays within the body, the more probable it is to serve as the nidus for undesirable tissue reactions that could delay and interfere with normal wound healing,[1,2] predisposition to wound infection,[3–15] the formation of suture granuloma and sinus[16–28] and calculi,[29–34] tissue adhesion,[35,36] thrombogenicity,[37–43] and anastomotic stricture.[44,45] Existing experimental evidence suggests that the extent of inflammatory reaction that a wound closure biomaterial elicits is related to the level of strength that a wound can reach. This, in turn, makes wound closure biomaterials like sutures more or less liable to "cut out." For example, Everett reported that sutures that generate a marked tissue response are more likely to cut out and weaken wound strength because an excessive inflammatory reaction may lead to edema and the subsequent weakening of the surrounding tissues with disruption of collagen fibers.[1] Barham et al. reported that the wound strength in the rectus muscle of rabbits is greater when closed with polyglycolide (Dexon) than with chromic catgut.[2] By 90 days, the Dexon-sutured wound had begun to plateau near a maximum strength, while chromic catgut-sutured wounds reached a lower wound strength than those sutured with Dexon.

The incidences of these undesirable tissue reactions reported in the literature indicate the importance of a timely shortening of the presence of the mass of wound closure biomaterials in tissues after the biomaterial serves its intended function. Although existing absorbable wound closure biomaterials, in general, are better than nonabsorbable ones to achieve such a goal, some absorbable sutures like PDS and Maxon developed in the 1980s, may not have the advantage of Dexon and Vicryl absorbable sutures (in terms of the rate of mass absorption) due to their prolonged mass retention (about 6 to 8 months *in vivo*).

An ideal wound closure biomaterial or device, thus, should have the following properties:

- Handle comfortably and naturally
- Cause minimum tissue reaction
- Have adequate tensile strength and knot security
- Be unfavorable for bacterial growth and easily sterilized
- Be nonelectrolytic, noncapillary, nonallergenic, and noncarcinogenic

As a result of recent progress in the field of wound closure biomaterials and devices, medical professionals are faced with an increasing challenge in selecting the proper wound closure biomaterials from a vast number of available biomaterials. The traditional way of choosing wound closure biomaterials, particularly with suture materials (largely based on habit and the surgeon's training background), is gradually becoming inappropriate. Although the principle for wound closure biomaterials selection is to choose those biomaterials and devices that provide the most secure wound approximation for an adequate time with minimal adverse effect on the normal wound healing process, Bennett recently listed many factors to consider in suture selection.[46] They are: presence of infection, tissue characteristics, wound location, tension on wound edges, age and medical condition of patient, cosmoses, color, speed, and cost. Some guidelines Bennett suggested are that sutures should not be used in tissues that tear easily or lack vascular supply; softer sutures like silk would be more comfortable for patients than stainless steel, monofilament nylon, or polypropylene sutures for mucosal or intertriginous wounds; a larger caliber suture should be used if wound edges are under great tension.

There are several review publications on the subject of wound closure biomaterials,[46–58] but due to page limitation, most have limited scope. The purpose of this book is to comprehensively and system-atically review all available information on wound closure biomaterials and devices in the literature. It is our hope that such a comprehensive review will not only assist medical professionals in their selection of these biomaterials and devices, but will also provide scientists and researchers with a coherent understanding of this field and useful information for the future design of even better wound closure devices. All aspects of wound closure biomaterials, their classification, type, and chemical, physical, mechanical, biological, and biodegradation properties along with surgical techniques in a few critical branches of surgery will be covered. However, the emphasis will be on suture materials because they are the most frequently used and studied.

REFERENCES

1. Everett, W.G., Suture materials in general surgery, *Progr. Surg.*, 8, 14, 1970.
2. Barham, R.E., Butz, G.W., and Ansell, J.S., Comparison of wound strength in normal, radiated, and infected tissues closed with polyglycolic acid and chromic catgut sutures, *Surg. Gynecol. Obstet.*, 146, 901, 1978.
3. Elek, S.D. and Conen, P.E., The influence of staphylococcus pyogenes for man; a study of the problems of wound infection, *Br. J. Exp. Pathol.*, 38, 573, 1957.
4. Edlich, R.F., Panek, P.H., et al., Physical and chemical configuration of sutures in the development of surgical infection, *Ann. Surg.*, 177, 679, 1973.
5. Paterson-Brown, S., Cheslyn-Curtis, S., Biglin, J., et al., Suture materials in contaminated wounds: a detailed comparison of new suture with those currently used, *Br. J. Surg.*, 74, 734, 1987.
6. Alexander, J.W., Kaplan, J.Z., and Altemeier, W.A., Role of suture materials in the development of wound infection, *Ann. Surg.*, 165, 192, 1967.
7. Blomstedt, B. and Osterberg, B., Suture materials and wound infection: an experimental study, *Acta Chir. Scand.*, 144, 269, 1978.
8. Osterberg, B. and Blomstedt, B., Effect of suture materials on bacterial survival in infected wounds: an experimental study, *Acta Chir. Scand.*, 145, 431, 1979.
9. Varma, S., Johnson, L.W., Ferguson, H.L., et al., Tissue reaction to suture materials in infected surgical wounds — A histopathologic evaluation, *Am. J. Vet. Res.*, 42, 563, 1981.
10. Torsello, G.B., Sandmann, W., et al., Experimental studies with absorbable and non-absorbable sutures in infected canine arterial anastomoses, *J. Vasc. Surg.*, 3, 135, 1986.
11. Cameron, A.E., Parker, C.J., Field, E.S., et al., A randomised comparison of polydioxanone (PDS) and polypropylene (Prolene) for abdominal wound closure, *Ann. R. Coll. Surg. Engl.*, 69, 113, 1987.
12. McHenry, M.C., Longworth, D.L., Rehm, S.J., Keys, T.F., Moon, H.K., Cosgrove, D.M., and Loop, F.D., Infections of the cardiac suture line after left ventricular surgery, *Am. J. Med.*, 85, 292, 1988.
13. Bucknall, T.E., Teare, L., and Ellis, H., Infectivity of suture materials used in abdominal wound closure, *Eur. Surg. Res.*, 13(1), 64, 1981.
14. Corder, A.P., Schache, D.J., Farquharson, S.M., and Tristram, S., Wound infection following high saphenous ligation. A trial comparing two skin closure techniques: subcuticular polyglycolic acid and interrupted monofilament nylon mattress sutures, *J. R. Coll. Surg. Edinburgh*, 36, 100, 1991.
15. Ananthakrishnan, N., et al., Bacterial adherence to cotton and silk sutures, *Natl. Med. J. India*, 5, 217, 1992.
16. Bucknall, T.E. and Ellis, H., Abdominal wound closure — A comparison of monofilament nylon and polyglycolic acid, *Surgery*, 89, 672, 1981.
17. Corman, M.L., Veidenheimer, M.C., and Coller, J.A., Controlled clinical trial of three suture materials for abdominal wall closure after bowel operations, *Am. J. Surg.*, 141, 510, 1981.
18. Bartone, F., Shore, N., Newland, J., et al., The best suture for hypospadias?, *Urology*, 29, 517, 1987.
19. Murphy, J.R., Shay, S.S., Moses, F.M., Braxton, J., Jaques, D.P., and Wong, R.K.H., Suture granuloma masquerading as malignancy of the biliary tract, *Dig. Dis. Sci.*, 35, 1176, 1990.
20. Katz, P.G., Crawford, J.P., and Hackler, R.H., Infected suture granuloma simulating mass of urachal origin: case report, *J. Urol.*, 135, 782, 1986.
21. Gleeson, M.J. and McMullin, J.P., Suture granuloma simulating a cholangiocarcinoma, *Br. J. Surg.*, 74, 1181, 1987.

22. Impieri, M., Suture granuloma of the greater omentum simulating tumor, *Ann. Chir.*, 40, 313, 1984.

23. Eldridge, P.R. and Wheeler, M.H., Stitch granulomata after thyroid surgery, *Br. J. Surg.*, 74, 62, 1987.

24. Nirankari, V.S., Karesh, J.W., and Richards, R.D., Complications of exposed monofilament sutures, *Am. J. Opthalmol.*, 95, 515, 1983.

25. Scheidler, D.M., Foster, R.S., Bihrle, R., Scott, J.W., and Litwiller, S.E., Anastomotic suture granuloma following radical retropubic prostatectomy, *J. Urol.*, 143, 133, 1990.

26. Lynch, T.H., Waymont, B., Beacock, C.J., Michael, D., and Wallace, A., Paravesical suture granuloma: a problem following herniorrhaphy, *J. Urol.*, 147, 460, 1992.

27. Pearl, G.S. and Someren, A., Suture granuloma simulating bladder neoplasm, *Urology*, 15, 304, 1980.

28. Fink, G. et al., Suture granuloma simulating lung neoplasm occurring after segmentectomy, *Thorax*, 48, 405, 1993.

29. Kaminski, J.M., Katz, A.R., and Woodward, S.C., Urinary bladder calculus formation on sutures in rabbits, cats, and dogs, *Surg. Gynecol. Obstet.*, 146, 353, 1978.

30. Gorham, S.D., Anderson, J.D., Monsour, M.J., et al., The *in vitro* assessment of a collagen/vicryl (polyglactin) composite film together with candidate suture materials for use in urinary tract surgery. II. Suture deposition of urinary salts, *Urol. Res.*, 16, 111, 1988.

31. Kirby, B.M., Knoll, J.S., Manley, P.A., and Miller, L.M., Calcinosis circumscripta associated with polydioxanone suture in two young dogs, *Vet. Surg.*, 18, 216, 1989.

32. Morris, M.C., Baquero, A., Redovan, E., Mahoney, E., and Bannett, A.D., Urolithiasis on absorbable and nonabsorbable suture materials in the rabbit bladder, *J. Urol.*, 135, 602, 1986.

33. Stacey-Clear, A., McCathy, K.A., Hall, D.A., Pile-Spellman, E.R., Mrose, H.E., White, G., Cardenosa, G., Sawicka, J., Mahoney, E., and Kopans, D. B., Calcified suture material in the breast after radiation therapy, *Radiology*, 183, 207, 1992.

34. Davis, S.P., Stomper, P.C., Weidner, N., and Meyer, J.E., Suture calcification mimicking recurrence in the irradiated breast: a potential pitfall in mammographic evaluation, *Radiology*, 172, 247, 1989.

35. Vallfors, B., Hansson, H., and Svensson, J., Absorbable or nonabsorbable suture materials for closure of the dura mater, *Neurosurgery*, 9, 407, 1981.

36. Hurd, W.W. et al., Etiology of closure-related adhesion formation after wedge resection of the rabbit ovary, *J. Reprod. Med.*, 38, 465, 1993.

37. Friberg, L.G., Mellgren, G.W., Eriksson, B.D., et al., Subclavian flap angioplasty with absorbable suture polydioxanone (PDS). An experimental study in growing piglets, *Scand. J. Thorac. Cardiovasc. Surg.*, 21, 9, 1987.

38. Chiu, I.S., Hung, C.R., Chao, S.F., et al., Growth of the aortic anastomosis in pigs. Comparison of continuous absorbable suture with nonabsorbable sutures, 1, *J. Thorac. Cardiovasc. Surg.*, 95, 112, 1988.

39. Torsello, G., Schwartz, A., Aulich, A., et al., Absorbable polydioxanone suture for venous anastomoses: experimental studies using venography and transluminal angioscopy, *Eur. J. Vasc. Surg.*, 1, 319, 1987.

40. Pae, W.E., Waldhausen, J.A., Prophet, G.A., and Pierce, W.S., Primary vascular anastomosis in growing pigs: comparison of polypropylene and polyglycolic acid sutures, *J. Thorac. Cardiovasc. Surg.*, 81, 921, 1981.

41. Sauvage, L.R. and Harkins, H.N., Growth of vascular anastomoses: experimental study of influence of suture type and suture method with note or certain mechanical factors involved, *Bull. Johns Hopkins Hosp.*, 91, 276, 1952.

42. Tawes, R.L., Jr., Aberdeen, E., et al., The growth of an aortic anastomosis: an experimental study in piglets, *Surgery*, 64, 1122, 1968.

43. Dahlke, H., Dociu, N., and Thurau, K., Thrombogenicity of different suture materials as revealed by scanning electron microscopy, *J. Biomed. Mater. Res.*, 14, 251, 1980.

44. Gillatt, D.A., Corfield, A.P., May, R.E., et al., Polydioxanone suture in the gastrointestinal tract, *Ann. R. Coll. Surg. Engl.*, 69, 54, 1987.

45. Kawakami, K. et al., Modes of biliobiliaryanastomosis in relation to the healing process and occurrence of postoperative stricture, *Surg. Today*, 23, 51, 1993.

46. Bennett, R.G., Selection of wound closure materials, *J. Am. Acad. Dermatol.*, 18, 619, 1988.

47. Guttman, B. and Guttmann, H., Sutures: properties, uses, and clinical investigation, in *Polymeric Biomaterials*, Dumitriu, S., Ed., Marcel Dekker, New York, 1994, chap. 10.

48. Benicewicz, B.C. and Hopper, P., Polymers for absorbable surgical sutures, Part I., *J. Bioactiv. Compatible Polyms.*, 5, 453, 1990.

49. Jódar, M.R., Bel, P.E., and Suñé, A.J.M., Synthetic absorbable suture materials I. Properties and thread length., *Ciencia Pharm.*, 2(1), 47, 1992.

50. Jódar, M.R., Bel, P.E., and Suñé, A.J.M., Synthetic absorbable suture materials. II. Test of the diameter or caliber, *Ciencia Pharm.*, 2, 292, 1992.

51. Jódar, M.R., Bel, P.E., Suñé-Negre, J.M., and Suñé, A.J.M., Synthetic absorbable suture materials III. Tension strength test (Part 2), *Ciencia Pharm.*, 3(2), 88, 1993.

52. Stone, I.K., Suture materials, *Clin. Obstet. Gynecol.*, 31, 712, 1988.

53. Chu, C.C., Suture materials, in *Concise Encyclopedia of Medical & Dental Materials*, Williams, D.F., Ed., Pergamon Press, New York, 1990, 346.

54. Chu, C.C., Suture materials, in *Encyclopedia of Materials Science and Engineering*, vol. 6, Beaver, M.B., Ed., Pergamon Press, New York, 1986, 4826.

55. Chu, C.C., The degradation and biocompatibility of suture materials, *Crit. Rev. Biocompat.*, 1, 261, 1985.

56. Chu, C.C., Survey of clinically important wound closure biomaterials, in *Biocompatible Polymers, Metals, and Composites,* Michael Szycher, Ed., Sponsored by Society for Plastics Engineers, Technomic, Westport, CT, 1983.

57. Chu, C.C., Biodegradable suture materials: intrinsic and extrinsic factors affecting biodegradation phenomena, in *Encyclopedic Handbook of Biomaterials and Bioengineering*, Part A: Materials, Vol. 1, Wise, D.L., Altobelli, D.E., Schwartz, E.R., Yszemski, M., Gresser, J.D., and Trantolo, D.J., Eds., Marcel Dekker, 1995, 543-688.

58. Chu, C.C., Degradation and biocompatibility of synthetic absorbable suture materials: general biodegradation phenomena and some factors affecting biodegradation, in *Biomedical Applications of Synthetic Biodegradable Polymers,* Hollinger, J., Ed., CRC Press, Boca Raton, FL, 1995, 103.

Chapter 2

Wound Healing and Inflammatory Response to Biomaterials

P. H. Lin, M. K. Hirko, J. A. von Fraunhofer, and H. P. Greisler

CONTENTS

I. INTRODUCTION

In the past few years, there has been a dramatic increase in the number of implantable biomaterials. These biomedical devices, constructed from a variety of materials and designed to perform many different functions, are today routinely implanted throughout the body. The underlying efficacy of a device is dependent upon not only its mechanical properties, such as physical shape, size, strength, and chemical nature, but also the tissue bed in which it is placed.[1] The implantation of biomaterials initiates both an inflammatory reaction to injury as well as mechanisms to induce healing.[2-4] Implantation of nonresorbable biomaterials, for instance, can cause a permanent alteration in the microenvironment surrounding the implant and in the tissues into which they are implanted. The extent to which the inflammatory reaction and healing mechanisms are activated is a measure of the host reactions to the biomaterial and ultimately may lead to: (1) impairment of functional capacity or (2) permanent biocompatibility of the biomedical device.

Implanted biomaterials elicit both local and systemic responses.[5] Examples of local tissue responses include inflammation, necrosis, and neoplastic transformation. Because the implantation of a bioprosthetic device generally leads to a surgical tissue defect, the local tissue response is the result of the influence of the device on the normal wound-healing process. Systemic responses to biomaterials include end-organ destruction, distant carcinogenicity, and adverse allergic/immunological reactions. An understanding of the biological response to biomaterials is essential for the effective utilization of medical devices. Although this chapter discusses wound healing, its primary focus is on the cell biology of inflammatory responses educed by biomaterial implantation along with their effect on the processes of wound healing and biocompatibility.

II. BIOLOGICAL TISSUES

At its simplest, tissue may be defined as a layer or group of similarly specialized cells that conjointly perform certain functions. There are many different types of tissues throughout the body and they differ markedly in composition, structure, strength, and function. There are, for example, very obvious differences between dental enamel, bone, and soft tissue such as skin. In this chapter, attention is directed primarily toward the soft tissues. Nevertheless, there are still marked differences in the structure and composition of the soft tissues as well as in their functions, and the latter, as well as such parameters as tensile strength and tear resistance, are determined in large part by the inherent properties of the tissue. An indication of the relative strengths of a variety of soft tissues is given in Table 2.1. It should be noted, however, that the strength and other properties of the same tissue are subject to individual

8

8

Table 2.1 Relative Tensile
Strength of Soft Tissues

Bladder	Weak
Cecum	Weak
Duodenum	Strong
Fascia	Strong
Ileum	Strong
Intestine	Weak
Respiratory tract	Weak
Skin	Strong

variation and, indeed, for the same person there can be wide variations in the properties of the same type of tissue in different areas of the body, e.g., skin. Further, the mechanical properties of tissue vary with patient age, gender, race, and health status, a common phenomenon being the "brittle bones" of elderly people. The healing propensity of soft tissue and the rate of healing after injury are generally not related to the strength of the tissue before injury. Thus the intestines generally have low tensile strength but heal quickly, while skin and fascia, which have high tensile strengths, heal more slowly.

The healing of wounds and incisions is a complex dynamic process that can be separated into a series of phases (see Figure 2.1 and Table 2.2), each characterized by the integrated actions of different cells. In the initial phase of wound healing, there is an inflammatory response that induces an outpouring of tissue fluids into the wound, an increased blood supply to the wound, and cellular and fibroblast proliferation. This inflammatory response is discussed in detail in the following sections. Phase I occurs over a period of 1 to 5 days. In the second phase of wound healing, roughly from day 5 to day 14, there is increased collagen formation and deposition within the wound, together with formation of fibrin and fibronectin through fibroblastic activity, and the wound closure/contraction commences. There is also formation of granulation tissue together with recanalization of lymphatics and bud formation by blood vessels. Phase II gradually merges into Phase III, day 14 onward, and there is reorganization and maturation (crosslinking) of the collagen fibers together with deposition of fibrous connective tissue, the latter resulting in scar formation. There is increased wound contraction together with revascularization, although the formation of new blood vessels decreases with progressive maturation of the collagen. It should be noted, as indicated above, the rate of wound healing varies with the type of tissue undergoing repair and is also dependent upon numerous other factors.

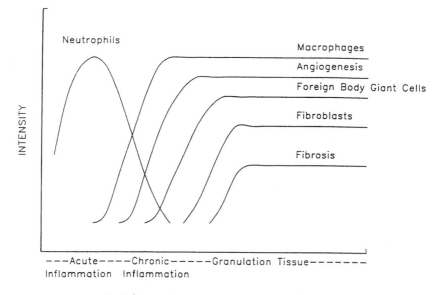

Figure 2.1 Inflammatory response to biomaterials.

Table 2.2 Phases
in Wound Healing

Phase I
Inflammation
Cellular proliferation
Phase II
Collagen synthesis
Phase III
Collagen remodeling
Collagen maturation

Complications in wound healing and their attendant delays commonly result from two primary causes, infection and mechanical effects. The infectious causes of delayed wound healing are commonly cellulitis or abscess formation, while mechanical failures most frequently involve dehiscence or hernia, the two effects often operating independently of each other although there can be a cause-and-effect relationship.[6,7]

The healing process outlined above and in Table 2.2 and Figure 2.1 is commonly referred to as *healing by primary intention* or *primary union* and occurs when there is no infection, minimal edema (swelling) or fluid discharge, and the wound edges are approximated. Under such conditions, scar formation is minimized and wound healing occurs rapidly and without incident. However, where there is infection, severe trauma, poor approximation of the tissues, or tissue loss, the wound may not heal by primary union and the healing process is both prolonged and more complex. Under such circumstances, the process is known as *healing by secondary intention,* and the wound may be left open with healing occurring from within the wound outward. Granulation tissue (see Sections III.C and V) forms within the wound and affects closure, although the wound is usually characterized by granulation and scar tissue. Finally, when two surfaces or edges of granulation tissue are approximated, the situation is known as *delayed primary closure* or *healing by third intention.* This approach is used for contaminated and/or infected wounds or if there is extensive tissue loss due to trauma, typically from accident-related injuries and wounding. Again, the wound is left open after extensive cleaning and debridement of dead or severely damaged tissue, with wound healing occurring through formation of granulation tissue deep within the wound. Subsequently, the skin edges and deeper tissues are approximated. Wound healing will be addressed again when granulation tissue is discussed in Section III.C.

III. INFLAMMATION AND WOUND HEALING

The implantation of bioprosthetic devices into tissues by either surgical or transcutaneous catheter techniques involves the creation of a tissue defect or wound. The subsequent inflammatory response is dependent both on the size of the wound as well as the physical and chemical nature of the implanted device. An early stage in the process of wound healing involves the initiation of the inflammatory response. Just as the initiation and the magnitude of inflammation are modulated by the physical and chemical properties of the biomaterial, the resolution of the inflammatory process is likewise dependent upon these characteristics. For example, a biomaterial may leach corrosive substances from its structural matrix and interfere with the surrounding stroma needed for wound repair. These chemical and physical attributes will determine the overall scope of the wound healing process and hence the biocompatibility of the implant.

Inflammation is qualitatively separated into acute and chronic inflammation. Although these designations are somewhat simplistic and arbitrary, they assist in identifying some of the important aspects of the inflammatory process and serve as valuable teaching tools. In reality, an inflammatory response should be considered more as a continuous spectrum of cellular events with overlapping histologic characteristics. The temporal sequence of inflammatory reaction and healing response following implantation of a biomaterial is illustrated in Figure 2.2. The normal foreign body reaction appears to persist for the life of the implant. However, the components of the normal foreign body reaction to the implant may vary. The chemical and physical properties of the biomaterial may be responsible for the variations in the intensity and duration of the inflammatory and wound healing responses.

Acute inflammation represents a stereotypic response, generally of short duration and lasting less than a week. It is characterized by an increased capillary permeability which results in the exudation of

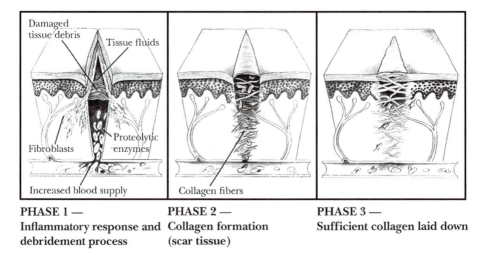

PHASE 1 —
Inflammatory response and
debridement process

PHASE 2 —
Collagen formation
(scar tissue)

PHASE 3 —
Sufficient collagen laid down

Figure 2.2 Three phases of tissue response to injury.

plasma proteins and emigration of polymorphonuclear neutrophilic leukocytes (PMN) to the site of inflammation. Chronic inflammation is of longer duration and is histologically associated with macrophages, lymphocytes, proliferation of connective tissues, deposition of matrix proteins, and capillary neogenesis. During the chronic inflammatory response, one often observes macrophages surrounding the biomaterial to form foreign body giant cells. These giant cells act to surround and "wall off" the biomaterial, remaining in the immediate vicinity for the duration of the implantation.

A. ACUTE INFLAMMATION

Acute inflammation is of relatively short duration, lasting from minutes to days, depending on the extent of tissue injury caused by the surgical implantation of the biomaterial. The main characteristics of acute inflammation are the exudation of fluid and plasma proteins (edema) and the emigration of leukocytes, predominantly neutrophils. During the implantation of a biomedical material, there is vascular and cellular damage exposing collagen and basement membrane to circulating platelets.[8] As a result, these platelets release their phospholipids to stimulate the intrinsic pathway of coagulation, while injured cells release thromboplastin to activate the extrinsic pathway of coagulation.

The aggregating platelets also release a variety of proteases, growth factors, and chemotactic substances that play roles in the activation of the complement pathway, recruitment of leukocytes, and the initiation of cellular proliferation.[9] During the acute phase of inflammation, the leukocytes degrade and ingest bacteria, immune complexes, and cell debris through the release of lysosomal enzymes and proteases (Table 2.3). However, the release of these enzymes and toxic free radicals from neutrophils can perpetuate the inflammatory process.[2]

Table 2.3 Neutrophil Products

Neutral proteases	**Prostaglandins**
Collagenase	**Platelet-activating factor**
Gelatinase	**Oxygen metabolites**
Elastase	Superoxide anion
Cathepsin D	Hydroxyl radicals
	Hydrogen peroxide
Lysosomal components	Hypochlorous acid
Cationic proteins	
Leukotriene B4	

From Shankar, R. and Greisler, H.P., in *Implantation Biology*, CRC Press, Boca Raton, 1994, 70.

The recruitment of leukocytes, particularly neutrophils and monocytes, to the site of implantation is one of the striking events in inflammation. Investigations on this topic have reported that leukocyte stimulation follows a series of processes that include margination, adhesion, emigration, phagocytosis, and extracellular release of leukocyte products.[10] This recruitment is also initiated and controlled by specific mechanisms involved in endothelial-leukocyte recognition. These mechanisms regulate not only the type of leukocyte that is stimulated, but also the stage of the inflammatory response and the site of recruitment.[11] Examples are recruitment of eosinophils to the site of allergic reactions and neutrophils to biomaterial-induced acute inflammation.

Recruitment of leukocytes is a dynamic process mediated by expression of specific cell surface adhesion molecules on endothelial cells (EC) and leukocytes.[12] Mechanisms of interaction include stimulation of leukocyte adhesion molecules (C5a, leukotriene B4), stimulation of endothelial adhesion molecules (interleukin 1, IL-1), or both effects (tumor necrosis factor, TNF).[13] A single adhesion receptor may be involved in multiple endothelial cell-leukocyte interactions. For example, E-selectin (ELAM-1) has been found to bind to neutrophils, T-lymphocytes, and monocytes *in vitro*.[14]

Shortly after the implantation of the biomaterial, circulating neutrophils interact with the capillary endothelium at the tissue injury site. The process of neutrophil adhesion to endothelial cells is initiated by the "rolling" of the neutrophil within the capillaries along the affected region. Antibodies to the neutrophil's L-selectin (LECAM) inhibit this "rolling" or "margination," [15] suggesting a role of L-selectin in the initial "rolling" phase of neutrophil-endothelial cell interaction. Cell culture studies have indicated that L-selectin perhaps participates in these interactions by presenting the appropriate neutrophil ligands to the E- and P-selectin on the vascular endothelium.[16] While neutrophils in circulation constitutively possess high levels of L-selectin and thus can interact with agonist-stimulated endothelial cells to initiate the process of adhesion, endothelial cells lining the blood vessels express E-selectin, intercellular adhesion molecule 1 (ICAM-1) and vascular cell adhesion molecule 1 (VCAM-1) only when stimulated by agonists such as bacterial lipopolysaccharides (LPS), cytokines like IL-1 and TNF, as well as the coagulation protease thrombin.[11,17–20]

Following the initial "rolling" phase, neutrophils shed their cell surface L-selectin[21] and undergo an upregulation of the surface expression of leukocyte adhesion receptor CD 11b/CD18, which is an activation-dependent receptor.[12,22] Inflammatory mediators such as cytokines and TNF have been found to stimulate a rapid increase in CD11b/CD18 on the leukocyte surface and enhance leukocyte adhesion to endothelium.[13] Recent studies involving antibody identification confirm that such neutrophil activation occurs *in vivo* at the site of inflammation.[21] The expression of activation-dependent adhesion receptors is now considered responsible for the stable attachment of neutrophils to endothelial cells, which will lead to transendothelial migration of neutrophils to the site of inflammation. Once lipid modulators and chemotactic peptides stimulate neutrophil adhesion to endothelial cells, the adhesive process should be rapid and have the capacity for regulation. *In vitro* studies with cultured endothelial cells have shown that neutrophil adhesion to endothelial cells can be induced within the first 2 min. Furthermore, this stimulation can be downregulated by removing the agonists.[23–26]

Neutrophil and endothelial cell expression of adhesion receptors, alone, is not enough to recruit neutrophils to the inflammatory site. The unidirectional migration of neutrophils toward the site of inflammation is also a function of various chemotactic stimuli. The most potent chemotactic stimuli to neutrophils are bacterial products,[27] components of the complement system (especially C5a[28]), products of the lipoxygenase pathway such as leukotriene B4,[29] platelet factor 4,[30] and cytokines such as IL-8.[31,32] Similar to leukocyte adhesion to endothelial cells, leukocyte chemotaxis is also mediated by the existence of specific leukocyte receptors for different chemotactic agents. Furthermore, at higher concentrations chemotactic agents initiate leukocyte activation, which leads to leukocyte degranulation and secretion.[2] Chemotactic agents can also increase the adhesiveness of neutrophils to endothelial cells by activation of adhesion receptors on endothelium.[33]

Additionally, plasma proteins that are adsorbed onto the biomaterial can act as chemotactic stimuli to neutrophils. Reports indicate that plasma and tissue proteins begin to adsorb onto the biomaterial nearly instantaneously following implantation.[34] This protein adsorption is a function of the following: concentration of protein in circulation, its diffusion coefficient, and the nature of the biomaterial such as its hydrophobicity, charge distribution, etc.[35,36] The net result of this complicated process is the emigration of neutrophils from between the endothelial cells to the subendothelial space.

In order for the neutrophils to reach the inflammatory region, they still have to travel through the basement membrane and intervening interstitial connective tissue. The exact mechanism by which this is accomplished is poorly understood. The process of migration via the connective tissue matrix resembles the biochemical processes associated with tumor cell invasion.[37] The first step in neutrophil penetration of basement membrane is adhesion of the neutrophil to the membrane glycoproteins, especially laminin.[38,39] Along with functioning as an attachment factor, laminin also has been shown to act as a neutrophil chemotactic agent, particularly when studied utilizing *in vitro* Boyden chamber experiments.[38] Next, neutrophils move through the basement membrane and connective tissue by secreting proteolytic enzymes that degrade the matrix components in the immediate microenvironment. The final phase involves the locomotion of the neutrophil through extracellular matrix. This neutrophil locomotion appears to be three-dimensional, the path of movement aligned to the direction of matrix fibers.[40-42]

Following recruitment of leukocytes to the area of inflammation, neutrophils begin to actively phagocytose bacteria and, when possible, the foreign material. Although the biomaterials in most instances cannot be phagocytosed due to their size, some aspects of phagocytosis do occur. Neutrophils attach to the biomaterial, especially when it is coated by naturally occurring serum factors called opsonins.[43] The two major opsonins are immunoglobulin G (IgG) and the complement-activated fragment C3b. Both neutrophils and macrophages possess specific adhesion receptors for these opsonins. Because of the size disparity between the biomaterial surface and the attached cells, "frustrated phagocytosis" may occur.[43,44] This process does not involve intracellular incorporation of the biomaterial but does result in the release of several lysosomal enzymes, proteases, and free radicals in an attempt to degrade the biomaterial. The amount of the lytic agents released by the neutrophil is dependent on the size, texture, and composition of the biomaterial particles.[45] In fact, the larger the particle, the greater is the secretion of leukocyte products. This suggests that the size of the implant and the proportion of particles in the implant that may be phagocytosed may modulate the degree of inflammatory response provoked by a particular biomaterial implant.

B. CHRONIC INFLAMMATION

Acute inflammation can take any one or a combination of the following courses:

1. Be totally resolved if the injury is mild and/or superficial
2. Induce formation of scar tissue if the original injury included substantial tissue destruction and/or when the inflammation occurs in the nonregenerative tissue
3. Result in abscess formation if there is an unresolved bacterial infection
4. Enter the chronic inflammatory phase

Chronic inflammation is characterized by mononuclear cell infiltration, primarily macrophages, lymphocytes, and plasma cells, with proliferation of fibroblasts and connective tissue elements, and capillary neogenesis. The progression of acute to chronic inflammation in tissues implanted with foreign biomaterials involves: (1) the chemical and physical nature/properties of the specific biomaterials; and (2) movement of the biomaterial at the implant site.[45]

Lymphocytes and plasma cells are involved primarily in immune reactions and play a key role in antibody production and delayed hypersensitivity responses. Although these cells are also present in nonimmunologic inflammatory reactions, their role is far from clear. Further, the interactions between biomaterials and lymphocytes are largely unknown. Lymphocytes can be activated by the presence of antigens. Activated lymphocytes can secrete lymphokines such as γ-interferon and interleukin-2 (IL-2) that stimulate monocyte chemotaxis, as well as macrophage activation and differentiation. Conversely, products of activated macrophages can influence the proliferation of both B- and T-lymphocytes.

Biologically, macrophages are perhaps the most important cell type in chronic inflammation. Macrophages appear at the site of biomaterial implantation, secondary to their role in the response to surgical injury, as well as in response to the "foreign" nature of the biomaterial itself. First, biochemical activation within the injured tissues chemotactically attracts neutrophils, followed by previously circulating monocytes. Bioactive molecules that serve to attract monocytes from the peripheral blood to the site of inflammation are listed in Table 2.4. Once at the site of inflammation, monocytes differentiate into macrophages. As a rule, macrophages can be seen adhering to the biomaterial within 24 hours after implantation.[46] The magnitude of macrophages attracted to the biopolymer is in part dependent on the texture of its surface. The roughened surface of abraded Teflon® attracts more macrophages than the smooth surface of polypropylene.[46] On the other hand, Behling and Spector[47] failed to notice any difference in the number of macrophages adhering to a variety of biopolymers. Most noticeably, while implants with roughened surfaces had a higher percentage of foreign body giant cells, smooth-surfaced implants contained primarily fibrous tissue and macrophages.

Table 2.4 Monocyte Chemotactic Factor

Coagulation factors	**Inhibitors of enzymes**
Coagulation factors V, VII, IX, and X	α_2-Macroglobulin
Thromboplastin	α_1-Antitrypsin
Prothrombin	Lipocortin
Components of the complement pathway	**Growth factors**
C1	Platelet-derived growth factor
C3	Transforming growth factor-β
C4	β Fibroblast growth factor
C5	
Factor B	**Oxygen metabolites**
Factor D	Superoxide anion
Properdin	Hydrogen peroxide
C3b inactivator	Hydroxyl anion
	Hypochlorous acid
Enzymes	**Cytokines**
Acid glycosidases	Interleukin-1
Acid phosphatase	Tumor necrosis factor
Acid proteases	Colony stimulating factor (CSF)
Arginase	
Collagenase	**Lipids**
Cytolytic proteinases	PGE2
Elastase	PGF2α
Lysozyme	Prostacyclin
Phospholipase A2	Thromboxane A2
Plasminogen activator	Leukotriene B, C, D, and E
	Platelet-activating factor
	Mono- and Di-HETES

From Shankar, R. and Greisler, H.P., in *Implantation Biology*, CRC Press, Boca Raton, 1994, 74.

To test the inflammatory responses induced by biomaterials, the cage implant system[20] is most often used. This system allows the sequential examination of the exudate surrounding the implant without the need to sacrifice the animal. Utilizing this investigation tool, Merchant et al.[48] have shown that monocytes and macrophages follow the appearance of neutrophils in the exudate and that macrophages have a preferential adsorption to the biomaterial. Neutrophils have a relatively shorter presence (hours to days) and disappear from the exudate more rapidly than macrophages, which remain for days to weeks or longer in the presence of a foreign body or infection. Eventually macrophages become the predominant cell type in the exudate, resulting in a chronic inflammatory response.

During the process of adhesion to, and/or phagocytosis of, biomaterials and their degradation products, macrophages become activated. Macrophage activation leads to release of bioactive agents, which have the potential to either degrade the biomaterial or compromise its functional capacity. In examining biological activity, it has been shown that macrophages are capable of producing a variety of growth factors, cytokines, chemotactic agents, proteases, arachidonic acid metabolites, oxygen-free radicals, complement components, and coagulation factors (Table 2.5). These secreted products may have a wide spectrum of effects from cell proliferation to cell death, and contribute to the chronic inflammatory response. IL-1, for instance, is a regulatory protein produced by macrophages, which has multiple effects on both the inflammatory and immune responses.[49] IL-1 is an important mediator of the inflammatory process because of its regulation of fibroblast growth, proliferation, and protein synthesis. By stimulating fibroblast activity, IL-1 induces the synthesis of the fibroblast product collagen,[50–52] and has also been shown to induce the proliferation of endothelial and smooth muscle cells.[49,53,54] These bioactive characteristics of IL-1 also indicate its importance as a biological mediator in terms of the biocompatibility of implanted materials.

Cellular proliferation at the implant site, which leads to both the wound healing as well as fibrous cap formation around the biomaterial, is predominantly a growth factor-mediated event. Macrophages add to this form of healing by secreting peptide growth factors such as platelet-derived growth factor

Table 2.5 Macrophage Products

C5a	Marder et al., 1985[148]
Collagen fragments	Postlethwait and Kong, 1976[149]
Elastin Fragments	Senior et al., 1980[150]
Endothelial cell products	Berliner et al., 1986[151]
Fibrinopeptides	Kay et al., 1973[152]
Fibronectin fragments	Norris et al., 1973[153]
Formyl methionyl peptides	Snyderman and Fudman, 1980[154]
Interleukin-1	Bevilaqua et al., 1985[155]
Interleukin-8	Matsushima and Oppenheim, 1989[156]
Kallikrein	Galin and Kaplan, 1974[157]
Monocyte chemotactic peptide 1 (MCP-1)	Valente et al., 1984[158]
N-acetylmuramyl-L-alanyl-D-isoglutamine	Ogawa et al., 1983[159]
Plasminogen activator	Galin and Kaplan, 1974[157]
Platelet factor 4	Devel et al., 1981[160]
Platelet-derived growth factor	Devel et al., 1982[62]
Smooth muscle cell products	Jauchem et al., 1982[161]
Thrombin	Bar-Shavit, 1983[162]
Leukotriene B4	Ford-Hutchinson et al., 1980[29]

Adapted from Shankar, R. and Greisler, H.P., in *Implantation Biology*, CRC Press, Boca Raton, 1994, 73.

(PDGF), fibroblast growth factor (FGF), and transforming growth factor β (TGF-β).[55–59] Secretion of these growth factors by activated macrophages will stimulate the growth of the endothelial cells, smooth muscle cells, and fibroblasts surrounding the biomaterial. PDGF is a potent mitogen for cells of mesenchymal origin, including smooth muscle cells and fibroblasts.[60,61] Additionally, it is also chemotactic to monocytes[62] and smooth muscle cells.[63] FGF is mitogenic to endothelial cells, smooth muscle cells, and fibroblasts and is an important promoter and regulator of angiogenesis.[58,64] While polymers such as Dacron®, ePTFE, and lactide/glycolide biopolymers stimulate the production of these growth factors,[65,66-68] it is unclear whether there is a preferential production of a specific growth factor by a particular biomaterial. It is probable that the biochemical composition of a biomaterial along with its construction and physical characteristics, as well as the site of implantation, may modulate the relative synthetic activities of specific growth factors by macrophages.

Attempts to downregulate the chronic inflammatory response through the use of steroids have been tried. However, their use to downregulate the acute and chronic inflammatory responses also may lead to inhibition of fibrous tissue formation, which may be deleterious to the overall healing of a biomaterial implant site.[69]

Greisler et al.[66] and Schwarcz et al.[70] reported differences in cellular responses elicited by different vascular graft implants including PG910, Dacron, and ePTFE grafts. In both dog and rabbit models, they noted a greater regeneration of smooth muscle-like myofibroblasts and endothelial cells in response to lactide/glycolide copolymers than were seen with either Dacron or ePTFE grafts. Phagocytosis of the bioresorbable graft material by macrophages was followed by a transinterstitial capillary and myofibroblast ingrowth. The resultant inner capsule was lined with endothelial cells functionally capable of prostacyclin production.[66,70] The kinetics of the endothelial cell and myofibroblast ingrowth paralleled the kinetics of macrophage infiltration and phagocytosis. When the graft was fully resorbed, the endothelialization and the myofibroblast ingrowth were complete and the macrophages disappeared. Dacron, which was not phagocytosed, failed to stimulate as extensive a transinterstitial capillary infiltration.[67]

To determine the mechanisms involved in the macrophage-induced resorption of PG910, Greisler et al.[68] cultured rabbit peritoneal macrophages in the presence of Dacron and PG910 and showed that PG910 stimulated macrophages to produce more mitogen into the conditioned media than did Dacron or control cultures with neither biomaterial, and this mitogenic activity was due to the release of basic FGF from the cultured macrophages. Dacron, on the other hand, induced more TGF-β production from macrophages, which might explain in part the suppression of the neointimal cellular ingrowth.[71] Aside from being a negative growth modulator at some concentrations, TGF-β is also a potent stimulator of matrix protein synthesis by fibroblasts and smooth muscle cells.[72] Thus, the ability of certain biopolymers to stimulate macrophages to secrete enhanced amounts of TGF-β may also play a role in tissue remodeling and wound healing (Section VI).

Macrophages also produce cytokines in response to biomaterial exposure. Cytokines such as IL-1 and TNF are potent cellular growth modulators and stimulators of adhesion receptors on endothelial cells that bind neutrophils and monocytes.[18,19,73,74] IL-1 is induced by exposure of human monocytes in culture to Dacron and polyethylene polymers, causing increased fibroblast proliferation and matrix protein formation.[75]

When considering the tissue inflammatory reactions attributed to implanted biomaterials, macrophages must be considered as multipotential regulators. Macrophages can play a complex role involving chemotactic factors, cytokines, growth factors, prostaglandins, coagulation, and complement factors. The complex interaction of these various bioactive macrophage products leads to wound healing and cellular ingrowth.

C. GRANULATION TISSUES

While chronic inflammation is generally a result of persistent inflammatory stimuli with the presence of macrophages and lymphocytes, the foreign body reaction and the development of granulation tissue may be considered to be the normal wound healing response to biomaterial implants. Within hours to days of biomaterial implantation, the healing response is initiated by the action of monocytes and macrophages, followed by proliferation of fibroblasts and vascular endothelial cells at the implant site, leading to the formation of granulation tissue, the hallmark of healing. Granulation tissue derives its name from the pink granular appearance on the surface of healing wounds, with its characteristic histologic features including the proliferation of new small blood vessels and fibroblasts. Depending on the extent of the inflammatory response, granulation tissue may appear as early as 3 to 5 days after implantation of a biomaterial.

The formation of small blood vessels, by budding or sprouting of preexisting vessels, is a process called angiogenesis or neovascularization.[75–77] This process involves proliferation, maturation, and organization of endothelial cells into capillary tubes.[78] These new capillary vessels have leaky endothelial junctions, allowing the passage of red blood cells and proteins into the extravascular space. This contributes to the typical edematous appearance of new granulation tissue.[79] Fibroblasts also proliferate in developing granulation tissue and are active in synthesizing collagen and proteoglycans. In the early stages of granulation tissue development, proteoglycans predominate. Later, however, collagen, especially type III collagen, predominates and forms the fibrous capsule. The majority of the large fibroblastoid cells in granulation tissue acquire features of smooth muscle cells and are called myofibroblasts. They contain large amounts of contractile proteins in their cytoplasm and are considered to be responsible for the wound contraction seen during the development of granulation tissue.

Extracellular matrix (ECM) components surrounding the biomaterial surfaces are involved in angiogenesis during granulation tissue formation and subsequent fibrous capsule development. Macrophages, in addition to their active role in phagocytosis and wound debridement, release several cytokines which further modify growth factor production and the extracellular matrix environment at the site of tissue remodeling.[80] Granulation tissue is composed of many mesenchymal and nonmesenchymal cell types with an extensive neovasculature embedded within a loosely assembled extracellular matrix composed of collagens, fibronectin, and proteoglycans. Pathologic conditions related to wound healing events, such as hypertrophic scars, have been found to exhibit elevated fibronectin levels.[81] Heparin has been noted to affect the angiogenesis process. Heparin enhances the migration of capillary endothelial cells *in vitro*, potentiates the action of FGF, which is a family of potent angiogenic factors, as well as protecting FGF from enzymatic degradation in biologic matrices.[82–84] Heparin may play a dual role in granulation tissue formation since heparin/hydrocortisone complexes have been found to inhibit angiogenesis.[85] Furthermore, heparin alone has been noted to inhibit vascular smooth muscle cell growth.[86] Application of fibronectin to wound sites results in increased wound closure and increased wound strength. These observations have led to the clinical application of fibronectin for enhanced healing of corneal and cutaneous ulcers.[87–93]

The extent of injury or defect created by the surgical implantation of a biomaterial can significantly affect the wound healing response. As stated earlier, wound healing by primary union (or first intention) is the healing of clean, surgical incisions in which the wound edges are approximated by surgical sutures. This type of healing occurs without significant bacterial contamination and with a minimal loss of tissue. Wound healing by secondary union (or second intention) occurs when there is a large tissue defect that must be filled or when there is extensive loss of cells and tissue. In wound healing by secondary intention, regeneration of parenchymal cells cannot completely reconstitute the original architecture. Abundant granulation tissue grows in from the margin of the tissue defect to complete the repair. This frequently results in larger areas of fibrosis or scar formation.

IV. FOREIGN BODY REACTION

The foreign body reaction to biomaterials, a distinctive pattern of chronic inflammation, is composed of both foreign body giant cells and the components of granulation tissue, which consist of macrophages, fibroblasts, and capillaries in varying amounts, depending upon the biocompatibility of the implanted materials. These foreign body giant cells are multinucleated and are believed to be formed at the site of inflammation from the fusion of macrophages. Adams[94] suggested that the formation of giant cells is the final step in the maturation/differentiation process of monocytes. *In vitro* monocyte and macrophage culture studies have indicated that in the presence of a foreign substance macrophages may coalesce to form giant cells[95] and retain many of the biochemical properties of macrophages.[96]

Giant cell formation at the site of implantation of the foreign body can be evoked *in vivo*. Mariano and Spector[97] showed that giant cells were formed at the site of implantation when glass cover slips were implanted subcutaneously. They suggested that the incoming new monocyte/macrophages recognize the existing wound macrophages as metabolically inefficient and, as a direct result, differentiate into giant cells. The composition of foreign body reaction may be influenced by the form and topography of the surface of the implanted biomaterial. Giant cells are also believed to be formed preferentially in response to certain polymers such as roughened polycarbonate and hydrophobic materials.[75] Relatively flat and smooth surfaces, such as those found on breast prostheses, have a foreign body reaction composed of a layer of macrophages one to two cells in thickness.[98] Relatively rough surfaces, such as those found on the outer surfaces of expanded polytetrafluoroethylene vascular grafts, have a foreign body reaction composed of macrophages and foreign body giant cells at the surface.

The foreign body reaction that consists of macrophages and foreign body giant cells may persist for the life of the implant.[98,99] Nonetheless, it is unclear whether they become quiescent after a time or continue to be activated, releasing their lysosomal constituents. The giant cells at the site of the foreign body may play a role in wound healing by virtue of the functional capacities of these cells. The presence of an implant with its foreign body reaction may lead to a fibrous encapsulation surrounding the biomaterial, thereby isolating the implant from the local tissue environment.

V. FIBROSIS OR FIBROUS ENCAPSULATION

The end-stage healing response to biomaterials generally is fibrosis or fibrous encapsulation,[100–102] which is the formation of a dense and fibroconnective tissue scar. Depending on the extent of tissue damage caused by the implanted material, there may be a prolonged inflammatory response with extensive tissue repair including excess proliferation of mesenchymal cells and an abundant deposition of extracellular matrix. During this phase of the repair process, macrophages continue to phagocytize and produce cytokines that attract leukocytes and mesenchymal cells, such as fibroblasts and smooth muscle cells, to the implant site and in many cases may activate them to produce additional cytokines. Some of the cytokines, known as fibrogenic cytokines, may initiate a cascade of events that trigger the continued proliferation of fibroblasts and/or stimulate the production of connective tissue which ultimately leads to fibrosis.[80,103] These fibrogenic cytokines, including IL-1, TNF-α, PDGF, FGF, and TGF-β, are produced by the activated macrophages, but also to varying degrees by other cell types such as lymphocytes, endothelial cells, and fibroblasts themselves. Some of these cytokines that promote fibrous growth are also mitogenic and chemotactic for endothelial cells (e.g., FGF), and thus promote capillary growth *in vivo*.[104,105] Angiogenesis is an important component of fibrous tissue formation, as it provides the essential nutrient support for cellular proliferation and metabolism.

Another important feature mediated by fibrogenic cytokines is the upregulation of collagen synthesis, which promotes connective tissue deposition, thus leading to fibrous tissue formation. Studies of collagen synthesis in response to fibrogenic cytokines has focused on types I and III collagen, which are the predominant connective tissue elements altered in many fibrotic disorders. Types I and III collagen represent 80 and 20%, respectively, of the total collagen synthesized by fibroblasts.[101] The synthesis of these collagens can be increased significantly by both macrophage-derived growth factors and lympho-cyte-derived mediators, including fibroblast-activating factors (FAFs).[106] TGF-β has been shown to stimulate the expression of collagen and fibronectin genes as well as the production and release of extracellular matrix proteins.[80]

The body's attempt to repair local damage induced by the implant involves two distinct processes: (1) regeneration, which is the replacement of injured tissue by parenchymal cells of the same type; and (2) replacement by granulation tissue that constitutes the fibrous capsule.[2] Important cellular adaptations include atrophy (decrease in cell size or function), hypertrophy (increase in cell size), hyperplasia (increase in cell number), and metaplasia (change in cell type). Other adaptations that may affect tissue repair include a change by cells from producing one family of proteins to another (phenotypic change), or marked overproduction of protein. These adaptations may contribute to the pathophysiology of chronic inflammation and fibrosis.

VI. GROWTH FACTORS AFFECTING WOUND HEALING

It has long been known that, in the absence of pathology, physiological wound healing follows a sigmoidal curve[107] with the healing tissue asymptotically approaching the strength of uninjured tissue, if it ever does. Although significant wound tear strength is normally achieved within 28 days, it can take weeks, months, and even longer for the healed tissue to regain its original strength. The cellular processes involved in wound healing and their control by autocrine and/or paracrine factors released into the wound area by various cells have been discussed in previous sections. The role of these factors, typically platelet-derived growth factor (PDGF), transforming growth factor-beta (TGF-β), fibroblast growth factor (FGF) and epidermal growth factor (EGF), in wound healing has been addressed by several workers.[108–110] However, wound healing can be delayed, or enhanced, by such factors as the physical status of the patient, surgical technique, the incision procedure, and the suture material and suturing technique.[111-114]

Multiple studies have examined the effects of these growth factors on various wound healing models. Brown et al.[115] demonstrated in a rabbit model that there was an increased rate of epithelialization in split-thickness dermal wounds and partial-thickness burns when EGF was applied topically on a daily basis. EGF-supplemented wound chambers in rats accumulated more collagen and glycoaminoglycans than unsupplemented chambers and, in addition, demonstrated increased cellularity.[116] The breaking strength of intestinal wounds exposed to EGF was higher 5 d after wounding than that of unsupplemented wounds.[117] Supplemental EGF accelerates collagen accumulation in a polytetrafluoroethylene (PTFE) model in diabetic rats[118] and reverses the healing impairment produced by systemic methylprednisolone when injected into a sponge model in rats.[119]

FGF has also been extensively studied in animal models. Basic FGF (bFGF) has been demonstrated to accelerate epithelialization when applied topically to a rabbit ear wound[120] or a partial-thickness pigskin model.[121] It has been demonstrated to increase cellularity and collagen content when injected into a subcutaneous sponge model in rats.[121] Dermal wounds in guinea pigs treated with bFGF-containing collagen sponges demonstrated increased breaking strength as compared with unsupplemented controls.[122] bFGF has also been demonstrated to increase the breaking strength of incisional wounds in rats on days 5 to 7 when injected into incisional wounds in rats.[123] Topical bFGF can overcome impairments in wound contraction in rats produced by infection[124] or diabetes.[125]

PDGF has been demonstrated to be an effective wound supplement in animal models. It has been shown to increase the rate of epithelialization in a rabbit ear model.[120] Subcutaneous sponges in rats injected daily with PDGF demonstrated greater cellularity and a higher collagen content at 7 d than uninjected controls.[126] When PDGF was placed into incisional wounds in rats in a collagen vehicle, wound breaking strength was increased as compared with control wounds for up to 7 weeks after wounding.[127–129] Incisional wounds in irradiated rats had higher wound breaking strengths at days 7 and 12 when supplemented with PDGF in a collagen vehicle at the time of wounding.[130]

TGF-β has frequently been used as a wound supplement. Though it does not appear to stimulate epithelialization in a rabbit ear model,[120] it does stimulate collagen synthesis.[131] It is a potent stimulant of collagen synthesis and angiogenesis when injected subcutaneously into the necks of newborn mice.[132] TGF-β-containing Schilling chambers placed subcutaneously in rats contained more cells and collagen 5 and 9 d after placement than control chambers.[133] Incisional wounds left open in guinea pigs that were treated with TGF-β-containing sponges accumulated more granulation tissue at day 8 than non-TGF-β-treated wounds.[134] When TGF-β was placed into incisional wounds in rats in a collagen vehicle, wound breaking strength was increased over controls between days 3 and 14.[135] TGF-β supplements can overcome an Adriamycin®-induced wound healing impairment in rats when placed either in subcutaneous Schilling wound chamber[136] or in incisional wounds.[137] Lower dose TGF-β-supplemented linear incisions in irradiated skin developed greater breaking strength 7 d after wounding than untreated wounds.[138] TGF-β supplementation can also reverse a glucocorticoid-induced healing deficit in rats in incisional wounds on day 7 when applied to the wounds in a collagen vehicle.[139]

Other growth factors have in general been less well studied. TNF-α-supplemented subcutaneous polyvinyl sponges in rats contained more collagen 14 d after placement than unsupplemented sponges.[140]

TNF-α increased wound breaking strength in incisional wounds in normal and Adriamycin-treated rats on day 11 when administered with a collagen vehicle.[141] TNF-α has been demonstrated to stimulate epithelialization.[142] Interleukin-2, when administered in rats intraperitoneally via an osmotic pump, produced greater wound breaking strength in dorsal incisional wounds at day 10 and greater collagen content in subcutaneously placed polyvinyl sponges.[143] It has also been demonstrated to reverse an Adriamycin-induced healing deficit in incisional wounds in rats.[144]

Abnormal wound healing can be caused by a number of different factors, commonly malnutrition, vitamin deficiencies, diseases such as diabetes and uremia, as well as by systemic treatment with certain drugs. In particular, cytotoxic chemotherapeutic drugs used in the treatment of malignant neoplasms (antineoplastic agents) and various steroids are known to have varying effects on wound fibroplasia.[111,115–117,145-147] Generally, decreased wound tear strength (WTS) and wound tear energy (WTE) values are found with patients undergoing chemotherapy for postoperative treatment of neoplasms.[111,147] In other words, therapeutic doses of cytotoxic agents retard the early phases of wound fibroplasia. *In vivo* animal studies showed that while the presence of a tumor will decrease WTS and WTE, treatment with therapeutic doses of a chemotherapeutic drug to which the tumor responds results in a significant improvement in wound strength at 21 d.[111] However, treatment with therapeutic doses of a chemotherapeutic drug that the tumor does not respond to has no effect on wound strength.

The method of surgical incision has been shown to affect WTS (Figure 2.3).[112] The conventional steel scalpel has certain advantages, notably convenience, low cost, and ready availability, but its use requires good manual dexterity and, usually, a separate procedure to coagulate bleeding from small vessels. Various thermal knives have been developed in recent years; these devices are easy to use, rapid in action, and will coagulate tissue and vessels during surgery. WTS following surgical incisions with different instruments showed that the conventional steel scalpel resulted in greater wound tensile strengths than those achieved with thermal knives, suggesting that thermal injury during surgery delays wound healing.[112] Finally, it has been found that the tautness of the suture used to approximate a healing wound can have a marked effect on wound healing.[113] Clearly, it is necessary to have good initial mechanical closure of a wound in order to reduce the risk of infection and encourage healing by primary union. However, achieving a secure knot (see Chapter 6) may result in excessive tension being applied to the first throw of the suture, particularly with certain of the newer, more "slippery" synthetic sutures. The possible impairment of wound healing by excessive suture tension has been demonstrated and it was found that "loosely" approximated wound edges had significantly greater WTS and WTE values than "tightly" sutured edges (Figure 2.4).[113] In this particular study, the "tightly" sutured wound was one in which the edges were approximated by a 1=1=1 knot configuration with maximum tension applied to the first throw. In contrast, in the "loosely"-sutured wound, a rod of 3.14 mm^2 cross-sectional area was laid beside the incision while the suture was placed in the same manner as for the "tight" wound, and then was removed subsequently to relieve the tension across the wound. The marked difference in wound strength for the loose and tight wound closures is very clear from Figure 2.4. Although hydroxyproline (the marker amino acid for collagen) assays for the two types of wound showed no differences, scanning electron microscopy demonstrated greater proliferative activity in the loosely approximated wounds.[113]

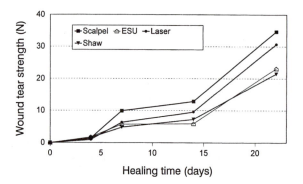

Figure 2.3 Effect of surgical incision method on wound tear strength in newtons.

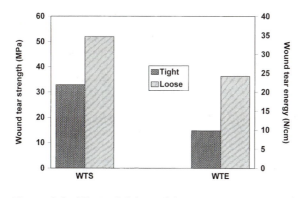

Figure 2.4 Effect of tight and loose sutures on wound strength.

VII. SUMMARY

This chapter discusses the process of wound healing and the multiplicity of factors that can adversely affect the course of this event. The application of PDGFs, notably EGF and TGF-β, to accelerate wound healing is noted, particularly the ability of the latter to reverse the impaired wound healing caused by antitumor agents. Surgical influences on wound healing, such as the method of surgical incision and the tension applied across a wound by suture, are also discussed.

REFERENCES

1. Spector, M., Cease, C., and Tong-Li, X., The local tissue response to biomaterials, *Crit. Rev. Biocompat.*, 5, 269, 1989.
2. Cotran, R.S., Kumar, V., and Robbin, S.L., Inflammation and repair, in *Robbin's Pathologic Basis of Disease*, W.B. Saunders, Philadelphia, 1989, 39.
3. Callin, J.I., Goldstein, I.M., and Syderman R., *Inflammation: Basic Principles and Clinical Correlates*, 2nd ed., Raven Press, New York, 1992.
4. Cohen, I.K., Diegelmann, R.F., Lindblad, W.J., Eds., *Wound Healing: Biochemical and Clinical Aspects*, W.B. Saunders, Philadelphia, 1992.
5. Black, J., *Biological Performance of Materials*, Marcel Dekker, New York, 1981.
6. Corman, M.L., Veidenheimer, M.C., and Coller, J.A., Controlled clinical trial of three suture materials for abdominal wall closure after bowel operations, *Am. J. Surg.*, 141, 510, 1981.
7. Richards P.C., Balch C.M., and Aldrete J.S., Abdominal wall closure: a randomized prospective study of 571 patients comparing continuous versus interrupted suture techniques, *Ann. Surg.*, 197, 238, 1983.
8. Hunt, T.K. and Van Winkle, W., Jr., Normal repair, in *Fundamentals of Wound Management*, Hunt, T.K. and Dunphy, J.E., Eds., Appleton-Century-Crofts, New York, 1979, 2.
9. Terkeltaub, R.A. and Ginsberg, M.H., Platelets in response to injury, in *The Molecular and Cellular Biology of Wound Repair*, Clark, R.A.F. and Henson, P.M., Eds., Plenum Press, New York, 1988, 38.
10. Jutila, M.A., Leukocyte traffic to sites of inflammation, *APMIS*, 100, 191, 1992.
11. Butcher, E.C., Leukocyte-endothelial cell recognition. Three (or more) steps to specificity and adversity, *Cell*, 67, 1033, 1991.
12. Springer, T.A., Adhesion receptors of the immune system, *Nature*, 346, 423, 1991.
13. Cotran, R.S. and Pober, J.S., Cytokine-endothelial interaction in inflammation, immunity, and vascular injury, *J. Am. Soc. Nephrol.*, 1, 225, 1990.
14. Picker, L.J., Kishimoto, T.K., Smith, C.W., Warnock, R.A., and Butcher, E.E., Elam-1 is an adhesion molecule for skin-homing T-cell, *Nature*, 349, 796, 1991.
15. Von Adrian, U.H., Chambers, J.D., McEvoy, L., Bargatze, R.F., Arfors, K.E., and Butcher, E.E., Two step models of leukocyte-endothelial cell interactions in inflammation: distinct roles for LECAM-1 and the leukocyte beta 2 integrins *in vivo*, *Proc. Natl. Acad. Sci. U.S.A.*, 88, 7538, 1991.
16. Picker, L.J., Warnock, R.A., Burns, A.R., Doerschuk, C.M., Berg, E.L., and Butcher, E.C., The neutrophil selectin LECAM-1 presents carbohydrate ligands to the vascular selectins ELAM-1 and GMP-140, *Cell*, 66, 921, 1991.
17. Smith, C.W., Kishimoto, T.K., Abbassi, O., Hughes, B., Rothlein, R., McIntire, I.V., Butcher, E.C., and Anderson, D.C., Chemotactic factors regulate lectin adhesion molecule 1 (LECAM-1)-dependent neutrophil adhesion to cytokine-stimulated endothelial cells *in vitro*, *J. Clin. Invest.*, 87, 609, 1991.

18. Bevilacqua, M.P., Stengelin, S., Gimbrone, M.A., Jr., and Sedd, B., Endothelial leukocyte adhesion molecule-1: an inducible receptor for neutrophils, related to complement regulatory proteins and lectins, *Science*, 243, 1160, 1989.

19. Shankar, R., de la Motte, C.A., and Dicorlerto, P.E., 3-Deazaadenosine inhibits thrombin-stimulated platelet-derived growth factor production and endothelial-leukocyte adhesion molecule-1 mediated monocytic cell adhesion in human aortic endothelial cells, *J. Biol. Chem.*, 267, 9376, 1992.

20. Jurgensen, C.H., Huber, C.H., Zimmerman, T.P., and Worlberg, G., 3-Deazaadenosine inhibits leukocyte adhesion and ICAM-1 biosynthesis in tumor necrosis factor-stimulated human endothelial cells, *J. Immunol.*, 144, 653, 1990.

21. Kishimoto, T.K., Jutila, M.A., Berg, E.L., and Butcher, E.C., Neutrophil Mac-1 and Mel-14 adhesion proteins inversely regulated by chemotactic factors, *Science*, 245, 1238, 1989.

22. Larson, R.S. and Springer, T.A., Structure and function of leukocyte integrins, *Immunol. Rev.*, 114, 181, 1990.

23. Harlan, J.M., Leukocyte-endothelial interactions, *Blood*, 65, 513, 1985.

24. Geng, J.G., Bevilacqua, M.P., Moore, K.L., McIntyre, T.M., Porescott, S.M., Kim, J.M., Bloss, G.A., Zimmerman, G.A., and McEver, R.P., Rapid neutrophil adhesion to activate endothelium mediated by GMP-140, *Nature*, 343, 757, 1990.

25. Zimmerman, G.A., McIntyre, T.M., and Prescott, S.M., Thrombin stimulates neutrophil adherence by an endothelial cell-dependent mechanism: characterization of the response and relationship to platelet-activating factor synthesis, *Ann. NY Acad. Sci.*, 485, 349, 1986.

26. Zimmerman, G.A., McIntyre, T.M., and Prescott, S.M., Thrombin stimulates the adherence of neutrophils to human endothelial cells, *J. Clin. Invest.*, 76, 2235, 1985.

27. Showell, H.J., Freer, R.J., Zigmond, S.H., Shiffman, E., Aswanikumar, S., Corcoran, B.A., and Becker, E.L., The structure-activity relations of synthetic peptides as chemotactic factors and inducers of lysosomal enzyme secretion for neutrophils, *J. Exp. Med.*, 143, 1154, 1976.

28. Snyderman, R., Gewwurz, H., and Megenhagen, C.E., Interactions of the complement system with endotoxin lipopolysaccharide: generation of a factor chemotactic for polymorphonuclear leukocytes, *J. Exp. Med.*, 128, 259, 1968.

29. Ford-Hutchinson, A.W., Bray, M.A., Doig, M.V., Shipley, M.E., and Smith, M.J.H., Leukotriene B, a potent chemo-kinetic and aggregating substance released from polymorphonuclear leukocytes, *Nature*, 286, 264, 1980.

30. Devel, T.F., Senior, R.M., Chang, D., Griffin, G.L., Hendrickson, R.L., and Kaiser, E.T., Platelet factor 4 is chemotactic for neutrophils and monocytes, *Proc. Natl. Acad. Sci, U.S.A.*, 78, 4584, 1981.

31. Djeu, J.Y., Matsushima, K., Oppenheim, J.J., Shiotsuki, K., and Blanchard, D.K., Functional activation of human neutrophils by recombinant monocyte-derived neutrophil chemotactic factor, *J. Immunol.*, 144, 2205, 1990.

32. Libby, P. and Hasson, G.K., Involvement of the immune system in human artherogenesis. Current knowledge and unanswered questions, *Lab. Invest.*, 64, 5, 1991.

33. Tonnesen, J.G., Smedly, L.A., and Henson, P.M., Neutrophil-endothelial cell interaction: modulation of neutrophil adhesiveness induced by complement fragments C5a and C51 des arg and formyl-methionyl-leucyl-phenylalanine *in vitro*, *J. Clin. Invest.*, 74, 1581, 1984.

34. Greisler, H.P., Vascular graft healing-interfacial phenomena, in *New Biologic and Synthetic Vascular Prosthesis*, R.G. Landes Company, Austin, Texas, 1991.

35. Vroman, L., Methods of investigating protein interaction on artificial and natural surfaces, *Ann. NY Acad. Sci.*, 516, 300, 1987.

36. Roohk, H.V., Pick, J., Hill, R., Hung, E., and Bartlett, R.H., Kinetics of fibrinogen and platelet adherence to biomaterials, *Trans. Am Soc. Artif. Intern. Organs*, 22, 1, 1976.

37. Liotta, L.A., Tumor invasion and metastasis. Role of the basement membrane, *Am. J. Pathol.*, 117, 339, 1984.

38. Terranova, V.P., DiFlorio, R., Hujanen, E.S., Lyall, R., Liotta, L.A., Thorgeirsson, U., Siegel, G.P., and Schiffmann, E., Laminin promotes rabbit neutrophil motility and attachment, *J. Clin. Invest.*, 77, 1180, 1986.

39. Yoon, P.S., Boxer, L.A., Mayo, L.A., Yang, A.X., and Wicha, M.S., Human neutrophil laminin receptors. Activation-dependent receptor expression, *J. Immunol.*, 138, 259, 1987.

40. Wilkinson, P.C. and Lackie, J.M., The influence of contact guidance on chemotaxis of human neutrophil leukocytes, *Exp. Cell Res.*, 145, 255, 1983.

41. Grinnell, F., Migration of human neutrophils in hydrated collagen lattices, *J. Cell Sci.*, 58, 95, 1982.

42. Brown, A.F., Neutrophil granulocytes: adhesion and locomotion on collagen substrata and in collagen matrices, *J. Cell Sci.*, 58, 445, 1982.

43. Henson, P.M., Mechanisms of exocytosis in phagocytic inflammatory cells, *Am. J. Pathol.*, 101, 494, 1980.

44. Henson, P.M., The immunologic release of constituents from neutrophil leukocytes: II. Mechanisms of release during phagocytosis, and adherence to nonphagocytosable surfaces, *J. Immunol.*, 107, 1547, 1971.

45. Anderson, J.M., Mechanism of inflammation and infection with implanted devices, *Cardiovasc. Pathol.*, 2(Suppl. 3), 335, 1993.

46. Salthouse, T.N., Some aspects of macrophage behavior at the implant surface, *J. Biomed. Mater. Res.*, 18, 395, 1984.

47. Behling, C.A. and Spector, M., Quantitative characterization of cells at the interface of long-term implants of selected polymers, *J. Biomed. Mater. Res.*, 20, 653, 1986.

48. Merchant, R., Anderson, J.M., Phua, K., and Hiltner, A., *In vivo* biocompatibility studies. II. Biomer: preliminary cell adhesion and surface characterization studies, *J. Biomed. Mater. Res.*, 18, 309, 1984.

49. Dinarello, C.A., Interleukin 1, *Rev. Infect. Dis.*, 6, 51, 1984.

50. Schmidt, J.A., Mizel, S.B., Cohen, D., and Green, I., Interleukin 1: a potential regulator of fibroblast proliferation, *J. Immunol.*, 128, 2177, 1982.

51. Hibbs, M.S., Postlethwait, A.E., Mainardi, C.L., Seyer, J.M., and Kang, A.H., Alterations in collagen production in mixed mononuclear leukocyte-fibroblast cultures, *J. Exp. Med.*, 157, 47, 1983.

52. Grinnell, F., Fibronectin and wound healing, *Am. J. Dermatopathol.*, 4, 185, 1982.

53. Martin, B.M., Gimbrone, M.A., Jr., Unanue, E.R., and Cotran, R.S., Stimulation of nonlymphoid mesenchymal cell proliferation by a macrophage-derived growth factor, *J. Immunol.*, 126, 1510, 1981.

54. Martin, B.M., Gimbrone, M.A., Jr., Unanue, E.R., and Cotran, R.S., Macrophage factors: their role in proliferation of smooth muscle, fibroblasts, and endothelium, in *Plasma and Cellular Modulatory Proteins*, Bing, D.H. and Rosenbaun, R.A., Eds., Center for Blood Research, Inc., Boston, 1981, 83.

55. Nathan, C.F., Secretory products of macrophages, *J. Clin. Invest.*, 79, 319, 1987.

56. Shimokado, K., Raines, E.W., Madtes, D.K., Barrett, T.B., Benditt, E.P., and Ross, R., A significant part of macrophage-derived growth factor consists of at least two isoforms of PDGF, *Cell*, 43, 277, 1985.

57. Baird, A., Mormede, P., and Bohen, P., Immunoreactive fibroblast growth factor in cells of peritoneal exudate suggests its identity with macrophage derived growth factor, *Biochem. Biophys. Res. Commun.*, 126, 358, 1985.

58. Sunderkotter, C., Boebler, M., Schulze-Osthoff, K., Bharadwaj, R., and Sorg, C., Macrophage derived angiogenic factors, *Pharmacol. Ther.*, 51, 195, 1991.

59. Assoian, R.K., Fleuredelys, B.E., Stevenson, H.C., Miller, P.J., Madtes, D.K., Raines, E.W., Ross, R., and Sporn, M.B., Expression and secretion of type B transforming growth factor by activated macrophages, *Proc. Natl. Acad. Sci. U.S.A.*, 84, 6020, 1987.

60. Rutherford, R.B. and Ross, R., Platelet factors stimulate fibroblasts and smooth muscle cells quiescent in plasma serum to proliferate, *J. Cell Biol.*, 69, 196, 1976.

61. Ross, R., Glomset, J.A., Kariya, B., and Harker, L., A platelet-dependent serum factor that stimulates the proliferation of arterial smooth muscle cells *in vitro*, *Proc. Natl. Acad. Sci. U.S.A.*, 71, 1207, 1974.

62. Deuel, T.F., Senior, R.M., Huang, J.S., and Griffin, G.L., Chemotaxis of monocytes and neutrophils to platelet-derived growth factor, *J. Clin. Invest.*, 69, 1046, 1982.

63. Raines, E.W., Bowen-Pope, D.F., and Ross, R., Platelet-derived growth factor, in *Handbook of Experimental Pharmacology*, Vol. 95, Sporn, M.B. and Roberts, A.B., Eds., Springer-Verlag, New York, 1990.

64. Burgess, W.H. and Maciag, T., The heparin-binding (fibroblast) growth factor family of proteins, *Annu. Rev. Biochem.*, 58, 575, 1989.

65. Greisler, H.P., Ellinger, J., Schwarcz, T.H., Golan, J., Raymond, R.M., and Kim, D.U., Arterial regeneration over polydioxanone prostheses in the rabbit, *Arch. Surg.*, 122, 715, 1987.

66. Greisler, H.P., Endean, E.D., Klosak, J.J., Ellinger, J., Dennis, J.W., Buttle, K., and Kim, D.U., Polyglactin 910/polydioxanone biocomponent totally resorbable vascular prostheses, *J. Vasc. Surg.*, 7, 697, 1988.

67. Greisler, H.P., Schwarcz, T.H., Ellinger, J., and Kim, D.U., Dacron inhibition of arterial regenerative activity, *J. Vasc. Surg.*, 3, 747, 1986.

68. Greisler, H.P., Dennis, J.W., Endean, E.D., Ellinger, J., Friesel, R., and Burgess, W.H., Macrophage/biomaterial interaction: the stimulation of endothelialization, *J. Vasc. Surg.*, 9, 588, 1989.

69. Craddock, P.R., Fehr, J., Dalmasso, A.P. Brigham, K.L., and Jacob, H.S., Hemodialysis leukopenia: pulmonary vascular leukostasis resulting from complement activation by dialyzer cellophane membranes, *J. Clin. Invest.*, 59, 879, 1977.

70. Schwarcz, T.H., Nussbaum, M.L., Ellinger, J., and Greisler, H.P., Inner capsule prostaglandin content of vascular prostheses, *Surg. Forum*, 37, 441, 1986.

71. Greisler, H.P., Henderson, S.C., and Lam, T.M., Basic fibroblast growth factor production *in vitro* by macrophages exposed to Dacron and Polyglactin 910, *J. Biomater. Sci.*, 4, 415, 1993.

72. Roberts, A.B. and Sporn, M.B., Regulation of endothelial cell growth, architecture and matrix synthesis by TFG-β, *Am. Rev. Respir. Dis.*, 140, 126, 1989.

73. Dicorleto, P.E. and de la Motte, C.A., Role of cell surface carbohydrate moieties in monocytic cell adhesion to endothelium *in vitro*, *J. Immunol.*, 143, 3666, 1989.

74. Dicorleto, P.E. and de la Motte, C.A., Thrombin causes increased monocytic-cell adhesion to endothelial cells through a protein kinase C-dependent pathway, *Biochem. J.*, 265, 71, 1989.

75. Ziats, N.P., Miller, K.M., and Anderson, J.M., *In vitro* and *in vivo* interactions of cells with biomaterials, *Biomaterials*, 9, 5, 1988.

76. Maciag, T., Molecular and cellular mechanisms of angiogenesis, in *Important Advances in Oncology*, DeVita, V.T., Hellman, S., and Rosenberg, S., Eds., J.B. Lippincott, Philadelphia, 1990, 85.

77. Thompson, J.A., Anderson, K.D., and DiPietro, J.M., Site-directed neovessel formation *in vivo*, *Science*, 241, 1349, 1988.

78. Ausprunk, D.H., Tumor angiogenesis, in *Chemical Messengers of the Inflammatory Process*, Houck, J.C., Ed., Elsevier/North Holland, Amsterdam, 1979, 317.

79. Schoefl, G.I., Studies of inflammation. III. Growing capillaries; their structure and permeability, *Virchows Arch. Pathol. Anat.*, 337, 97, 1963.

80. Sporn, M.B. and Roberts, A.B., Peptide growth factors are multifunctional, *Nature*, 332, 217, 1988.

81. Kischer, C.W., Shetlar, M.R., and Chvapil, M., Hypertrophic scars and keloids. A review and new concept concerning their origin, *Scanning Electron Micros.*, 4, 1699, 1982.

82. Azizkhan, R.G., Azizkhan, J.C., and Zetter, B.R., Mast cell heparin stimulates migration of capillary endothelial cells *in vitro*, *J. Exp. Med.*, 152, 931, 1980.

83. Folkman, J., Klagsbrun, M., and Sasse, J., A heparin-binding angiogenic protein — basic fibroblast growth factor — is stored within basement membrane, *Am. J. Pathol.*, 130, 393, 1988.

84. Thornton, S.C., Mueller, S.N., and Levine, E.M., Human endothelial cells: use of heparin in cloning and long term serial cultivation, *Science*, 223, 1296, 1984.

85. Folkman, J., Langer, R., and Linhardt, R.J., Angiogenesis inhibition and tumor regression caused by heparin or a heparin fragment in the presence of cortisone, *Science*, 221, 719, 1983.

86. Castellot, J.J., Jr., Wright, T.C., and Karnovsky, M.J., Regulation of vascular smooth muscle cell growth by heparin and heparin sulfates, *Semin. Thromb. Hemosta.*, 13, 489, 1987.

87. Saba, T.M. and Jaffe, E., Plasma fibronectin (opsonic glycoprotein): its synthesis by vascular endothelial cells and role in cardiopulmonary integrity after trauma as related to reticuloendothelial function, *Am. J. Med.*, 68, 577, 1986.

88. Saba, T.M., Blumenstock, F.A., and Shah, D.M., Reversal of opsonic deficiency in surgical, trauma, and burn patients by infusion of purified human plasma fibronectin, *Am. J. Med.*, 80, 229, 1986.

89. Nishida, T., Nakagawa, S., and Manabe, R., Clinical evaluation of fibronectin eyedrops on epithelial disorders after herpetic keratitis, *Ophthalmology*, 92, 213, 1985.

90. Kono, I., Matsumoto, Y., and Kano, K., Beneficial effect of topical fibronectin in patients with keratoconjunctivitis sicca in Sjogren's syndrome, *J. Rheumatol.*, 12, 487, 1985.

91. Spigelman, A.V., Deutsch, T.A., and Sugar, J., Application of homologous fibronectin to persistent human corneal epithelial defects, *Cornea*, 6, 128, 1987.

92. Berman, M., Manseau, E., and Law, M., Ulceration is correlated with degradation of fibrin and fibronectin at the corneal surface, *Invest. Ophthalmol. Vis. Sci.*, 24, 1358, 1983.

93. Phan, T.M., Foster, C.S., and Boruchoff, S.A., Topical fibronectin in the treatment of persistent corneal epithelial defects and trophic ulcers, *Am. J. Ophthalmol.*, 104, 494, 1987.

94. Adams, D.O., The granulomatous inflammatory response: a review, *Am. J. Pathol.*, 84, 164, 1976.

95. Murch, A.R., Grounds, M.D., Marshall, C.A., and Papadimitriou, J., Direct evidence that inflammatory multinucleate giant cells form by fusion, *J. Pathol.*, 137, 177, 1982.

96. Schlesinger, L., Musson, R.A., and Johnson, R.B., Jr., Functional and biochemical studies of multinucleated giant cells from the culture of human monocytes, *J. Exp. Med.*, 159, 1289, 1984.

97. Mariano, M. and Spector, W.G., The formation and properties of macrophage polykaryons (inflammatory giant cells), *J. Pathol.*, 113, 1, 1974.

98. Chambers, T.J. and Spector, W.G., Inflammatory giant cells, *Immunobiology*, 161, 283, 1982.

99. Rae, T., The macrophage response to implant materials, *Crit. Rev. Biocompat.*, 2, 97, 1986.

100. von Recum, A.F., *Handbook of Biomaterials Evaluation. Scientific, Technical, and Clinical Testing of Implant Materials*, MacMillan, New York, 1986.

101. Clark, R.A.F. and Henson, P.M., *The Molecular and Cellular Biology of Wound Repair*, Plenum Publishing, New York, 1988.

102. Hunt, T.K., Heppenstall, R.B., and Pines E., *Soft and Hard Tissue Repair*, Praeger Scientific, New York, 1984.

103. Kovacs, E.J., Fibrogenic cytokines: the roles of immune mediators in the development of fibrosis, *Immunol. Today*, 12, 17, 1991.

104. Folkman, J. and Klagsbrun, M., Angiogenic factors, *Science*, 235, 442, 1987.

105. Ford, H.R., Hoffman, R.A., Wing, E.J., Magee, M., McIntyre, L., and Simmons, R.L., Characterization of wound cytokines in the sponge matrix model, *Arch. Surg.*, 124, 1422, 1989.

106. Wahl, S.M., Hunt, D.A., Allen, J.B., Wilder, R.L., Paglia, L., and Hand, A.R., Bacterial cell wall induced hepatic granulomas: an *in vivo* model of T-cell-dependent fibrosis, *J. Exp. Med.*, 163, 884, 1986.

107. Douglas D.M., Wound healing and management, *Williams and Wilkins*, Baltimore, 1963.

108. Assoian R.K., Grotendorst G.R., Miller D. M., and Sporn M.B., Cellular transformation by coordinated action of three peptide growth factors from human platelets, *Nature*, 308, 804, 1984.

109. Postlethwait, A. E., Keski-Oja J., Moses H. L., and Kang A. H., Stimulation of the chemotactic migration of human fibroblasts by transforming growth factor-13, *J. Exp. Med.*, 165, 251, 1987.

110. Brown, G.L., Curtsinger, L.J., White, M., Mitchell, R.O., Pietsch, J., Nordquist, R., von Fraunhofer, J.A., and Schultz, G.S., Acceleration of tensile strength of incisions treated with EGF and TGF-beta, *Ann. Surg.*, 208, 788, 1988.

111. Bland, K.I., Palin, W.E., von Fraunhofer, J.A., Morris, R.R., Adcock, R.A., and Tobin, G.R., II, Experimental and clinical observations of the effects of cytotoxic chemotherapeutic drugs on wound healing, *Ann. Surg.*, 199, 782, 1984.

112. Sowa, D.E., Masterson, B.J., Nealon, N., and von Fraunhofer, J.A., Effects of thermal knives on wound healing, *Obstet. Gynecol.*, 66, 436, 1985.

113. Stone, I.K., von Fraunhofer, J.A., and Masterson, B.J., The biomechanical effects of tight suture closure on fascia, *Surg. Gynecol. Obstet.*, 163, 448, 1986.

114. Richards, P.C., Balch, C.M., and Aldrete, J.S., Abdominal wall closure: a randomized prospective study of 571 patients comparing continuous versus interrupted suture techniques, *Ann. Surg.*, 197, 238, 1983.

115. Brown, G.L., Curtsinger, L., III, Brightwell, J.R., et al., Enhancement of epidermal regeneration by biosynthetic epidermal growth factor, *J. Exp. Med.*, 198, 1319, 1986.

116. Laato, M., Niinikoski, J., and Lebel, L., Stimulation of wound healing by epidermal growth factor, *Ann. Surg.*, 203, 379, 1986.

117. Kingsnorth, A.N., Vowles, R., and Nash, J.R., Epidermal growth factor increases tensile strength in intestinal wounds in pigs, *Br. J. Surg.*, 77, 409, 1990.

118. Hennessey, P.J., Black, C.T., and Andrassy, R.J., EGF increases short-term type I collagen accumulation during wound healing in diabetic rats, *J. Pediatr. Surg.*, 25, 893, 1990.

119. Laato, M., Heino, J., Kahari, V.M., et al., Epidermal growth factor prevents methylprednisolone-induced inhibition of wound healing, *J. Surg. Res.*, 47, 354, 1989.

120. Mustoe, T.A., Pierce, G.F., and Morishima C., Growth factor-induced acceleration of tissue repair through direct and inductive activities in a rabbit dermal ulcer model, *J. Clin. Invest.*, 87, 694, 1991.

121. Fiddes, J.C., Hebda, P.A., and Hayward, P., Preclinical wound-healing studies with recombinant human basic fibroblast growth factor, *Ann NY Acad. Sci.*, 638, 316, 1991.

122. Marks, M.G., Doillon, C., and Silver, F.H., Effects of fibroblasts and basic fibroblast growth factor on facilitation of dermal wound healing by type I collagen matrices, *J. Biomed. Mater. Res.*, 25, 683, 1991.

123. McGee, G., Davidson, J.M., and Buckley, A., Recombinant basic fibroblast growth factor accelerates wound healing, *J. Surg. Res.*, 45, 145, 1988.

124. Hayward, P., Hokanson, J., Heggers, J., et al., Fibroblast growth factor reverses the bacterial retardation of wound contraction, *Am. J. Surg.*, 163, 288, 1992.

125. Tsuboi, R. and Rifkin, D.B., Recombinant basic fibroblast growth factor stimulates wound healing in healing-impaired db/db mice, *J. Exp. Med.*, 172, 245, 1990.

126. Lepisto, J., Laato, M., and Miinikoski, J., Effects of homodimeric isoforms of platelet-derived growth factor (PDGF AA and PDGF BB) on wound healing in rats, *J. Surg. Res.*, 53, 596, 1992.

127. Pierce, G.F., Mustoe, T.A., Altrock, B.W., et al., Role of platelet derived growth factor in wound healing, *J. Cell. Biochem.*, 45, 319, 1991.

128. Pierce, G.F., Mustoe, T.A., Senior, R.M., et al., In vivo incisional wound healing augmented by platelet-derived growth factor and recombinant c-sis gene homodimeric proteins, *J. Exp. Med.*, 167, 974, 1988.

129. Pierce, G.F., Mustoe, T.A., Lingelbach, J., et al., Platelet-derived growth factor and transforming growth factor-β enhance tissue repair activities by unique mechanisms, *J. Cell. Biol.*, 109, 429, 1989.

130. Mustoe, T.A., Purdy, J., Gramates, P., et al., Reversal of impaired wound healing in irradiated rats by platelet-derived growth factor-BB, *Am. J. Surg.*, 158, 345, 1989.

131. Pierce, G.F., Tarpley, J.E., and Yanagihara, D., Platelet-derived growth factor (BB homodimer), transforming growth factor-β1, and basic fibroblast growth factor in dermal wound healing, *Am. J. Pathol.*, 140, 1375, 1992.

132. Roberts, A.B., Sporn, M.B., and Assoian, R.K., Transforming growth factor type-β: rapid induction of fibrosis and angiogenesis in vivo and stimulation of collagen formation in vitro, *Proc. Natl. Acad. Sci. U.S.A.*, 83, 4167, 1986.

133. Sporn, M.B., Roberts, A.B., and Shull, J.H., Polypeptide transforming growth factors isolated from bovine sources and used for wound healing in vivo, *Science*, 219, 1329, 1983.

134. Ksander, G.A., Ogawa, Y., Chu, G.H., et al., Exogenous transforming growth factor-β2 enhances connective tissue formation and wound strength in guinea pig dermal wounds healing by secondary intent, *Ann. Surg.*, 211, 288, 1990.

135. Mustoe, T.A., Pierce, G.F., Thomason, A., et al., Accelerated healing of incisional wounds in rats induced by transforming growth factor-β, *Science*, 237, 1333, 1987.

136. Lawrence, W.T., Sporn, M.B., Gorschboth, C., et al., The reversal of an Adriamycin induced healing impairment with chemoattractants and growth factors, *Ann. Surg.*, 203, 142, 1986.

137. Curtsinger, L.J., Pietsch, J.D., and Brown, G.L., Reversal of Adriamycin-impaired wound healing by transforming growth factor-β, *Surg. Gynecol. Obstet.*, 168, 517, 1989.

138. Bernstein, E.F., Harisiadis, L., Salomon, G., et al., Transforming growth factor-β improves healing of radiation-impaired wounds, *J. Invest. Dermatol.*, 97, 430, 1991.

139. Pierce, G.F., Mustoe, T.A., and Lingelbach, J., Transforming growth factor-β reverses the glucocorticoid-induced wound-healing deficit in rats: possible regulation in macrophages by platelet-derived growth factor, *Proc. Natl. Acad. Sci. U.S.A.*, 86, 2229, 1989.

140. Regan, M.C, Kirk, S.J., and Hurson, M., Tumor necrosis factor inhibits in vivo collagen synthesis, *Surgery*, 113, 173, 1993.

141. Mooney, D.P., O'Reiley, M., and Gamelli, R.L., Tumor necrosis factor and wound healing, *Ann. Surg.*, 211, 124, 1990.

142. Schultz, G.S., White, M., and Mitchell, R., Epithelial wound healing enhanced by transforming growth factor-alpha and vaccinia growth factor, *Science*, 235, 350, 1987.

143. Barbul, A., Knud-Hansen, J., and Wasserkrug, H.L., Interleukin 2 enhances wound healing in rats, *J. Surg. Res.*, 40, 315, 1986.

144. DeCunzo, P., MacKenzie, J.W., Marafino, B.J., et al., The effect of interleukin-2 administration on wound healing in Adriamycin-treated rats, *J. Surg. Res.*, 49, 419, 1990.

145. Cohn, I., Jr., Slack, N.H., and Fisher, B., Complications and toxic manifestations of surgical adjuvant chemotherapy for breast cancer, *Surg. Gynecol. Obstet.*, 127, 1201, 1968.

146. Cohen, S.C., Gabelnick, H.L., Johnson, R.K., and Goldin, A., Effects of antineoplastic agents on wound healing in mice, *Surgery*, 78, 238, 1975.
147. Palin, W.E., von Fraunhofer, J.A., Tobin, G.R., II, and Bland, K.I., Effects of cytotoxic chemotherapeutic drugs on wound fibroplasia in normal and tumor-bearing rats, *Surg. Forum*, 34, 568, 1983.
148. Marder, S.R., Chenoweth, D.E., Goldstein, I.M., and Perez, H.D., Chemotactic responses of human peripheral blood monocytes to the complement-derived peptides C5a and C5 des-Arg, *J. Immunol.*, 134, 3325, 1985.
149. Postlethwait, A.E. and Kang, A.H., Collagen and collagen peptide-induced chemotaxis of human blood monocytes, *J. Exp. Med.*, 143, 1299, 1976.
150. Senior, R.M., Griffin, G.L., and Meecham, R.P., Chemotactic activity of elastin-derived peptides, *J. Clin. Invest.*, 66, 859, 1980.
151. Berliner, J.A., Territo, M., Alamada, L., Carter, A., Shafonsky, E., and Fogelman, A.M., Monocyte chemotactic factor produced by large vessel endothelial cells *in vitro*, *Arteriosclerosis*, 6, 254, 1986.
152. Kay, A.B., Pepper, D.S., and Ewart, M.R., Generation of chemotactic activity for leukocytes by the action of thrombin of human fibrinogen, *Nature*, 243, 56, 1973.
153. Norris, D.A., Clark, R.A.F., Swigart, L.M., Huff, J.C., Weston, W.L., and Howell, S.E., Fibronectin fragment(s) are chemotactic for human peripheral blood monocytes, *J. Immunol.*, 129, 1612, 1982.
154. Snyderman, R. and Fudman, E.J., Demonstration of a chemotactic factor receptor on macrophages, *J. Immunol.*, 124, 2754, 1980.
155. Bevilaqua, M.P., Pober, J.S., Wheeler, M.E., Cotran, R.S., and Gimbrone, M.A., Jr., Interleukin-1 acts on cultured human vascular endothelium to increase the adhesion of polymorphonuclear leukocytes, monocytes and related leukocytes, *J. Clin. Invest.*, 76, 20003, 1985.
156. Matsushima, K. and Oppenheim, J.J., Interleukin-8 and MCAF: novel inflammatory cytokines inducible by IL-1 and TNF, *Cytokine*, 1, 2, 1989.
157. Galin, J.I. and Kaplan, A.P., Mononuclear cell chemotactic activity of kallikrein and plasminogen activator and its inhibition by C1 inhibitor and alpha 2-macroglobulin, *J. Immunol.*, 113, 1928, 1974.
158. Valente, A.J., Fowler, S.R., Sprague, E.A., Kelley, J.L., Suenran, C.A., and Schwartz, C.J., Initial characterization of a peripheral blood mononuclear cell chemoattractant derived from cultured arterial smooth muscle cells, *Am. J. Pathol.*, 117, 409, 1984.
159. Ogawa, T., Kotani, S., Kusumoto, S., and Shiba, T., Possible chemotaxis of monocytes by *N*-acetylmuramyl-L-alanyl-D-isoglutamine, *Infect. Immunol.*, 39, 449, 1983.
160. Deuel, T.F., Senior, R.M., Chang, D., Griffin, G.L., Henrikson, R.L., and Kaiser, E.T., Platelet factor 4 is chemotactic for neutrophils and monocytes, *Proc. Natl. Acad. Sci. U.S.A.*, 78, 4584, 1981.
161. Jauchem, J.R., Lopez, M., Sprague, E.A., and Schwartz, C.J., Mononuclear cell chemoattractant activity from cultured arterial smooth muscle cells, *Exp. Mol. Pathol.*, 37, 167, 1982.
162. Bar-Shavit, R., Kahn, A., Fenton, J.W., and Wilner, G.D., Chemotactic response of monocytes to thrombin, *J. Cell Biol.*, 96, 282, 1983.

Chapter 3

Surgical Needles

J. A. von Fraunhofer and C. C. Chu

CONTENTS

I. INTRODUCTION

The surgical needle, to which the suture is attached, has the primary function of introducing the suture through the tissues to be brought into apposition. Thereafter, the tissues are maintained in apposition by the suture until physiologic healing of the wound has occurred. Ideally, the needle has no role in wound healing, but inappropriate needle selection can prolong the operating time and/or damage tissue integrity leading to such complications as tissue necrosis, wound dehiscence, bleeding, leakage of anastomoses, and poor tissue apposition. Clearly, needle selection is an important factor in suturing and the progress of wound healing.

The use of needles to place sutures is time-honored and there are references to their use as early as 3000 B.C.[1,2] Since then, both the mode of needle usage and methods of suture attachment have changed with advances in surgical procedures and developments in needle design and configuration as well as with changes in the suture material. An excellent review of the historical development of surgical needles has been published by Trier.[1] In earlier times, it was common to insert the "needle" through the wound edges and then wind the suture material in figure-8 loops across the wound to bring the edges into apposition. With primitive peoples, sharpened bones, wood, and even thorns were used as the needle[1,2] and this suturing technique, using metal pins, was often used in the last century, particularly for repair of cleft lips. Late in the 19th century eyed surgical needles, adapted from domestic sewing needles, were developed and this innovation was followed somewhat later by the development of the eyeless or swaged needle. Eyed needles are still used in general and veterinary surgery, primarily with larger suture sizes, but the eyeless needle is now becoming the instrument of choice for virtually all other surgical procedures.

Clearly, for maximum effectiveness, the surgical needle must be able to carry the suture material through tissue with minimal trauma and to achieve this aim, needles are required to satisfy a number of criteria (Table 3.1).

Table 3.1 Needle
Selection Criteria

Minimal tissue trauma
High sharpness (acuity)
Corrosion resistance
High strength
Stable shape
Proper balance
Abrasion resistance
Smooth profile

0-8493-4964-8/97/$0.00+$.50
© 1997 by CRC Press, Inc.

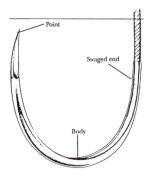

Figure 3.1 Surgical needle components. (Courtesy of Ethicon, Inc., Somerville, NJ.)

The needle necessarily must be sharp to ensure easy and rapid tissue penetration and, on passage through tissue, not cause undue trauma. The latter criterion is achieved, in part, by fabricating needles from corrosion- and abrasion-resistant materials and providing the needle with a smooth, scratch-free surface finish to minimize frictional effects. A properly balanced needle is important for ease of use and secure handling with the needle holder.

Surgical needles are customarily used with needle holders and, during use, are required to penetrate a variety of tissues and exogenous materials so that the needle itself must have high strength in order to resist bending or distortion. Needles are commonly fabricated from stainless steel, a material that has high strength, is readily available, presents few manufacturing problems, can be polished to a smooth finish, and is relatively inexpensive. The gripping action of needle holders and the repeated grip-release action during surgical procedures can damage the needle surface so that wear and abrasion resistance is a necessary prerequisite for surgical needles.

A wide variety of surgical needles exist but all types have basically three components: the point, the body, and the eye, swage or attachment end, Figure 3.1. Differences between needles arise from variations and modifications within these basic parameters.

II. NEEDLE DIMENSIONS

For many years, the standard alloy for most surgical applications was the low carbon type 316L stainless steel with the approximate composition: Fe, 64.97 to 71.97%; Cr, 16 to 18%; Ni, 10 to 14%; Mo, 2 to 3%; and C, 0.03%. This austenitic stainless steel possesses satisfactory characteristics for surgical applications, notably good strength, flexibility, uniform properties, and good corrosion resistance. This alloy was superseded for surgical needle fabrication by the high strength martensitic ASTM 42000 and ASTM 42020 nickel-free stainless steels and these alloys were the "standard" for needle manufacture for several years. In recent years, however, there has been increasing use of ASTM 45500 stainless steel for needle manufacture. ASTM 45500 has a lower level of chromium but does contain 7.5 to 9.5% nickel. The compositions of these 400-series stainless steels are shown in Table 3.2 and their physical properties are summarized in Table 3.3. The higher strength ASTM 45500 steel wire is used in the fabrication of compound curved tapercut needles (see Section III) where advantage is taken of the higher strength to fabricate needles in finer gauges with a greater length of taper section while the needles still carry the same suture size. A further advantage of using a higher strength steel for needle manufacture is that stronger needles are less subject to deformation during tissue penetration. Newer generations of surgical needles, particularly those of complex geometry and the laser-drilled swages, are increasingly fabricated from the higher strength ASTM 45500 stainless steel.

Wires used to manufacture needles are specified by diameter (inches or millimeters) or by gauge, such as the British standard wire gauge (SWG), the USP system, or the Brown and Sharpe (B&S) gauge. The approximate correlations between these various wire sizes are shown in Table 3.4.

Ideally, the wire size used to fabricate the needle is as close as possible to the diameter of the suture which will be attached to it. If the suture has a larger diameter (gauge) than the needle, then there is a risk of increased drag when pulling the suture through the hole created in tissue by the needle.

The size of a surgical needle is determined by four dimensions, the length, the chord, the radius, and the diameter (Figure 3.2). The needle length is the distance measured along the needle from the attachment end to the point. The needle radius is the distance from the center of the circle to the body of the needle if the needle curvature were to be extended to a complete circle. The chord is the linear distance between the needle point and the attachment end while the needle diameter is the gauge or

Table 3.2 Compositions (wt %) of Stainless Steel Alloys

Alloy	Cr	Ni	Mn	P	S	Si	Ti	Co and Ta	Cu	Mo	Fe
42000	12–14	0	1.00*	0.04 *	0.03*	1*	0	0	0	0	Bal
42020	12–14	0	1.25*	0.06 *	0.15^	1*	0	0	0	0.6*	Bal
45500	11–12.5	7.5–9.5	0.50*	0.04 *	0.03*	0.5*	0.8–1.4	0.1–0.5	1.5–2.5	0.5*	Bal

Note:*, maximum amount; ^, minimum level; Bal, balance.

Data from Thacker, J. G., Rodeheaver, G. T., Towler, M. A., and Edlich, R. F., *Am. J. Surg.*, 157, 334, 1989.

Table 3.3 Properties of Stainless Steels

Property	ASTM 42000	ASTM 42020	ASTM 45500
Specific gravity	7.7	7.6	7.8
Modulus of elasticity (GPa)	200	200	200
Yield strength (MPa)	1441	1360	2317
Tensile strength (MPa)	2055	1940	2482

Data from Thacker, J. G., Rodeheaver, G. T., Towler, M. A., and Edlich, R. F., *Am. J. Surg.*, 157, 334, 1989.

Table 3.4 Wire Dimensions

Diameter (mm)	Diameter (in.)	Standard wire gauge (SWG)	Brown and Sharpe (B&S)	USP
0.079–0.102	0.0031–0.004	44–42	40–38	6–0
0.142	0.0056	39	35	5–0
0.160–0.203	0.0063–0.008	38	34–32	4–0
0.254	0.010	33	30	3–0
0.320	0.0126	30	28	2–0
0.404	0.0159	27	26	0
0.455	0.0179	26	25	1
0.511	0.0201	25	24	2
0.574	0.0226	24	23	3
0.643	0.0253	23	22	4
0.813	0.0320	21	20	5
0.914	0.0360	20	19	6
1.016	0.0400	19	18	7

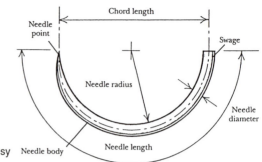

Figure 3.2 Anatomy of a surgical needle. (Courtesy of Ethicon, Inc., Somerville, NJ.)

thickness of the wire from which the needle was fabricated. Needle curvature is specified in degrees of the subtended arc and, typically, needle curvatures are $^1/_4$, $^3/_8$, $^1/_2$, or $^5/_8$ of a circle.

Some surgical needles are treated with silicone or polytetrafluoroethylene (PTFE) to reduce surface friction. Although the use of surface coatings to reduce friction and wear is common in many industrial applications, such coatings may present problems with surgical needles. Typically, the repeated gripping and release action of needle holders constitutes a severe wear test for a surface coating while the abrasion and friction that a needle would normally experience during surgical use would exacerbate any problems associated with coating damage or detachment. The latter can introduce problems in some surgical procedures and ophthalmic needles in particular are generally uncoated to avoid the possibility of vision impairment due to debris deposition in the cornea.

III. THE NEEDLE-SUTURE ATTACHMENT

The attachment end of the surgical needle may have three different configurations, namely closed eye, French (split or spring) eye, or swaged (eyeless). Closed eye needles are very similar to the common or household sewing needle although the shape of the eye may be round, square, or oblong. The disadvantage of closed eye needles is that sutures have to be tied through the eye, thereby increasing the bulk of suture that has to be drawn through the tissues. Further, tying sutures to needles is a tedious and time-consuming process in the operating room. The French eye needle is slitted from inside the eye toward the distal end of the needle, the slit being provided with ridges to hold the suture in place. The advantage of the French eye needle is that the suture can readily be snapped into or out of the eye, thereby simplifying suture attachment. However, it is possible during surgery for the needle to become detached from the suture and possibly lost within deep wounds. Accordingly, eyed needles are infrequently used in most surgical procedures although they are still used for veterinary surgery with the larger gauge sutures.

Virtually all surgical needles used in modern surgery are swaged, with the suture being bonded to the needle to form a continuous unit although the security of suture attachment does vary with the suture size and the needle diameter. Swaged needles have the great advantage that the suture is supplied with the needle attached in sterile packets so that immediate tissue suturing is possible while the risk of contamination of the needle or suture is greatly reduced. Swaged needles are manufactured in two configurations, the channel swage and the drilled swage. For larger diameter needles, a hole is drilled in the distal end of the needle and the suture is held in place by an adhesive. With smaller gauge needles, a U-shaped channel is cut in the end of the needle and after placement of the suture, the needle body is crimped or closed around the suture to hold it securely in place. The pull-out force to detach the suture from the needle is some 30 to 83% of the tensile failure load of the suture itself.[4]

Recently, laser-drilled needles have become available and these are manufactured by laser drilling a hole in the distal end of the needle body parallel to the axis of the needle.[5,6] The suture is retained within the hole held by an adhesive. Compared to the channel swage, the laser-drilled needle has a smoother outer circumference while the length of the laser-drilled suture swage is shorter than that required for the channel swage. These are significant advantages, particularly the latter since it permits the surgeon to hold the needle closer to the distal end.

Table 3.5 Shapes of Surgical Needle Bodies and Surgical Applications

Needle body shape	Applications
Straight	Skin closure, G.I. tract, oral and nasal cavity, pharynx, tendon
Half-curved	Skin closure
$1/_4$ circle	Eye, microsurgery
$3/_8$ circle	Skin closure, eye, fascia, nerve, vessels, dura, G.I. tract, periosteum, muscle, myocardium, G.U. tract, tendon, pleura
$1/_2$ circle	Eye, muscle, biliary tract, G.I. tract, G.U. tract, respiratory tract, skin, oral and nasal cavity, pharynx, peritoneum
$5/_8$ circle	G.U. tract, cardiovascular system, oral and nasal cavity
Compound curved	Anterior segment of eye, oral surgery, plastic surgery, vascular surgery

The laser-drilled swage needle is finding rapid acceptance by surgeons because the size differential between needle and suture, that is the needle:suture diameter ratio, is smaller than for the traditional crimped or channel needle. This reduced needle:suture diameter ratio has been reported to facilitate surgical suturing and aid in wound healing.[5] The pull-out force for detaching the suture from the needle is the same or slightly greater for the laser-drilled needle than for the channel swage.[5,6]

IV. THE NEEDLE BODY

The needle body is the portion that is grasped by a needle holder during suturing procedures and, as indicated above, there should be a close correspondence between needle diameter and suture gauge to minimize any drag effects. Needle bodies are supplied in a variety of shapes or curvatures which provide the needle with certain characteristics and, consequently, different surgical uses, as summarized in Table 3.5. It should be noted that manufacturers will supply a variety of suture materials with an assortment of needle shapes, but it is generally not possible to obtain all suture materials attached to every type of needle. Accordingly, the surgeon has to select the suture–surgical needle combination that best suits the clinical requirements of the intended procedure and his personal preferences.

The straight needle may be preferred for suturing more accessible tissue, typically the skin, when suturing often can be performed without using needle holders. The two principal types of straight needle are the straight-cutting Keith needle, used for skin closure of abdominal wounds, and the Bunnell (BN) needle, which has a taper-point and is used for tendon repair and gastrointestinal tract suturing. Straight needles are used also in some microsurgical procedures, such as nerve and vessel repair, and in some types of ophthalmic surgery.

The half-curved or ski-shaped needle was used for skin closure, but its awkward shape and handling difficulty has resulted in this shape of needle being used very infrequently in modern surgery.

The most frequently used needles are curved and the curvatures are usually $1/_4$, $3/_8$, $1/_2$, or $5/_8$ of the arc of a circle, that is, a curvature of 90, 135, 180, and 225°. Curved needles are favored in surgery because they more predictable in their passage through tissue but, as a result of the curvature, they require the use of needle holders. The $3/_8$-circle (135°) needle is well adapted for skin closure, its primary application, and can be manipulated reasonably easily for suturing large and superficial wounds. The wide manipulation arc of the needle, however, mitigates against its use for deep cavities or where there is restricted access. The $1/_2$-circle (180°) needle was designed for suturing in restricted access or confined areas, but the $5/_8$ (225°) needle is often preferable for suturing in deep cavities such as the pelvis and for applications in intraoral, G.U. tract, and cardiovascular surgery.

Recently, compound curved needles have been introduced into surgery.[7–10] This type of needle has a short, relatively straight point with a curved distal section so that there are two separate and distinct needle radii. Typically, the needle has an 80° curvature at the needle tip that converts to a 45° curvature for the rest of the body. In ophthalmic surgery, the compound curved needle has certain advantages. The steep curve of the tip permits short, deep, and very accurate insertions into the tissue and allows the suture to be placed at equal distances either side of the incision while maintaining good visibility as the needle body is pushed through tissue. Equidistant suture placement is particularly important in plastic surgery and ophthalmology since accurate positioning will reduce the risk of unequal tension across the wound, a necessary requirement for esthetic results in plastic surgery and in ophthalmology, typically corneal-scleral surgery, to ensure that the eye maintains good and defect-free vision. Since its introduction, the compound curved needle appears to have definite appeal to various surgical specialties that benefit from the greater precision and accuracy in tissue approximation.[7-10] It is possible that needles with a variety of compound curvatures will be available in the future, particularly since the higher strength ASTM 45500 stainless steel permits needles to be fabricated in a variety of shapes, chord lengths, and diameters without sacrificing needle strength.

The cross section of the needle body varies with the type of needle, such as blunt, cutting, reverse cutting, and so forth. This is discussed in the next section.

V. NEEDLE POINTS

Surgical needle points fall into three broad categories: blunt, tapered, and cutting. Blunt needles have a rounded tip and an oval cross section; these needles are used for blunt dissection, friable tissue, intestine, kidney, liver, spleen, and fascia. Tapered needles have a sharp tip and an oval cross section, but do not cut tissue. Rather, they pierce and spread tissue and are used to effect passage through a variety of tissues that are less resistant to penetration or where the smallest possible hole is required such as for internal anastomoses. In contrast, cutting needles have sharpened points and edges to permit passage through tissue that is tough or resistant to penetration, typically skin, muscle, and tendon. There are four types of cutting needles: conventional, reverse, tapercut, and side cutting or spatulate.

Conventional cutting needles have oval bodies with triangular points and three cutting edges; two cutting edges are at the sides of the point and the third is on the concave side of the needle curvature. The triangular point smoothes out to a flattened or oval body with both straight and curved needles. The disadvantage of the conventional cutting needle is that it may cut out of tissue by virtue of the fact that the inside (concave) cutting edge cuts toward the wound or incision edge on passage through tissue. There have been various advances in the design of the conventional cutting needle, notably narrower points, thinner wire diameters, and flattened sides to facilitate gripping with needle holders while reducing the bending tendency of finer diameter wires. Nevertheless, the risk of needle cut out can be a problem during surgery and to overcome this difficulty reverse cutting needles were developed.

The reverse cutting needle has a similar configuration to the conventional cutting needle, namely a triangular point with two lateral cutting edges but the third cutting edge is situated on the outer or convex side of the needle point. This configuration provides the needle with greater strength, reduces the risk of needle cut out, and moves the penetration hole away from, rather than toward, the incision. These needles are designed for use with tougher, more penetration-resistant tissues such as skin and mucosa. They are also favored in situations where reduced tissue trauma and minimized scar tissue formation are required, typically cosmetic and ophthalmic surgery. A significant advance on this type of needle has been the development of combination taper point and reverse cutting point needles, known as tapercut needles. These needles are available with the compound curved body.[7-10]

Tapercut needles have a reverse cutting edge tip and a tapering point and, in one proprietary form, have three cutting edges that extend approximately 0.8 mm back from the trocar point and then merge into a round taper body.[7,11] These needles are widely used with dense, fibrous connective tissue, particularly where there is a need for a reduced risk of separation of parallel connective tissue fibers.

Side cutting or spatulate needles are manufactured by flattening the outer convex surface of the body to produce a body that is trapezoidal or hexagonal in cross-section, the so-called cobra head design. This needle has cutting edges only on the sides, which significantly reduces the risk of tissue cut out that can occur with other cutting needles. This type of needle and its variations, which are designed to have up to four cutting edges, are favored for ophthalmic surgery since the needle can separate thin layers of corneal or scleral tissue and pass between the plane separating them.

It should be noted that surgical needles often are provided with ribbing on the inner and /or outer surfaces or on both sides of the needle body to increase needle security within the needle holder. The needle cross section may have several configurations, but the more common appear to be a square ribbed body, a flat ribbed body with rounded sides, or a triangular ribbed body.

VI. NEEDLE ACUITY

The most important biomechanical performance parameters for surgical needles are acuity or sharpness, bending resistance, and ductility and these subjects are discussed in the next two sections. Needle acuity would appear, at first sight, to be the most important biomechanical parameter since the needle is required to penetrate tough or fibrous tissue without undue trauma, creating a pathway through which the body of the needle and the attached suture will then pass. Clearly, surgical needles must be sharp to enable them to readily penetrate tissue without causing undue trauma. Further, the relative ease of tissue penetration with a sharp needle facilitates surgical dexterity while reducing the risk of needle bending or deformation during use since less force has to be applied to a sharp needle. However, quantification of needle acuity is difficult.

Most acuity studies[3-15] involve determining the force required to force the needle through a suitable target material, with acuity defined[4,5] as 100× the reciprocal of the force required to penetrate the target material. However, it should be noted that the penetration resistance of the target medium will strongly influence the measured acuity. Thus, while acuities of the same order of magnitude will be obtained by different workers for the same type of needle,[3-5] there may be small differences in the reported values due to the use of different target materials. The target materials for acuity measurements typically have been synthetic skin and membrane products such as Medpar®, a laminated film of Mylar® and polyethylene,[3,6,7,10-12] and Porvair®[6,9,13] as well as thin films of rubber.[4,5] One study showed that a cuticular needle had an acuity of the order of 2.5 to 3.0, that is, a force of 30 to 40 g was required to penetrate a thin rubber membrane, while the same wire diameter plastic surgery needle had an acuity of 5 to 10, that is, it required only 10 to 20 g to penetrate the same target material.[3,5] Other workers, using synthetic membranes, have shown comparable values, namely an acuity of 5.4 for a cuticular needle and an acuity of 10.0 for a plastic surgery needle of the same dimensions using Medpar as the target material.[3] The recently introduced compound curved tapercut needles fabricated from ASTM 45500 stainless steel also demonstrated comparable acuities[7-12] for penetration of Medpar. Acuity values determined using Porvair as the target material were lower for some types of vascular surgery needle[9] although other studies demonstrated very high acuities, 15 to 29, for penetration of microsurgical spatula needles into the same target material.[13]

Clearly, the acuity of finer gauge and very sharp needles is greater than that of larger gauge and blunter needles, but a number of factors actually determine needle sharpness (Table 3.6) and many of these factors act in concert to influence acuity. It is difficult, therefore, to isolate or specify which factor has the greatest effect on needle acuity, particularly when comparing needles produced by different manufacturers or even needles from the same manufacturer which have slight differences in dimension or design. Nevertheless, it is possible to indicate the effect of many of these factors on needle acuity.

Table 3.6 Factors in Needle Acuity

Composition of the wire
Wire physical properties
Diameter of the wire
Design of the needle
Type of needle point
Manufacturing process
Needle surface finish

The greater acuity of thinner gauge needles is clear from the literature,[3-12] and the data given in Tables 3.7 and 3.8. Needle acuity increases as the needle wire diameter decreases and, in fact, it has been shown[4] that acuity is linearly dependent upon wire diameter according to the relationship

$$\text{Acuity} = k - k^1 \cdot d$$

where k and k^1 are constants and d is the wire diameter. A correlation coefficient of 0.83 was found for the equation

$$\text{Acuity} = 16 - 22 \cdot d$$

An even higher value of the correlation coefficient, r = 0.98, was found for an exponential relationship

$$\text{Acuity} = k \cdot e^{k^1 \cdot d}$$

and the values of k and k^1 were found to be 0.67 and 7.1, respectively.[4]

Table 3.7 Acuity Constants for Surgical Needles

Equation	Constant k	Constant k¹
Acuity vs. wire diameter $A = k - k^1 \cdot d$	16	22
Acuity vs. wire diameter $A = k \cdot e^{k^1 \cdot d}$	0.7	7
Acuity vs. surface hardness $A = k - k^1 \cdot (MHv)$	236	0.4

Table 3.8 Needle Acuity Values

Needle designation	Needle diameter (mm)	Manufacturer	ASTM Alloy	Sharpening process	Acuity
CE4	0.58	Davis & Geck	42000	Machine grinding	5.00[3]
PRE4	0.58	Davis & Geck	42020	Hand honed	6.54[3]
RE5	0.58	Deknatel	42000	Hand honed	3.68[3]
ED5	0.58	Deknatel	42020	Hand honed	5.23[3]
RE2	0.58	Deknatel	42020	Hand honed	5.76[3]
FS2	0.58	Ethicon	42000	Machine grinding	5.47[3], 2.73[4]
PS2	0.58	Ethicon	45500	Electrohoned	8.91[3], 7.73[4]
PS4	0.58	Ethicon	45500	Electrohoned	10.00[3]
P-12	0.54	McGhan	—	—	13.37[3]
S-33	0.50	McGhan	—	—	9.76[3]
PRE2	0.43	Davis & Geck	42020	Hand honed	7.54[3]
RE3	0.43	Deknatel	42020	Hand honed	5.48[3]
P3	0.43	Ethicon	45500	Electrohoned	11.96[3]

From Thacker, J.G., Rodeheaver, G.T., Towler, M.A., and Edlich, R.F., *Am. J. Surg.*, 157, 334, 1989; von Fraunhofer, J.A., Storey, R.J., and Masterson, B.J., *Biomaterials*, 9, 281, 1988.

Likewise, and as anticipated, greater needle acuity has been found for needles fabricated from wires with enhanced physical properties.[3] Since there is a direct correlation between the tensile strength and surface hardness of materials, it follows that needle acuity will increase with wire surface hardness (MHv) and a relationship of the form

$$\text{Acuity} = k - k^1 \cdot (MHv)$$

has been observed, where the constants k and k¹ have the respective values of 235.7 and 0.39, with a correlation coefficient of 0.97.[4] It is probable that these constants for both relationships can be "rounded" to the values given in Table 3.7.

The effect of surface finish on acuity can be seen from the data in Table 3.8. The differences in acuity of needles of nominally the same diameter and similar compositions that have been sharpened by machine grinding, hand honing, and electrohoning are evident. A smoother surface finish coupled with the finer point that may be achieved with electrohoning will provide the surgical needle with a greater acuity. Likewise, silicone treatment of the needle surface will enhance the sharpness of the needle and this has been confirmed in studies of the acuity of biopsy needles.[16]

Needle acuity is strongly influenced by the type of needle point and, particularly, the taper ratio of the point, the latter being defined as the ratio of the length of the cutting edges to the width of the needle where the cutting edges stop.[12,15] Irrespective of the type of point, it has been demonstrated that for needles of the same size and comparable point geometries, higher acuities are associated with larger taper ratios.[12,15] Differences in needle point geometry, such as those existing between standard and compound curved taper point needles, have no effect on needle acuity,[8,9] provided there are no other differences between the needles such as wire diameter, composition, or physical properties. Large differences exist in needle acuity when the needle geometries differ.[12,13,15]

Accurate prediction of surgical performance from *in vitro* acuity values is difficult for two reasons, both deriving from the acuity measurement technique. Most acuity studies report the initial force required to penetrate the target but the maximum penetration force is of greater significance. The latter is the

Table 3.9 Effect of Repeat Penetrations on Needle Acuity

Needle designation (attached suture)	Wire diameter (mm)	Initial acuity	Acuity after 10 penetrations	Acuity decrease
FS2 (5-O suture)	0.57	2.74	2.00	27.0%
PS2 (4-O suture)	0.49	5.18	3.85	25.7%
PS3 (5-O suture)	0.48	6.33	5.83	7.9%
PC3 (5-O suture)	0.40	8.29	9.93	−19.8%

Data from von Fraunhofer, J.A., Storey, R.J., and Masterson, B.J., *Biomaterials*, 9, 281, 1988.

force required to pass the body of the needle through the target material and it may be 50 to 100% greater than the initial penetration force.[7,11] Determination of the maximum penetration force is a difficult experimental procedure and requires specialized test facilities so that there are few reports of the values of this parameter. Nevertheless, it is reasonable to assume that the observation of lower maximum penetration forces being associated with greater needle acuities[7,11] is a general rule for surgical needles. However, one study showed that there was no statistically significant difference in the acuities (initial penetration forces) for a tapercut and a reverse cutting edge needle, but there was a large difference in the maximum penetration forces. The maximum penetration force for the reverse cutting edge needle was 15.2 g while that for the tapercut needle was 21.6 g. This 50% difference in maximum penetration forces is related to the relative lengths of the two cutting edges. The tapercut needle has relatively short cutting edges so that it only cuts a small hole in the target material, which provides greater resistance to passage of the needle body. In contrast, the longer cutting edge of the reverse cutting edge needle cuts a larger hole in the target, thereby reducing the resistance to passage of the needle body.

The second problem with using acuity values to predict surgical performance arises from the fact that in surgical use, the needle and attached suture are passed through tissue several times before the suture is tied off, while in acuity tests, there may be only a single passage of the needle through the target material. In fact, it has been shown that repeat penetration of a target material by a surgical needle will generally result in a decrease in acuity. This "blunting" action of repeated use is common with all cutting and drilling instruments, and this is clearly shown by the data in Table 3.9 where needle acuity decreases with increasing number of penetrations.[4] However, in one case the acuity actually increased with repeat penetrations of the test medium, suggesting either some form of self-sharpening or removal of small asperities on the needle with repeated passage into the target material.

VII. NEEDLE BIOMECHANICS

Two important factors in needle biomechanics are the resistance to bending and needle ductility,[6–8,10,11,13,14,17] characteristics that have important clinical implications. Strong needles possess greater deformation resistance and, consequently, there should be reduced trauma when used to create a pathway for the suture. The corollary to this is that surgical accuracy is reduced when weak needles that may be more susceptible to bending are used in tough tissue.[2,14]

A specialized test apparatus has been developed to evaluate needle bending resistance[14] and this device has been used in several studies,[6–8,10,11,13,14] the measured parameters being the yield moment and the ultimate moment. The system incorporates a clamp that holds the needle at a constant moment arm while rotating it at a constant angular speed (1.5°/s) against a fulcrum attached to a load cell transducer. The device generates a force-deflection curve from which three parameters, the yield moment, the ultimate moment, and the ductility, are determined. The force deflection curve for curved surgical needles shows an initial linear elastic region followed by nonlinear increasing plastic deformation region and, accordingly, yield moment is determined using the 2% offset strain method common in tensile testing of nonferrous metals. The ultimate moment is defined as the greatest bending moment on the curve. Refinement of the testing method resulted in the development of an index of elastic deformation, which is the quotient of the yield moment divided by the angular degree of deformation. The index of elastic deformation relates the magnitude of the yield moment to the angular needle deformation and, other things being equal, a higher index of elastic deformation indicates a greater resistance to deformation. Finally, the needle resistance to breakage or ductility is determined by measuring the work required to fracture the needle by cyclic bends through an arc of 90°.

The literature reports many studies of the biomechanical properties of surgical needles,[6–8,10,11,13,14] and many of these parameters are summarized in Table 3.10. The most important determinants of the yield

Table 3.10 Mean Values of Biomechanical Parameters of Surgical Needles

Needle designator	Wire diameter (mm)	Yield moment (N·cm)	Ultimate moment (N·cm)	Work (N·cm)	Index of elastic deformation
D&G CE4	0.58	3.2[a]	5.5[a]	—	11.8[a]
Ethicon FS2	0.58	3.6[a]	5.9[a]	—	14.8[a]
Deknatel RE5	0.58	4.5[a]	6.2[a]	—	18.3[a]
Deknatel ED5	0.58	3.0[a]	6.2[a]	—	13.2[a]
D&G PRE4	0.58	3.0[a]	6.0[a]	—	11.2[a]
Ethicon PS2	0.58	5.7[a], 7.5[b]	8.1[a], 9.4[b]	27.3[b]	18.5[a]
Deknatel RE2	0.58	2.8[a]	6.1[a]	—	13.1[a]
Ethicon PS4	0.58	4.9[a]	9.0[a]	—	16.8[a]
Deknatel RE3	0.43	1.5[a]	3.9[a]	—	6.6[a]
D&G PRE2	0.43	0.9[a]	2.6[a]	—	3.8[a]
Ethicon P3	0.43	2.1[a]	3.8[a]	—	7.0[a]
Ethicon V-7	0.58	6.2[b], 5.9[c]	8.4[b], 9.2[c]	27.6[b], 27.3[c]	—
Ethicon V-7 (compound curved)	0.58	6.0[c]	9.0[c]	30.4[c]	—

[a] Data from Abidin, M.R., Towler, M.A., Rodeheaver, G.T., Thacker, J.G., and Edlich, R.F., *J. Biomed. Mater. Res. App. Biomater.*, 23, 129, 1989.
[b] Data from Hoard, M.A., Bellian, K.T., Powell, D.M., and Edlich, R.F., *J. Oral Maxillofac. Surg.*, 49, 1198, 1991.
[c] Data from Hoard, M.A., Franz, D.A., Bellian, K.T., and Edlich, R.F., *J. Oral Maxillofac. Surg.*, 50, 484, 1992.

and ultimate moments are the needle diameter, the wire material, and, possibly, the needle manufacturer.[14] Both the yield and ultimate moments are significantly lower for smaller needles (0.43 mm) than for 0.58-mm needles.[14] Likewise, the yield and ultimate moments are greater for needles manufactured from ASTM 45500 alloy than those fabricated from ASTM 42000 and 42020 alloys, while it appears that electrohoning may provide some enhancement of the two biomechanical moments.[14] It also has been suggested[13,14] that differences in manufacturing and honing/surface grinding techniques, together with the wire material, used by the needle manufacturers may also contribute to differences in the yield and ultimate moments, as well as work to fracture, of the various types of surgical needles. However, it has been shown that needle geometry does not affect the biomechanical parameters, as found when the compound curved taperpoint and standard tapercut needles are compared.[7,8,10] These needles, manufactured from the same alloy (ASTM 45500) and with the same diameter but differing in their geometries, showed little or no differences in sharpness, yield moment, ultimate moment, or work to fracture.[7,8,10] These studies demonstrated that the changed geometry, which improved surgical performance, has no adverse effects on biomechanical properties. In fact, the altered geometry results in a proportionately greater resistance to bending because of the reduced bending moment. Similarly, the clinical advantages of differences in needle point geometry, such as the different configurations of the tapercut and standard reverse cutting edge needle, have no effect on the needle biomechanical parameters. Thus, although the tapercut needle has a greater chord and overall length and radius of curvature than the reverse cutting edge needle but shorter cutting edges, there are no differences in needle acuity (i.e., the initial penetration force), yield moment, ultimate moment, or work to fracture.[11] Similar findings have been reported for spatula needles.[13] Interestingly, comparison of channel and laser-swaged needles clearly demonstrated that the yield moment and work to fracture were markedly greater for the laser-swaged needle.[6]

It follows from the above that the majority of surgical needles have adequate biomechanical properties for surgical use although it appears, other things being equal, that needle characteristics may be strongly dependent upon the needle manufacturer. Certain factors can enhance the biomechanical properties of needles, notably laser-drilled swages and the use of higher strength wires for needle manufacture. Other factors such as needle or point geometry, however, have little effect on the biomechanical parameters.

VIII. NEEDLE HOLDERS

Surgical needles have been used for centuries, but it appears that surgeons usually held the needle between their fingers, with the use of needle holders only becoming relatively common in the 19th century.[1] The actual origins of the needle holder are unknown but it has been suggested[1] that they might have developed through modification of artery forceps. Notwithstanding its origins, the needle holder was developed to hold the needle as it is inserted through tissue and so providing a clear field of operation while reducing the risk of injury to adjacent tissues as well as to the surgeon's fingers. As a result, the primary requirement for a needle holder is the ability to securely grasp the needle and to permit accurate and precise manipulation of the needle within the surgical field. However, quantification of these attributes is difficult and the first reported study of the performance of needle holders was only published in 1986[18] although there have been numerous references within the literature to personal preferences regarding the selection and design of needle holders.[1] Since this first study, the literature on needle holders has grown and there is increased emphasis on achieving a scientific basis for their selection.[19,20]

There is a great variety of needle holders, most of which are named after their inventors who designed these instruments to fulfill certain clinical requirements and/or personal preferences. Accordingly, needle holders are named after their original designers or their clinical usage, for example, Mathieu, Castroviejo, Gillies, Webster, Halsey, DeBakey, Halsey, Mayo-Hegar, Crile Wood, Tucker, microvascular, and many others. It would be a daunting task to describe each needle holder in even general terms, particularly when nominally the same needle holder from different manufacturers may vary in dimensions and often in design details. Accordingly, the focus of this section is primarily the biomechanics of needle holders rather than needle holder design considerations per se although some basic factors will be covered.

As stated earlier, the needle holder is used to hold the surgical needle while it is inserted through tissue and, in essence, the needle holder is a pair of first-class levers rotating on a common fulcrum. The jaws are distal to the fulcrum and the remaining portions of the levers are the handles and these usually terminate in ringlets through which the surgeon places a finger tip. A locking or ratchet mechanism is usually provided on the holder shanks, close to the ringlets, so that once the needle is grasped and the ratchets are engaged, the needle remains securely gripped by the spring force of the ratchet mechanism until the interlocked ratchets are released. The ratchet mechanism usually has three interlocking teeth so that the spring force can be increased incrementally as the opposing ratchets interlock.

The force applied at the jaw interface, P_j, is directly related to the force applied at the rings, P_r, by the length of the shank from the fulcrum to the ringlet force application point, L_r, and the distance of the needle holding point in the jaws to the fulcrum, L_j:

$$P_j = P_r \cdot L_r / L_j$$

and the mechanical advantage of the needle holder is given by L_r/L_j. The clamping moment, P_r, characteristic of the needle holder, determines the stress applied to the needle.

Since a wide variety of needle sizes, corresponding to the suture gauges, are used in surgery, needle holders likewise are available in a variety of sizes. Further, depending upon the precise surgical procedure and the operating site, long or medium length needle holders with short handles are required. Clearly, needle holders used for larger needles will have correspondingly heavier jaws and clamping actions than those for smaller gauge needles. Likewise, needle holders used within deeper wounds will have longer handles than those used for suturing cutaneous wounds. It follows from this overview that the needle holder should possess such characteristics as strength, corrosion resistance, wear/abrasion-resistant jaws, accurately meeting jaws on closure, and, usually but not always, a locking mechanism to clamp the jaws together and handles with finger rings. Finally, needle holders are available in a variety of jaw designs and surface finishes (Figure 3.3). Since the surgeon requires precise control of the needle during its insertion and subsequent passage through tissue, any reduction in needle control will have a negative impact. For example, slippage or wobbling of the needle within the needle holder adversely affects control and, consequently, the surface finish and security of the jaws are important considerations for needle holders, as indicated in Table 3.11. Needle holder jaws may be plain, notched, serrated, or provided with inserts that are smooth or carry teeth. The inserts may be tool steel or latterly, tungsten carbide. Profiled jaws provide a more secure grip on the needle, but there is an attendant risk of damage to the needle, and possibly the suture, if too great a pressure is applied. Smooth jaws may be less favored in certain procedures by surgeons since it is possible for the needle to rotate or twist within the needle holder jaws during clinical use and even for the needle to slip from between the jaws.

Needle holder security, defined as the torque required to rotate and to twist the needle in the needle holder, is determined by a number of factors, notably the design of the needle holder, the size of the needle holder, the number of handle ratchet interlocks, and the type of jaws, especially their shape and surface topography. Needle holder security is evaluated by means of an universal testing machine and a special clamping and pulley jig that permits determination of the rotational and twisting moments.[18-20] Studies on the Ryder and Mayo-Hegar needle holders with three different types of jaw facings and

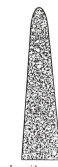
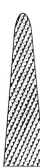

Figure 3.3 Surgical needle holder jaw faces. (Courtesy of Ethicon, Inc., Somerville, NJ.)

Smooth jaws   Jaws with tungsten carbide particles   Jaws with teeth

Table 3.11   Design Factors for Needle Holder Jaws

Length	Long, short
Width	Narrow, wide
Profile	Flat, convex, concave
Surface	Smooth, slotted, serrated, granular

ratchet settings at 1, 2, and 3 notches showed that the needle holding security is significantly greater when the jaws have teeth, compared to smooth jaws, while, in general, greater security was found for jaws with 3600 teeth per square inch compared to 2500 teeth per square inch. For smooth jaws and those with 2500 teeth per square inch, increasing the number of ratchet interlocks from 1 to 3 resulted in a 50 to 60% increase in the rotational and twisting moments, with the ratchet effect being rather less for jaws with 3600 teeth per square inch.[18] It should be mentioned that these effects will vary with the type of needle holder and a corollary of the greater security of toothed jaws and increased ratchet interlocking is the risk of damage, typically flattening, of the needle body. Needle security is also influenced by the needle body ribbing, with the greatest security being found in the order square ribbed > flat ribbed > triangular ribbed, although needle holder design does influence the measured needle security.

A recent development in needle holder design is to provide the jaw inserts with a bonded metal coating containing tungsten carbide particles. These jaws provide a secure grip on the surgical needle while apparently diminishing the risk of damage to the needle.[21] Another development has been the modification of the jaw design. Conventional needle holder jaws are flat and since the majority of surgical needles are curved, these flat jaws may bend and flatten the needle when large forces are applied.[19] These considerations resulted in the development of atraumatic needle holders that have inserts with apposable convex and concave clamping surfaces with a 6-mm radius of curvature so that when closed, the jaw inserts approximate the circular curvature of surgical needles.[22] Biomechanical studies of the new jaw inserts showed that the clamping force and needle security (rotational and twisting moments) were the same, at all three ratchet settings, for both flat and curved jaw needle holders. In contrast, the clamping moment of the curved jaw needle holder was not measurable regardless of ratchet setting and needle diameter while the flat jaw needle holder exhibited a clamping moment that increased with ratchet setting and needle diameter. The greater clamping moment of the flat jaw needle holder resulted in permanent deformation of the needle when the clamping moment exceeded the yield moment of the needle, as in the case of smaller diameter surgical needles. No needle damage was observed with the curved jaw needle holder, a significant advantage when these devices are used for smaller diameter needles.

A trend of growing momentum in health care is the increasing use of disposable items in all aspects of surgery, including disposable emergency wound care kits. The latter contain disposable Webster surgical needle holders and a recent study has reported the biomechanical performance of these devices.[23] Disposable Webster needle holders from three different manufacturers were found to be very similar in their dimensions and, correspondingly, in their mechanical advantages, but they differed significantly in their clamping moments. In fact, the clamping moments of two disposable Webster needle holders were of sufficient magnitude to irreversibly deform smaller diameter (0.35-mm) surgical needles. It was noted that the clamping force could be adjusted by slight bending of one handle of the needle holder.

Table 3.12 Mechanical Advantage and Clamping Moment for Various
Needle Holders

Needle holder	Mechanical advantage	Clamping moment (N·cm)	Ref.
Crile-Wood	4.40	3.67	20
Crile-Wood - PS4 needle-ratchet 3	—	3.27	22
Crile-Wood - RB1 needle-ratchet 3	—	2.28	22
DeBakey	4.54	3.28	20
Halsey	3.71	2.17	20
Mayo-Hegar	4.73	5.63	20
Microvascular	4.62	2.66	20
Webster disposable 1-ratchet 3	3.34	3.57	23
Webster disposable 2-ratchet 3	3.02	10.07	23
Webster disposable 3-ratchet 3	3.49	7.97	23

The values of mechanical advantage and clamping moment for several different needle holders are given in Table 3.12.

The studies discussed above clearly indicate the need for the establishment of performance standards and biomechanical quantification of needle holders to reduce the risk of surgical needle damage, and its consequent unpredictable trajectory in tissue. In particular, if the yield moments of surgical needles and the clamping moments of needle holders were specified, then it would be possible to match these items in the surgical situation to reduce the risk of irreversible needle deformation.

A further consideration is the possible damage to a suture by the needle holder if the latter is used to tie the suture, with smooth jaws or those with shallow serrations being preferred to reduce the risk of suture damage. It has been shown[24] that tungsten carbide inserts with teeth within the needle holder jaws produced distinct morphological changes in nylon sutures that resulted in markedly reduced tensile strengths. In contrast, smooth tungsten carbide inserts did not cause suture damage. It was noted that the effect of the number of teeth on the inserts was most marked with larger size monofilament sutures and far less with smaller gauge and braided materials.[24] These considerations apparently resulted in the development of a new needle holder jaw face specifically designed to provide security of needle clamping but with reduced risk of needle and suture damage.[21] This design comprises a stainless steel jaw metallurgically bonded with tungsten carbide particles so that the jaw face has a fine granular textured surface. Studies have shown that the bonded jaw surface provided better needle security than smooth jaws but less than that obtained with needle holder jaws with teeth; however, in contrast to needle holder jaws with teeth, compression of monofilament sutures between the metallurgically bonded jaws did not damage the suture material or reduce its strength.[21]

IV. SUMMARY

The surgical needle, to which the suture is attached, has the primary function of introducing the suture through the tissues to be brought into apposition. Although the needle should have no role in wound healing, inappropriate needle selection can prolong the operating time and/or damage tissue integrity. For maximum effectiveness, the surgical needle must be able to carry the suture material through tissue with minimal trauma, and, accordingly, needles are required to satisfy a number of criteria, notably strength, corrosion resistance, proper balance, and high acuity.

Suture attachment to the surgical needle may be through an eye, swaging, or laser-drilled holes, the latter being preferred because the suture and needle diameters are closer in diameter. Curved needles and, latterly, compound curved needles are the instruments of choice since they provide greater accuracy in suture placement. Cutting and reverse cutting needles points are common, the latter often preferred in surgical practice since the risk of cut-out is reduced. The adoption of newer, higher strength alloys permits the fabrication of narrower gauge needles with greater acuities than hitherto. Further, newer stainless steel alloys allow manufacturers greater design possibilities with regard to the needle taper ratio and the length of the cutting edge while these higher strength alloys improve the biomechanical properties of surgical needles. Surface finish and the honing method affect needle acuity, with greatest acuities being obtained through electrohoning.

Surgical needles are used in conjunction with needle holders and the design parameters and properties of these devices are discussed. Many designs and sizes of needle holders are available, but they may vary markedly in needle security, even between needle holders of nominally the same design but from different manufacturers. Jaw design markedly influences needle security and developments such as teethed jaw inserts, curved inserts, and jaws with a bonded metal coating containing tungsten carbide particles have markedly improved needle security. Biomechanical studies of needle holders indicate that the clamping moment of some jaws may be sufficient to permanently deform the needle when the clamping moment exceeded the yield moment of the needle. However, the adoption of curved jaw needle holders significantly reduces the risk of this. It has been shown that the yield moments of surgical needles and the clamping moments of needle holders should be matched to reduce the risk of irreversible needle deformation during surgical procedures. Further, the risk of damage to a suture by the needle holder, if used to tie the suture, is reduced with new tungsten carbide jaw inserts without detriment to needle security.

REFERENCES

1. Trier, W.C., Considerations in the choice of surgical needles, *Surg. Gynecol. Obstet.*, 149, 84, 1979.
2. Aston, S.J., The choice of suture material for skin closure, *J. Dermatol. Surg.*, 2, 57, 1976.
3. Thacker, J.G., Rodeheaver, G.T., Towler, M.A., and Edlich, R.F., Surgical needle sharpness, *Am. J. Surg.*, 157, 334, 1989.
4. Von Fraunhofer, J.A., Storey, R.J., and Masterson, B.J., Characterization of surgical needles, *Biomaterials*, 9, 281, 1988.
5. Von Fraunhofer, J.A. and Johnson, J.D., A new surgical needle for periodontology, *Gen. Dentist.*, 40, 418, 1992.
6. Ahn, L.C., Towler, M.A., McGregor, W., Thacker, J.G., Morgan, R.F., and Edlich, R.F., Biomechanical performance of laser-drilled and channel taper point needles, *J. Emerg. Med.*, 10, 601, 1992.
7. Hoard, M.A., Franz, D.A., Bellian, K.T., and Edlich, R.F., A new compound curved tapercut needle for oral surgery, *J. Oral Maxillofac. Surg.*, 50, 484, 1992.
8. Cook, T.S., Towler, M.A., Girard, P., McGregor, W., Devlin, P.M., and Edlich, R.F., A new, compound curved needle for skin and skin-graft closure, *J. Burn Care Rehabil.*, 13, 650, 1992.
9. Tribble, C.G., Moody, F.P., Girard, P., Towler, M.A., McGregor, W., Bellian, K.T., and Edlich, R.F., A new, compound-curved needle for vascular surgery, *Am. Surg.*, 58, 458, 1992.
10. Edlich, R.F., Zimmer, C.A., Morgan, R.F., Becker, D.G., Thacker, J.G., Bellian, K.T., and Powell, D.M., A new, compound-curved needle for microvascular surgery, *Ann. Plastic Surg.*, 27, 339, 1991.
11. Hoard, M.A., Bellian, K.T., Powell, D.M., and Edlich, R.F., Biomechanical performance of tapercut needles for oral surgery, *J. Oral Maxillofac. Surg.*, 49, 1198, 1991.
12. Bellian, K.T., Thacker, J.G., Tribble, C.G., Powell, D.M., Becker, D.G., Zimmer, C.A., Morgan, R.F., and Edlich, R.F., Biomechanical performance of tapercut cardiovascular needles, *Am. Surg.*, 57, 591, 1991.
13. Wu, M.M., Morgan, R.F., Thacker, J.G., and Edlich, R.F., Biomechanical performance of microsurgical spatula needles for the repair of nail bed injuries, *J. Emerg. Med.*, 11, 187, 1993.
14. Abidin, M.R., Towler, M.A., Rodeheaver, G.T., Thacker, J.G., and Edlich, R.F., Biomechanics of curved surgical needle bending, *J. Biomed. Mater. Res. Appl. Biomat.*, 23, 129, 1989.
15. McClung, W.L., Thacker, J.G., Edlich, R.F., Allen, R.C., and Rodeheaver, G.T., Biomechanical performance of ophthalmic surgical needles, *Ophthalmology*, 99, 232, 1992.
16. Von Fraunhofer, J.A. and Malangoni, M.A., The acuity of biopsy needles, *Biomaterials*, 10, 68, 1989.
17. Abidin, M.R., Towler, M.A., Nochimson, G.D., Rodeheaver, G.T., Thacker, J.G., and Edlich, R.F., A new quantitative measurement for surgical needle ductility, *Ann. Emergency Med.*, 18, 64, 1989.
18. Thacker, J.G., Borzelleca, D.C., Hunter, J.C., McGregor, W., Rodeheaver, G.T., and Edlich, R.F., Biomechanical analysis of needle holding security, *J. Biomed. Mater. Res.*, 20, 903, 1986.
19. Edlich, R.F., Towler, M.A., Rodeheaver, G.T., Becker, D.G., Lombardi, S.A., and Thacker, J.G., Scientific basis for selecting surgical needles and needle holders for wound closure, *Clin. Plast. Surg.*, 17, 583, 1990.
20. Edlich, R.F., Thacker, J.G., McGregor, W., and Rodeheaver, G.T., Past, present and future for surgical needles and needle holders, *Am. J. Surg.*, 166, 522, 1993.
21. Abidin, M.R., Dunlapp, J.A., Towler, M.A., Becker, D.G., Thacker, J.G., McGregor, W., and Edlich, R.F., Metallurgically bonded needle holder jaws; a technique to enhance needle holding security without sutural damage, *Am. Surg.*, 56, 643, 1990.
22. Towler, M.A., Chen, N.C., Moody, F.P., McGregor, W., Thacker, J.G., Rodeheaver, G.T., and Edlich, R.F., Biomechanics of a new atraumatic surgical needle holder, *J. Emerg. Med.*, 9, 477, 1991.
23. Francis, E.H., III, Towler, M.A., Moody, F.P., McGregor, W., Himmel, H.N., Rodeheaver, G.T., and Edlich, R.F., Mechanical performance of disposable surgical needle holders, *J. Emerg. Med.*, 10, 63, 1992.
24. Stamp, C.V., McGregor, W., Rodeheaver, G.T., Thacker, J.G., Towler, M.A., and Edlich, R.F., Surgical needle holder damage to sutures, *Am. Surg.*, 54, 300, 1988.

Chapter 4

Classification and General Characteristics of Suture Materials

C. C. Chu

CONTENTS

The purpose of this chapter is to provide readers with an organized overview of commercially available suture materials in terms of the commonly used classification: absorbability in biological tissues, size, physical configuration (monofilament vs. multifilaments), type of coating materials used to facilitate handling properties, and, finally, the four major characteristics of suture materials and their performance. Such an organized view should provide an overall picture of the suture materials having a vast difference in chemical, physical/mechanical, and biological characteristics without being lost in details.

I. ABSORBABLE VS. NONABSORBABLE

In terms of their performance, suture materials are generally classified into two broad categories: absorbable and nonabsorbable. Absorbable suture materials lose their entire tensile strength within 2 to 3 months; those that retain their strength longer than 2 to 3 months are nonabsorbable. The absorbable suture materials are catgut (collagen sutures derived from sheep intestinal submucosa), reconstituted collagen, polyglycolide (PGA), poly(glycolide-lactide) random copolymer (Vicryl®), poly-*p*-dioxanone (PDS®, PDSII®), poly(glycolide-trimethylene carbonate) block copolymer (Maxon®), poly(glycolide-ε-caprolactone) (Monocryl®), and Glycolide-Trimethylene Carbonate block copolymer (Biosyn®). The nonabsorbable sutures are divided into the natural fibers (i.e., silk, cotton, and linen), and man-made fibers (i.e., polyethylene, polypropylene, polyamide, polyester, poly(tetrafluoroethylene) (Gore-Tex®), and stainless steel). Table 4.1 summarizes all commercial suture materials that are available mainly in the United States and Europe and the Pacific rim, their generic and trade names, physical configurations, and manufacturers.[1]

II. SUTURE SIZE

Suture materials are also classified according to their size. Currently, two standards are used to describe the size of suture materials: United States Pharmacopoeia (USP) and European Pharmacopoeia (EP).[1] Table 4.2 summarizes both EP and USP standards. The USP standard is more commonly used. In the USP standard, the size is represented by a combination of two Arabic numerals: a 0 and any number other than 0, like 2-0 (or 2/0). The higher the first number, the smaller the suture material. Sizes greater than 0 are denoted by 1,2,3, etc. This standard size also varies with the type of suture material.

Table 4.1 A List of Commercially Available Suture Materials

Generic name	Trade name	Physical configuration	Surface treatment	Manufacturer*
Natural Absorbable Sutures				
Catgut	Catgut or surgical gut	Twisted multifilament	Plain and chromic	A, E, D/G, SSC
Catgut	Surgigut®	Twisted multifilament	Plain and chromic	USS
Catgut	Softgut®	Twisted multifilament	Glycerin-coated	D/G
Reconstituted collagen	Collagen	Twisted multifilament	Plain and chromic	E
Synthetic Absorbable Sutures				
Polyglycolide	Dexon "S"®	Braided multifilament	None	D/G
Polyglycolide	Dexon Plus®	Braided multifilament	Poly(oxyethylene-oxypropylene)	D/G
Polyglycolide	Dexon II®	Braided multifilament	Polycaprolate	D/G
Polyglycolide	Medifit®	Braided multifilament	None	JPS
Poly(glycolide-L-lactide) (polyglactin 910)	Vicryl®	Braided multifilament	Polyglactin 370 and calcium stearate	E
Poly(glycolide-L-lactide)	Polysorb®	Braided multifilament	Coated	USS
Poly-p-dioxanone	PDS II®	Monofilament	None	E
Poly(glycolide-co-trimethylene carbonate)	Maxon®	Monofilament	None	D/G
Poly(glycolide-co-ε-caprolactone) (poliglecaprone 25)	Monocryl®	Monofilament	None	E
Glycomer 631	Biosyn®	Monofilament	None	USS
Nonabsorbable Sutures				
Silk	Surgical Silk®	Braided multifilament	Tru-permanizing	E
Silk	Dermal®	Twisted multifilament	Tanned gelatin (or other proteins)	E
Silk	Virgin Silk®	Twisted multifilament	—	E
Silk	Silk	Braided multifilament	Silicone	E, D/G
Silk	Sofsilk®	Braided multifilament	Coated	USS
Silk	Silk	Braided multifilament	Paraffin wax	SSC
Cotton	Surgical cotton	Twisted multifilament	—	E
Cotton	Cotton	Twisted multifilament	—	D/G
Linen	Linen	Twisted multifilament	—	SSC, E
Polyester	Ethibond®	Braided multifilament	Polybutylate	E
Polyester	Mersilene®	Braided multifilament	—	E
Polyester	Ethiflex®	Braided multifilament	Teflon	E
Polyester	Dacron®	Braided multifilament	None	D/G
Polyester	Ti-Cron®	Braided multifilament	Silicone	D/G
Polyester	Surgidac®	Braided and monofilament	Coated with braid	USS
Polyester	Silky Polydek®	Braided multifilament	Teflonized	SSC
Polyester	Sterilene®	Braided multifilament	Teflonized	SSC
Polyester	Tevdek®	Braided multifilament	Teflonized	SSC
Polyester	Astralen®	Braided multifilament	Teflonized	A
Polyester	Polyviolene®	Braided multifilament	—	L
Polyester	Mirafil®	Monofilament	—	BM
Polyester	Novafil®	Monofilament	None	D/G
Polyamide (nylon 6 and 66)	Ethilon®	Monofilament	—	E
Polyamide (nylon 6 and 66)	Nurolon®	Braided multifilament	Coated	E
Polyamide (nylon 66)	Surgilon®	Braided multifilament	Silicone	D/G
Polyamide (nylon 66)	Dermalon®	Monofilament	None	D/G
Polyamide (nylon 66)	Bralon® monosof®	Braided monofilament	Coated	USS
Polyamide	Sutron®	Monofilament	—	SSC
Polyamide (nylon 6)	Supramid®	Core-sheath	—	A
Polypropylene	Prolene®	Monofilament	—	E
Polypropylene	Surgilene®	Monofilament	None	D/G

Table 4.1 (continued)   A List of Commercially Available Suture Materials

Generic name	Trade name	Physical configuration	Surface treatment	Manufacturer*
Polypropylene	Surgipro®	Monofilament	None	USS
Poly(tetrafluoroethylene	Gore-Tex®	Monofilament	None	Gore
Stainless steel	Surgical stainless steel	Mono- or twisted multifilament	—	E
Stainless steel	Flexon®	Twisted multifilament	—	D/G
Stainless steel	Stainless steel	Mono- or twisted multifilament	—	D/G
Stainless steel	Steel	Monofilament	—	USS
Stainless steel	Stainless steel	Mono- or twisted multifilament	—	A, SSC

Note: A, Astra; E, Ethicon; L, Look; D/G, Davis & Geck; SSC, Societe Steril Catgut; BM, Braun Melsungen; JPS, Japan Medical Supplies; USS, US Surgical; Gore, W.L. Gore and Associates.

Table 4.2   Suture Size Classification

USP size codes		EP size codes	Suture diameter (mm)	
Nonsynthetic absorbable materials	Nonabsorbable and synthetic absorbable materials	Absorbable and nonabsorbable materials	Min.	Max.
	11/0	0.1	0.01	0.019
	10/0	0.2	0.02	0.029
	9/0	0.3	0.03	0.039
	8/0	0.4	0.04	0.049
8/0	7/0	0.5	0.05	0.069
7/0	6/0	0.7	0.07	0.099
6/0	5/0	1	0.10	0.14
5/0	4/0	1.5	0.15	0.19
4/0	3/0	2	0.20	0.24
3/0	2/0	2.5	0.25	0.29
2/0	0	3	0.30	0.39
0	1	4	0.40	0.49
1	2	5	0.50	0.59
2	3	6	0.60	0.69
3	4	7	0.70	0.79
4	5	8	0.80	0.89
5	6	9	0.90	0.99
6	7	10	1.00	1.09

In the EP standard, the code number ranges from 0.1 to 10. The corresponding minimum diameter (mm) can be easily calculated by taking the code number and dividing by 10. The EP standard does not separate natural from synthetic absorbable sutures as the USP standard does.

Because a range of diameters is permitted for each USP suture size, the tensile strength (force/cross-sectional area) of sutures of the same USP size may be different from each other. For example, two polypropylene sutures of the same USP size from two different manufacturers having the same tensile breaking load may have different tensile strengths because of a possible difference in suture cross-sectional area due to slightly different diameters. The polypropylene suture with a smaller diameter may have a higher tensile breaking strength than the one with a larger diameter. A recent study by von Fraunhofer et al. reported that some types of sutures have consistently less variability in diameter than others.[2] They found that Prolene has the greatest variability in diameter, particularly in the 2/0 and 3/0 sizes, among six tested sutures (chromic catgut, Softgut®, Dexon® Plus, Vicryl, PDS, and Prolene®) of USP sizes ranging from 3/0, 2/0, 1/0, to 1. However, Prolene has overall the lowest diameter at all four USP sizes.[2] Softgut, a glycerin-coated catgut from Davis & Geck, has a significantly greater diameter than the other five sutures tested at all four USP sizes. The diameters of chromic gut, Dexon Plus, Vicryl,

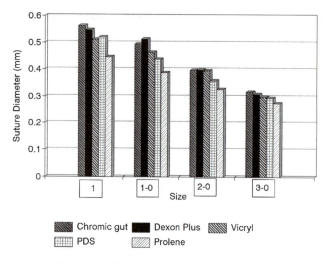

Figure 4.1 Variation in suture diameter of five sutures in four different USP sizes. (Data from von Fraunhofer, J.A., Storey, R.S., Stone, I.K., and Masterson, B.J., *J. Biomed. Mater. Res.*, 19, 595, 1985. With permission.)

and PDS are comparable at most USP sizes, as shown in Figure 4.1, although PDS is a monofilament and the rest are multifilaments.

III. MONOFILAMENT VS. MULTIFILAMENT

In terms of the physical configuration of suture materials, they can be classified into monofilament, multifilament, twisted, and braided. Suture materials made of nylon, polyester, and stainless steel are available in both multifilament and monofilament forms. Catgut, reconstituted collagen, and cotton are available in twisted multifilament form, while PGA, Vicryl, silk, polyester-based, and polyamide-based suture materials are available in the braided multifilament configuration. PDS, Maxon, Monocryl, Biosyn, polypropylene, and poly(tetrafluoroethylene) suture materials exist in monofilament form only. Stainless steel metallic suture materials can be obtained in either monofilament or twisted multifilament configurations. Another unique physical configuration of suture material is available in polyamide (nylon 6) and has the trade name Supramid®, which has a twisted core covered by a jacket of the same material.

IV. COATING MATERIALS

Suture materials are frequently coated to facilitate their handling properties, particularly a reduction in tissue drag when passing through the needle tract and the ease of sliding knots down the suture during knotting (i.e., knot tie-down). Although nonabsorbable beeswax, paraffin wax, silicone, and poly(tetrafluoroethylene) are the traditional coating materials, new coating materials have been reported, particularly those that are absorbable. This is because the coating materials used for absorbable sutures must be absorbable, and traditional nonabsorbable coating materials like wax are not appropriate for absorbable sutures.[3–5] Furthermore, absorbable coating materials should have better tissue biocompatibility because of the lack of chronic tissue reaction.

The trend is to develop coating materials that have a chemical property similar to the suture to be coated. There are basically two types of absorbable coating materials: water soluble and insoluble. Water-insoluble coating materials have chemical constituents similar to those of the suture, and they are broken down by hydrolysis. They remain on the suture surface longer than water-soluble coatings. A typical example is polyglactin 370 used for Vicryl suture. Dexon II sutures have a polycaprolate coating that is water insoluble. Water-soluble coating materials dissolve promptly to reveal the uncoated suture after wound closure. A typical example is poloxamer-188 found on Dexon Plus. Their merits are described later. Multifilament sutures are more commonly provided with coating materials than monofilament sutures. For example, multifilament Vicryl and Dexon Plus or II have coating materials applied, while monofilament PDS and Maxon sutures have no coatings.

Dexon Plus, however, is coated with a surfactant (Pluronic® F-68 from BASF), which is poly(oxyethylene-co-oxypropylene).[5] Because this surfactant coating material (Poloxamer-188) is quite water

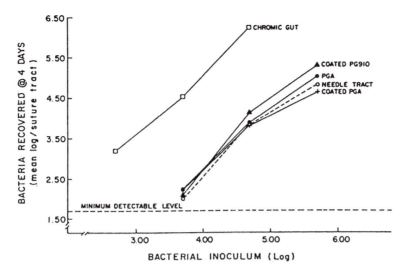

Figure 4.2 The amount of *S. aureus* recovered from the implant site at day 4 of various sutures as a function of the concentration of bacterial inoculum. The results indicate the level of influence of suture materials on the resistance of tissue to infection. The higher the recovered bacteria from a suture, the higher propensity of that suture to lower the resistance of tissue to infection. (From Rodeheaver, G.T., Foresman, P.A., Brazda, M.T., and Edlich, R.F., *Surg. Gynecol. Obstet.*, 164, 17, 1987. With permission.)

soluble and easily removed by water in tissue after wound closure, the coated Dexon suture should become uncoated after completing wound closure. Rodeheaver et al. reported that this temporary coating material for absorbable sutures is nontoxic to experimental animals, improves the handling property, and offers a better resistance to infection.[6-8] As described in Chapter 8, the role of sutures in wound infection is a major concern, and the development of antimicrobial sutures would be very beneficial.

Figures 4.2 and 4.3 illustrate the potential benefit of poloxamer-188 surfactant coating material on the resistance to infection of female Swiss-Webster mice subdermal tissue.[6] The effect of the poloxamer-188-coated PGA (Dexon Plus), PG910 (Vicryl without poloxamer-188 coating material), chromic catgut, and their corresponding uncoated controls on the resistance of host tissue to infection was assessed by the number of bacteria (*S. aureus* and *E. coli*) present in the suture implantation site at the end of 4 d of postimplantation. Dexon Plus consistently showed a lower number of *S. aureus* present in the suture site than the uncoated Dexon "S" over the range of inoculum concentration of 3.7 to 5.7 on a log scale; however, the difference was not statistically significant ($p > 0.05$). In contrast, chromic catgut sutures significantly ($p < 0.01$) inhibited the host tissue defense against wound infection induced by both *S. aureus* and *E. coli* over the range of inoculum concentration. Thus, Rodeheaver et al. concluded that both coatings used on these two synthetic absorbable sutures do not retard the local host defense mechanism against microorganisms and thus would not increase the risk of wound infection.[6]

Although coating of suture materials facilitates easy passage through tissue and handling property, it frequently results in poor knot security. For example, Dexon Plus and coated Vicryl require four or five square throws to form secure square knots, while the uncoated Dexon and Vicryl sutures form secure knots with only two throws (1=1).[7,9] Water-soluble coating materials like poloxamer-188, found on Dexon Plus, do not suffer from the adverse effects of water-insoluble coating materials on knot security. Table 4.3 illustrates this potential advantage.[6] The table shows the effect of time of hydration in saline solution of both poloxamer-188-coated Dexon Plus and polyglactin 370/calcium stearate-coated Vicryl sutures on the percent of 15 two-square-throw (1=1) knots that were secure (defined as a knot that failed at knot break with ears still intact). The most significant finding is that Dexon Plus showed a consistent increase in percent of knot security with the duration of hydration and reached 100% after 2 h hydration *in vivo*, while the polyglactin 910 coated with non-water-soluble material had 0% knot security over the entire duration of hydration (0.5 to 240 h). The reason for this observation is that the dissolution of water-soluble poloxamer-188 coating material revealed the underneath substrate, i.e., uncoated PGA suture. It is known that uncoated PGA sutures form secure 1=1 knots.[9] The coating for Vicryl is not water soluble and thus the coated Vicryl suture exhibited 0% knot security even at the end of 240 h hydration in saline.

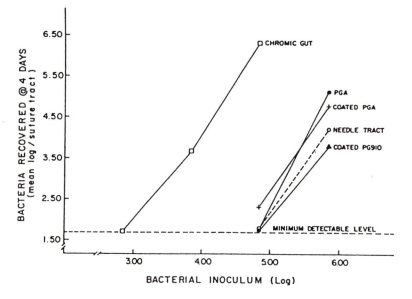

Figure 4.3 The amount of *E. coli* recovered from the implant site at day 4 of various sutures as a function of the concentration of bacterial inoculum. The results indicate the level of influence of suture materials on the resistance of tissue to infection. The higher the recovered bacteria from a suture, the higher propensity of that suture to lower the resistance of tissue to infection. (From Rodeheaver, G.T., Foresman, P.A., Brazda, M.T., and Edlich, R.F., *Surg. Gynecol. Obstet.*, 164, 17, 1987. With permission.)

Table 4.3 Influence of Moisture on the Security of Two-Throw Square Knots Tied with Coated Synthetic Absorbable Sutures

	Knot security,[a] %			
	Coated polyglycolide		Coated polyglactin 910	
Exposure time, hr	*In vitro*	*In vivo*	*In vitro*	*In vivo*
0	0	0	0	0
0.5	60	100	0	0
1.0	87	100	0	0
2.0	100	100	0	0
24.0	100	100	0	0
240.0	100	—	0	—

[a] Percentage of 15 knots that went to knot break.

From Rodeheaver, G.T., Foresman, P.A., Brazda, M.T., and Edlich, R.F., *Surg. Gynecol. Obstet.*, 164, 17, 1987. With permission.

There is, however, one technical concern about using water-soluble coating material in actual wound closure. Suture materials are frequently soaked in saline after their removal from packages before wound closure. Some or the bulk of water-soluble coating materials might be removed by this routine soaking practice. Thus, it is important to minimize the time of soaking when dealing with water-soluble coated suture materials.

Besides the approach of using water-soluble coating materials to improve knot security and handling properties, there are several other patented procedures and materials reported recently to improve either knot tie-down performance or knot security .[10-13] In general, a coating designed to improve knot tie-down would reduce knot security. It is difficult to achieve both. There are very few reported treatments that would achieve these two contradictory and mutually exclusive properties. One of them is the use of a combination of both coating and textured yarns reported by Kawai et al.[10] The coating materials used by Kawai et al. included sucrose fatty acid ester, beeswax, paraffin wax, poly(oxy-ethylene-co-oxypropylene), polyglactin 370, gelatin, silicone, and poly(tetrafluoroethylene). Textured

Table 4.4 Knot Tie-Down and Knot Security of 3/0 PGA Sutures with Textured Yarns and Various Coating Materials

	50-g load		100-g load		
	K.R.	**R.V.**	**K.R.**	**R.V.**	**Knot Security**
Textured suture					
Uncoated	220g	112g	410g	123g	33.4 cycles to untie a knot
Coat A	180	10	330	20	57.4
Coat B	180	11	280	26	46.1
Coat C	200	13	360	17	35.2
Nontextured suture					
Uncoated	230	108	400	129	13.8 cycles to untie a knot
Coat A	190	10	350	22	10.9
Coat B	200	10	300	23	9.8
Coat C	180	12	340	18	6.1

Note: K.R. = knotting resistance; R.V. = roughness value.

From Kawai et al., U.S. Patent 4,983,180, 1991.

Table 4.5 Characterization and Absorption of Suture Coating from Copolymers of ε-Caprolactone and Glycolide at Various Composition Ratios

Characterization			
Copolymer composition caprolactone/glycolide/GA[a]	90/5/10 by mole	90/8/4 by mole	90/10/0 by mole
Intrinsic viscosity of copolymer in HFIP, dl/g	0.19	0.31	0.28
Melting Point[b]	41–44°C	42–40°C	35–45°C
Absorption[c]			
Percent nonhydrolyzed copolymer[d] at			
2 d	19.79	25.76	77.23
2 d (repeat)	15.82	35.23	81.80

[a] Glycolic acid.
[b] Determined by hot-stage microscopy.
[c] *In vitro* hydrolysis at 100°C (sterile water)
[d] Determined by measuring weight loss of copolymer after the indicated number of days.

From Bezwada et al., U.S. Patent 4,994,074, 1991.

yarns were achieved by standard texturing processes employed in the textile industry, and they include false-twist, knit-deknit, stuffing box, and crimping gear methods. Table 4.4 illustrates both the effect of coating/textured and textured alone on knot tie-down and knot security at both 50 and 100 g load conditions. A lower knotting resistance and knot roughness value indicate a better (easier) knot tie-down. Knot security was assessed by the number of cycles required to completely loosen a knot, and hence the larger the number of cycles, the better the knot security. The data in Table 4.4 show that a combination of coating (using any of the existing suture coating materials) and textured yarns improves both knot tie-down and knot security considerably.[10] The coating without texturing of yarns improves knot tie-down, but adversely reduces knot security.

Other recently reported absorbable but not water-soluble coating materials that could improve knot tie-down and knot security are high molecular weight polycaprolactone (copolymer of at least 90% by weight of caprolactone and 10% at most of other biodegradable monomers like glycolide, lactide, and their derivatives[11,12]) or a random copolymer of 25 to 75% by weight of glycolide and the remaining trimethylene carbonate.[13] Table 4.5 lists the chemical, physical, and absorption properties of one formula of the absorbable coating of ε-caprolactone and glycolide copolymer,[12] while Table 4.6 lists the physical and mechanical properties of these 2/0 absorbable coated Vicryl sutures.[12] The observed improved knot tie-down and knot security was attributed to deep penetration and even distribution of the coating materials into the interstices of suture filaments. The patented random copolymer of glycolide and

Table 4.6 Physical and Mechanical Properties of 2/0 Vicryl Sutures Coated with Copolymers of ε-caprolactone and Glycolide at Various Composition Ratios

	Caprolactone/glycolide/GA.[a] Copolymer, 90/5/10 by mole IV (0.19 dl/g)		Caprolactone/glycolide/GA.[a] Copolymer, 90/8/4 by mole IV (0.31 dl/g)		Caprolactone/glycolide/GA.[a] Copolymer, 90/10/0 by mole IV (0.28 dl/g)	
	10% sol.	15% sol.	10% sol.	15% sol.	10% sol.	15% sol.
Diam. (mils)	12.6	12.7	12.8	12.7	12.9	12.9
Tissue drag[b] (g)	18.34	22.13	22.13	17.00	32.25	14.54
Wet roughness tie-down[c] (g)	310.32	353.98	137.89	113.41	149.66	124.40
Percent elong[d]	17.7	18	16.6	17.3	17.6	17.3
Dry knot tensile[d] (psi)	73,800	72,600	73,800	69,500	71,900	68,800
Wet knot tensile[d] (psi)	75,400	71,800	73,000	71,000	71,900	70,400
Dry strength tensile[d] (psi)	124,300	121,600	116,600	119,200	112,500	113,200

[a] Glycolic acid.

[b] Tissue drag is a measure of the relative smoothness of the suture while passing through tissue, and is determined by using an Instron Tensile Tester and a recording device.

[c] Tie-down measured on a Table-Model Instron Tensile tester as described in U.S. Patent No. 3,942,532.

[d] Tensile properties of elongation determined generally according to the procedures outlined in U.S. Patent No. 4,838,267. Wet tensile properties were measured after immersing the coated suture in water at 25°C for 24 hrs.

From Bezwada et al., U.S. Patent 4,994,074, 1991.

trimethylene carbonate coating material was suggested to have the advantages of not flaking off from the substrate sutures because of its high molecular weight and low glass transition temperature and of retaining its lubricant property even when the coated suture is wet.

Most of the coating materials described above are for synthetic sutures. There is relatively little research and development of new coating materials for natural absorbable sutures like catgut and reconstituted collagen sutures. Gaillard recently reported that the widely reported relatively poor *in vivo* biocompatibility and performance of collagen-based sutures could be improved by using biodegradable polymeric coating materials instead of the conventional chromium salts.[14] The rationale behind his approach is that a biodegradable protective coating could temporarily shield the substrate catgut sutures from enzymatic biodegradation during the early stage of wound healing so that the coated catgut sutures should be able to not only retain better strength in this critical period of wound healing, but also delay and reduce the well-known adverse tissue reactions by delaying the onset of enzymatic biodegradation beyond the initial stage of wound healing. It is well known that the rapid loss of tensile strength during the early stage of wound healing is one of the most important concerns for catgut sutures. By varying the composition and thickness of coating materials, Gaillard believed that a range of biodegradation properties of coated catguts could be achieved for a variety of clinical purposes. The use of synthetic biodegradable polymers as the coating for catgut sutures would also eliminate the known toxicity of chromium salts and improve knot tie-down and security. Gaillard's recipe for the biodegradable protective coating consists of biodegradable linear polyesters like glycolide or lactide reinforced with urea and urethane linkages. In order to improve the bonding of this type of coating material to the collagen substrate, linear aliphatic polyesterdiols were capped with di- or polyisocyanates that have $-N=C=O$ functional groups which could chemically bond to $-NH_2$ groups from amino acids like lysine or $-OH$ groups from amino acids like hydroxyproline in collagen. The di- or polyisocyanate-capped polyesterdiol coating materials could be completely biodegraded from about 10 h to 3–4 weeks, depending on the type of polyesterdiol and polyisocyanate and coating conditions.

V. CHARACTERISTICS OF SUTURE MATERIALS

Because of the fibrous nature of suture materials and their role in wound closure, they are characterized and evaluated by four characteristics: physical and mechanical properties, handling properties, biological properties, and biodegradation properties. Table 4.7 summarizes individual properties under each of the four categories. It is important to recognize that these characteristics are interrelated. For example,

Table 4.7 Four Major Categories of the Characteristics of Suture Materials

Physical/mechanical	Handling	Biocompatibility	Biodegradation

USP vs. EP size (diameter)
Mono vs. multifilament
Tensile breaking strength and
  elongation
Modulus of elasticity
Bending stiffness
Stress relaxation and creep
Capillarity
Swelling
Coefficient of friction
	Pliability
	Packaging
	  memory
	Knot tie-down
	Knot slippage
	Tissue drag
		Inflammatory reaction
		Propensity toward wound
		  infection, calculi formation,
		  thrombi formation,
		  carcinogenicity, and allergy
			Tensile breaking
			  strength and mass
			  loss profiles
			Biocompatibility
			  of degradation
			  products

Table 4.8 Mechanical Properties of Absorbable Sutures[a]

Class (chemical name)	Commercial name	Break strength straight pull (MPa)	Break strength knot pull (MPa)	Elongation to break (%)	Young's modulus (GPa)
Catgut		310–380	110–210	15–35	2.4 (358,000)[b]
Regenerated collagen					
Poly(p-dioxanone)	PDS, PDSII	450–560	240–340	30–38	1.2–1.7 (211,000)[b]
Poly(glycolide-co-trimethylene carbonate)	Maxon	540–610	280–480	26–38	3.0–3.4 (380,000)[b]
Poly(glycolide-co-lactide) or polyglactin 910	Vicryl	570–910	300–400	18–25	7–14
Polyglycolide-co-ε-caprolactone or poliglecaprone 25	Monocryl	(91,000)[b]	(45,700)[b]	39[b]	(113,000)[b]
Poly(glycolic acid) or polyglycolide	Dexon S Dexon Plus	760–920	310–590	18–25	7–14
Glycomer 631[c]	Biosyn	3.7–4.4 kg	2.4–2.9 kg	44–47	145–190 kpsi

[a] Mechanical properties presented are typical for sizes 0 through 3-0 but may differ for finer of larger sizes. Partial source: Casey, D.J. and Lewis, O.G., in *Handbook of Biomaterials Evaluation: Scientific, Technical, and Clinical Testing of Implant Materials*, Von Recum, A.F., Ed., Macmillan Publishing, New York, 1986, chap. 7.

[b] Data in parentheses are in psi units of 2/0 size; from Bezwada, R.S. et al., *Biomaterials*, 16, 1141, 1995.

[c] 3/0 size. Data from Roby, M.S., et al., US Patent, 5,403,347, April 4, 1995.

capillarity of a suture material under physical/mechanical characteristics is closely related to its ability to transport bacteria, which is a biological characteristic. The modulus of elasticity under physical/mechanical characteristics is frequently used to relate to pliability of sutures under handling characteristics. A brief description of each of those essential properties is given below, and the properties are listed in Tables 4.8 through 4.12. The wide range of data in those tables indicates the complexity of the issues and the difficulty of drawing general conclusions. Nevertheless, the information in those tables should provide readers with an overall view of the various essential properties of suture materials. Readers should be aware of the fact that the data in the tables would vary, depending on specific clinical and/or physical environments that suture materials are subject to and on constant refining of manufacturing processes by suture manufacturers. The details of each of the four major characteristics are described in following chapters.

A. PHYSICAL/MECHANICAL CHARACTERISTICS

The category of physical and mechanical characteristics is probably the most important one in terms of suture function, i.e., close wounds and carry physiologic load during healing. They include those related to strength, stiffness, viscoelasticity, coefficient of friction, compliance, size, form (monofilament or multifilament), fluid absorption and transport, etc. Strength includes knotted and unknotted (straight pull) tensile strength, modulus of elasticity (relating to stiffness), elongation at break, and toughness (refers to the area under the stress-strain curve and relates to the ability of a material to absorb impact energy). As shown later in Chapters 5 and 6, there is a wide variety of mechanical properties among

Table 4.9 Mechanical Properties of Nonabsorbable Sutures[a]

Class (chemical name)	Commercial name	Break strength straight pull (MPa)	Break strength knot pull (MPa)	Elongation to break (%)	Young's modulus (GPa)
Cotton and linen	Cotton	280–390	160–320	3–6	5.6–10.9
Silk	Silk, Surgical Silk, Dermal®, Virgin Silk	370–570	240–290	9–31	8.4–12.9
Polypropylene	Surgilene®, Prolene®	410–460	280–320	24–62	2.2–6.9
Nylon 66 and nylon 6	Surgilon®, Dermalon®, Nurolon®, Ethilon®, Supramid®	460–710	300–330	17–65	1.8–4.5
Poly[(tetramethylene ether)terephthalate-co-tetramethylene terephthalate]	Novafil®	480–550	290–370	29–38	1.9–2.1
Poly(butylene terephthalate)	Miralene®	490–550	280–400	19–22	3.6–3.7
Poly(ethylene) terephthalate	Dacron®, Ethiflex®, Ti-Cron®, Polydek®, Ethibond®, Tevdek®, Mersilene®, Mirafil®	510–1,060	300–390	8–42	1.2–6.5
Polytetrafluoroethylene	Gore-Tex	1859[b]	1437[b]	33[c]	—
Stainless steel	Flexon®, Stainless steel, Surgical S.S.	540–780	420–710	29–65	200

[a] Mechanical properties presented are typical for sizes 0 through 3-0 but may differ for finer or larger sizes.
[b] CV-4 size in kg/cm². Data from Hertweck, S.P., von Fraunhofer, J. A., et al., *Biomaterials*, 9, 324, 1988.
[c] CV-4 size from Dang, M. C., Thacker, J. G., et al., *Arch. Surg.*, 125, 647, 1990.

Data partially from Casey, D.J. and Lewis, O.G., in *Handbook of Biomaterials Evaluation : Scientific, Technical, and Clinical Testing of Implant Materials*, Von Recum, A.F., Ed., Macmillan Publishing, New York, 1986, chap. 7.

Table 4.10 Relative Tissue Reactivity to Sutures

		Nonabsorbable	Absorbable
M	▲	Silk, cotton	Catgut
O	│	Polyester coated	Dexon and Vicryl
S	│	Polyester uncoated	Maxon, PDS, Monocryl, Biosyn
T	│	Nylon	
		Polypropylene, Gore-Tex	

Data partially from Bennett, R. G., *J. Am. Acad. Dermatol.,* 18(4), 619, 1988.

existing commercial suture materials. The strength property is the most frequently reported and studied physical/mechanical characteristic of suture materials. Because strength is expressed in terms of the cross-sectional area of the material, it is normalized based on the dimension of the material and hence could be used to compare sutures having different chemical structure and/or sizes. Tensile breaking force, however, does not take into account suture size (i.e., diameter). Thus, a larger size suture, say polypropylene, would have a higher tensile breaking force than the same suture of a smaller size even though the two sutures may have the same tensile strength. Therefore, a meaningful comparison of tensile breaking force of several sutures should be done under same suture size (diameter) and form. In addition, knotted tensile strength or breaking force is frequently lower than for the unknotted suture. Strength values are obtained in either dry or wet conditions. The ASTM testing conditions that stipulate the cross-head speed, gage length, temperature (21 ± 1°C), and humidity (65 ± 2%) of the testing room should be followed, if possible, for obtaining and reporting strength data. Among these physical and mechanical properties, viscoelasticity, bending stiffness, and compliance are the least studied and understood and are worthy of brief comments below.

Table 4.11 General Comparison of Absorbable Sutures[a]

Trade name	Configuration	Tensile strength	Tissue reactivity	Handling	Knot security	Memory	Absorption	Degradation mode	Comments
Collagen (plain)	Twisted	Poor (0% at 2–3 weeks)	Moderate	Fair	Poor	Low	Unpredictable (12 weeks)	Proteolytic	Less impure than surgical gut
Collagen (chromic)	Twisted	Poor (0% at 2–3 weeks)	Moderate	Fair	Poor	Low	Unpredictable (12 weeks)	Proteolytic	Less impure than surgical gut
Surgical gut (plain)	Twisted	Poor (0% at 2–3 weeks)	High	Fair	Poor	Low	Unpredictable (12 weeks)	Proteolytic	May be ordered as "fast-absorbing gut" (Ethicon) for percutaneous sutures
Surgical gut (chromic)	Twisted	Poor (0% at 2–3 weeks)	Moderately high	Fair	Fair	Low	Unpredictable (14–80 d)	Preteolytic	Darker, more visible (Davis & Geck); mild or extra chromatization (Davis & Geck)
Coated Vicryl	Braided	Good (50% at 2–3 weeks)	Low	Better	Fair	Low	Predictable (80 d)	Hydrolytic	Clear, violet, coated
Dexon "S"	Braided	Good (50% at 2–3 weeks)	Low	Fair	Good	Low	Predictable (90 d)	Hydrolytic	Uncoated
Dexon Plus	Braided	Good (50% at 2–3 weeks)	Low	Better	Fair	Low	Predictable (90 d)	Hydrolytic	Clear, green, coated
PDS	Monofilament	Better (50% at 5–6 weeks)	Low	Fair	Poor	High	Predictable (180 d)	Hydrolytic	Violet, clear
Maxon	Monofilament	Better (50% at 4–5 weeks)	Low	Fair	Fair	High	Predictable (210 d)	Hydrolytic	Green, clear
Monocryl	Monofilament	Good (50% at 1–2 weeks)	Low	Good	Fair	Low	Predictable (119 d)	Hydrolytic	Gold
Biosyn	Monofilament	Good (50% at 2–3 weeks)	Low	Good	—	Low	Predictable (90–110 d)	Hydrolytic	Second lowest in modulus of elasticity

Partial Source: Bennett R.G., *J. Am. Acad. Dermatol.*, 18(4) Part 1:619, 1988, and Roby, M.S. et al., US Patent 5,403,347, April 4, 1995.

Table 4.12 General Comparison of Nonabsorbable Sutures

Generic or trade name	Configuration	Tensile strength	Tissue reactivity	Handling	Knot security	Memory	Comments
Cotton	Twist	Good	High	Good	Good	Poor	Obsolete
Silk	Braid	Good	High	Very good	Good	Poor	Predisposes to infection; does not tear tissue; Davis & Geck suture is silicone treated; Ethicon is waxed
Ethilon	Monofilament	High	Low	Poor	Poor	High	Cuts tissue; nylon 6,6; black, clear, or green
Dermalon	Monofilament	High	Low	Poor	Poor	High	Nylon 6,6
Supramid	Monofilament or braid	High	Low	Poor	Poor	High	Nylon 6
Nurolon	Braid	High	Moderate	Good	Fair	Fair	May predispose to infection; black or white; waxed; nylon 6,6
Surgilon	Braid	High	Moderate	Fair	Fair	Fair	Nylon 6,6
Prolene	Monofilament	Fair	Low	Poor	Poor	High	Very low coefficient of friction; cuts tissue; blue or clear
Surgilene	Monofilament	Fair	Low	Poor	Poor	High	—
Dermalene	Monofilament	Good	Low	Poor	Poor	High	—
Novafil	Monofilament	High	Low	Fair	Poor	Low	Blue or clear
Mersilene	Braid	High	Moderate	Good	Good	Fair	Green or white
Dacron	Braid	High	Moderate	Good	Good	Fair	Green or white
Polyviolene	Braid	High	Moderate	Good	Good	Fair	Green or white
Ethibond	Braid	High	Moderate	Good	Good	Fair	Green or white
Ti-Cron	Braid	High	Moderate	Poor	Poor	Fair	—
Polydek	Braid	High	Moderate	Good	Good	Fair	—
Tevdek	Braid	High	Moderate	Poor	Poor	Fair	—
Gore-Tex	Monofilament	Fair/poor	Low	Very good	Fair	Poor	No packaging memory, and knot construction has virtually no effect on breaking strength
Stainless steel	Monofilament, twist, or braid	High	Low	Poor	Good	Poor	May kink

Data partially from Bennett, R.G., *J. Am. Acad. Dermatol.,* 18(4), 619, 1988.

Viscoelasticity relates to the ability of materials to change either their dimension under a constant force (i.e., creep) or their strength under a constant dimension (i.e., stress relaxation). This ability is believed to be related to the quality of a suture to hold a wound. For example, a suture with a high creep phenomenon will become "relaxed" after the recession of wound edema, which could lead to a suture knot loop becoming too loose to appose the wound edges properly. Viscoelasticity of suture materials is also the least studied and understood.[15,16]

Bending stiffness is a complex mechanical phenomenon and it closely relates to the handling characteristics of suture materials, particularly knot security. There are very little reported data describing bending stiffness of sutures. Most reported stiffness-of-sutures data were derived from the modulus of elasticity obtained from a tensile strength test. Because making a knot involves bending suture strands, those stiffness data based on modulus of elasticity do not adequately represent the quality of knot strength, security, and tie-down. There are two reported studies of the bending stiffness of sutures.[17,18]

Chu et al.'s study of bending stiffness was based on the force required to bend a suture to a predetermined angle.[17] The measured bending force was converted to flexural stiffness in pounds per square inch according to an ASTM formula. A commercial bending stiffness tester (Taber V-5 model 150B from Teledyne Taber) was used to obtain the required data. Sutures with a braided structure were generally more flexible than those of a monofilament structure, irrespective of their chemical constituents. Coated sutures had a significantly higher bending stiffness than the corresponding uncoated ones. This is particularly true when polymers rather than wax or silicone were used as the coating material. This increase in bending stiffness is attributable to the loss of mobility of constituent fibers under bending force. An increase in suture size significantly increased their stiffness, and the magnitude of increase depended on the chemical constituents of the suture. The large porous volume inherent in Gore-Tex® monofilament suture was the reason for its lowest flexural stiffness.

The flexural stiffness of sutures was also found to depend on the duration of bending during the stiffness test. In general, monofilament sutures exhibited the largest time-dependent stiffness. This was most pronounced with the Gore-Tex suture, which lost half of its initial stiffness after 1 min. Most braided sutures also showed less time dependence in their stiffness. Nylon sutures did not exhibit this time-dependent phenomenon regardless of their physical form. The present quantitative bending stiffness data were consistent with other reported semiquantitative stiffness data based on torsional mode testing described below.[18]

The second reported bending stiffness study of a few sutures (Tomita, et al.[18]) used the technique reported by Scott and Robbin.[19] In principle, a constant weight was attached to each end of a suture of fixed length (25.5 cm) and the distance between these two ends was measured after 1 min loading. Stiffness coefficient (G) was calculated by the formula

$$G = TD^2/8$$

where T is the applied force in dynes and D is the stiffness index, which is the average distance between the two parallel ends of a suture. Bending stiffness data from Tomita et al. generally agree with the Chu et al. data that braided sutures are generally more flexible than monofilaments, and Gore-Tex suture has the lowest bending stiffness. The details of bending stiffness of suture materials are described in Chapter 6.

Suture compliance is a mechanical property that closely relates to the ease with which suture elongates under a tensile force. It is believed that the level of suture compliance should contribute to the compliance of tissues at the anastomotic site. Suture compliance is particularly important in surgery where there is a tubular anastomosis, such as vascular anastomoses. There is only one reported study that examined the effect of suture compliance on the compliance of arterial anastomotic tissues closed with sutures.[20] Compliance mismatch between a vascular graft and host tissue has long been suggested as one of the several factors contributing to graft failure.[21] Compliance mismatch at the anastomotic site is a major component of overall compliance mismatch associated with vascular grafts. Since sutures are the only foreign materials at the anastomotic site, it is expected that a wide range of suture compliance might result in different levels of anastomotic compliance.

Megerman et al. very recently tested this hypothesis by using two 6/0 sutures with a vast difference in suture compliance: Novafil® and Prolene®.[20] Novafil is an elastomeric suture made from polybutester and is characterized by a high elongation at low tensile force, low modulus of elasticity, and high hysteresis, while Prolene suture has a relatively higher modulus of elasticity, low elongation at low tensile force, and low hysteresis. These differences in suture compliance are shown in Figure 4.4.[20] In a clinical condition of minimal tubular compliance and diameter mismatch like artery–artery anastomoses, a far more compliant anastomosis was achieved with Novafil (5.9 ± 2.0%) than with Prolene (3.3 ± 0.6%) suture. Compliance (C) was calculated with the following formula:

$$C = (D_{sys} - D_{dias})/(P_{sys} - P_{dias})/D_{dias}$$

where D and P are diameter and pressure, respectively, and are reported in units of percent diameter change per 100 mm Hg pressure, and "sys" is systolic and "dias" is diastolic. Thus, arterial anastomoses closed with a more compliant suture like Novafil produced arterial anastomotic compliance on average over 75% more than those closed with the less compliant Prolene suture. Megerman et al., however, pointed out that no advantage (of using a more compliant suture) was observed under two conditions. First, if the tensile force applied during knotting exceeds the level at which a compliant suture behaves like a noncompliant suture. For example, Novafil suture loses its compliance when the applied tensile load is >125 g, as shown in Figure 4.4. Under this circumstance, Novafil suture is no more compliant than Prolene suture. Also, the above holds if there is a mismatch in tubular compliance or diameter, such as the anastomosis between a vein and artery. This is because compliance of an anastomosis must not exceed that of the stiffer vessel or graft.[22] In addition to the mechanical characteristics of suture materials, techniques of suture closure have also been reported to affect anastomotic compliance.[23].

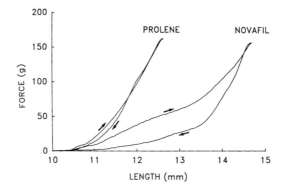

Figure 4.4 Tensile force-elongation curves of 6/0 Novafil and Prolene sutures. Arrows indicate order in which tensile force was applied and released. (From Megerman, J., Hamilton, G., Schmitz-Rixen, T., and Abbott, W.M., *J. Vasc. Surg.*, 18(5), 827, 1993. With permission.)

Capillarity of a suture describes the ease with which liquid is transported along the suture strand and is an inherent physical property of multifilament sutures due to their available interstitial space. Capillarity is thus related to the ability of a suture to transport or spread microorganisms. Bucknall reported that braided nylon suture could take up three times as many microorganisms as monofilament nylon.[24] There are two methods to evaluate the capillarity of sutures: qualitative, according to USP XVII,[25] and quantitative, as developed by Blomstedt et al.[26] The former method determines whether a 0.1% methylene blue dye solution could transport through a suture of fixed length under a weight of 2 g to reach the end marked by white cotton within 8 h. If the cotton becomes blue within 8 h, the suture is classified as capillary, otherwise, it is noncapillary

Table 4.13 summarizes capillarity data of some size 0 sutures according to the USP XVII qualitative method.[26] None of the monofilament sutures exhibited capillarity, while braided polyester (Mersilene®), twisted polyamide with cover (Supramid®), and twisted linen showed capillarity. It was surprising that braided silk with wax coating and catgut (plain and chromic) did not have any capillarity. It appears that wax treatment on silk was able to reduce capillarity. Although the qualitative USP XVII method is a fast and easy way to evaluate suture capillarity, it does not distinguish the rate of capillarity.

Blomstedt et al. developed a quantitative method to determine the rate of capillarity of sutures.[26] The method is based on conductivity via capillarity of suture strands when they are wet. Figure 4.5 shows the results from the Blomstedt et al. quantitative study of the rate of capillarity of those sutures having capillarity based on the USP XVII qualitative method (Table 4.13).[26] There was a more than tenfold difference in the rate of fluid transport (the slope of the curve) among the three sutures having capillarity based on the USP XVII method. For example, Supramid, Mersilene, and twisted linen had the rate constants 0.24, 0.04, and 0.01 cm²/sec, respectively.

Table 4.13 Capillarity of Different Suture
Materials According to the USP XVII Method

Material	Capillarity
Polypropylene, monofilament	–
Polyamide, monofilament	–
Polyamide, braided waxed	–
Polyamide, twisted with cover	+
Polyester, braided	+
Linen, twisted	+
Silk, braided waxed	–
Catgut, plain	–
Catgut, chromic	–

Note: + = capillary; – = noncapillary.

From Blomstedt, B. and Osterberg, B., *Acta Chir. Scand.*,
143, 67, 1977.

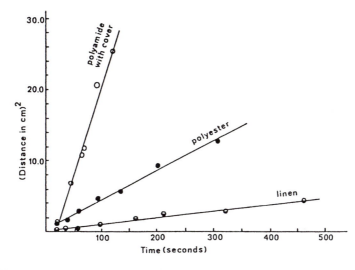

Figure 4.5 Fluid transport rate curves of suture materials with capillary. (From Blomstedt, B. and Osterberg, B., *Acta Chir. Scand.*, 143, 67, 1977. With permission.)

Fluid absorption of sutures, a property relating to capillarity, may also be responsible for the spread of microorganisms in tissues. Table 4.14 summarizes the level of absorption of saline and blood plasma of several sutures.[26] In general, both the chemical nature and physical structure of the sutures determine the level of fluid absorption; however, it appears that the chemical nature is more important than the physical structure of the sutures for the wide range of fluid absorption. Synthetic sutures have much lower fluid absorption capability than natural sutures because the former are more hydrophobic than the latter. Within each type (i.e., synthetic or natural) of suture, multifilament sutures have a higher fluid absorption than their monofilament counterparts because of the additional capillarity effect associated with multifilament sutures. Among the sutures tested, plain and chromic catgut sutures showed the highest level of fluid absorption in both saline and blood plasma media. Obviously, bulk fluid absorption in addition to surface fluid absorption is required to reach such a high level of fluid absorption. The protein nature of catgut sutures provides many bonding sites for fluid molecules to attach and such attachments are not limited to the surface of catgut suture. In contrast, almost all absorbed fluid in synthetic sutures was retained on the surface of sutures.

B. HANDLING CHARACTERISTICS
Handling characteristics describe those properties that relate to the "feel" of suture materials by surgeons during wound closure. It is the category of suture characteristics that is the most difficult to evaluate

Table 4.14 Absorption of Saline and Blood Plasma
in Different Suture Materials

Material	Fluid absorption in percent of strand dry weight ± S.E.	
	Saline (n = 20)	Blood plasma (n = 20)
Polypropylene, monofilament	0.4 ± 0.1	0.2 ± 0.1
Polyamide, monofilament	7.8 ± 0.1	10.1 ± 0.2
Polyamide, braided waxed	11.9 ± 0.5	16.1 ± 0.4
Polyamide, twisted with cover	23.6 ± 0.3	27.8 ± 0.8
Polyester, braided	13.9 ± 0.4	16.0 ± 0.3
Linen, twisted	84.5 ± 1.2	92.2 ± 1.3
Silk, braided waxed	59.5 ± 1.0	65.2 ± 0.7
Catgut, plain	96.8 ± 0.5	100.1 ± 0.7
Catgut, chromic	85.2 ± 0.7	100.1 ± 0.8

From Blomstedt, B. and Osterberg, B., *Acta Chir. Scand.*, 143, 67, 1977.

objectively. These characteristics include pliability (or stiffness), knot tie-down, knot security, packaging memory, surface friction, viscoelasticity, tissue drag, etc. They are directly and indirectly related to physical/mechanical characteristics. For example, the term "pliability" of a suture is a subjective description of how easily a person could bend it and hence relates to the surgeon's "impression" of a suture during knot tying. It is directly related to the bending modulus of a suture and indirectly to coefficient of friction. Packaging memory, another handling property that indirectly relates to pliability, is the ability of sutures to retain kinks after being unpacked. The ability to retain such kinks after unpacking would make surgeons' handling of sutures more difficult during wound closure, particularly when tying a knot. This is because sutures with high memory, like nylon, polypropylene, PDS, and Maxon, tend to untie their knots as they try to return to their kinked form. Thus, packaging memory should be as low as possible. In general, monofilament sutures have more packaging memory than braided ones. The three exceptions are the newly available Monocryl, Biosyn, and Gore-Tex sutures, which were reported to have exceptionally low packaging memory. The easiest means to evaluate packaging memory of sutures is to hang them in air and measure the time required to straighten out the kinks from packaging.

Knot tie-down and security describe how easily a surgeon can slide a knot down to the wound edge and how well the knot will stay in position without untying or slippage. These handling characteristics relate to surface and mechanical properties of sutures. A relatively smooth surface like a monofilament or coated braided suture would have a better knot tie-down than a suture with a rough surface such as an uncoated braided suture, if everything else is equal. The coefficient of friction of sutures also relates to knot tie-down and security. A linear relationship between knot security and coefficient of friction was reported by Herman.[27] A high coefficient of friction would make knot tie-down difficult but would lead to a more secure knot. This is because a high-friction suture could provide additional frictional force to hold the knot together. This high-friction suture surface also makes the passage of suture strands difficult during knot tie-down. It thus appears that knot tie-down and knot security are two contradictory requirements. There is no reported standard test for evaluating knot tie-down capacity.

However, Tomita et al. recently reported a method to objectively quantify the knot tie-down capacity of 2/0 silk, polyester sutures, Gore-Tex, and an experimental ultrahigh molecular weight polyethylene suture (Nesplon®).[18] Their method was based on the technique developed by Kobayashi.[28] The pullout friction test would measure the frictional resistances produced by both surface friction and cross-sectional deformation of sutures when tying and holding a knot securely. In principle, a suture thread was wound around a sponge tube, tied with a square knot, and placed in a tensile testing machine, as shown in Figure 4.6. As the lower jaw descends at a rate of 30 mm/min, the suture would exert a wringing force on the sponge and the tie-down capacity would be reflected by the magnitude of this wringing force. Figure 4.7 is a typical result of such a suture tie-down test. The variations in resistance (peak and valley) from 30 to 60 s were an indication of tie-down roughness and were regressed to a simple linear curve by the least-square method. Table 4.15 summarizes the knot tie-down resistance and roughness as well as knot security of the four tested sutures. The two monofilament sutures (Gore-Tex and UHMW-PE [Ultrahigh Molecular Weight Polyethylene]) as a group had a much lower knot tie-down resistance than the braided sutures (Surgical Silk® and Ethibond®). A higher contact surface area among braided suture strands may be responsible for the high resistance to knot sliding. Silk suture was found to have the largest difference between static (for knot security) and dynamic (for knot tie-down) resistances. These silk data are consistent with their well-known excellent handling characteristics.

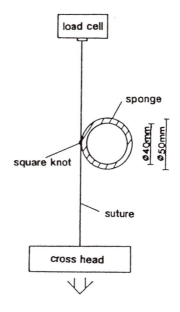

Figure 4.6 Schematic drawing of testing the suture tie-down capacity, according to the Kobayashi technique. (From Tomita, N., Tamai, S., Morihara, T., Ikeuchi, K., and Ikada, Y., *J. Appl. Biomater.*, 4, 61, 1993. With permission.)

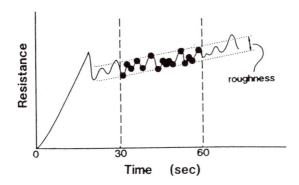

Figure 4.7 A typical result of a suture tie-down test based on the Kobayashi technique. (From Tomita, N., Tamai, S., Morihara, T., Ikeuchi, K., and Ikada, Y., *J. Appl. Biomater.*, 4, 61, 1993. With permission.)

Table 4.15 Knot Properties of Sutures (USP-2 Standard)

Suture material	Knot security[a]	Tie-down resistance ($\times 10^3$ N) (n = 3)	Tie-down roughness ($\times 10^3$ N) (n = 3)
Silk	3	11.7 ± 0.4	0.58 ± 0.14
PET	3–4	12.7 ± 3.6	2.2 ± 0.40
Gore-Tex (CV2)	—	3.6 ± 0.4	0.15 ± 0.01
UHMW-PE	6	7.3 ± 1.5	1.1 ± 0.60

[a] Number of throws required to achieve a secured knot defined as the one that broke without slipping more than 10 mm.

From Tomita, N., Tamai, S., Morihara, T., et al., *J. Appl. Biomater.*, 4, 61, 1993. With permission.

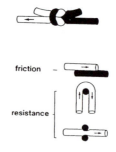

Figure 4.8 Schematic drawing of the contribution of both surface friction and the resistance resulting from cross-sectional deformity of sutures (including both bending and contraction deformation) to knot security. (From Tomita, N., Tamai, S., Morihara, T., Ikeuchi, K., and Ikada, Y., *J. Appl. Biomater.*, 4, 61, 1993. With permission.)

The high knot tie-down resistance of braided sutures also led to their higher knot security as evident from the lower number of throws that were required to achieve a secure knot (defined as one that broke without slipping more than 10 mm, as given in Table 4.15. Tomita et al. attributed the high knot security of these braided sutures to not only the surface friction force, but also to the resistance resulting from cross-sectional deformity of sutures (including both bending and contraction deformation), as schematically illustrated in Figure 4.8.

Recently, Tomita et al. reported that the slope of a logarithmic plot of a cross-sectional stress relaxation vs. time closely related to the degree of difference between static and dynamic resistance of sutures.[29] The cross-sectional relaxation was measured by compressing two sutures that were perpendicular to each other. Only silk and Gore-Tex sutures exhibited similar patterns in a plot of the slope of the cross-sectional relaxation vs. relaxation load and the plot of the difference between static and dynamic resistances vs. relaxation load. Ethibond and Nesplon sutures, however, did not have such a maximum pattern in the cross-sectional relaxation plot. Thus, Tomita et al. attributed the magnitude of the difference of static and dynamic resistance of a suture to its cross-sectional plasticity. The details of stress relaxation of suture materials are given in Chapter 6.

Tissue drag describes how easy it is to pull a suture through tissue during wound closure and suture removal. Hence it gives an indication of the extent of tissue tear in needle holes. Obviously, tissue drag should be maintained at a minimum for easy passage of sutures through tissue, which is reflected in a surgeon's "feel" about a suture. Tissue drag is closely related to both the surface physical roughness and coefficient of friction of a suture. In general, coated or monofilament suture materials have less tissue drag than their uncoated or braided counterparts. This is because a coating material can smooth a rough surface and also change the coefficient of friction.

There are very few reported studies that examine the relationship between the structure/physical configuration of sutures and tissue drag.[30,31] These published studies focus on the evaluation of suture withdrawal stress and work after predetermined periods of implantation. It is known that healing around a suture in a wound would lead to ingrowth of fibrous connective tissues into the interstitial space of the suture. This tissue ingrowth could exert a significant resistance during suture withdrawal. Table 4.16 summarizes the maximum suture withdrawal stress (g/cm) and work (g-cm/cm) of six commercial sutures subdermally implanted in dogs for up to 14 d.[30] Mode II, which used the test sutures to close three 1-in.-long cutaneous incisions via short curved needle and continuous stitch, was a better model for simulating clinical trauma proximal to the suture location. In general, monofilament sutures (e.g., nylon, polypropylene, and polyethylene) showed significantly lower maximum withdrawal stress values than multifilament braid sutures like silk (plain or silicone coated) and Tevdek® (a Teflon-coated polyester). Plain silk had the highest maximum withdrawal stress (146.9 g/cm) among the six types of sutures. The duration of implantation appeared not to exert a strong effect. The data of withdrawal work were consistent with the maximum withdrawal stress. A subsequent detailed analysis of the withdrawal stress profile vs. length of suture withdrawn in cutaneous tissues of pigs indicated an unique pattern.[31] A sharp maximum withdrawal stress along the length of suture withdrawn was the most characteristic pattern for silicone-coated silk sutures over all three periods of implantation (1, 2, and 3 weeks), while the synthetic monofilament polyethylene, polypropylene, and nylon as well as Tevdek sutures showed relatively flat withdrawal stress curves (less profound maximum withdrawal stress) with the length of suture withdrawn.

C. BIOCOMPATIBILITY

Biocompatibility of suture materials describes how sutures, which are foreign materials to the body, could affect surrounding tissues and how the surrounding tissues could affect the properties of sutures.

Table 4.16.A Maximum Withdrawal Stress (g/cm[a])

Suture size	A: Silk/Plain		B: Silk/Silicone		C: PE/Teflon		D: Nylon		E: Polyethylene		F: Polypropylene	
	Mode I	Mode II	Mode I	Mode II	Mode I	Mode II	Mode I	Mode II	Mode I	Mode II	Mode I	Mode II
2-0	36.2	146.9[b]	25.5	118.1[b]	14.2	85.3[b]	10.3	34.4	13.8	49.3	13.2	45.3
4-0	20.8	146.9[b]	12.5	118.1[b]	9.3	85.3[b]	8.6	73.7	5.7	35.5	5.5	32.4
6-0	17.4	146.9[b]	6.3	118.1[b]		85.3[b]	6.6					

Table 4.16.B Withdrawal Work (g-cm/cm)

Suture size	A: Silk/Plain		B: Silk/Silicone		C: PE/Teflon		D: Nylon		E: Polyethylene		F: Polypropylene	
	Mode I	Mode II	Mode I	Mode II	Mode I	Mode II	Mode I	Mode II	Mode I	Mode II	Mode I	Mode II
2-0	3.9	47.1[b]	3.7	40.6[b]	2.7	43.8[b]	3.6	13.2	4.1	33.5	4.1	22.3
4-0	3.8	47.1[b]	2.6	40.6[b]	2.7	43.8[b]	3.4	32.7	2.4	15.1	2.4	10.6
6-0	1.4	47.1[b]	1.4	40.6[b]		43.8[b]	3.1					

[a] Averages for all implant duration periods.
[b] No trend with suture size.

From Homsy, C.A., McDonald, K.E., and Akers, W.W., *J. Biomed. Mater. Res.*, 2, 215, 1968. With permission.

Thus, biocompatibility is a two-way relationship. The extent of tissue reactions to sutures depends largely on the chemical nature of sutures and their degradation products if they are absorbable. Sutures from natural sources like catgut and silk usually provoke more tissue reactions than synthetic ones. This is due to the availability of enzymes to react with natural biopolymers. In addition to the most important chemical factors, physical form and the amount and stiffness of suture materials have been reported to elicit different levels of tissue reactions. For example, a stiff suture would result in stiff projecting ends in a knot where cut. These stiff ends could irritate surrounding tissues through mechanical means, a problem associated with some monofilament sutures, but generally not found in braided multifilament sutures.

Because the quantity of a buried suture relates to the extent of tissue reaction, it is well known that in surgery one should use as little suture material as possible, such as a smaller knot or a smaller size, to close wounds. The use of a smaller size of suture for wound closure without detriment to the provision of adequate support to wounds and cutting through wound tissue is due to the square relationship between diameter (D) and volume (V) ($V = \pi D^2 \times$ length), which suggests that a slight increase in suture size or diameter would increase its volume considerably.

There are two basic means to study biocompatibility of suture materials: cellular response and enzyme histochemistry. The former is the most frequently used and provides information about the type and density of inflammatory cells at a suture site. The latter provides information on what these inflammatory cells would do and is based on the fact that any cellular response is always associated with the presence of a variety of enzymes and is particularly useful in the study of the mechanism of absorption of absorbable sutures. In the cellular response approach, histological stains with a variety of dyes like the most frequently used H & E are the standard methods of evaluation of cellular activity at the suture sites. Figure 4.9 is a typical example of histological photomicrographs of PDS and Maxon sutures at 35 d postimplantation in a variety of tissues.[32] In addition to a qualitative description of cellular activities, tissue response could be graded by the most frequently used and accepted method of Sewell et al. or its modification.[33] A detailed description of the grading system of Sewell et al. is given in Chapter 8.

Most biocompatibility studies of suture materials have been performed in rat gluteal muscle. This implantation site has given a very consistent and reproducible cellular response for valid comparisons, even though it is not a common site for suture in surgery. However, Walton recently raised the question of using this common test procedure, particularly in orthopedic surgery.[34] His arguments were based on the observed inflamed nature of the postoperative synovial tissue and the mechanically stressed nature of the suture. A detailed description of Walton's findings is given in Chapter 7.

The second means for the study of suture biocompatibility is the use of enzyme histochemistry. It is a more objective, quantitative, consistent, and reproducible method than cellular response, which is based on a more subjective histological evaluation. Enzyme histochemistry is, however, more tedious and requires more sophisticated facilities and better experience. The data obtained would provide additional insight into the functions of those cells appearing during various stages of wound healing. The enzymatic activity of a suture implant site is quantified by microscopic photometry of a cryostat section of the tissue. Figure 4.10 is a typical finding of an enzyme histochemical study of suture biocompatibility.[35-37] The high level of cellular response to silk suture observed from histological study is confirmed in this enzyme histochemical study. Enzyme histochemistry is also useful for studying the biodegradation mechanism of absorbable sutures because not only are natural absorbable sutures degraded through the enzymatic route, but also the degradation products must be metabolized via enzyme activity.

The normal tissue reaction to sutures has three stages, characterized by the appearance of a variety of inflammatory cells.[35,37-39] They are initial infiltration of polymorphonuclear leukocytes, lymphocytes, and monocytes during the first 3 to 4 d (i.e., acute response); appearance of macrophages and fibroblasts from day 4 to day 7; and beginning maturation of fibrous connective tissue formation with chronic inflammation after the 7th to the 10th day. During the first 7 d postimplantation, there is virtually no difference in normal tissue reaction between synthetic absorbable and nonabsorbable sutures. However, a slightly higher inflammatory reaction to synthetic absorbable sutures could persist for an extended period until they are completely absorbed and metabolized, while synthetic nonabsorbable sutures, in general, are characterized with a minimal chronic inflammatory reaction with a thin fibrous connective tissue capsule surrounding the sutures usually by 28 d postimplantation.

Due to this normal tissue reaction, fibrous and/or epidermic tissue ingrowth into sutures may pose a problem during the removal of sutures, particularly for those sutures placed through the cutaneous surface due to the ingrowth of epidermis in addition to fibrous connective tissue. This problem is particularly profound in multifilament sutures because of the available interstitial space within these sutures for tissue infiltration. The formation of a perisutural cuff due to a downgrowth of epidermis along the suture path

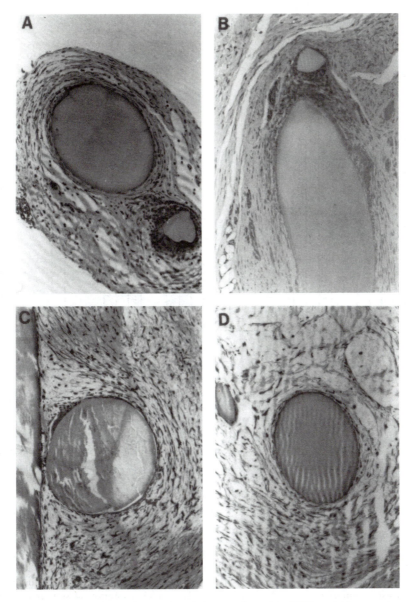

Figure 4.9 Light histological photomicrographs of tissue adjacent to PDS and Maxon sutures 3 and 5 d postimplantation in a variety of tissues of New Zealand White rabbits (magnification × 130). (A) peritoneum/PDS; (B) fascia/PDS; (C) peritoneum/Maxon; and (D) fascia/Maxon. (From Metz, S.A., Chegini, N., and Masterson, B.J., *J. Gynecol. Surg.*, 5(1), 37, 1989. With permission.)

has been found to be responsible for 70 to 85% of the force required to remove the suture.[30,31,38] Among the multifilament sutures, silk is the worst offender as described in the previous section. A very recently reported U.S. patent disclosed an approach of using composite suture to reduce tissue ingrowth of silk suture through encapsulation of the silk suture with biocompatible polymeric resin. The details of this composite silk suture are given in Chapter 12.

In addition to the normal tissue reactions to sutures, there are several adverse tissue reactions that are suture and site specific. Some examples include urinary stone or calci formation, granuloma formation, thrombogenicity, propensity toward wound infection and recurrence of tumor after radical surgery, and allergy. The detailed description of these adverse effects is given in Chapter 8.

Monofilament sutures are considered to be a better choice than multifilament ones in closing contaminated wounds. This is because not only do multifilament sutures elicit more tissue reactions, which may lessen tissue ability to deal with wound infections, but also multifilament sutures have a capillary

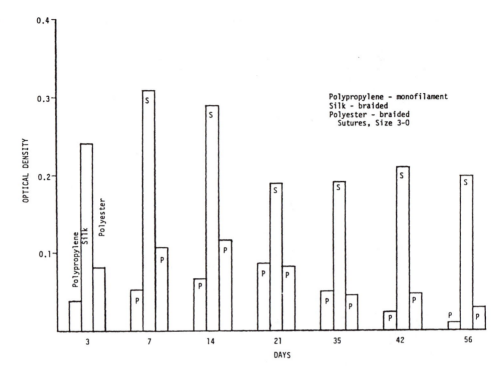

Figure 4.10 Enzyme histochemical evaluation of macrophage hydrolase activity of monofilament polypropylene and braided silk and polyester sutures. (From van Winkle, W. and Salthouse, T.N., *Biological Response to Sutures and Principles of Suture Selection*, Ethicon, Somerville, NJ, 1976. With permission.)

effect that could transport microorganisms from one region of the wound to another. The reason multifilament sutures generally elicit more tissue reactions than their monofilament counterparts is that inflammatory cells are able to penetrate the interstitial space within a multifilament suture and invade each filament. Such an invasion by inflammatory cells, well evident in histological pictures, could not occur in monofilament sutures. Thus, the available surface area of a suture to tissue should bear a close relationship to the level of tissue reaction that a suture could elicit.

D. BIODEGRADATION AND ABSORPTION CHARACTERISTICS

Absorbable sutures require consideration of their biodegradation and absorption, factors that are not relevant for most nonabsorbable sutures. This unique biodegradation characteristic is also responsible for the fact that absorbable sutures do not elicit permanent chronic inflammatory reactions found with nonabsorbable sutures. The most important characteristics in biodegradation and absorption of sutures are the strength and mass loss profiles and biocompatibility of degradation products. Although there is a wide range of strength and mass loss profiles among the available absorbable sutures, they have one common characteristic: strength loss always occurs much earlier than mass loss, as shown in Figure 4.11. This suggests that absorbable sutures retain a large portion of their mass in tissue while they have already lost all their designated function to provide support for the wound tissue. Thus, an ideal absorbable suture should have matched mass loss and strength loss profiles. As described in detail in Chapter 7, such an ideal absorbable suture is not available because of the inherent relationship between strength and fiber structure.

The observed wide range of strength and mass loss profiles among the available absorbable sutures is attributable not only to the chemical differences among the absorbable sutures, but also to a variety of intrinsic and extrinsic factors, such as pH, electrolytes, stress applied, temperature, γ-irradiation, microorganisms, and tissue type, to name a few. The details of the effects of these factors on the biodegradation properties of synthetic absorbable sutures have been reviewed recently by Chu[41–43] and are discussed in Chapter 7.

The biocompatibility of degradation products is usually not a problem because all existing absorbable sutures are made from the well-known biocompatible glycolide and lactide and their derivatives. However, biocompatibility of degradation products also depends on the rate of their accumulation in the surrounding

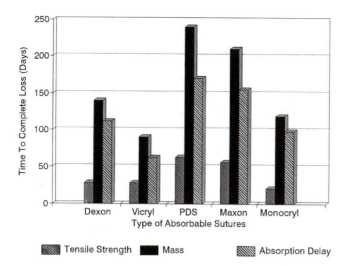

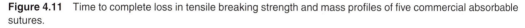

Figure 4.11 Time to complete loss in tensile breaking strength and mass profiles of five commercial absorbable sutures.

tissues. This implies that the ability of the surrounding tissues to actively metabolize degradation products is essential. Such a metabolism depends on the extent of blood circulation in the tissue. A well-vascularized tissue could remove degradation products as fast as they are released from an absorbable suture and subsequently metabolized, which could minimize tissue reactions to degradation products.

Due to their ability to release degradation products, absorbable sutures have recently been studied as a vehicle to deliver a variety of biochemicals like growth factors to facilitate wound healing or antibiotics to combat wound infection. This new approach would increase the value of absorbable sutures and extend their function beyond the traditional role of wound closure. Again, details are given in Chapter 12.

Biodegradation properties are usually examined *in vitro* and/or *in vivo*. In the *in vitro* environment, the most commonly used medium is physiological saline phosphate buffer of pH 7.44 at 37°C. However, other buffers like Tris or other body fluids like urine, bile, and synovial fluids have been used. Occasionally, microorganisms were deliberately incorporated into these media to examine the effect of microorganisms on biodegradation properties of absorbable sutures. In the *in vivo* environment, unstressed absorbable sutures are normally implanted in rat gluteal muscle for predetermined periods of implantation. As briefly described above in Section V.C, Walton raised the question that the use of unstressed sutures and gluteal muscle site might not represent the real clinical environment that absorbable sutures normally experience.[34] The sutures retrieved at various periods of immersion or implantation are then subject to evaluation of their mechanical and physical properties to assess their changes with time. The degree of absorption *in vivo* is evaluated by the change in suture cross-sectional area, while the level of tissue reaction is assessed by either the histological method and/or enzyme histochemistry previously described in Section V.C.

VI. SUMMARY

A systematic classification of suture materials based on absorbability, size, physical form, and coating materials is described. Absorbability is the most common way to classify sutures. When specifying a suture, size is the most important feature. Both USP and European size classifications were given, although the majority of the literature uses the USP size classification. Sutures could also be classified based on the physical form of their constituent fibers, monofilament vs. multifilament. Most multifilament sutures are braided; a few are twisted. The trend of research is to provide monofilament sutures with similar physical/mechanical properties of braided ones. Most sutures are also coated to facilitate their handling properties; however, coating frequently results in poor knot security. Thus, the direction of research is to develop coating materials that would improve the handling properties of sutures without detriment to knot properties.

The performance of suture materials depends on their four general characteristics (physical/mechanical, handling, biocompatibility, and biodegradation). These four characteristics and their interrelationships are introduced for providing an overall framework of the required properties of suture materials. This introduction is followed by a far more detailed description of these general characteristics of suture materials in subsequent chapters of the book.

REFERENCES

1. Chu, C.C., Survey of clinically important wound closure biomaterials, in *Biocompatible Polymers, Metals, and Composites,* Szycher, M., Ed., Technomic Publishing, Lancaster, PA, 1983.
2. von Fraunhofer, J.A., Storey, R.S., Stone, I.K., and Masterson, B.J., Tensile strength of suture materials, *J. Biomed. Mater. Res.,* 19, 595, 1985.
3. Conn, J., Jr. and Beal, J.M., Coated Vicryl synthetic absorbable sutures, *Surg. Gynecol. Obstet.,* 140, 377, 1975.
4. Mattei, F.V., Absorbable coating composition for sutures, U.S. Patent 4,201,216, Ethicon, 1980.
5. Casey, D.J. and Lewis, O.G., Absorbable and nonabsorbable sutures, in *Handbook of Biomaterials Evaluation: Scientific, Technical, and Clinical Testing of Implant Materials,* von Recum, A.F., Ed., Macmillan Publishing, New York, 1986, chap. 7.
6. Rodeheaver, G.T., Foresman, P.A., Brazda, M.T., and Edlich, R.F., A temporary nontoxic lubricant for a synthetic absorbable suture, *Surg. Gynecol. Obstet.,* 164, 17, 1987.
7. Rodeheaver, G.T., Thacker, J.G., Owen, J., et al., Knotting and handling characteristics of coated synthetic absorbable sutures, *J. Surg. Res.,* 35, 525, 1983.
8. Rodeheaver, G.T., Kurtz, L., Kircher, B.J., and Edlich, R.F., Pluronic F-68: a promising new skin wound cleanser, *Ann. Emerg. Med.,* 9, 572, 1980.
9. Rodeheaver, G.T., Thacker, J.G., and Delich, R.F., Mechanical performance of polyglycolide and polyglactin 910 synthetic absorbable sutures, *Surg. Gynecol. Obstet.,* 153, 835, 1981.
10. Kawai, T., Matsuda, T., and Yoshimoto, M., Coated sutures exhibiting improved knot security, U.S. Patent 4,983,180, Japan Medical Supply, 1991.
11. Messier, K.A. and Rhum, J.D., Caprolactone polymers for suture coating, U.S. Patent 4,624,256, Pfizer Hospital Products Group, Inc., 1986.
12. Bezwada, R.S., Hunter, A.W., and Shalaby, S.W., Copolymers of ε-caprolactone, glycolide and glycolic acid for suture coatings, U.S. Patent 4,994,074, Ethicon, Inc., 1991.
13. Wang, D.W., Casey, D.J., and Lehmann, L.T., Surgical suture coating, U.S. Patent 4,705,820, American Cyanamid, 1987.
14. Gaillard, B.D., Sheathed surgical suture filament and method for its preparation, U.S. Patent 4,506,672, Assut S.A. Switzerland, 1985.
15. Von Fraunhofer, J.A. and Sichina, W.J., Characterisation of surgical suture materials using dynamic mechanical analysis, *Biomaterials,* 13, 715, 1992.
16. Metz, S.A., von Fraunhofer, J.A., and Masterson, B.J., Stress relaxation of organic suture materials, *Biomaterials,* 11, 197, 1990.
17. Chu, C.C. and Kizil, Z., Quantitative evaluation of stiffness of commercial suture materials, *Surg. Gynecol. Obstet.,* 168, 233, 1989.
18. Tomita, N., Tamai, S., Morihara, T., Ikeuchi, K., and Ikada, Y., Handling characteristics of braided suture materials for tight tying, *J. Appl. Biomater.,* 4, 61, 1993.
19. Scott, G.V. and Robbin, C.R., Stiffness of human hair fibers, *J. Soc. Cosmet. Chem.,* 29, 469, 1978.
20. Megerman, J., Hamilton, G., Schmitz-Rixen, T., and Abbott, W.M., Compliance of vascular anastomoses with polybutester and polypropylene sutures, *J. Vasc. Surg.,* 18, 827, 1993.
21. Abbott, W.M., Megerman, J., Hasson, J.E., L'Italien, G., and Warnock, D., Effect of compliance mismatch upon vascular graft patency, *J. Vasc. Surg.,* 5, 376, 1987.
22. Hasson, J.E., Megerman, J., and Abbott, W.M., Increased compliance near vascular anastomoses, *J. Vasc. Surg.,* 2, 419, 1985.
23. Hasson, J.E., Megerman, J., and Abbott, W.M., Suture technique and para-anastomotic compliance, *J. Vasc. Surg.,* 3, 591, 1986.
24. Bucknall, T.E., Factors influencing wound complications: a clinical and experimental study, *Ann. R. Coll. Surg.,* 65, 71, 1983.
25. United States Pharmacopeia, 17th revision, 1965, 693.
26. Blomstedt, B. and Osterberg, B., Fluid absorption and capillarity of suture materials, *Acta Chir. Scand.,* 143, 67, 1977.
27. Herman, J.B., Tensile strength and knot security of surgical suture materials, *Am. Surg.,* 37, 209, 1971.
28. Kobayashi, H., Suture materials (Japanese), GEKA Mook No. 4, Tokyo, Kinbara Syuppan, 1976, pp.1-14.
29. Tomita, N., Tamai, S., Ikeuchi, K, and Ikada, Y., Effects of cross-sectional stress-relaxation on handling characteristics of suture materials, *Bio-Med. Mater. Eng.,* 4(1), 47, 1994.
30. Homsy, C.A., McDonald, K.E., and Akers, W.W., Surgical suture — Canine tissue interaction for six common suture types, *J. Biomed. Mater. Res.,* 2, 215, 1968.
31. Freeman, B.S., Homsy, C.A., Fissette, J., and Hardy, S.B., An analysis of suture withdrawal stress, *Surg. Gynecol. Obstet.,* 131(3), 441, 1970.

32. Metz, S.A., Chegini, N., and Masterson, B.J., In vivo tissue reactivity and degradation of suture materials: a comparison of Maxon and PDS, *J. Gynecol. Surg.*, 5, 37, 1989.

33. Sewell, W.R., Wiland, J., and Craver, B.N., A new method of comparing sutures of bovine catgut with sutures of bovine catgut in three species, *Surg. Gynecol. Obstet.*, 100, 483, 1955.

34. Walton, M., Strength retention of chromic gut and monofilament synthetic absorbable suture materials in joint tissues, *Clin. Orthop. Related Res.*, 242, 303, 1989.

35. Van Winkle, W. and Salthouse, T.N., *Biological Response to Sutures and Principles of Suture Selection*, Ethicon, Somerville, NJ, 1976.

36. Salthouse, T.N. and Matlaga, B.F., Significance of cellular enzyme activity at nonabsorbable suture implant sites: silk, polyester and polypropylene, *J. Surg. Res.*, 19, 127, 1975.

37. Salthouse, T.N., Biocompatibility of sutures, in *Biocompatibility in Clinical Practice,* Vol. 1, Williams, D.F., Ed., CRC Press, Boca Raton, FL, 1981.

38. Bennett, R.G., Selection of wound closure materials, *J. Am. Acad. Dermatol.*, 18, Part 1, 619, 1988.

39. Madsen, E.T., An experimental and clinical evaluation of surgical suture materials, I and II, *Surg. Gynecol. Obstet.,* 97, 73, 1953.

40. Ordman, L.J. and Gillman, T., Studies in the healing of cutaneous wounds, *Arch. Surg.* 93, 857, 1966.

41. Chu, C.C., Degradation of synthetic wound closure polymeric materials: theories and experimental findings, in *Biomedical Applications of Synthetic Biodegradable Polymers,* Hollinger, J., Ed., CRC Press, Boca Raton, FL, 1995, pp. 103–128.

42. Chu, C.C., Biodegradable suture materials: Intrinsic and extrinsic factors affecting biodegradation phenomena, in *Handbook of Biomaterials and Applications*, Vol. 1, Part III, Wise, D.L., Altobelli, D.E., Schwartz, E.R., Yszemski, M., Gresser, J.D., and Trantolo, D.J., Eds., Marcel Dekker, 1995, 543–688.

43. Chu, C.C., The degradation and biocompatibility of suture materials, in *CRC Critical Reviews in Biocompatibility,* vol. 1, issue 3, Williams, D.F., Ed., CRC Press, Boca Raton, FL, 1985, pp. 261–322.

Chapter 5

Chemical Structure and Manufacturing Processes

C. C. Chu

CONTENTS

This chapter describes the chemical/physical structure, the basic processes of manufacturing, and some essential properties of suture materials. The information given should provide readers with some basic knowledge of the molecular and chemical structure of suture materials. Such fundamental knowledge of the basic structure of suture materials is essential for appreciation and understanding of their mechanical, biological, and biodegradation properties to be described in subsequent chapters.

I. ABSORBABLE SUTURE MATERIALS

Currently, there are two natural absorbable and six synthetic absorbable sutures that are commercially available. The natural absorbable sutures are all based upon collagen and they are catgut and reconstituted collagen. Synthetic absorbable sutures are all based on polyglycolide and its copolymers: Dexon®, a polyglycolide homopolymer; Vicryl®, a glycolide-L-lactide random copolymer of 90 to 10 molar ratio; PDS®, a poly-*p*-dioxanone; Maxon®, a glycolide-trimethylene carbonate block copolymer; Monocryl®, a copolymer of glycolide and ε-caprolactone; and Biosyn®, a triblock copolymer of glycolide and trimethylene carbonate. There are other names used to represent the above commercial absorbable sutures. For example, PGA, polyglactin 910, polyglyconate, poliglecaprone 25, and Glycomer 631 have been used to represent Dexon, Vicryl, Maxon, Monocryl, and Biosyn, respectively. Figure 5.1 shows the appearance of these absorbable sutures.

In addition to the above commercial synthetic absorbable sutures, there are a few new synthetic absorbable sutures that have been introduced outside the U.S.A. or/and under FDA review. An example is LTS®, which is similar to Monocryl, made from poly(ε-caprolactone) homopolymer.[1] Chitin suture, a polysaccharide introduced and marketed in Japan in the late 1980s, has not been commercially sold in the U.S. yet. These emerging suture materials are described in Chapter 12.

A

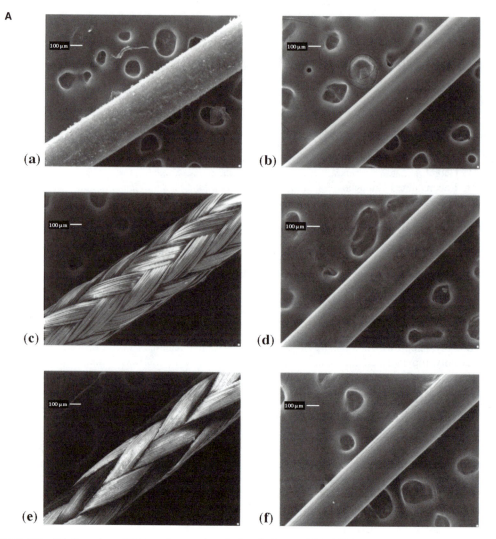

(a) (b)

(c) (d)

(e) (f)

Figure 5.1 (A) Scanning electron micrographs of absorbable sutures: (a) chromic catgut (2/0 surgical gut), (b) Maxon®, (c) Dexon®, (d) Monocryl®, (e) Vicryl®, (f) PDSII®.

A. CATGUT

Multifilament twisted plain catgut was described as early as 175 A.D. The basic constituent is collagen. Collagen is a protein consisting of three polypeptides interweaved in a left-hand triple-helical structure. Each polypeptide chain has the general amino acid sequence of $(-Gly-X-Y-)_n$, where X is frequently proline (Pro) and Y is frequently hydroxyproline (Hyp).[2] Table 5.1 lists the essential amino acid contents of a typical collagen in tendon.[2] One important and unique aspect of collagen is its essential electrical neutrality under physiological conditions due to the approximate equal number of acidic (glutamic and aspartic acids) and basic (lysine and arginine) side groups.[3] Because pKs for amino and carboxyl groups are about 10 and 4, respectively, the electrostatic interactions among the acidic and basic groups are expected to be significantly disturbed at pH either <4 or >10.[4] Thus, any pH change would lead to a weakening of the inter- or intramolecular electrostatic interactions in collagen fibers. Such a weakening in fiber structure due to pH change is evident in the observed swelling of the fibers, which would be ultimately reflected in the observed accelerated loss of strength and mass of catgut sutures at highly acidic or alkaline conditions (described in Chapter 7). The use of intermolecular crosslinking agents like formaldehyde or glutaldehyde could stabilize fiber structure against the pH-induced change.

Li recently listed three factors that could stabilize the triple-helical structure of a collagen molecule.[2] The first factor is the geometrical stabilization factor which provides a tight fit of the amino acids within the triple-helix coil structure. In order to maintain such a tight space-filling triple helix structure, a

B

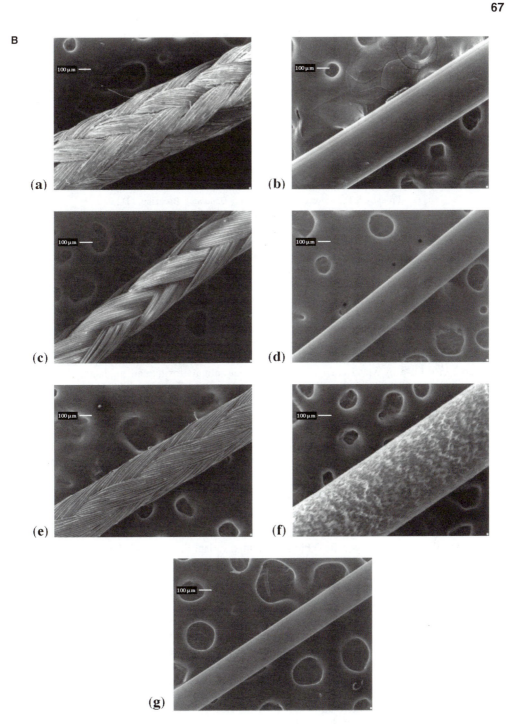

Figure 5.1 (Continued) (B) Scanning electron micrographs of nonabsorbable sutures: (a) 1/0 silk (Davis & Geck), (b) polypropylene (2/0 Prolene®), (c) polyester (2/0 Mersilene®), (d) monofilament nylon (2/0 Ethilon®), (e) multifilament nylon (2/0 Nurolon®), (f) expanded polytetrafluoroethylene (Gore-Tex®), (g) stainless steel (3/0 Surgical Steel®).

glycine unit must be present as every third amino acid residue. The second factor is the formation of intermolecular hydrogen bonds between the backbone NH_2 and $>C=O$ groups. The third factor is the interference of water molecules with the above-described intermolecular hydrogen bonds.

Collagen molecules are synthesized in endoplasmic reticulum of cells like fibroblasts by enzymatic regulated stepwise polymerization. These procollagen molecules are then released into the extracellular

Table 5.1 Amino Acid Content of Collagen

Amino acids	Content, residues/1000 residues[a]
Gly	334
Pro	122
Hyp	96
Acid polar (Asp, Glu, Asn)	124
Basic polar (Lys, Arg, His)	91
Other	233

[a] Reported values are average values of 10 different determinations for tendon tissue.

From Li, S.T., in *Biomedical Engineering Handbook*, Bronzino, J.D., Ed., CRC Press, 1995. With permission.

space followed by enzymatic cleavage at both head (COOH-terminal domain) and tail (NH_2-terminal domain) of the procollagen molecule. After the enzymatic cleavage, the remaining procollagen helical domain segments called tropocollagen (about 3000 Å) assemble into microfibrils of about 50 to 300 nm in diameter with the characteristic periodic bands seen under electron microscopy. These microfibrils aggregate in parallel to form fibrils, which bundle together to form collagen fibers. It is important to know that the organization of collagen molecules in a microfibril is tissue specific.[2]

Although 14 different types of collagen have been identified, the majority of collagen biomaterials is based on type I collagen because of its greater abundance. Since there are very few differences in the structure of type I collagen due to species, this extensive similarity in structure may be attributed to the acceptable broad use of type I collagen obtained from animals for human implantation. The detailed structure and properties of collagen biomaterials have recently been reviewed by Li.[2]

Catgut suture is derived from the submucosa of sheep intestines or serosa of bovine intestine. The jejunum and ileum portions of the intestine of sheep or beef are split into two or more longitudinal ribbons, and then the mucosa muscularis and other unwanted layers are removed by chemical and mechanical treatments. The remaining portion is treated in diluted formaldehyde to block the -OH and -NH_2 groups on collagen in order to increase the strength and the resistance to enzyme attack. Several ribbons are then twisted into strands, dried, machine ground, and polished by a centerless grinder to a correct and smooth size. This grinding and polishing process can produce unpredictable amounts of weak points and local tearing of fibrils. Thus, fibrils could fray during use. Reproducible strength is also difficult to achieve.

The resulting untreated catgut suture is called plain catgut. If the plain catgut is further tanned in a bath of chromium trioxide, it is called chromic catgut, a variant first developed by Lister in 1840. There are two types of chromicizing processes: Tru and surface chromicizings. The former is done to each ribbon before it is spun into strands while the latter is conducted on the finished strand. This treatment changes the color of plain catgut from a yellowish tan shade to a darker shade of brown. Depending on the concentration of the chromic bath and duration of chromicizing, mild and extra chromic catgut are available. Of course, the degrees of absorption and tissue response are also affected by the severity of the tanning process. Chromic catgut suture is generally more resistant to absorption and causes less tissue reaction than plain catgut suture. Catgut sutures are packaged in alcohol solution like ethanol or isopropanol to retain their flexibility and the packages are sterilized by either Co^{60} γ-irradiation or ethylene oxide.

Recently, Davis & Geck introduced a glycerin-coated chromic catgut (Softgut®) to eliminate the need for alcohol in packaging catgut and to improve handling qualities.[5] The glycerin-treated chromic catgut sutures have a smoother and more uniform surface appearance than untreated catgut, and, as a result of glycerin treatment, the sutures are thicker. There were some complications like pains at 10 d, dyspareunia at 3 months, and persistent dyspareunia at 3 years associated with this glycerin-coated chromic catgut in the repair of perineal wounds.[6] The effect of the glycerin treatment of chromic catgut suture on its *in vivo* performance and knot security is discussed in Chapters 7 and 8. Davis & Geck, Ethicon, and Deknatel all have plain gut and chromic gut sutures. There are no trade names of catgut sutures associated with a particular suture manufacturer.

B. RECONSTITUTED COLLAGEN

Collagen can be reconstituted either from enzymatic digestion of native collagen-rich tissues or via the extraction of these tissues with salt solutions. Reconstituted collagen, however, exhibits various polymorphic

Table 5.2 Properties of Glycolide Polymorphs

	Alpha	Beta
Stability range	42–82.5°C (m.p.)	Below 42°C
Crystal system	Orthorhombic	Monoclinic
Refractive index		
nα	1.486	1.430
nβ	1.506	1.555
nγ	1.620	1.568
Vapor pressure mm at 20°C	0.04	0.02

From Frazza, E.J. and Schmitt, E.E., *J. Biomed. Mater. Res. Symp.*, 1, 43, 1971. With permission.

aggregated forms that are different from the native collagen. Piez reported that the formation of polymorphic aggregates of collagen depends on the environment for reconstitution.[7] For example, under either a high concentration of neutral salts or nonaqueous solution, collagen molecules aggregate into random arrays without specific regularities.[2] There are two other well-known polymorphic forms of collagen: fibrous-long-spacing (FLS) and segment-long-spacing (SLS). The FLS collagen is formed by randomly aligning molecules in a head-to-tail, tail-to-tail, or head-to-head orientation without overlap. The SLS collagen is formed by collagen molecules where all heads are aligned in parallel.

Reconstituted collagen sutures are prepared from bovine long flexor tendons. The tendon is cleaned, frozen, sliced, treated with ficin, and then swollen in dilute cyanoacetic acid. The resulting viscous gel is extruded through a spinneret into an acetone bath for coagulation. The coagulated fibril is stretched, twisted, and dried or treated with chromic salts before twisting and drying. These sutures are similar in appearance to catgut. They are made only in fine sizes, and thus are almost exclusively used in microsurgery.

C. POLYGLYCOLIDE (DEXON®)

Polyglycolide (PGA) with the $-[CH_2-COO]_n$ repeating chemical unit was the first synthetic absorbable suture, introduced in the early 1970s.[8–10] It was developed by Davis & Geck under the trade name Dexon. There are a variety of Dexon sutures. Dexon "S" is an uncoated PGA suture, while the recently available Dexon Plus and Dexon II have coating materials to facilitate handling properties, knot performance, and smooth passage through tissue. Dexon Plus is coated with a copolymer of poly(oxyethylene-oxypropylene), while Dexon II has a polycaprolate coating. Recently, PGA sutures made by companies other than Davis & Geck have been introduced, such as Medifit® from the Japan Medical Supply Co.

PGA suture is polymerized from the cyclic dimer of α-hydroxyacetic acid, more commonly called glycolic acid. Glycolic acid exists in sugar beets, unripe grapes, and wheat and barley leaves. Most higher plants utilize glycolic acid in photorespiration. On heating, glycolic acids form cyclic dimers, called glycolide, more readily than other hydroxy acids due to the formation of stable, ring-strain free six-member ring anhydrides. Glycolide could be prepared either by pyrolysis of the low molecular weight polymer obtained from the thermal dehydration of glycolic acid[8,11–14] or through the elimination of sodium chloride from sodium monochloroacetate.[13] Glycolide exists in two polymorphic forms, α and β, depending on the crystallization temperature (T_c) during purification.[8] The α form obtained at 42°C $< T_c <$ 82.5°C is thermodynamically stable and less sensitive to moisture than the β isomer, which is stable below 42°C. Thus, the α isomer is preferred for the preparation of high molecular weight PGA. Table 5.2 and Figure 5.2 summarize the physical properties of these two types of glycolide.

PGA can be polymerized either directly or indirectly from glycolic acid. The direct polycondensation produces a polymer of M_n less than 10,000 because of the requirement of a very high degree of dehydration (99.28% up) and the absence of monofunctional impurities.[14,15] For PGA of molecular weight higher than 10,000 it is necessary to proceed through the ring-opening polymerization of the cyclic dimers of glycolic acid.

Numerous catalysts are available for this ring-opening polymerization. They include organometallic compounds and Lewis acids.[13,15] Chujo et al. reported that anionic polymerization catalysts like KOH and pyridine result in brittle and highly colored PGA with low yields, while protonic acids like sulfuric acid yield brittle and highly colored PGA in high yield.[13] For biomedical applications, stannous chloride dihydrate or trialkyl aluminum are preferred. The mechanism of polymerization is believed to be cationic melt polymerization if stannous chloride dihydrate (in the presence of alcohol) is used, or nucleophilic

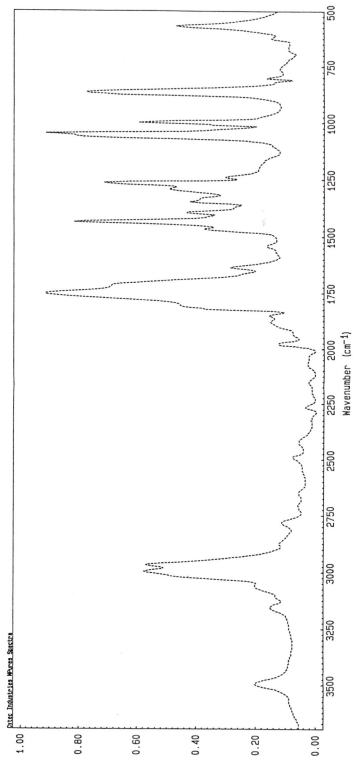

Figure 5.2 Infrared spectra of α and β forms of glycolide. (From Frazza, E. J. and E.E. Schmitt, *J. Biomed. Mater. Res. Symp.*, 1, 43, 1971.)

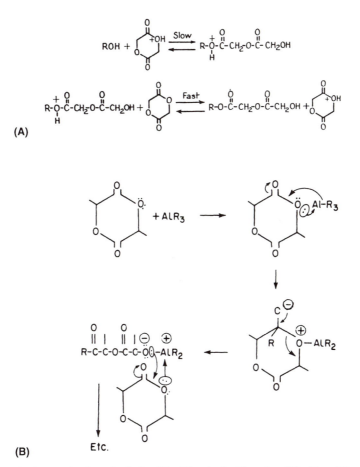

Figure 5.3 Polymerization mechanism of polyglycolide: (A) cationic, (B) nucleophilic. (From Wise, D. L., Fellmann, T.D., Sanderson, J.E., and Wentworth, R.L., in *Drug Carriers in Biology and Medicine*, New York, Academic Press, 1979, 237; Frazza, E. J. and Schmitt, E.E., *J. Biomed. Mater. Res. Symp.*, 1, 43, 1971. With permission.)

attack of a carbanion on one of the glycolide carbonyls if the trialkyl aluminum is used, as shown in Figure 5.3.[8,16] The kinetics of polymerization in the presence of antimony trifluoride catalyst follow the following equation:[13]

$$R = - d[M]/dt = k[C][M] \qquad (1)$$

where [C] is the initial catalyst concentration and [M] is the unreacted monomer concentration. The above equation indicates that the polymer yield increases linearly with polymerization time up to about 100% and is independent of the temperature of polymerization and the quantity of catalyst. The high activation energy (20.7 kcal/mol) and the low heat of polymerization (6.3 kcal/mol) could be due to the relatively small ring-strain of the glycolide.[13] Frequently, an alcohol-like lauryl alcohol is added into the polymerization to control the molecular weight. No polymer could be obtained by γ-irradiation under any conditions.

The resulting PGA polymer having M_w from 20,000 to 140,000 is suitable for fiber extrusion and suture manufacturing. Table 5.3 lists the available chemical and physical properties of a typical PGA.[8,17–21] Dexon suture fibers are made through the melting spinning of PGA chips. The fibers are stretched to several hundred percent of their original length at a temperature above its glass transition temperature (about 36°C), heat-set for improving dimensional stability and inhibiting shrinkage, and subsequently braided into final multifilament braid suture forms of various sizes. Tables 5.4 and 5.5 list physical and mechanical properties of a typical PGA fiber and 2/0 size Dexon suture. Before packaging, all Dexon sutures are subject to heat under vacuum to remove residual unreacted monomers or very low molecular

Table 5.3 Chemical and Physical Properties of Polyglycolide

Melting temperature	224–226°C,[8,19] 215–217°C[21]
Glass transition temperature	36°C[8]
Density	1.5–1.64 g/cm[13,21]
Specific volume (1/density)	0.5952 cm^3/g
Specific gravity	1.548[21]
Specific gravity (100% crystalline)	1.707[21]
Specific gravity (100% amorphous)	1.50[21]
Heat of fusion (100% crystalline)	49.34 cal/g[17]
Unit cell	Orthorhombic[19]
	a = 5.22 Å, b = 6.19 Å, c = 7.02 Å
Crystalline structure	Planar zigzag chain molecules form a
	sheet structure parallel to ac plane[19]
Solvent	Hexafluoroisopropanol (HFIP)
Molecular weight	20–145,000[8,15]
Inherent viscosity	0.5–0.6 dl/g[8]
Intrinsic viscosity	0.6–1.6 dl/g[9,12]
Mark-Houwink constant K in HFIP	10^{-4}dl/g[12]
Mark-Houwink constant a in HFIP	0.8[12]

Note: Superscripts correspond to reference numbers.

Table 5.4 Polyglycolide Fiber Properties

Diameter	15–25 μm
Tenacity	5–10 g/denier
	100–200,000 psi
Knot/straight tenacity	50–80%
Elongation	15–35%

From Frazza, E.J. and Schmitt, E.E., *J. Biomed. Mater. Res. Symp.*, 1, 43, 1971. With permission.

Table 5.5 Mechanical Property of 2/0 Size Dexon Sutures

Tensile breaking strength (GPD)	Tensile breaking elongation (%)	Yield stress (GPD)	Yield strain (%)	Modulus of elasticity (GPD)	Specific work of rupture (N/TEX) × 10^{-2}	Flexural stiffness[a] (kg/cm^2)
6.30	22.6	0.80	1.9	55	6.63	1.15 × 10^2

Note: GPD, gram per denier.

[a] Chu, C.C. and Kizil, Z., *Surg. Gynecol. Obstet.*, 168, 233, 1989.

From Chu., C.C., *Ann. Surg.*, 193(3), 365, 1981. With permission.

weight volatile oligomers according to a patented procedure.[22,23] Dexon sutures are sterilized by ethylene oxide because of the well-known adverse effect of γ-irradiation, i.e., accelerated loss of tensile strength (refer to Chapter 7).

PGA was found to exhibit an orthorhombic unit cell with dimensions a = 5.22 Å, b = 6.19 Å, and c (fiber axis) = 7.02 Å. The planar zigzag-chain molecules form a sheet structure parallel to the ac plane, as shown in Figure 5.4, and do not have the polyethylene type arrangement.[19] The molecules between two adjacent sheets orient in opposite directions. The tight molecular packing and the close approach of the ester groups might stabilize the crystal lattice and contribute to the high melting point of PGA (224 to 227°C). The specific gravities of PGA are 1.707 for a perfect crystal and 1.50 in a completely amorphous state.[21] The heat of fusion of 100% crystallized PGA is reported to be 12 kJ/mol or 45.7 cal/g.[17] A recent study of injection molded PGA discs reveals their IR spectroscopic characteristics.[24] As shown in Figure 5.5, the four bands at 850, 753, 713, and 560 cm^{-1} are associated with the amorphous regions of the injection-molded PGA discs and could be used to assess the extent of hydrolysis. Peaks associated with the crystalline phase include those at 972, 901, 806, 627, and 590 cm⁻¹. Two broad intense peaks at 1142 and 1077 cm⁻¹ can be assigned to C-O stretching modes in the ester groups and oxymethylene groups, respectively. These two peaks appear to be associated mainly with ester and oxymethylene groups originating in the amorphous domains. Hydrolysis could cause both of these C-O stretching modes to substantially decrease in intensity.[24]

The healing of the sutured wound is profoundly affected by the approximating force exerted by a suture loop, which, in turn, is determined by several physicomechanical factors. Besides the well-known factors, such as tensile properties and knotting regimen, the stress relaxation characteristics of the suture

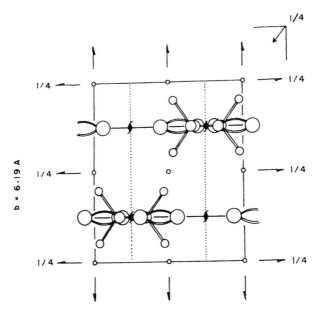

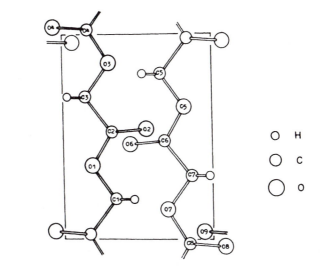

Figure 5.4 Crystal structure of polyglycolide. (From Chatani, Y., Suehiro, K., Okita, Y., Tadokoro, H., and Chujo, K., *Die Makromol. Chem.*, 113, 215, 1968. With permission.)

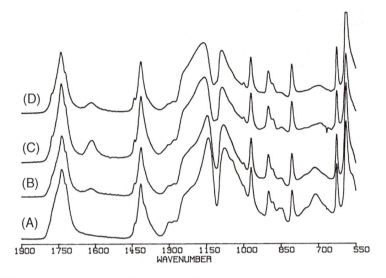

1900   1750   1600   1450   1300   1150   1000   850   700   550
WAVENUMBER

Figure 5.5 FTIR spectra of injection-molded polyglycolide disc as a function of hydrolysis time. (A) 0 d control; (B) 55 hrs; (C) 7 d; (D) 21 d. (From Chu, C.C., Zhang, L., and Coyne, L., *J. Appl. Polym. Sci.*, 56, 1275, 1995. With permission.)

that affect the postplacement approximating force applied by the suture loop is probably the least-known mechanical property in sutures. Recent work done by von Fraunhofer et al. has demonstrated that the tautness of the suture across a healing wound can significantly affect the healing process, and, in particular, it was shown that healing wounds exhibit greater tear strengths and tear energies when tied with loose sutures than tight sutures.[25] Thus, the development of some means to improve the course of wound healing through reduction of the suture approximating force across a wound is clearly beneficial. The use of the inherent viscoelastic properties of polymeric suture fibers, i.e., stress relaxation, to reduce the approximating force within the suture during wound healing appears to be a plausible solution. Based on these viscoelastic properties, von Fraunhofer et al. suggested that Dexon, Vicryl, and silk sutures may be best suited for ligation since these materials retain a high degree of stiffness over a long period of time and thus should minimize the risks of delayed hemorrhage. On the other hand, Prolene and, to a degree, PDS exhibit moduli that change with time and may give better results during the normal healing process since these materials tend to relax significantly with respect to time.[26] The details of this viscoelastic property of several commonly used suture materials are described in Chapter 6.

D. POLY(GLYCOLIDE-LACTIDE) COPOLYMER (VICRYL®)

The glycolide-L-lactide random copolymer suture material (Vicryl), sometimes called polyglactin 910 with $[CH_2-COO]_{90}-[CH(CH_3)-COO]_{10}-$ as the repeating unit, is also copolymerized in the same fashion as PGA. For biomedical use, Lewis acid catalysts are preferred.[15] For suture use, the glycolide-L-lactide copolymers must have a high concentration of glycolide monomer for achieving proper mechanical and degradation properties. Multifilament braided Vicryl sutures contain a 90/10 molar ratio of glycolic to L-lactic acid and is coated with 2 to 10% of a 50:50 mixture of an amorphous polyglactin 370 (a 65/35 mole ratio of lactide-glycolide copolymer) and calcium stearate. Vicryl sutures are sterilized by ethylene oxide like other synthetic absorbable sutures.

Figure 5.6 illustrates the changes in percent crystallinity with the mole percent of glycolide in the glycolide/L-lactide copolymer.[27] The data suggest that the mole percent of glycolide must be greater than 70% to achieve crystalline characteristics. As described in Chapter 7, synthetic absorbable sutures must have some level of crystallinity to achieve a proper tensile strength and its retention during hydrolytic degradation for wound closure use. This is because very low crystalline or totally amorphous biodegradable polymers would degrade too fast to be useful as wound closure biomaterials. Figure 5.7 illustrates such a relationship between the rate of degradation *in vivo* and the composition of glycolide to L-lactide.[28] A comparison between Figures 5.6 and 5.7 indicates that a copolymer with L-lactide composition between 25 and 75% is totally amorphous and hence would degrade the fastest. For this reason, 90:10 molar ratio of glycolide to L-lactide has been used as the optimal comonomer ratio for suture use. If

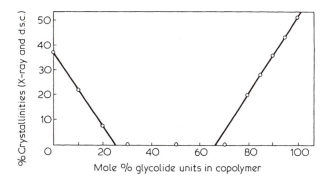

Figure 5.6 Percent of level of crystallinity for GA/LA copolymers as a function of glycolide (or lactide) composition determined by X-ray and DSC measurements. (From Reed, A.M. and Gilding, D.K., *Polymer*, 20, 1459, 1979. With permission.)

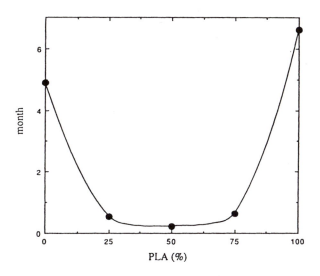

Figure 5.7 The effect of glycolide to lactide composition on the *in vivo* degradation rate of polyglactin implanted under the dorsal skin of rat. The degradation rate was expressed in terms of the time for 50% weight loss of the implant. (From Miller, P.A., Brady, J.M., and Cutright, D.E., *J. Biomed. Mater. Res.*, 11, 719, 1977. With permission.)

DL- instead of L-lactide is used as the comonomer, however, the U-shaped relationship between the level of crystallinity and glycolide composition disappears. This is because polylactide from 100% DL-lactide composition is totally amorphous.

Lactic acid, due to its one asymmetric carbon, has two optical isomers, L(+) and D(–). It is present as either an intermediate or an end product in carbohydrate metabolism. The six-membered cyclic dimers of lactic acid, called lactides, are also optically active. They exist in L(–), D(+), and meso forms. Vicryl absorbable copolymer suture is polymerized from L(–) lactide rather than other optical or racemic isomers. Copolymer sutures from glycolide and DL racemic lactide can shrink up to 50% due to higher amorphous contents, while the copolymer sutures prepared from either pure D- or L-lactide isomer exhibit very low shrinkage.[29] The sheet crystalline structure of PGA is disturbed in the lactide-glycolide copolymer because the methyl group in lactide comonomer affects the chain packing along the b axis.[19] The broadening of the X-ray reflections in the copolymer demonstrates this. Such disorder in the b direction (the direction in which sheets stack) of the copolymer might contribute to the difference in the biodegradation phenomena between the copolymer and the homopolymer PGA sutures. Table 5.6 lists the physical properties of the 2/0 size copolymer suture, Vicryl.[29] ATR infrared spectra of Vicryl sutures appear similar to PGA and are shown in Figure 5.8. IR bands associated with molecules in the amorphous domains of the copolymer suture are 560, 710, 850, and 888 cm^{-1}, while 590, 626, 808, 900, and 972 cm^{-1} are associated with the crystalline domains. Like PGA, these IR bands could be used to assess the extent of hydrolysis.

Table 5.6 Physical and Mechanical Properties of 2/0 Vicryl Suture

Inh. vis. (dL/g)	Crystallinity (%)	Density (g/cm³)	Crystallite (110/020/002)	Orientation f(φ)	Long period (Å)	Tensile force (kg)	Modulus of elasticity (kg/cm²)	Specific work of rupture (N/TEX)×10⁻²	T_m (°C)	T_g (°C)	Flexural stiffness (kg/cm²)
1.373	40	1.537	69/ 40/ 82	0.966	87	5.13	23.25	5.46[a]	198.1[b]	36–45	3.21×10² [c]

[a] Data from Chu., C.C., *Ann. Surg.*, 193(3), 365, 1981.

[b] Data from Fredericks, R.J., Melveger, A.J., and Dolegiewitz, L.J., *J. Polym. Sci. Polym. Phys. Ed.*, 22, 57, 1984.

[c] Data from Chu, C.C., and Kizil, Z., *Surg. Gynecol. Obstet.*, 168, 233, 1989.

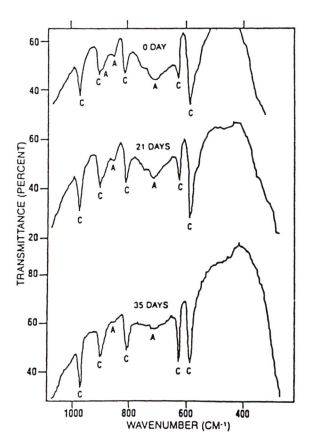

Figure 5.8 ATR IR spectra of 2/0 Vicryl suture upon hydrolysis. A — amorphous peaks; C — Crystalline peaks. (From Fredericks, R.J., Melveger, A.J., and Dolegiewitz, L.J., *J. Polym. Sci. Polym. Phys. Ed.*, 22, 57, 1984. With permission.)

E. POLY-*p*-DIOXANONE (PDS®, PDSII®)

Before the availability of PDS monofilament absorbable suture, synthetic absorbable sutures were available only in braided form in large size (Dexon and Vicryl) because their high density of ester functional groups makes these two sutures rigid in larger size (e.g., 2/0) monofilament form. There is a strong need to have monofilament absorbable sutures of relatively large size but flexible because monofilament sutures have generally less tissue dragging and tearing when they pass through tissues and exhibit less tissue reaction than the corresponding braided suture. Monofilament sutures, in general, do not provide capillary wicking of fluids, which would minimize the spread of wound infection, if any. One chemical method to provide some molecular flexibility without leaving the glycolide family is to reduce the density of ester functional group in Dexon so that the frequency of hydrogen bonding could be reduced for less rigid molecules. These flexible molecules would allow the manufacturing of monofilament absorbable sutures like PDS with acceptable flexibility.

PDS suture with the repeating unit [-O-(CH$_2$)$_2$-OCH$_2$CO-] is the first commercially available monofilament absorbable suture that derives from the glycolide family. It is a poly(ester-ether). This relatively new synthetic degradable monofilament suture is polymerized from *p*-dioxanone monomers. The monomer, 1,4-dioxanone-2,5 dione or *p*-dioxanone, is obtained from the reaction of chloroacetic acid with metallic sodium dissolved in a large excess of ethylene glycol.[30] The resulting *p*-dioxanone is purified by multiple redistillation and crystallization. Fiber-grade high molecular weight PDS polymer is made from the ring-opening polymerization of highly purified (>99%) in the presence of organometallic catalysts, such as Et$_2$Zn or zirconium acetylacetonate, as shown in Figure 5.9.[25] The resulting polymer has an inherent viscosity of 0.70 (0.1% polymer solution in tetrachloroethane at 25°C) and a degree of crystallinity of 37%. Poly-*p*-dioxanone polymer has T$_g$ = –16 to –10°C and T$_m$ = 110 to 115°C. Monofilament PDS suture is made from the melt-spinning of the dried polymer chips through a spinneret into monofilaments of any desired suture diameter.[30] The extruded fibers are then drawn about five times

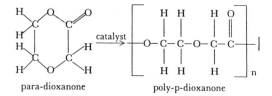

Figure 5.9 PDS polymerization process.   para-dioxanone   poly-p-dioxanone

at T > 43°C and heat-set to orient the molecules for better physical and mechanical properties. The drug/cosmetic violet dye #2 is added to make violet colored PDS sutures. A 2/0 size PDS suture has an inherent viscosity of 0.64 and a degree of crystallinity of 30%.

Recently, an enhanced version of PDS suture (PDSII) has been introduced for improving its flexibility and handling characteristics. PDS and PDSII are chemically identical, but PDSII suture differs from PDS in fiber morphology resulting from different fiber spinning conditions. PDSII suture is made by subjecting the melt-spun PDS fibers to a short period of annealing at a temperature above T_m of PDS (about 125°C).[32] This additional heated drawing treatment, not used in PDS suture, partially melts the surface layer of PDS fibers and subsequently modifies the near-surface crystalline structure of PDS monofilament suture. Thus, a distinctive skin-core morphology that the PDS suture does not have is observed in the PDSII suture, as shown in Figure 5.10.[32] The core of the PDSII suture has a more highly ordered and larger spherulitic crystal structure than the surrounding annular area characterized by smaller crystals, while the untreated PDS suture shows a relatively even crystalline structure throughout its cross section. Table 5.7 illustrates the crystalline properties of PDSII and the untreated PDS sutures of 2/0, 4/0, and 6/0 sizes.[32] The larger crystals in PDSII are evident in their larger breadth (L). Table 5.8 summarizes mechanical properties of PDSII and PDS sutures over a wide range of sizes. In general, PDSII sutures have a lower modulus of elasticity.

PDS sutures are sterilized by ethylene oxide the same way as other synthetic absorbable sutures and no coating is used. Table 5.9 summarizes essential physical and mechanical properties of a 2/0 size PDS suture.[31,33] Based on the PDS chemical structure, i.e., ether and ester linkages separated by a methylene group (CH$_2$), PDS is expected to be sensitive to oxidative, photooxidative, and γ-irradiation degradation.

Recently, there have been a few varieties of PDS-related copolymers reported in the literature that may have potential use as wound closure biomaterials.[34–37] A copolymer of PDS and PGA (20%) has an absorption profile similar to Dexon and Vicryl sutures, but it has compliance similar to PDS. A copolymer of PDS and PLLA (15%) results in a more compliant suture than homopolymer PDS but with similar absorption profiles as PDS. A detailed description of the variety of PDS related copolymers is given in Chapter 12.

F. POLY(GLYCOLIDE-TRIMETHYLENE CARBONATE) COPOLYMER (MAXON®)

Another commercially available monofilament absorbable suture, Maxon, is made from block copolymer of glycolide and 1,3-dioxan-2-one (trimethylene carbonate or GTMC). It consists of 32.5% by weight (or 36 mol%) of trimethylene carbonate with the repeating unit $[-OCH_2CO-]_{67}[-O(CH_2)_3OCO-]_{33}$.[38,39] Maxon is a poly(ester-carbonate). The polymerization process of Maxon suture is divided into two stages. The first stage is the formation of middle block, which is a random copolymer of glycolide and 1,3-dioxan-2-one (trimethylene carbonate). Diethylene glycol is used as an initiator and stannous chloride dihydrate (SnCl$_2$·2H$_2$O) serves as the catalyst. The polymerization is conducted at about 180°C. The weight ratio of glycolide to trimethylene carbonate in the middle block is 15:85. After the synthesis of the middle block, the temperature of the reactive bath is raised to about 220°C to prevent the crystallization of the copolymer and additional glycolide monomers as the end blocks are added into the reaction bath to form the final triblock copolymer. The chemical reaction is shown in Figure 5.11. The undyed Maxon has a natural clear appearance, while green-colored Maxon is dyed by green DG#6 with <0.3% by weight. Maxon suture is sterilized by ethylene oxide and no coating is used. Table 5.10 summarizes essential physical and mechanical properties of 2/0 size Maxon.[20,38]

G. GLYCOLIDE-ε-CAPROLACTONE COPOLYMER (MONOCRYL®)

Monocryl is a copolymer suture of glycolide and ε-caprolactone. Due to the proprietary nature of this new synthetic absorbable suture, its chemical properties, detailed polymerization routes, and other related essential properties are sparse at the present time. However, the generic copolymerization process between glycolic acid and ε-caprolactone was recently reported by Fukuzaki et al. in Japan as shown in Figure 5.12A.[40,41] The resulting copolymers were low molecular weight biodegradable copolymers of glycolic acid and various

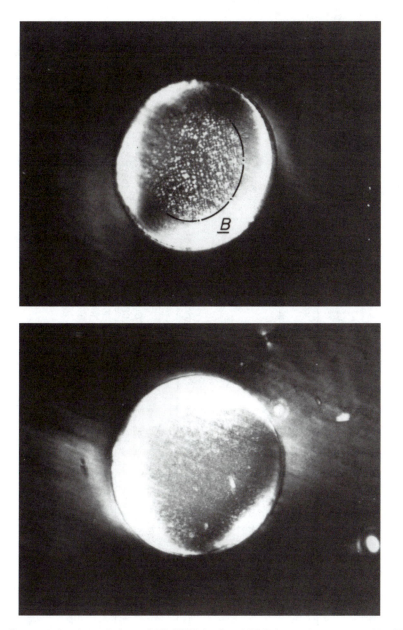

Figure 5.10 Cross-sectional morphology of 6/0 PDSII (top) and PDS (bottom) sutures at ×430. (From Broyer, E., U.S. Patent 5,294,395, Ethicon, Inc., 1994.)

lactones for potential drug delivery purpose. The composition of lactone ranged from as low as 15 to as high as 50 mol% and the average molecular weight ranged from 4510 to 16,500. The glass transition temperature ranged from 18 to –43°C, depending on the copolymer composition and molecular weight.

Monofilament Monocryl suture is a segmented block copolymer consisting of both soft and hard segments. The purpose of having soft segments in the copolymer is to provide good handling property like pliability, while the hard segments are used to provide adequate strength. Monocryl is made in a two-stage polymerization process.[42] In the first stage, soft segments of prepolymer of glycolide and ε-caprolactone are made. This soft segmented prepolymer is further polymerized with glycolides to provide hard segments of polyglycolide. Monocryl has a composition of 75% glycolide and 25% ε-caprolactone and should have a higher molecular weight than those glycolide/ε-caprolactone copolymers reported by Fukuzaki et al. for adequate mechanical properties required by sutures. Figure 5.12B illustrates the chemical structure of Monocryl suture.[42]

Table 5.7 A Comparison of the Crystalline Properties of Two Types of Poly(*p*-Dioxanone) Sutures of a Variety of Sizes

Suture size	PDS II X_e	PDS II L	PDS II l_s	PDS II F_h	PDS X_e	PDS L	PDS l_s	PDS F_h
2/0	0.52	78	95	106	0.47	64	96	229
4/0	0.55	72	97	208	0.52	61	97	213
6/0	0.56	76	97	180	0.51	71	99	213

Note: X_e is the relative crystallinity; L is an estimate of the breadth in angstroms of individual crystallites using the Debye-Scherrer equation $L = \lambda/\beta\cos\theta$; l_s is a measure of the long-range crystalline structure determined by small-angle radiation scatter in Å; F_h is a measure of the long-range crystallite perfection in the chain direction along the fiber axis as indicated by crystalline peak width in angstroms at half-height.

From Broyer, E., U.S. Patent 5,294,395, Ethicon, Inc., 1994.

Table 5.8 A Comparison of the Physical/Mechanical Properties of Two Types of Poly-*p*-Dioxanone Sutures of a Variety of Sizes

Nominal suture size	PDS II Diameter (mils)	PDS II Gurley stiffness	PDS II Tensile St. (psi × 10^{-3})	PDS II Modulus of elasticity (psi × 10^{-3})	PDS II Ten. St./Mod. Elast.	PDS Diameter (mils)	PDS Gurley stiffness	PDS Tensile St. (psi × 10^{-3})	PDS Modulus of elasticity (psi × 10^{-3})	PDS Ten. St./Mod. Elast.
2	23.3	240	63.7	210	0.30	23.8	364	72.5	336	0.22
1	20.8	149	—	—	—	19.6	169	75.7	318	0.24
0	18.4	85	69.1	200	0.35	17.0	118	71.8	323	0.22
2/0	14.1	30	70.2	198	0.35	13.6	54	73.4	337	0.21
3/0	12.0	16	74.2	204	0.36	11.6	23	75.3	333	0.23
4/0	8.4	5.6	—	—	—	8.7	7.0	82.3	354	0.23
5/0	6.6	1.8	82.6	199	0.43	6.9	2.6	77.2	334	0.23
6/0	4.4	0.2	—	—	—	4.4	0.2	89.6	322	0.28
7/0	0.4	0.04	—	—	—	0.4	0.04	—	351	—

From Broyer, E., U.S. Patent 5,294,395, Ethicon, Inc., 1994.

Table 5.9 Physical and Mechanical Properties of 2/0 PDS Suture

Molecular weight (M_w)	Heat of fusion (ΔH) (cal/g)	Glass transition temperature (T_g) (°C)	Melting temperature (T_m) (°C)	Birefringence	d spacing (Å)	Crystallite size (Å)	Tensile breaking force (kg)	Elong. to break (%)	Flexural stiff. (kg/cm²)
63,120[a]	19.02	−10	104.7	4.96×10^{-3}	4.05	78	5.76	82.13	1.00×10^{4} [b]

[a] Data from Lin, H.L., Chu, C.C., and Grubb, D., *J. Biomed. Mater. Res.*, 27(2), 153, 1993.
[b] Data from Chu, C.C. and Kizil, Z., *Surg. Gynecol. Obstet.*, 168, 233, 1989.

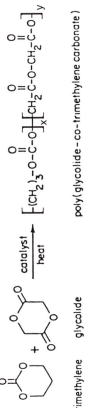

Figure 5.11 Maxon suture polymerization process. x = 33% by weight and y = 67% by weight.

Table 5.10 Physical and Mechanical Properties of 2/0 Maxon Suture

Intrinsic viscosity (dl/g)	Heat of fusion (Cal/g)	Melting temp. (°C)	Glass trans. temp. (°C)	Surface wettability (dyn/cm)	Tensile breaking load (kg)	Breaking elongation (%)	Modulus of elasticity (psi)	Flexural stiffness (kg/cm²)
1.60	10.15	206.7	20	72.4[a]	5.76	32[b]	500,000[b]	4.48×10^{3} [c]

[a] Data from Zhang, L., Loh, I.H., and Chu, C.C., *J. Biomed. Mater. Res.*, 27, 1425, 1993.
[b] Data from Katz, A., Mukherjee, D.P., Kaganov, A.L., and Gordon, S., *Surg. Gynecol. Obstet.*, 161, 213, 1985.
[c] Data from Chu, C.C. and Kizil, Z., *Surg. Gynecol. Obstet.*, 168, 233, 1989.

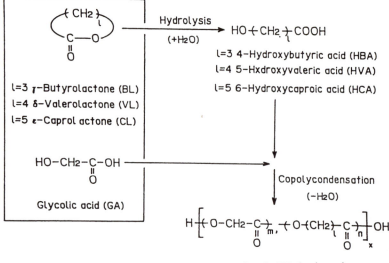

Figure 5.12A Reaction scheme for direct copolycondensation of glycolic acid (GA) and various lactones in the presence of water without catalysts at 200°C. (From Fukuzaki, H., Yoshida, M., Asano, M., Kumakura, M., Mashimo, T., Yuasa, H., Imai, K., Yamandka, H., Kawaharada, U., and Suzuki, K., *J. Biomed. Mater. Res.*, 25, 315, 1991. With permission.)

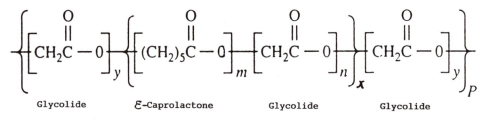

Figure 5.12B Monocryl® suture chemical structure.

The most unique aspect of Monocryl monofilament suture is its pliability as claimed by Ethicon.[42] The force required to bend a 2/0 suture is only about 2.8×10^4 lb/in^2(193 MPa) for Monocryl, while the same size PDSII and Maxon monofilament sutures require about 3.9 and 11.6×10^4 lb/in^2 (269 to 800 MPa) force, respectively (please refer to Chapter 6 for details). This inherent pliability of Monocryl is due to its low glass transition temperature resulting from the ε-caprolactone comonomer unit. Its T_g is expected to be between 15 and –36°C. Unlike Maxon and PDSII, Monocryl suture appears to have less out-of-package memory which improves its handling characteristics.

H. GLYCOLIDE-TRIMETHYLENE CARBONATE TRIBLOCK COPOLYMER (BIOSYN®)

The latest addition to the arsenal of synthetic absorbable sutures is a triblock copolymer, Glycomer 631 (Biosyn) from U.S. Surgical.[43] This block copolymer consists of glycolide (60%), dioxanone (14%), and trimethylene carbonate (26%), with glycolide being the predominant component. The center block is a random copolymer of 1,3 dioxanone-2-one (65% by weight) and 1,4 dioxane-2-one (35% by weight). The two ends of this center block are capped by a block polymer consisting mainly of glycolide (>50%) that could be copolymerized with lactide, trimethylene carbonate, p-dioxanone or ε-caprolactone.

The purpose of using triblock polymer chemistry to design Biosyn is to make synthetic absorbable monofilament sutures having good handling properties, such as flexibility, without compromising other mechanical properties, like knot strength and security and biodegradation properties. As we described in Chapter 4, sutures must be bent for packaging. Before use, the packaged suture material must be straightened out upon its removal from the package after a long period of shelf life. The ability to remove the kinks from a suture is a very important handling characteristic that surgeons always encounter during wound closure.

Table 5.11A A Comparison of Mechanical Properties of 3/0 Size Biosyn and Maxon Sutures

Physical Property	Biosyn	Maxon
Diameter (mm)	0.29	0.293
Knot-pull strength (kg)	2.4	2.9
Young's modulus (kpsi)	145	425
Straight-pull strength (kg)	3.7	3.9
Strain energy 0–5% (kg-mm)	0.84	1.6
Strain energy 0–10% (kg-mm)	2.76	5.19
Elongation (%)	44	30
Tensile strength (kg/mm²)	55.3	56.2

Data from Roby, M.S. et al., U.S. Patent 5,403,347, April 4, 1995.

Table 5.11B Physical and Mechanical Properties of 3/0 New Absorbable Block Copolymer Monofilament Suture

Physical Property	Example 1	Example 2
Diameter (mm)	0.3	0.29
Knot-pull strength (kg)	2.9	2.4
Young's modulus (kpsi)	190	145
Straight-pull strength (kg)	4.4	3.7
Strain energy 0–5% (kg-mm)	1.28	0.84
Strain energy 0–10% (kg-mm)	3.89	2.76
Elongation (%)	47	44
Tensile strength (kg/mm²)	60.6	55.3

From Roby, M.S. et al., US Patent 5,403,347 April 4, 1995.

Biosyn has the next lowest modulus of elasticity (145×10^3 psi) among all existing synthetic absorbable suture materials, and its strain energy at both 5 and 10% strain (0.84 and 2.76 kg-mm, respectively), was about $^1/_2$ of the corresponding size Maxon sutures.[43] Table 5.11 lists the important mechanical properties of 3/0 Biosyn and their comparison with Maxon sutures. The rate of tensile strength loss of Biosyn sutures is similar to Vicryl suture *in vitro* with about 8% of its original tensile breaking strength remaining at the end of 28 days. Because of its very new status, there is extremely little published information about Biosyn.

II. NONABSORBABLE SUTURE MATERIALS

A. SILK

Silk is one of the three major fibrous proteins (the others are wool and collagen). Silk fiber is semicrystalline and has two major constituents: a fiber protein called fibroin and the gummy substance called sericin that holds the fibers together. As it is spun by the silkworm, silk fiber consists of two triangular filaments stuck together with sericin. Tables 5.12 and 5.13 show the amino acid composition of silk fibroin and sericin.[44] The most significant feature of the amino acid composition of silk fibroins is the high concentration of glycine, alanine, and serine. Together, these three small size amino acids take up about 80 to 85% of the total amino acids in *Bombyx mori* and *Anaphe pernyi*. Such a high concentration of these three amino acids having small and simple side groups in silk fibroins permits the arrangement of polypeptide molecules into an orderly and crystalline manner and is responsible for the desirable mechanical, physical, and chemical properties of silk fibers. The amino acids with bulky side groups like tyrosine consist of a small portion of silk fibroins and cannot be accommodated within the three-dimensional, ordered crystalline structure. Thus, disordered amorphous regions coexist with the crystalline ones. Silk fibers have about a 60% level of crystallinity.[45,46] As described later, this arrangement of crystalline to amorphous domains in fibroin bears an important relationship to properties such as moisture absorption and biodegradation, which occur mainly in the amorphous regions of silk. Cross-sectional views of silk fiber show a somewhat irregular triangular shape.

Table 5.12 Amino Acid Composition of Silk Fibroins (Residues/1000 Residues)

	B. mori				A. pernyi	A. moloneyi
	Fiber	Fiber	Gland	Gland	Fiber	Fiber
Gly	446.0	447.6	433.0	452.0	265	424
Ala	294.0	287.0	347.0	296.0	441	530
Val	22.0	20.3	16.0	21.0	7	21
Leu	5.3	4.5	2.4	4.5	8	2
Ile	6.6	5.9	4.6	6.2	—	1
Ser	121.0	116.1	103.0	89.5	118	3
Thr	9.1	9.5	7.2	5.7	1	2
Asp	13.0	16.2	13.9	16.9	47	5
Glu	10.2	12.4	10.6	11.9	8	3
Lys	3.2	3.1	3.4	2.9	1	1
Arg	4.7	4.9	4.5	3.7	26	1
His	1.4	1.7	1.9	1.5	8	2
Tyr	51.7	53.9	47.9	42.6	49	1
Phe	6.3	6.2	6.8	6.0	6	1
Pro	3.6	4.2	3.5	N.d.	3	2
Trp	1.1	4.3	—	N.d.	11	—
Met	1.0	—	—	—	—	—
(Cys)$_2$	2.0	0.47	0.8	N.d.	—	—
		Gly > Ala			Gly < Ala	

From Robson, R M., in *Fiber Chemistry*, Lewin, M. and Pearce, E.M., Eds., *Handbook of Fiber Science and Technology*, Vol. IV, Marcel Dekker, New York, 1985, chap. 7. With permission.

Table 5.13 Amino Acid Composition of Silk Sericins (Residues/1000 Residues)

	B. mori		Tussah	
			A. pernyi	A. mylitta
	Cocoon	Gland	Cocoon	Cocoon
Gly	127.0	147	149.9	149.1
Ala	55.1	43	27.8	27.3
Val	26.8	36	11.9	7.9
Leu	7.2	14	9.9	5.5
Ile	5.5	7	8.0	3.9
Ser	319.7	373	226.3	232.1
Thr	82.5	87	149.6	131.6
Asp	138.4	148	122.5	141.5
Glu	58.0	34	67.4	60.3
Lys	32.6	24	14.7	20.1
Arg	28.6	36	54.5	61.1
His	13.0	12	25.0	24.1
Tyr	34.0	26	49.2	43.3
Phe	4.3	3	6.0	24.7
Pro	5.7	7	19.1	10.9
Trp	—	N.d.	—	—
Met	0.5	N.d.	1.3	Trace
(Cys)$_2$	1.4	5	1.8	Trace

From Robson, R.M., in *Fiber Chemistry*, Lewin, M. and Pearce, E.M., Eds., *Handbook of Fiber Science and Technology*, Vol. IV, Marcel Dekker, New York, 1985, chap. 7. With permission.

In contrast to wool and the other α-keratins, silk from *B. mori* has a trace amount of cystine indicating that the early assumption that silk fibroins do not have cystine is questionable. It was suggested that this trace amount of cystine is responsible for the secondary structure of silk fibroins. A wide range of

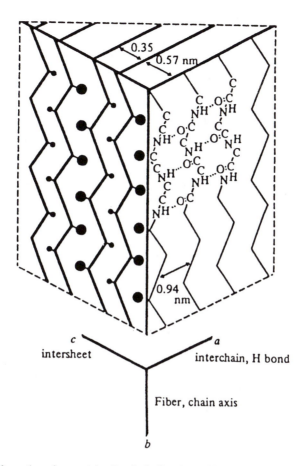

Figure 5.13 The conformation of a crystal unit cell of silk polypeptide chains. (From Marsh, R.E., Corey, R.B., and Pauling, L., *Biochem. Biophys. Acta*, 16, 1, 1955. With permission.)

molecular weight of silk fibroins has been reported due to the difficulty in obtaining a homogeneous preparation without degradation or aggregation. Recently, more consistent values from 350,000 to 370,000 Da have been reported.[44]

The molecular conformation of *B. mori* silk fibroins in the crystalline region assumes the β-pleated sheet configuration as shown in Figure 5.13.[44,47] Within each pleated sheet, close to fully extended polypeptide chains are arranged antiparallel (e.g., either two adjacent chains run in opposite directions or fold back) with the axis of the chains parallel to the fiber axis and intermolecular H-bonds between the >C=O and >NH functional groups of adjacent chains. The Gly residues lie on one side of the sheet and the Ser and Ala on the other. The fibroin molecules are about 1400 Å long and tend to be oriented parallel to the fiber axis. Each pleated sheet is parallel to the ab plane. The unit cell has the following dimensions: a (interchain) = 9.4 Å, b (fiber axis) = 6.97 Å, and c (intersheet) = 9.2 Å. Intersheets are held together through hydrophobic bonds.

Sericin is the gummy protein that holds fibroin filaments together in cocoon silk and consists of about 25% of the cocoon by weight. Sericin has more distinctive amino acid compositions than fibroin, as shown in Table 5.13. In *B. mori* sericin, Gly, Asp, and Ser together comprise two thirds of the total amino acid residues. The hydrophilic nature of sericin derives from the high concentration of amino acids with side polar groups like -OH and -COOH. Sericin has relatively more cystine than fibroin. In most silk sutures, except Virgin Silk for microsurgery, sericin is removed. The presence of sericin could be identified by a mixture of dyes: C.I. Acid Blue 40 and C.I. Acid Orange 56.[48] A yellow-red is associated with silk with >10% sericin, while a blue indicates <10% sericin.

All silks are not, however, chemically identical. Different silkworm species produce fibrous proteins that contain different sequences and proportions of amino acids. These compositional differences in turn influence the mechanical properties of the fibers. The most common form of silk, produced by the silkworm *B. mori* from which most silk sutures are made, has a predominant six-residue sequence Gly-Ser-Gly-Ala-Gly-Ala, which repeats itself for long distances along the chain. This sequence accounts for a large proportion of the amino acid residues that are present. The identity of the silkworm species used for making silk suture materials is not publicly available, but is suspected to be the most common silkworm, *B. mori*.

The process of making silk sutures has not been disclosed by the manufacturer. It is believed, however, that the raw silk fibers from the cocoon are cleaned first by removing the natural waxes and sericin (called degumming). The cleaned silk fibers are then either twisted or braided to form the suture strand. Silk has a relatively high standard moisture regain of 11%. Various types of surface treatments are used to render it noncapillary, serum proof, incapable of the ingrowth of tissues, or all of these. Wax or silicone has been used as the coating material. Tissue ingrowth is prevented by encasing the twisted silk fibers in a nonabsorbing coating of tanned gelatin or other protein substances. The trade name of this specially treated silk suture is Dermal from Ethicon. Other trademarks of silk sutures are braided Surgical Silk (Ethicon), twisted Virgin Silk (Ethicon), and braided Protein Silk (Davis & Geck). With the very fine size silk sutures for microsurgery and ophthalmology, the sericin component of the virgin silk is not removed during manufacturing processing. Figure 5.14 illustrates the SEM view of the irregular triangular cross sections of degummed *B. mori* silk fibers. The highly fibrillar structure of silk fibers is also evident in the internal fibrillar structure through longitudinally split of silk fiber, as shown in Figure 5.15. Silk sutures are sterilized either by Co^{60} γ-irradiation or ethylene oxide.

The mechanical properties of silk closely correlate with the fraction of bulky side groups present and thus with the crystalline:amorphous ratio as well as the conformational arrangement of chain segments in the amorphous domains. Earland and Robins[49] and Zuber[50] reported that peptide chain segments located in the amorphous domains are connected among themselves and to the crystallites via disulfide and ester linkages and hydrogen and ionic bonds where they are appropriate. As described in detail in Chapter 6, silk sutures have relatively very high modulus of elasticity. This high elastic modulus is attributed to the strong inter- and intramolecular interactions among peptide chain segments in the amorphous domains as well as interactions between these randomly oriented amorphous and highly ordered crystalline peptide chain segments through various types of H-bonds, ionic bonds, and ester and disulfide linkages. If silk sutures are stretched beyond their yield point, these inter- or intramolecular bonds would be broken first and randomly oriented amorphous peptide chain segments are thus allowed to be extended. At this phase of the stress-strain curve, a characteristic of low modulus yield plateau is evident. The degree of yield plateau depends on the strength and amount of inter- and intramolecular forces among the amorphous peptide chain segments and between the amorphous and crystalline peptide chain segments. Weaker inter- and intramolecular forces would result in a pronounced yield plateau.

The macromolecular structure of silk fibers is also responsible for their well-known loss of tensile strength *in vivo*. Any loss of fiber tensile strength could be attributed to either the scission of primary bonds in the backbone macromolecules or/and the breakage of secondary bonds like H-bonds due to a reactive species like water. The moisture regain of a typical silk fiber is about 9.9% due to the high concentration of polar side groups in amino acid residues. Water molecules absorbed by silk fibers reside in the amorphous domains and compete with the amino acids in the amorphous chain segments for inter- and intramolecular interactions.[44] This competition by water molecules leads to a more open amorphous structure by the replacement of relatively strong inter- and intramolecular interactions in the amorphous domains with water. As a result, a lower tensile strength is observed. The observed *in vivo* strength loss of silk sutures might be a combination of the scissions of both primary and secondary bonds; however, the breakage of secondary bonds within silk fibers in water probably plays a more important role than the scission of primary bonds. This is because the high crystallinity level found in most silk fibers should retard the diffusion of relatively large proteolytic enzymes[51] and hence render silk fibers resistant to proteolytic enzymatic hydrolysis.

Because of the undesirable *in vivo* loss of tensile strength and somewhat higher tissue reactions and ingrowth to silk sutures, Shalaby et al. recently reported the impregnation of silk with hydrophobic thermoplastic elastomers to improve the performance of silk sutures.[52] The rationale behind the approach is to provide an inert barrier between silk sutures and surrounding tissue so that tissue reactions and cellular invasion could be minimized. This modified silk suture was prepared by treating a multifilament silk suture with a solution of a highly flexible, hydrophobic, and deformable polymer in a solvent and heating the moving suture to obtain a continuous impregnation of the silk with the elastomer. This elastomer with a molecular weight >10,000 Da is a segmented polyether-ester and consists of soft segments, poly(polyoxytetramethylene) terephthalate (POTMT), and crystallizable hard segments, polybutylene terephthalate. The elastomer has 5 to 50% by weight of the composite silk suture. *In vivo*

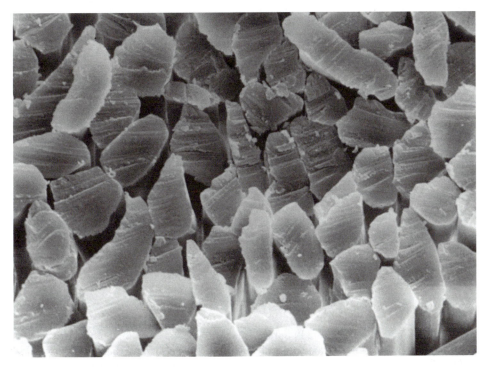

Figure 5.14 SEM view of the cross sections of degummed *B. mori* silk fibers. (From Robson, R.M., in *Fiber Chemistry*, Lewin, M. and Pearce, E.M., Eds., *Handbook of Fiber Science and Technology*, Vol. IV, Marcel Dekker, New York, 1985, chap. 7. With permission.)

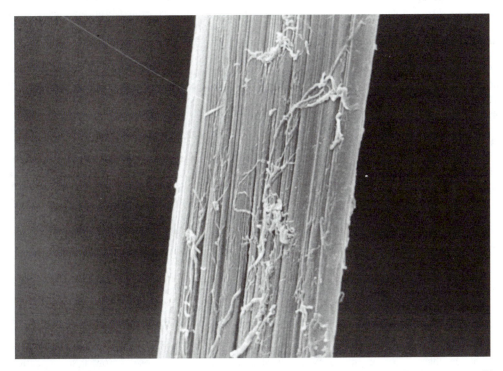

Figure 5.15 Longitudinally split tussah silk filament revealing the characteristic internal fibrillar structure. (From Robson, R.M., in *Fiber Chemistry*, Lewin, M. and Pearce, E.M., Eds., *Handbook of Fiber Science and Technology*, Vol. IV, Marcel Dekker, New York, 1985, chap. 7. With permission.)

Table 5.14 Mechanical and Biological Properties of Composite Silk Sutures in Sprague Dawley Rats

	Composite silk	Beeswax paraffin waxed silk control
Tensile strength retention (%)		
7	56.6	57.6
28	49.4	37.9
56	39.9	20.9
Sewell tissue reaction score[a]		
7	14.75	34.08
28	10.75	33.42
56	10.58	28.83
Cellular invasion (%)[b]		
7	9.58	66.67
28	5.00	100
56	2.92	100

[a] The higher the number, the worse the tissue reaction; 0, none; 1 to 8, minimal; 9 to 24, slight; 25 to 40, moderate; 41 to 56, marked; >56, extensive. From Sewell, Wiland, and Craver, *Surg. Gynecol. Obstet.*, 100, 483, 1955.
[b] Estimated based on the percent of suture invaded by cells.

From Shalaby, S.W. et al., U.S. Patent 4,461,298, 1984.

evaluation of this composite silk suture in Sprague Dawley rats, shown in Table 5.14, indicated that the impregnation of silk sutures indeed could not only provide better tensile breaking strength retention over a period of 56 d, but also significantly reduced tissue reactions and cellular invasion.

B. COTTON AND LINEN

Basically, there are three types of cotton, classified according to length: short staple ($3/_8$ to $3/_4$ in.), intermediate-length staple ($13/_{16}$ to $1 1/_4$ in.), and long staple fibers ($1 1/_2$ to $2 1/_2$ in.). Cotton sutures are made from twisted long staple fiber. The raw cotton fibers are first separated from their seeds (called ginning), cleaned, and blended to ensure a spun yarn of uniform quality. Then they go through carding and combing processes that continue to separate and align the fibers for evenness, smoothness, fineness, and strength. Slivers from the carder or the comber are finally processed through roving and spinning. The amount of twist and the size of the yarn are introduced and controlled during the spinning process. The purpose of twist is to maintain the integrity of the strand to keep it from fraying during use. The resulting cotton sutures are smoothed with starch and coated with wax. Cotton sutures are sold under the name of Cellulose from both Davis & Geck and Ethicon.

The cross-sectional shape of cotton fiber varies from a U-shape to a nearly circular form. The fiber has a natural twist called convolutions,[53] and a long staple cotton has about 30 twists per inch. This twist facilitates the spinning of cotton fiber. Cotton is 10 to 20% stronger when wet than dry, and its strength can be increased by a process called mercerization. Cotton is a relatively high-density fiber with a specific gravity of 1.54 (polyester, 1.38; nylon, 1.14). It absorbs moisture well and its moisture regain is 7 to 8%. Microorganisms such as fungi can grow on cotton fiber and eventually cause it to deteriorate.

Linen suture is made from twisted long staple flax fibers. The first step in preparing flax fibers is called retting, which loosens the bark from the stem, followed by breaking and scotching. The resulting flax fibers go through a hackled process before they are ready for spinning.

The properties of flax fiber are about the same as those of cotton, except for the wicking ability. Wicking ability, commonly known as the capillary effect, is important in suture design. Flax fiber has higher wicking ability than cotton, and hence liquid travels readily along the fiber.

The basic structural unit of cotton and flax is cellulose shown in Figure 5.16. The skeleton of the cellulose chain consists of successive β-linkages of glucose rings at C_1 and C_4 positions. The three OH-groups on each ring in the chain have an important influence on the properties of the cellulose molecule. They contribute to the high moisture absorbency and melting point. Due to the large number of H-bonds, the cellulose crystal is extremely stable. Since it decomposes before it melts, cellulose cannot be melt-spun, nor can it be dissolved in water or any ordinary solvents. Both cotton and linen sutures are sterilized by ethylene oxide. Cotton and linen are the two least frequently used suture materials for wound closure and hence they are the least important materials.

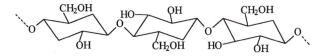

Figure 5.16 Chemical structure of cellulose.

C. POLYESTER BASED

They are three types of nonabsorbable polyester-based sutures: poly(ethylene terephthalate) (PET) based, poly(butylene terephthalate) (PBT) based, and the copolymer of poly(tetramethylene ether) terephthalate and poly(tetramethylene terephthalate) based (polybutester). PET-based polyester sutures are braided Dacron® and Ti-Cron® from Davis & Geck; Ethibond®, Mersilene®, and Ethiflex® from Ethicon; Surgidac® from US Surgical; Polydek® and Tevdek® from Deknatel; and monofilament Mirafil® from B. Braun. PBT-based polyester sutures are monofilament Miralene® from B. Braun. The monofilament copolymeric polybutester suture, Novafil® from Davis & Geck, is the most recent polyester-based suture.

PET sutures are made of polyethylene terephthalate, $HO-[OC-C_6H_4-COO-CH_2-CH_2-O]_n-H$, which in turn is polymerized from ethylene glycol, $HO-CH_2CH_2-OH$ and terephthalic acid, $HOOC(C_6H_4)COOH$ (or dimethyl terephthalate in the case of Terylene®). Polymerization is conducted in a vacuum at a high temperature. The first stage involves the formation of low molecular weight oligomers through ester interchange. The oligomers are then polycondensed further to build up high molecular weight polyester. The second stage is carried out at about 270°C and reduced pressure (0.5 torr). The resulting polyester chips are melt-spun into round cross-sectional-shaped filaments. The filaments are then hot-stretched (above $T_g = 69°C$) to about five times their original length. Further crystallization occurs during the hot drawing. Depending on the degree of drawing, polyester yarns of either normal strength or high tenacity can be obtained. The molecular weight of PET that is capable of making fibers is on the order of 20,000.

Unlike the simple zigzag planar structure of polyethylene and nylon, the PET molecule has an extended rectilinear shape, the plane of the benzene rings being planar as required by resonance and parallel to the (100) plane.[54] The -COO- group is out of the plane of the benzene rings by 12° and the ethylene glycol residue by 20°. Figure 5.17 shows the ordered (crystalline) structure of PET.[55] The chain repeat distance is 10.75Å, which is only slightly less than a fully extended chain molecule. In a stretched fiber the axes of the molecular chains are inclined in relation to the fiber axis in such a way that the (230) plane remains vertical and the inclination of the (001) plane to the fiber axis increases. For a fiber annealed at 210°C and relaxed, the angle between the fiber axis and the crystal axis is 5°.

The benzene ring, together with its two associated C-C bonds, forms a single rigid structure. Consequently, the chain is rigid and less flexible than nylon and polyethylene. This accounts for the slow rate of crystallization and high melting point (265°C). The melt-spun filaments are thus largely amorphous before drawing. The maximum rate of crystallization of amorphous PET occurs at 190°C. The stereochemical structure of the PET chain changes during crystallization. The ethylene glycol residues of crystalline and oriented amorphous PET chain acquire a transconfiguration, while the same residues in amorphous PET possess mainly gauche conformation with a small portion of transconformation.[56]

The molecular structure of PET is also winding-speed dependent during the melt spinning process. PET yarns wound at a speed <3000 m/min has a low level of crystallinity, while at a higher speed, an increasing higher level of crystalline structure develops but reaches a plateau at 7000 m/min.[57] The crystal unit is triclinic and the crystallite dimension depends on processing history. A range of crystal density from 1.455 to 1.515 g/cm^3 has been reported, but the amorphous density has a narrower range from 1.335 to 1.336 g/cm^3.

Recently, a monofilament copolyester suture (polybutester or Novafil®) has become available with the repeating unit $[-O(CH_2)_4-OCO-C_6H_4CO]_{84}-[O(CH_2CH_2CH_2CH_2)_n CO-(C_6H_4)-CO-]_{16}$. The $[-O(CH_2)_4-OCO-C_6H_4CO]$ unit serves as the hard segment, while the $[O(CH_2CH_2CH_2CH_2-)_n-CO-(C_6H_4)-CO-]$ unit serves as the soft segment with average molecular weight ranging from 500 to 3000. Polybutester suture is made from a block copolymer of poly(butylene terephthalate) as the hard segment and poly(tetramethylene ether) glycol terephthalate as the soft segment.[58] Novafil suture fibers made from polybutester copolymer are drawn in two stages from 6X to 8X at temperatures from 120 to 165°C to provide a desirable quality of tensile strength, knot strength and security, flexibility, fatigue life, and low tissue drag. The number average molecular weight ranges from 25 to 30,000. Figure 5.18 illustrates the chemical structure of Novafil polybutester suture.[59] The ratio of the hard and soft segments can be adjusted to achieve the desirable handling properties. Novafil suture has the ratio of hard to soft segments

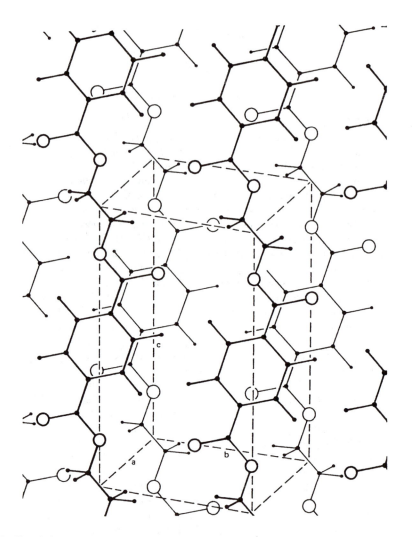

Figure 5.17 The chain arrangement in polyethylene terephthalate crystals. (From Daubeney, R.P., Bunn, C.W., and Brown, C.J., *Proc. R. Soc.*, 226A, 531, 1954. With permission.)

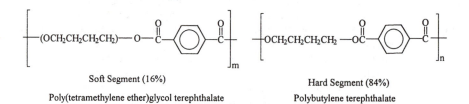

Soft Segment (16%)

Poly(tetramethylene ether)glycol terephthalate

Hard Segment (84%)

Polybutylene terephthalate

Figure 5.18 Chemical structure of polybutester (Novafil) suture.

of 84:16%.[59] Titanium dioxide, carbon black, or iron oxide could be used to color the suture. Novafil sutures could be sterilized by ethylene oxide or γ-irradiation; but it should not be sterilized by heat because the elastomeric property of the suture could be adversely affected.

Novafil suture has chemical structure very similar to Hytrel polyester elastomer manufactured by duPont. Due to the presence of both hard and soft segments, this copolyester exhibits a continuous two-phase domain microstructure. The crystalline domain consists of the short and hard segment of polybutylene terephthalate (84% in Novafil suture) and serves as the tie points that connect the noncrystalline domain consisting of mainly the soft poly (tetramethylene ether) glycol terephthalate long segments. Because of this unique morphology, this copolyester behaves like a thermally reversible network resembling that of conventionally crosslinked polymers. The copolymer melts at 211°C and would exhibit brittle behavior at a temperature < –90°F. This copolyester has good resistance to oils and chemicals; however, concentrated mineral acids and bases, phenols, cresols, and certain carboxylic acids and chlorinated solvents would attack the copolyester. Hytrel copolyester also needs protection from UV light. This suggests that Novafil suture may degrade if it is used in areas exposed to sunlight, such as in cataract surgery. As described in Chapter 7, long-term stability of Novafil sutures in ophthalmologic surgery has been reported to be a concern.

Because of its elastomeric character, Novafil has a distinctly different stress-strain behavior than PET-based polyester suture and other synthetic monofilament sutures like nylon and polypropylene. The stress-strain curve of Novafil suture exhibits a biphasic pattern, while both PET-based polyester sutures and polypropylene and nylon monofilament sutures show monophasic patterns.[59,60] Novafil suture elongates (to about 10%) easily under tension, followed by a steep rise in force required for further elongation. This mechanical behavior may be advantageous in management of wound edema because the suture loop would easily stretch upon wound edema instead of cutting through the edematous tissue. After the resolution of the edema, the Novafil suture loop is expected to return to its original diameter more easily than those sutures exhibiting monophasic stress-strain behavior. As a result of this elastomeric character, Novafil is expected to be less stiff than other monofilament sutures, as evident in the reported stiffness coefficient of Novafil (14.81 ± 1.14) which is about twofold less than equivalent size nylon-based (Dermalon) and polypropylene-based (Surgilene) monofilament sutures. The elastomeric characteristic of polybutester block copolymer also render Novafil less susceptible to package memory than polypropylene- and nylon-based monofilament sutures. The detailed mechanical properties of Novafil are given later in Chapter 6.

Although polyester-based sutures are not considered to be degradable and there is no reported clinical case of failed polyester sutures due to the hydrolytic scission of their ester linkages, the presence of these ester linkages inherently provides the opportunity for their eventual hydrolytic scissions. The relatively hydrophobic nature of the polyester sutures and their high glass transition temperature relative to body temperature are responsible for the observed *in vivo* stability of this class of suture materials. Under alkaline conditions, the hydrolytic degradation of polyester sutures is a surface phenomenon with very little change in molecular weight, and the rate of hydrolysis is inversely proportional to the diameter of fibers. This is because highly ionized reagents like NaOH cannot readily diffuse into the relatively nonpolar polyesters. Because fiber diameter would decrease with alkaline hydrolysis, tensile strength (force/cross-sectional area) of the fiber would not change. However, the rate of alkaline hydrolysis would increase significantly if the alkaline agent could readily diffuse into the fiber by the addition of chemicals like quaternary ammonium compounds to serve as a carrier for -OH anions. Collins et al. reported that heat-setting of PET fibers at a temperature $<T_m$ increased their hydrolytic resistance.[61] Under acidic conditions, bulk instead of surface hydrolysis could occur with a reduction of molecular weight but without the reduction of fiber diameter. This is because the small H^+ cations could diffuse into polyester fibers readily. Acid-catalyzed hydrolysis of polyester fibers is usually significantly slower than alkaline-catalyzed hydrolysis.

D. POLYAMIDE BASED

The most successful aliphatic polyamide that polymer scientists have synthesized is nylon. Nylon is polymerized either from polycondensation of a dicarboxylic acid and a diamine, or through a ring-opening polymerization of appropriate lactams. Although there are numerous types of nylon, such as nylon 3, 4, 5, 6, 7, 8, 9, 11, 12, 66, and 610, only 66 and 6 are used to make suture materials. The former is more popular in the United States, while the latter is used in Europe. The tradenames of nylon sutures are braided Surgilon® and monofilament Dermalon® with the repeating unit $[-NH(CH_2)_6-NHCO(CH_2)_4CO-]$ from Davis & Geck; braided Nurolon® and monofilament Ethilon® with the repeating unit $[-NH(CH_2)_5CO-]$ from Ethicon; monofilament Monosof® and braided Bralon® from US Surgical; and sheath-core structure Supramid® from S. Jackson. Surgilon nylon suture is coated with silicone, while Nurolon nylon suture is coated with wax. Bralon is coated with a proprietary material. All nylon sutures are sterilized with Co^{60} γ-irradiation.

Nylon 66 is made from adipic acid, $HOOC(CH_2)_4COOH$, and hexamethylene diamine, $H_2N(CH_2)_6NH_2$. These two chemicals, dissolved separately in methanol, are mixed and nylon salt, $H_3H^+(CH_2)_6NH_3^+ \, ^-OOC(CH_2)_4COO^-$, is precipitated. Equal moles of adipic acid and diamine are important for achieving high molecular weight nylon 66. Because of the increasing price of oil, alternative syntheses of raw materials for making nylon salt have been explored, including cereal products, notably bran and husks, and butadiene.[62]

Nylon salt is melted under an inert gas atmosphere to prevent discoloration. Acetic acid is added as a stabilizer during polycondensation. No catalyst is needed for polymerization; suitable conditions are 4 h at a temperature of 280°C. The molten polymer is extruded in ribbon form, which is quenched with cold water in order to reduce the crystal size, and then cut into chips. The extent of polymerization is determined by the residual moisture content. A vacuum should be applied if high molecular weight nylon is desirable.[63] Nylon 66 can also be made by interfacial polycondensation.[63] The reaction takes place at the interface between a diamine water solution and a dicarboxylic acid chloride in a water-insoluble solvent. The reaction is rapid and precise amounts of the reactants is unnecessary. This method results in high molecular weight nylon 66. Nylon 66 of molecular weight 12,000 to 20,000 is suitable for melt-spinning into fibers.

Nylon 6 is made from caprolactam. Two alternative methods are used.[62] The first method involves the liquefying and heating of caprolactam under high pressure. The resulting nylon 6 polymer chain consists of an average of 200 repeating units. The second method needs about 10% water and is carried out at a high temperature with a controlled release of steam. There are three reactions in the second method of polymerization: addition, condensation, and hydrolysis.[63]

The major chain growth mechanism of nylon 6 molecules is the addition reaction, while nylon 66 is made by condensation reaction. Thus, the polymerization of nylon 6 is expedited in the presence of aminocaproic acid. The second method is easier to control, but it takes longer than the first. Nylon 6 is also made anionically. The resulting polymer, however, has a very high molecular weight and is not as thermally stable as that made by the second method. Thus, it is not directly applicable to injection molding or extrusion.[63] Whichever polymerization method is used, nylon 6 contains about 10% extractable monomers and cyclic oligomers, which act as plasticizers and are preferably removed for biomedical uses by water washing or vacuuming.

The resulting nylon 66 or 6 chips are then melt-spun into a cooling chamber in which nylon filaments form. In the case of nylon 66, the filaments are run through a steam chamber to wet them before they are wound. This treatment eliminates the undesirable extension of the yarns after they reach equilibrium by absorbing moisture from the air. The wound yarn is further cold-drawn by stretching about 400% in order to acquire better strength. During this cold-drawing process, vegetable oil is applied to the yarn as a lubricant and is washed off afterwards.

In the case of nylon 6, the same process of melt-spinning as for nylon 66 is used except that the steam chamber is not suitable. The relatively high residual concentration of monomers in nylon 6 would make the filaments sticky and adhere to one another if steamed. The filaments are normally drawn to 350 to 400%. Higher drawing can be achieved if a stronger fiber is needed. It is well recognized in fiber technology that by increasing the draw ratio (the ratio of the speed of output and input feed rollers), the tensile strength and elastic modulus increase, while the elongation at break decreases. If the molecular weight of nylon 6 is between 20,000 and 25,000, hot-drawing is used.

Unlike PET, both nylon fibers are fairly crystalline when they are spun. The crystal structures of nylon 66 and 6 fall into three categories: α, β, and γ phases. Almost all the commercially important nylons exist in either the α or β phase.

Even-even polyamides such as nylon 66 exist mainly in the α phase, which is more stable than the β phase and is characterized by the progressive stacking of planar sheets (parallel to the ac plane) of H-bonded molecules to meet the requirement of completely strain-free H-bonding.[64] The molecules in the crystalline region are in the fully extended zigzag conformation and the adjacent molecules have the same directionality (parallel) for strain-free H-bonding, as shown in Figure 5.19. The structure is triclinic, with a=4.9 Å, b=5.4 Å, c (fiber axis) = 17.2 Å, and one chemical repeat per unit cell. The perpendicular distance between H-bonded sheets is 3.6 Å, while the normal distance between chains within a H-bonded planar sheet is 4.2 Å. The β phase is less stable than the α phase and cannot be reliably determined except in samples having a high degree of axial orientation. The formation of the β phase is thought to be due to the up-and-down staggering of successive H-bonded sheets. Others postulate initial stages of ordering and the presence of unrelated small crystallites.

Unlike nylon 66, H-bonded sheets of the α phase of nylon 6 involve adjacent molecules arranged in opposite directions (antiparallel) so that all the H-bonds are free of strain. Figure 5.19 illustrates these parallel and anti parallel chain conformations. Other even nylons from nylon 8 up, however, crystallize into the γ phase. H-bonds in the γ phase are between parallel molecules (like nylon 66). This forces the

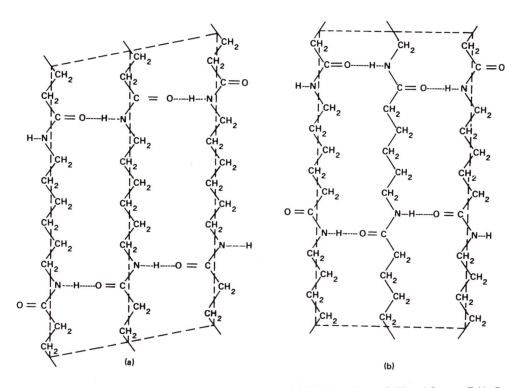

Figure 5.19 Ordered chain conformation for nylon 66 (a) and 6 (b). (From Bunn, C. W. and Garner, E. V., *Proc. R. Soc.*, A189, 38, 1947. With permission.)

chains to twist slightly in order to realize strain-free H-bonds and, hence, assume a puckered or pleated conformation. Consequently, the unit cell of the γ phase is about 2% shorter. Nylon 6 assumes the γ phase after an iodine treatment, while most chemically untreated nylon 6 exists predominantly in the α form.[65]

The unstable β and γ phases can be converted into the α phase by improving crystallinity and orientation, namely drawing and annealing.[65] The relative amount of the α to γ phases is also found to depend on the winding speed in the spinning process.[66] Indications are that the γ phase is mainly generated from orientation-induced nuclei at speeds higher than 2500 m/min. Drawing at high ratios facilitates a γ to α transition. Due to the complex morphology of nylon 6, crystallinity values from density measurement (which are based on the additivity of the amorphous and crystalline phases) are inaccurate.

Because of the inherent susceptibility of the amide linkage to hydrolytic degradation, nylon sutures have been reported to lose strength after implantation. Thus, nylon sutures should not be used for fastening implants. The details of the biodegradation properties of nylon sutures are given in Chapter 7.

E. POLYPROPYLENE

Polypropylene (PP) suture materials with the repeating unit [-CH$_2$-CH(CH$_3$)-] are made from isotactic polypropylene, which is polymerized from propylene with a Ziegler-Natta catalyst.[67] However, a syndiotactic PP suture has recently been reported by Liu et al. of US Surgical and the details of this new type of PP suture are given in Chapter 12. The Ziegler-Natta catalyst consists of a transition metal halide (e.g., TiCl$_3$) with a reducing agent (e.g., AlR$_3$). Ziegler-Natta catalyst systems are quite complex, and the exact structure of the catalysts cannot be determined precisely.[68,69] Many factors could influence the activity of the catalyst, such as the crystal structure, the molar ratio of the components, the aging of the complex, impurities, and the temperature of preparation.[69] The general polymerization kinetics are similar to other types of addition polymerization. The stereo regularity of the resulting polypropylene is controlled by the propagation step, which consists of repeated insertion of the propylene monomer into the carbon-transition metal bond through the polarization mechanism. This mechanism (Figure 5.20), normally called a bimetallic mechanism, provides for an active site that can complex an incoming propylene monomer and maintain the end group of the growing polymer chain in a position suitable for propagation. Other mechanisms, like the monometallic one, involving an active site in which the transition metal assumes an octahedral configuration, are also proposed.[70] It is, at present, difficult to distinguish the two mechanisms.

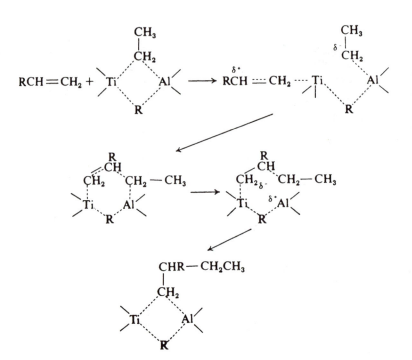

Figure 5.20 Bimetallic mechanism of polypropylene. (From Kaufman, H.S. and Falcetta, J.J., *Introduction to Polymer Science and Technology: An SPE Textbook,* Wiley-Interscience, New York, 1977, 92. With permission.)

PP usually has a wide range of molecular weight distribution (MWD) ranging from 2 to 12 polydispersity (ratio of M_w:M_n). Recently, a narrower MWD PP has become available and is called controlled rheology (CR) PP.[71] The intrinsic viscosity of PP is measured in decalin solvent at 137°C according to the following equation:

$$M_v = ([\eta] \times 10^4)^{1.25}$$

The melting and glass transition temperatures of PP are about 165 and –15°C, respectively.

PP sutures made from isotactic polypropylene have a molecular weight about 80,000 or melt-flow-rate between 3 and 35. The crystallinity is 50% before melt-spinning decreases to 33% after spinning and before drawing, and increases to 47% after drawing. Annealing increases the crystallinity further to 68%.[71] The currently available monofilament polypropylene sutures are Surgilene® from Davis & Geck, Prolene® from Ethicon, and Surgipro® from US Surgical. PP sutures, in general, do not have any coating material applied and they are sterilized by ethylene oxide because of their sensitivity toward Co[60] γ-irradiation sterilization.

Due to the steric position of the CH₃ group in propylene, either a regular (isotactic and syndiotactic) or irregular (atactic) chain configuration can result. If atactic, it cannot crystallize and is a grease. In the isotactic form (CH₃ group on the same side of the backbone), the chain cannot assume a planar zigzag form as polyethylene and nylon 66 do, because of the bulky size of -CH₃. As shown in Figure 5.21, the chain thus twists into a helix form with three chemical repeat units per turn and packs into a monoclinic unit cell. The helix form permits the best inter- and intramolecular packing of side groups. Within a limited temperature range and in the presence of certain foreign nuclei, isotactic polypropylene can be crystallized into a hexagonal unit cell.

The two major sources of PP-based sutures were Ethicon and Davis & Geck. However, the recent introduction of Surgipro by US Surgical brings some additional PP-based wound closure biomaterials to the surgical community. It is well known in the fiber industry that fibers having the same chemical basis do not warrant the same performance. This is because a wide range of physical, mechanical, and thermal properties of fibers could be achieved simply by altering their processing conditions.

Table 5.15 summarizes the physical, thermal, surface wettability, and mechanical properties of Surgipro and Prolene monofilament sutures.[72] In general, besides a few properties, the two types of PP

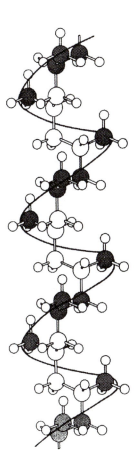

Figure 5.21 Ordered helix molecular conformation of isotactic polypropylene. (From Mandelkern, L., *In Introduction to Macromolecules*, Springer-Verlag, New York, 1972, p.49. With permission.)

sutures were similar in their properties. Except 4/0 Prolene, all other PP sutures had essentially the same level of crystallinity. However, a closer examination of other thermal properties (i.e., melting temperature) of both PP sutures revealed that Surgipro sutures were quite different from the corresponding Prolene. This difference in melting temperature and shape of the melting peaks imply that these two PP sutures, although chemically identical, have slightly different fiber morphology from each other due to slight differences in fiber processing technique, thermal history, and/or molecular weight of the raw materials. This difference in fiber morphology was also confirmed in thermally stimulated current (TSC) and interior morphology data as described below.

The interior morphology of these two types of PP sutures, from the peelback study (Figure 5.22),[72] is an additional difference between these two types of PP suture fiber. Although both types of PP sutures exhibited microfibrillar structure, Surgipro showed a single type of microfibrillar morphology that is uniformly distributed along the cross-sectional area of the fiber. In the Prolene sutures, however, there are two distinctive morphological domains arranged alternately along the lateral direction of the fiber: a region of less densely packed but fine microfibrils with many voids that are similar to Surgipro suture and an adjacent region of densely packed more coarse microfibrils with few voids. These two domains were separated by a band of solid mass that appeared morphologically distinctively different from either of the two domains located on both sides of the band. The band material looked more like the materials located on the surface of the fiber. This distinctive difference in interior fiber morphology between the two types of PP sutures suggests that these two types of PP sutures were made from slightly different fiber processing conditions, which would be reflected in their mechanical and thermal properties as described previously and below.

This visible interior morphological difference between Surgipro and Prolene suture fibers was also confirmed by TSC data, as shown in Figure 5.23.[72] A significant difference in TSC curves between Surgipro and Prolene suture fibers is evident in the figure. Surgipro suture had a much narrower peak than Prolene suture and the depolarization process of Prolene began at a much lower temperature than for the Surgipro suture. This implies that Surgipro suture has more homogeneous and uniform noncrys-

Table 5.15 A Comparison of Properties of Surgipro and Prolene Monofilament Sutures

Suture	Diameter (mm)	Linear density (g/1000 m)	Level of crystallinity (%)	Melting point (°C)	Specific wettability (dyn/cm)	Initial stiffness (Taber unit)	Tensile breaking load (kg)	Tensile breaking elongation (%)	Toughness (kg/cm)
					Property				
Prolene 0	0.39	109.4	49.5	155.3	20.78	0.45	4.642 ± 0.279	75.60 ± 14.8	8.76 ± 2.33
Prolene 4/0	0.20	27.2	43.8	143.0	21.60	0.06	1.498 ± 0.079	45.9 ± 5.95	1.97 ± 0.40
Surgipro 0-1*	0.38	112.0	50.7	153.8	21.44	0.39	4.027 ± 0.194	76.9 ± 19.7	9.54 ± 1.57
Surgipro 0-2*	0.42	113.1	50.7	156.7	21.04	0.45	4.124 ± 0.075	78.5 ± 5.4	10.21 ± 0.97
Surgipro 4/0-1*	0.19	27.1	51.2	151.0	21.76	0.04	1.077 ± 0.089	35.6 ± 5.93	2.09 ± 0.56
Surgipro 4/0-2*	0.20	27.3	51.5	151.5	21.67	0.03	1.336 ± 0.058	35.3 ± 3.3	2.20 ± 0.38

* The numbers 1 and 2 indicate different fiber manufacturing processes.

From Chu, C.C., Pratt, L., Zhang, L., Hsu, A., and Chu, A., *J. Appl. Biomater.*, 4, 169, 1993. With permission.

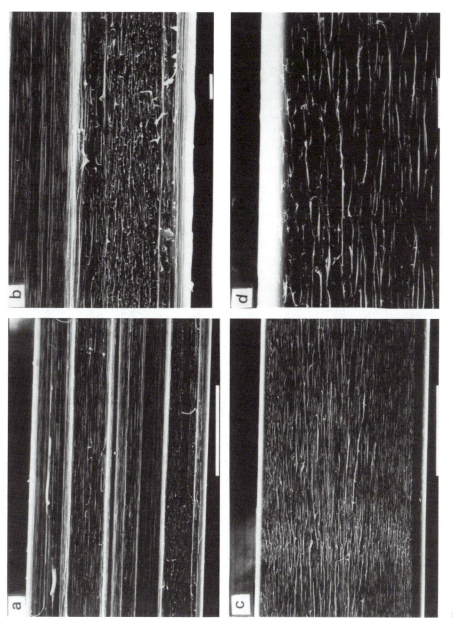

Figure 5.22 Interior morphology of 4/0 polypropylene sutures obtained from peelback technique: (a) Prolene at ×1000; (b) Prolene at ×360; (c) Surgipro at ×360; (d) Surgipro at ×2000. (From Chu, C.C., Pratt, L., Zhang, L., Hsu, A., and Chu, A., *J. Appl. Biomater.*, 4, 169, 1993. With permission.)

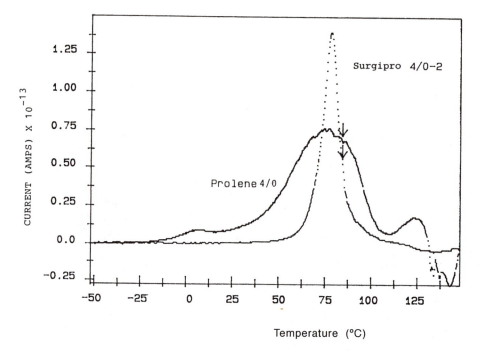

Figure 5.23 Thermally stimulated current study of 4/0 polypropylene sutures. (From Chu, C.C., Pratt, L., Zhang, L., Hsu, A., and Chu, A., *J. Appl. Biomater.*, 4, 169, 1993. With permission.)

talline domains in terms of chain segment length, conformation, and morphology than Prolene sutures. Surgipro's depolarization began at about 60°C and accelerated, reached a maximum rate at 78°C, and then decreased thereafter. The whole process occurred over a span of 28°C. On the other hand, Prolene suture exhibited two different stages of depolarization: a small one from –15 to 25°C and a larger one from 25 to 100°C. These two stages of depolarization suggested that Prolene suture fiber has two types of noncrystalline domains that coincided with their two different types of interior morphology observed by SEM (Figure 5.22). One of these two types of morphology dominated as illustrated by the SEM and the relative magnitude of the TSC peaks. Because of these two different types of morphology in Prolene, there were two TSC peaks: one at about 10°C and the other at 76°C. The bulk of the depolarization process, however, occurred in the stage between 25 and 100°C. The depolarization process of Prolene sutures occurred over more than 115°C. This suggests that there were small portions of the segments of Prolene molecules (judged by the small magnitude of the current output during the depolarization process) located in the noncrystalline domains that are slightly polarized when a DC current is applied so that they could depolarize very easily at a lower temperature. These small portions of the chain segments were believed to be slightly off from the fiber axis so a low DC current was sufficient to cause them to orient along the direction of the fiber axis (i.e., the polarization process). Subsequently, a lower temperature would depolarize (i.e., randomize) them. The bulk of the depolarization process occurred at a higher temperature and was believed to come from those noncrystalline chain segments that were initially oriented nearly perpendicular to the fiber axis so a higher temperature would be required to depolarize them.

The two distinctive fiber morphologies observed in Prolene fibers as demonstrated in the TSC curve were also reported by Kloos based on X-ray study.[73] Kloos showed that the fiber morphology of melt-spun PP fibers depends on molecular weight distribution. His wide- and small-angle X-ray data showed that PP fibers of broad molecular weight distribution exhibited two distinctive fiber morphologies with bimodal orientation: large lamellae with chain axis parallel to fiber axis, and smaller crystallites resident in the noncrystalline domains and oriented perpendicular to the fiber axis. PP fibers melt-spun from narrow molecular weight distribution, however, had only one morphology: fibrillar structure with all crystallites oriented in the fiber axis. Based on these reported data, it appears that Prolene suture fibers have a larger molecular weight distribution than Surgipro suture fibers. Further study is needed to confirm this prediction.

PP fibers are inherently unstable to both heat and light, but they are totally hydrolytically resistant due to the lack of ester or amide linkages. The heat and light instability arise from the high temperature for fiber spinning, which frequently results in the presence of oxygen-containing functional groups like >C=O in the molecule. This PP fiber instability may be the cause of the observed clinical failure of PP sutures in ophthalmology, as described in the Chapter 7.

F. POLYTETRAFLUOROETHYLENE (GORE-TEX®)

The most recently introduced nonabsorbable monofilament suture is Gore-Tex® made from a highly crystalline linear polytetrafluoroethylene (PTFE). This fully fluorinated thermoplastic polyolefin with the $[CF_2-CF_2]_n$ repeating unit is an addition polymer and is polymerized through a free radical polymerization route in aqueous dispersion under pressure with persulfates and hydrogen peroxide as initiators. The monomer (tetrafluoroethylene) is made from a two-step process: the fluorination of chloroform by HF to produce $CHClF_2$, which is subsequently dimerized by pyrolysis to form tetrafluoroethylene. PTFE has the highest enthalpy and entropy of polymerization (−156 kJ/mol and −112 J/mol-deg, respectively) in vinyl polymerization.[74] Its molecular weight can be as high as 5×10^6.

Due to the extremely stable C-F bond, PTFE has a very high melting temperature, 327°C, which makes the fabrication of PTFE very difficult. This difficulty is further compounded by a high viscosity above T_m due to restricted bond rotation and high molecular weight. Thus, PTFE is usually fabricated by a combination of heat and pressure, namely sintering, which is usually applied to metal and ceramics. PTFE powders are preformed at high pressure (2000 to 10,000 psi, 14 to 70 MPa) at room temperature and then sintered above their melting point (>365°C) for a brief period. The resulting products can subsequently be machined to the desirable shape and size. Microfibrous PTFE is made from wet-spinning of a mixture of an aqueous PTFE dispersion and cellulose xanthate to provide fibers that are subsequently sintered at 385°C by contact with a metal roll to develop fibers of low but useful strength.

PTFE is a highly crystalline polymer with the degree of crystallinity reaching as high as 93 to 98%. Its crystalline density is 2.30 g/cm³. Based on both X-ray diffraction data and calculated potential-energy profile, PTFE assumes a twisted zigzag helix structure with 13 monomer units in six turns at <19°C.[75] Figure 5.24 is an illustration of an ordered and twisted conformation of PTFE molecule.[55] This twisted helix conformation is slightly untwisted at >19°C (first order phase transition) as evidenced in the diffuse streaks of X-ray diffraction pattern. A further increase in temperature to above 30°C (second order transition) would result in additional diffuseness due to random angular displacement of chain molecules from their long axes. The helix chain conformation deviation from an extended zigzag polyethylene is due to the strong electronegativity of fluorine atoms, which repulse among themselves. The stiffness of the PTFE chain is high. PTFE has two T_g, -113°C and 127–130°C, depending on the type of crystalline forms which have different degree of interlocking fluorine atoms within the two types of helix structure. These cylindrical helices would pack together like parallel rods to form so-called conformationally disordered crystal (*condis*).

The most outstanding property of PTFE is its extreme resistance to the attack of chemicals and solvents. Only molten or liquid NH_3-dissolved alkali metals would attack PTFE through the removal of fluorine atoms. PTFE has a very low coefficient of friction (0.04 to 0.05), but poor abrasion resistance, and is completely unaffected by water. PTFE has very good electrical properties, with its dielectric constant as low as 2.0. PTFE is a weak polymer compared with other polyolefins. Molded PTFE, with a tensile strength about 5,200 psi (36 MPa), can be easily strained to beyond its elastic recovery point but it has high elongation (350 to 550%). However, the dry tenacity of PTFE fiber ranges from 0.9 to 2.0 g/denier with 25 to 31×10^3 psi (172 to 214 MPa) tensile strength with 19 to 140% elongation.[76] Upon radiation, PTFE would degrade rather than undergo crosslinking and its degradation occurs preferentially on the scission of backbone C-C bonds before C-F bonds. The presence of C-F bonds provides an easy detection of PTFE by IR at 8.2 to 8.3 μm absorption bands.

Monofilament suture made from PTFE (Gore-Tex), however, is different from molded PTFE in morphological structure. The Gore-Tex suture is an expanded PTFE characterized by two distinctive components: nodes held together by fine fibrils of 5 to 10 μm diameter and >17 μm long. The most unique property of Gore-Tex is its microporous structure with up to about nine billion pores per square inch. Hence, Gore-Tex suture has >50% air by volume. The pore size varies, but it is big enough for ingrowth of fibroblasts and leukocytes similar to that observed with Gore-Tex vascular grafts. The Gore-Tex suture does not follow USP size classification and is designated by CV (i.e., cardiovascular). The suture diameter is measured in its preexpanded dimension and the actual diameter of Gore-Tex suture is obviously much larger because it contains >50% air by volume. For example, CV-4 Gore-Tex suture has a similar diameter (0.35 mm) to 2/0 Prolene (0.303 mm).

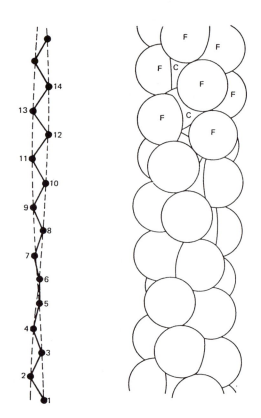

Figure 5.24 Ordered and twisted chain conformation of polytetrafluoroethylene. (From Bunn, C.W. and Howells, E.R., *Nature*, 174, 549, 1954. With permission.)

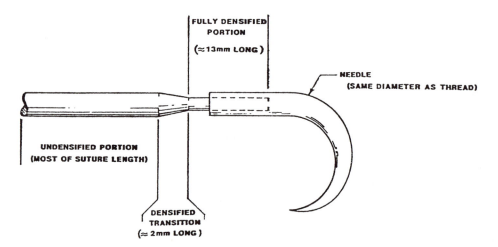

Figure 5.25 Schematic drawing of the needle-suture attachment technique for the Gore-Tex suture. (From Miller, C.M., Sangiolo, P., and Jacobson, J.J., II, *Surgery*, 101(2), 156, 1987. With permission.)

Because of the large pore volume, Gore-Tex suture has a unique property, namely a needle-to-suture-diameter ratio of 1.0 (Figure 5.25).[77] As shown in the figure, only the very short portion of a compressed Gore-Tex suture emerging from the needle orifice has a diameter smaller than the needle for its swage to a needle. The uncompressed portion of the suture retains the same diameter as the needle. The ability to achieve variable diameter through the length of a suture is attributed to the large air volume in Gore-Tex structure. Other commercial sutures have a needle-to-thread ratio >1.0, and frequently range from

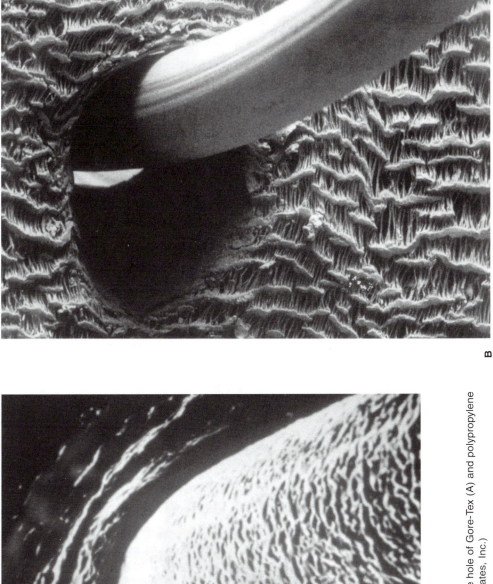

Figure 5.26 SEM photos showing the needle hole of Gore-Tex (A) and polypropylene (B) sutures. (Courtesy of W. L. Gore & Associates, Inc.)

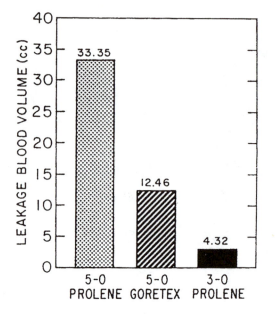

Figure 5.27 The needle hole leakage of blood volume of mongrel dogs' infrarenal aorta anastomosis closed by three synthetic monofilament sutures. (From Miller, C.M., Sangiolo, P., and Jacobson, J.J., II, *Surgery*, 101(2), 156, 1987. With permission.)

2.0 to 3.0. As a result of this high needle-to-suture-diameter ratio, the thread portion of a suture cannot fill up the hole generated by a needle in wound closure. Figure 5.26 illustrates a comparison between Gore-Tex and polypropylene sutures in their ability to fill up needle holes. Bleeding through this unfilled space at needle holes has been a common problem associated with sutures other than Gore-Tex. Miller et al. reported that a 5/0 Gore-Tex suture had about $1/3$ of the needle hole blood leakage of the same sized Prolene in the abdominal aorta of mongrel dogs, as shown in Figure 5.27.[77] Thus, Miller et al. recommended that Gore-Tex suture should be a better choice for wound closure in multiple arterial anastomoses like complicated extra-anatomic bypasses, fully heparinized patients, and aortic surgery where larger needle holes are made. The unique porous structure of Gore-Tex suture also results in very low bending stiffness.[78,79] Dang et al. reported that CV-4 Gore-Tex suture has a bending stiffness coefficient of 1.21, while a 2-0 size Prolene is more than 100 times stiffer with bending stiffness coefficient of 180.07.[78] Similar findings were reported by Chu et al.[79]

G. STAINLESS STEEL

The use of iron-based metallic sutures started as early as 1666. The most commonly used metallic suture now is stainless steel based. Stainless steel is an alloy of mainly iron, chromium, and nickel, but due to the wide range of possible alloy compositions, the incorporation of trace elements, and fabrications, there are many different grades of stainless steel. Table 5.16 lists some examples of stainless steels and their structure.[80] The three-digit classification in the table is based upon the main composition in the alloy stipulated by the American Iron and Steel Institute (AISI). Series 200 has mainly chromium, nickel, and manganese, Series 300 has mainly chromium and nickel, Series 400 has mainly chromium, and Series 500 has low chromium.

Only 304, 316, and 316L wrought stainless steels are used as sutures. Series 300 stainless steel has high chromium and nickel contents with an austenitic structure and is characterized by high corrosion resistance and ductility. The "L" in 316L stainless steel indicates extra low carbon content since a high level of carbon can result, under certain circumstances, in the precipitation of chromium as chromium carbides ($Cr_{23}C_6$), which would deplete the chromium content of the matrix, making the Cr depleted areas more susceptible to corrosion. Thus, the use of stainless steel with extra low carbon would reduce this undesirable precipitation effect. Presently, extra-low-carbon stainless steel is made by either electroslag-remelted (ESR) or vacuum-remelted (VM) processes. Different metallurgical processing conditions and finishing have a great effect on the mechanical properties and degree of corrosion resistance of stainless steel. This is because different types of grain structure, recrystallization, phase transforma-

Table 5.16 Representative Stainless Steel Compositions and Structure

Alloy designation	Composition (%)[a]									Structure
	Carbon	Manganese	Phosphorus	Sulfur	Silicon	Chromium	Nickel	Molybdenum	Others	
Wrought										
302	0.15	2.00	0.045	0.03	1.00	17.0–19.0	8.0–10.0			Austenitic
303	0.15	2.00	0.020	≤0.15	1.00	17.0–19.0	8.0–10.0	0.6[b]		Austenitic
304	0.08	2.00	0.045	0.03	1.00	18.0–20.0	8.0–10.5			Austenitic
305	0.12	2.00	0.45	0.30	1.00	17.0–19.0	10.5–13.0			Austenitic
316	0.08	2.00	0.045	0.03	1.00	16.0–18.0	10.0–14.0	2.0–3.0		Austenitic
316L	0.03	2.00	0.045	0.03	1.00	16.0–18.0	10.0–14.0	2.0–3.0		Austenitic
317	0.08	2.00	0.045	0.03	1.00	18.0–20.0	11.0–15.0	3.0–4.0		Austenitic
431	0.20	1.00	0.04	0.03	1.00	15.0–17.0	1.25–2.50			Martensitic
Precipitation hardenable 17-7 PH[c]	0.09	1.00	0.04	0.03	1.00	16.0–18.0	6.5–7.75		0.75–1.5 Al	Austenitic/martensitic
Cast										
CF-8M	0.08	1.50	0.04	0.04	2.00	18.0–21.0	9.0–12.0	2.0–3.0		Austenitic/ferritic

[a] Single values are maximum values unless otherwise noted.

[b] Optional

[c] Trademark of the Armco Steel Corporation.

From Sutow, E.J., in *Concise Encyclopedia of Medical and Dental Materials*, Williams, D.F., Ed., Pergamon Press, New York, 1990, 232. With permission.

tions, precipitation of carbide, cold-working, and surface modification may be obtained from various fabrication methods. Stainless steel sutures are fabricated from cold-worked mill products to enhance their mechanical properties so that the resulting wire would not fail during bending and twisting when tying knots. It is important, however, to ensure the generation of as few surface defects as possible during cold-work because an irregular surface could promote crevice and fretting corrosion and/or stress-concentration effects. Any debris from fabrication is removed by a process called passivation treatment in which the surface is treated with, typically, a strong acid like nitric acid. The acid treatment results in an oxide film on the surface, which is considered to be more stable than the natural air-formed film. Whether this passivated oxidative film should not be disturbed during subsequent handling is still debatable. Stainless steel is sterilized by heat or steam with heat. It was reported that steam sterilization also increases its resistance to corrosion.[80]

Currently the available stainless steel sutures are twisted Flexon® and monofilament Stainless Steel® from American Cyanamid, twisted or monofilament Surgical Stainless Steel from Ethicon and monofilament steel from US Surgical.

REFERENCES

1. Barber, F., Alan, J., and Click, N., The effect of inflammatory synovial fluid on the breaking strength of new "Long Lasting Absorbable sutures," *J. Arthroscop. Rel. Surg.*, 8, 437, 1992.
2. Li, S.T., Biologic biomaterials: tissue-derived biomaterials (collagen), in *Biomedical Engineering Handbook*, Bronzino, J.D., Ed., CRC Press, 1995, p. 627.
3. Li, S.T. and Katz, E.P., An electrostatic model for collagen fibrils. The interaction of reconstituted collagen with Ca⁺⁺, Na⁺, and Cl⁻, *Biopolymers*, 15, 1439, 1976.
4. Li, S.T., Golub, E., and Katz, E.P., Electrostatic properties of reconstituted collagen fibrils, *J. Mol. Biol.*, 98, 835, 1975.
5. Stone, I.K., von Fraunhofer, J.A., and Masterson, B.J., A comparative study of suture materials: chromic gut and chromic gut treated with glycerin, *Am. J. Obstet. Gynecol.*, 151, 1087, 1985.
6. Grant, A., Dyspareunia associated with the use of glycerol-impregnated catgut to repair perineal trauma. Report of a 3 year follow-up study, *Br. J. Obstet. Gynecol.*, 96, 741, 1989.
7. Piez, K.A., Molecular and aggregate structures of the collagens, in *Extracellular Matrix Biochemistry*, Piez, K.A. and Reddi, A.H., Eds., Elsevier, New York, 1984, 41.
8. Frazza, E.J. and Schmitt, E.E., A new absorbable suture, *J. Biomed. Mater. Res. Symp.*, 1, 43, 1971.
9. Schmitt, E.E. and Polistina, R.A., Surgical sutures, U.S. Patent 3,297,033, American Cyanamid, 1967.
10. Katz, A.R. and Turner, R.J., Evaluation of tensile and absorption properties of polyglycolide sutures, *Surg. Gynecol. Obstet.*, 131, 701, 1970.
11. Bischoff, G.A. and Walden, P., Uber das glycdid und seine homologen, *Berlin Chem. Ges. Ber.*, 26, 262, 1893.
12. Lowe, C.E., Preparation of high molecular weight polyhydroxyacetic ester, U.S. Patent 2,668,162, 1954.
13. Chujo, K., Kobayashi, H., Suzuki, J., Tokuhara, S., and Tanabe, M., Ring-opening polymerization of glycolide, *Die Makromol. Chem.*, 100, 262, 1967.
14. Filachione, E.M. and Fisher, C.H., Lactic acid condensation polymers — preparation by batch and continuous methods, *Ind. Eng. Chem.*, 36, 223, 1944.
15. Wise, D.L., Fellmann, T.D., Sanderson, J.E., and Wentworth, R.L., Lactic/glycolic acid polymers, in *Drug Carriers in Biology and Medicine*, Academic Press, New York, 1979, 237.
16. Cherdron, H., Ohse, H., and Korte, F., Homopolymerization of 4-, 6-, and 7-membered lactones with cationic initiators, *Makromol. Chem.*, 56, 179, 1962.
17. Brandrup, J. and Immergut, E.H., Eds., *Polymer Handbook*, 2nd ed., Wiley, New York, 1975.
18. Gliding, D.K., Reed, A.M., and Askill, I.N., Calibration in gel permeation chromatography: primary, universal and empirical methods, *Polymer*, 22, 505, 1981.
19. Chatani, Y., Suehiro, K., Okita, Y., Tadokoro, H., and Chujo, K., Structural studies of polyesters. 1. Crystal structure of polyglycolide, *Die Makromol. Chem.*, 113, 215, 1968.
20. Zhang, L., Loh, I.H., and Chu, C.C., A combined γ irradiation and plasma deposition treatment to achieve the ideal degradation properties of synthetic absorbable polymers, *J. Biomed. Mater. Res.*, 27, 1425, 1993.
21. Chujo, K., Kobayashi, H., Suzuki, J., and Tokuhara, S., Physical and chemical characteristics of polyglycolide, *Die Makromol. Chem.*, 100, 267, 1967.
22. Casey, D. and Lewis, O.G., Absorbable and nonabsorbable sutures, in *Handbook of Biomaterials Evaluation: Scientific, Technical, and Clinical Testing of Implant Materials*, von Recum, A., Ed., Macmillan Publishing, New York, 1986, 86.
23. Glick, A. and McPherson, J.B., Jr., Absorbable polyglycolide suture of enhanced in vivo strength retention, U.S. Patent 3,626,948, American Cyanamid, 1971.
24. Chu, C.C., Zhang L., and Coyne, L., Effect of irradiation temperature on hydrolytic degradation properties of synthetic absorbable sutures and polymers, *J. Appl. Polym. Sci.*, 56, 1275, 1995.

25. Stone, I.K., von Fraunhofer, J.A., and Masterson, B.J., The biomechanical effects of tight suture closure on fascia, *Surg. Gynecol. Obstet.*, 163, 448, 1986.

26. von Fraunhofer, A.J. and Sichina, W.J., Characterization of surgical suture materials using dynamic mechanical analysis, *Biomaterials*, 13, 715, 1992.

27. Reed, A.M. and Gilding, D.K., Biodegradable polymers for use in surgery — poly(glycolic)/poly(lactic acid) homo and copolymers: 1., *Polymer*, 20, 1459, 1979.

28. Miller, P.A., Brady, J.M., and Cutright, D.E., Degradation rates of oral resorbable implants (polylactates and polyglycolates): rate modification with changes in PLA/PGA copolymer ratios, *J. Biomed. Mater. Res.*, 11, 711, 1977.

29. Fredericks, R.J., Melveger, A.J., and Dolegiewitz, L.J., Morphological and structural changes in a copolymer of glycolide and lactide occurring as a result of hydrolysis, *J. Polym. Sci. Polym. Phys. Ed.*, 22, 57, 1984.

30. Doddi, N., Versfelt, C.C., Wasserman, D., Bioresorbable polydiozanone, in *Fiber-Forming Polymers, Recent Advances,* Robinson, J.S., Ed., Noyes Data Corp., Park Ridge, N.J., 1990, 341; U.S. Patent 4,052,988, 1977.

31. Ray, J.A., Doddi, N., Regula, D., Williams, J.A., and Melveger, A., Polydioxanone (PDS), a novel monofilament synthetic absorbable suture, *Surg. Gynecol. Obstet.*, 153, 497, 1981.

32. Broyer, E., Thermal treatment of theraplastic filaments for the preparation of surgical sutures, U.S. Patent 5,294,395, Ethicon, Inc., 1994.

33. Lin, H.L., Chu, C.C., and Grubb, D., Hydrolytic degradation and morphologic study of poly-p-dioxanone, *J. Biomed. Mater. Res.*, 27, 153, 1993.

34. Shalaby, S.W., Synthetic absorbable polyesters, in *Biomedical Polymers: Designed-to-Degrade Systems*, Shalaby, S.W., Ed., Hanser Publisher, New York, 1994, chap. 1.

35. Shalaby, S.W. and Koelmel, D.F., U.S. Patent 4,441,496, 1984.

36. Bezwada, R.S., Shalaby, S.W., and Newman, H.D., U.S. Patent 4,653,497, 1987.

37. Bezwada, R.S., Shalaby, S.W., Newman, H.D., and Kafrauy, A., U.S. Patent 4,643,191, 1987.

38. Katz, A., Mukherjee, D.P., Kaganov, A.L., and Gordon, S., A new synthetic monofilament absorbable suture made from polytrimethylene carbonate, *Surg. Gynecol. Obstet.*, 161, 213, 1985.

39. Casey, D.J. and Roby, M.S., Synthetic copolymer surgical articles and method of manufacturing the same, U.S. Patent 4,429,080, American Cyanamid, 1984.

40. Fukuzaki, H., Yoshida, M., Asano, M., Kumakura, M., Mashimo, T., Yuasa, H., Imai, K., Yamandka, H., Kawaharada, U., and Suzuki, K., A new biodegradable copolymer of glycolic acid and lactones with relatively low molecular weight prepared by direct copolycondensation in the absence of catalysts, *J. Biomed. Mater. Res.*, 25, 315, 1991.

41. Fukuzaki, H., Yoshida, M., Asano, M., Aiba, Y., and Kumakura, M., Direct copolymerization of glycolic acid with lactones in the absence of catalysts, *Eur. Polym. J.,* 26, 457, 1989.

42. Bezwada, R.S., Jamiolkowski, D.D., Erneta, M., Persivale, J., Trenka-Benthin, S., Lee, I.Y., Suryadevara, J., Yang, A., Agarwal, V., and Liu, S., Monocryl suture, a new ultra-pliable absorbable monofilament suture, *Biomaterials,* 16, 1141, 1995.

43. Roby, M.S., Bennett, S.L., Liu, E.K., Absorbable block copolymers and surgical articles fabricated therefrom, U.S. Patent 5,403,347, April 4, 1995.

44. Robson, R.M., Silk: composition, structure, and properties, in *Fiber Chemistry*, Lewin, M. and Pearce, E.M., Eds., Handbook of Fiber Science and Technology, Vol. IV, Marcel Dekker, New York, 1985, chap. 7.

45. Lucas, F. and Rudall, K.M., *Comprehensive Biochemistry*, Vol. 26B, Florkin, M. and Stotz, E.H., Eds., Elsevier, Amsterdam, 1968.

46. Fraser, R.D.B. and MacRae, T.P., *Conformation in Fibrous Proteins and Related Synthetic Polymers,* Academic Press, New York, 1973, 293.

47. Marsh, R.E., Corey, R.B., and Pauling, L., An investigation of the structure of silk fibroin, *Biochem. Biophys. Acta*, 16, 1, 1955.

48. Goto, S., Takeshige, F., Sumitani, K., and Ogasawara, M., *Teikoku Gakuen Kiyo*, 4, 31, 1978.

49. Earland, C. and Robins, S.P., Cystine residues in Bombyx mori and other silks, *Int. J. Protein Res.*, 5, 327, 1973.

50. Zuber, H., Silk fibroin III, *Kolloid-Z.*, 179, 100, 1961.

51. Mercer, E., The fine structure and biosynthesis of silk fibroin, *Aust. J. Sci. Res.*, 5, 366, 1952.

52. Shalaby, S.W., Stephenson, M., Schaap, L., and Hartley, G.H., Composite sutures of silk and hydrophobic thermoplastic elastomers, U.S. Patent 4,461,298, 1984.

53. Segal, L. and Wakelyn, P.J., Cotton fibers, in *Fiber Chemistry*, Lewin, M. and Pearce, E.M., Eds., Handbook of Fiber Science and Technology, Vol. IV, Marcel Dekker, New York, 1985, chap. 10.

54. Daubeny, R.P., Bunn, C.W., and Brown, C.J., The crystal structure of polyethylene terephthalate, *Proc. R. Soc.*, A226 (1167), 531, 1954.

55. Mandelkern, L., *Introduction to Macromolecules*, Springer-Verlag, New York, 1972.

56. Venkatesh, G.M., Bose, P.J., and Khan, A.H., Vibrational spectroscopic study of poly(ethylene terephthalate) crystallized by annealing in the oriented state, *J. Appl. Polym. Sci.*, 26, 223, 1981.

57. Heuvel, H.M. and Huisman, R., Effect of winding speed on the physical structure of as-spun poly(ethylene terephthalate) fibers, including orientation-induced crystallization, *J. Appl. Polym. Sci.*, 22, 2229, 1978.

58. Kaplan, D.S., Surgical suture derived from segmented polyether-ester block copolymers, U.S. Patent 4,246,904, American Cyanamid Co., 1981.

59. Rodeheaver, G.T., Borzelleca, D.C., Thacker, J.G., and Edlich, R.F., Unique performance characteristics of Novafil, *Surg. Gynecol. Obstet.*, 164, 230, 1987.

60. Von Fraunhofer, J.A., Storey, R.J., and Masterson, B.J., Tensile properties of suture materials, *Biomaterials*, 9, 324, 1988.

61. Collins, M.A., Zeronian, S.H., and Semmelmeyer, M., The use of aqueous alkaline hydrolysis to reveal the fine structure of poly(ethylene terephthalate) fibers, *J. Appl. Polym. Sci.,* 12, 2149, 1991.

62. Moncrieff, R.W., Nylon, in *Man-Made Fibres*, John Wiley & Son, New York, 1975, 333.

63. Kohan, M.I., Preparation and chemistry of nylon plastics, in *Nylon Plastics*, Kohan, M.I., Ed., Wiley-Interscience, New York, 1973, 13.

64. Bunn, C.W. and Garner, E.V., The crystal structure of two polyamides (nylons), *Proc. R. Soc.*, A189, 38, 1947.

65. Sbrolli, W., Nylon 6, in *Man-Made Fibers Science and Technology*, Vol. 2, Mark, Atlas and Cernia, Eds., Wiley-Interscience, New York, 1968, 229.

66. Heuvel, H.M. and Huisman, R., Effects of winding speed, drawing and heating on the crystalline structure of Nylon 6 yarns, *J. Appl. Polym. Sci.*, 26, 713, 1981.

67. Listner, G.J., Polypropylene monofilament sutures, U.S. Patent 3,630,205, Ethicon, 1971.

68. Goodman, M., *Topics in Stereochemistry*, Vol. 2, Allinger, N.L. and Eliel, E.L., Eds., Wiley-Interscience, New York, 1967, 73.

69. Kaufman, H.S. and Falcetta, J.J., *Introduction to Polymer Science and Technology: An SPE Textbook*, Wiley-Interscience, New York, 1977, 92.

70. Cossee, P., *The Stereochemistry of Macromolecules*, Vol. 1, Ketley, A.D., Ed., Marcel Dekker, 1967.

71. Wishman, M. and Hagler, G.E., Polypropylene fibers, in *Fiber Chemistry*, Lewin, M. and Pearce, E.M., Eds., Handbook of Fiber Science and Technology, Vol. IV, Marcel Dekker, New York, 1985, chap. 4.

72. Chu, C.C., Pratt, L., Zhang, L., Hsu, A., and Chu, A., A comparison of a new polypropylene suture with prolene, *J. Appl. Biomater.*, 4, 169, 1993.

73. Kloos, F., Dependence of structure and properties of melt spun polypropylene fibers on molecular weight distribution, *Polymer Science Symposium honoring Leo Mandelkern*, Florida State University, Tallahassee, FL, September 5, 1987.

74. Joshi, R. M. and Zwolinski, B.J., Heats of polymerization and their structural and mechanistic implications, in *Vinyl Polymerization*, Vol. 1, Part I, Ham, G.E., Ed., Marcel Dekker, New York, 1967.

75. Allcock, H.R. and Lampe, F.W., *Contemporary Polymer Chemistry*, Prentice-Hall, Englewood Cliffs, 1981, 46.

76. Billmeyer, F.W., Jr., *Textbook of Polymer Science*, 3rd ed., Wiley-Interscience, New York, 1984, 5033.

77. Miller, C.M., Sangiolo, P., and Jacobson, J.J., II, Reduced anastomotic bleeding using new sutures with a needle-suture diameter ratio of one, *Surgery*, 101, 156, 1987.

78. Dang, M.C., Thacker, J.G., Hwang, J.C.S., Rodeheaver, G.T., Melton, S.M., and Edlich, R.F., Some biomechanical considerations of polytetrafluoroethylene sutures, *Arch. Surg.*, 125, 647, 1990.

79. Chu, C.C. and Kizil, Z., Quantitative evaluation of stiffness of commercial suture materials, *Surg., Gynecol. Obstet.*, 168, 233, 1989.

80. Sutow, E.J., Iron-based alloys, in *Concise Encyclopedia of Medical and Dental Materials*, Williams, D.F., Ed., Pergamon Press, New York, 1990, 232.

Chapter 6

Mechanical Properties

J. A. von Fraunhofer and C. C. Chu

CONTENTS

Since the major function of suture materials is to hold the wound together until it heals, these materials experience the same kinds of mechanical forces as the wound does. It is often literally true that the life of a patient hangs by a tiny thread. Suture strength, however, is a complicated issue. Optimal utilization of suture materials is based on a proper match between tissue strength and suture strength, and two factors must be considered in this regard.

First, consider the kind of tissue. It is well recognized that the suture-holding strength of most soft tissues depends on the amount of fibrous tissue they have. Thus, the spinal cord and brain will scarcely support sutures due to their minimal amounts of fibrous connective tissue, while skin and fascia are the toughest of the soft tissues. The seromuscular coat of the intestinal wall is easily torn by sutures unless the tough, fibrous submucosa is sewn.

Second, consider the health of the sewn tissue. Tissues become friable with acute inflammation. If the suture is too tight, particularly with a fine suture, it could cut through the inflamed tissue.

The mechanical properties of fibrous polymers that are important for suture use include: (1) tensile properties; (2) tensile strength retention; (3) stiffness and flexibility; (4) viscoelasticity; and (5) knot strength and security. Each is discussed in detail in this chapter.

I. TENSILE PROPERTIES

Although the properties of knotted sutures are a better representation of the *in vivo* condition, tensile properties of straight sutures give a better fundamental characterization of different suture materials without the complications arising from the knot. There are many reported studies of mechanical properties of suture materials. However, most of those studies used relatively few sutures and only tensile breaking forces were reported. More thorough reports on the tensile properties of suture materials that cover the whole spectrum of sutures, such as stress-strain curves, elastic moduli, work of rupture, and stress-relaxation behavior, are sparse.[1,2] A comprehensive study of the tensile properties of seven commonly used suture materials, employing a new grip device, is the beginning of an awareness of the importance of such a fundamental characterization of suture materials.[1] The results of that study are summarized in Figure 6.1 and Table 6.1A.

It is evident from Figure 6.1 that a wide range of stress–strain relationships was observed in the seven commonly used sutures. Tenacity ranged from 3.43 GPD for silk, 4.3 GPD for Mersilene®, and 5.14 GPD for Prolene®, to 6.55 GPD for Vicryl®. The breaking strain ranged from 8.9% for Mersilene, 11.5% for silk, and 18.2% for Nurolon®, to 42.0% for Prolene. A summary of important mechanical properties of these sutures tested on both yarn and conventional grips is given in Table 6.1A.

Yield stress and strain are the correspondent stress and strain at the yield point on the stress–strain curve. Materials start to deform permanently after the yield point; they cannot recover their original

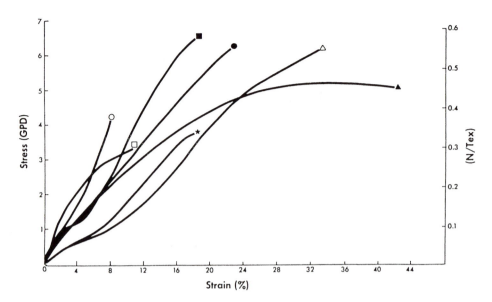

Figure 6.1   Stress-strain curves of 2/0 suture materials. (○) Mersilene; (●) Dexon; (□) Silk; (■)Vicryl; (n) Ethilon; (m) Prolene; (★) Nurolon. (Reproduced from Chu, C.C., *Ann. Surg.*, 193(3), 365,1981. With permission.)

Table 6.1A   Mechanical Properties of Suture Materials

Suture (2-0)	Mechanical Property					
	Yield Stress (GPD)	Breaking Stress (GPD)	Yield Strain (%)	Breaking Strain (%)	Modulus of Elasticity (GPD)	Specific Work of Rupture (N/Tex) × 10⁻²
Dexon	0.80 (0.77)	6.30 (6.2)	1.9 (1.9)	22.6 (26.3)	55 (53)	6.63
Vicryl	0.97 (0.98)	6.55 (6.28)	1.8 (1.9)	18.4 (20.8)	67.5 (64)	5.46
Mersilene	1.20 (1.25)	4.20 (4.08)	2.7 (2.9)	8 (8.2)	53 (47.5)	1.32
Silk	1.33 (1.22)	3.43 (3.35)	1.9 (1.90)	11.5 (13.1)	79.0 (78.5)	2.36
Nurolon	0.34 (0.325)	3.80 (3.75)	1.6 (1.8)	18.2 (21)	21.0 (19.5)	2.80
Ethilon	0.41 (0.38)	6.25 (5.88)	2.2 (2.4)	33 (37)	20.0 (19.0)	8.96
Prolene	0.52 (0.40)	5.14 (5.0)	1.2 (1.2)	42 (43.2)	58.5 (38.5)	14.69

Notes: Data from yarn grip tests, except those inside parentheses, which are from conventional grip tests. For those who are interested in N/Tex units, the conversion factor is 1 GPD = 0.08825 N/Tex.

From C.C. Chu, *Ann. Surg.*, 193(3), 365, 1981. With permission.

dimensions after the removal of the external force. The modulus of elasticity is equal to the slope of the stress–strain curve at the origin, and is a measure of the resistance to elongation and of the stiffness of the material before the yield point. The reciprocal of this property is called compliance. Suture materials thus can be grouped according to these mechanical properties. On the basis of yield stress, Nurolon, Ethilon®, and Prolene have the lowest yield stress (0.34 to 0.52 GPD), Dexon® and Vicryl are in the middle (0.80 to 0.97 GPD), while Mersilene and silk have the highest yield stress (1.20 to 1.33 GPD). When grouped on the basis of breaking stress, the order is different. Dexon, Vicryl, and Ethilon are then the strongest (6.30 to 6.25 GPD), Prolene is in the middle (5.14 GPD), while silk, Nurolon, and Mersilene are the weakest (3.43 to 4.30 GPD). In terms of breaking strain, Mersilene and silk exhibit the lowest values (8% and 11.5%, respectively), Vicryl and Nurolon have higher and similar values (18.4% and 18.2%, respectively), and Ethilon and Prolene possess the highest values (33% and 42%, respectively). These seven commonly used sutures also have wide ranges of moduli of elasticity. The order of increasing modulus of elasticity is Ethilon, Nurolon, Mersilene, Dexon, Prolene, Vicryl, and silk; the values range from 20 to 79 GPD. Dexon, Mersilene, and Prolene have close moduli of elasticity. The geometric form of sutures does not appear to have any significant effect on the modulus of elasticity as evidenced by

Table 6.1B Mean Tensile Properties of 2/0 Size Sutures that Have Recently Become Available Commercially (After 1984)

Suture	Failure Load (Kg)		Elongation at Break (%)	Work of Rupture (kg-cm)	Tensile Strength (kg/cm²)
	Straight	Knotted			
PDS II[a]	4.4 ± 0.2	—	35.7	18.07	—
Maxon[b]	7.09	4.41	4.39	15.92	6,056.5
Monocryl[c]	7.26	3.67	39		91,100
Novafil[b]	4.35	2.57	2.94	6.29	4,749.4
Gore-Tex[b] (CV-4)[d]	1.78	1.75	1.42	1.55	1,558.8
Biosyn[d]	3.7	2.4	44	2.76[e]	55.3[f]

[a] Unpublished data from Chu.
[b] Data from von Fraunhofer, J.A. et al., *Biomaterials*, 9, 324, 1988.
[c] Data from Bezwada, R.S. et al., *Biomaterials*, 16, 1995.
[d] 3/0 Size
[e] 0 to 10% in kg-mm
[f] kg/mm²

the small difference in elastic modulus between braided nylon (Nurolon) and monofilament nylon (Ethilon).

Specific works of rupture, W_s, of the seven suture materials are also given in Table 6.1A. W_s of fibrous materials is defined as: W_s = (work of rupture)/[(mass/unit length) × (initial length)]. Work of rupture (sometimes called toughness) is defined as the amount of energy needed to break a material and is represented by the area under the stress–strain curve. It measures the ability of a material to withstand sudden shocks of a given energy. The material will be broken if the amount of energy from a sudden shock exceeds the work of rupture of the material. In a clinical situation, coughing or vomiting by a patient will impose this kind of sudden shock on the suture material. In order to compare different materials, work of rupture should be normalized to take into account the various masses of different materials. Hence, specific work of rupture, which is the amount of energy needed to break a material of unit mass, should be used. There is a wide difference in specific work of rupture among the seven sutures, and the values range from 1.32 N/Tex for Mersilene to 14.69 N/Tex (Tex defined as weight in grams per kilometer of yarn) for Prolene — an almost tenfold difference. Specific works of rupture are about four times as great for sutures of the same chemical nature, but different geometrical configuration, such as Nurolon and Ethilon.

The shape of the stress–strain curves, along with the related mechanical properties extracted from the curves, provide important data for better characterization of suture materials. These shapes reveal a literal and overall discrimination of suture materials that is difficult to obtain by breaking strength and size specification alone. They are particularly helpful for discriminating between suture materials that have similar strengths or elongations. For example, although Dexon, Vicryl, and Ethilon behave similarly from the standpoint of breaking strength, these sutures exhibit very different stress–strain relationships, particularly in yield stress, breaking strain, and modulus of elasticity. Likewise, Nurolon and Vicryl have very similar breaking strains but show almost totally different stress–strain curves. Silk and Nurolon have similar values for the specific work of rupture, but different stress–strain characteristics. Mersilene, Dexon, and Prolene have similar moduli of elasticity, but their stress–strain curves are quite different. Even the same materials (e.g., nylon sutures: Ethilon and Nurolon) exhibit quite different stress–strain curves as a result of their different geometrical configurations. Suture materials can, thus, be classified into several broad categories: (1) relatively hard and brittle, such as Mersilene and silk; (2) relatively strong and ductile, such as Dexon, Vicryl, and Ethilon; (3) relatively weak but ductile and tough, like Prolene; and (4) relatively weak, ductile, and soft, like Nurolon.

These examples, and the data cited above, strongly suggest that suture materials having a few similar or even identical mechanical properties (i.e., breaking stress), are actually very different from each other in terms of overall performance. Therefore, more useful and complete information, such as stress–strain curves, could provide a better basis for discriminating between different suture materials for specific uses despite their nominal similarities. For example, judging from the mechanical properties alone, Nurolon and Ethilon, due to their low moduli and high strains, are considered to be less appropriate than other materials for suturing wounded tissues that are relatively inelastic and constrained, like bone and tendon. Prolene and Ethilon are believed to be suitable for closing tissues with large elongation capabilities, such as skin (789% ultimate elongation) and cardiac muscle (63.8%).

The difference in distensibility of different materials, however, can be compensated for by employing various suture techniques. For example, elongation of a suture material will not result in a wide separation of the wound cleft if a very short loop is used. Yield stress and strain data along with modulus of elasticity extracted from the stress–strain curves might also be important for sutures in closing surgical wounds having severe edema. Due to the swelling of these wounds, sutures will be elongated; the degree of elongation depends on the level of swelling. If the suture is elongated beyond its yield point, the suture is permanently deformed. When the edema is recessed (corresponding to the removal of external force), the suture might not be able to closely approximate the wound edge due to the inability of the suture to fully recover its original dimension. Since modulus of elasticity is a measure of the resistance of the material to deformation before the yield point, a suture having a high modulus of elasticity (hence, less compliance) is less likely to yield to the swelling pressure of the wound. Consequently, cutting through the sewn tissue may result.

Because suture materials stay either temporarily or permanently inside the body, they are subjected to various types and degrees of biodegradation, particularly in view of the hostile environment of the body. Due to the breakdown of molecules, suture materials often lose their original tensile strength with time. The retention of their tensile strength and the rate of tensile strength loss are vital factors in their usefulness in wound healing. For noncritical surgical conditions such as small vessel ligation or the coaptation of uncomplicated wounds in rapidly healing tissues, the rate of loss of tensile strength is probably of little importance. For more critical surgical wounds, however, differences in the rate of loss of tensile strength for suture materials may be highly significant, particularly in tissues slow to heal such as tendons and ligaments, and for those with neoplasia, hypoproteinemia, etc. In a few situations, suture materials must retain strength for the lifetime of the patient, e.g., a synthetic graft sutured to the aorta. Since the loss of tensile strength of a suture material depends on the animal species, type of tissue, size of suture material, and the testing condition, the reported data vary considerably. The details of strength retention of both absorbable and nonabsorbable sutures are given in Chapter 7.

After the comprehensive study of the tensile properties of seven commonly used sutures reported by Chu in 1980, there have been several chemically new commercial suture materials introduced, such as PDS®, Maxon®, Monocryl®, Biosyn®, Novafil®, and Gore-Tex®. Due to different testing conditions, size of suture materials, and unit of strength, it is almost impossible to compare the mechanical properties of these new sutures reported by different authors and labs with the tensile data of the Chu study. Thus, only a qualitative comparison of these newer suture materials with the above-mentioned seven commercial suture materials is given below. Table 6.1B summarizes the mean tensile properties of 2/0 Maxon, PDSII, Monocryl, Biosyn, Novafil, and Gore-Tex sutures. Among these five new suture materials introduced after 1984, Gore-Tex sutures appear to be the weakest in terms of straight pull force. The very high porous volume of Gore-Tex suture is the source for this weak tensile breaking force. It is surprising to know that the elongations at break for Maxon, Novafil, and Gore-Tex sutures are single digits and significantly lower than most sutures, which have double digits (Table 6.1A. vs. 6.1B). The reader should be aware of the fact that suture manufacturers constantly improve their processes of suture manufacturing (e.g., fiber spinning and raw materials) after their initial commercial introduction. Such revisions can lead to subsequent periodic changes, either significant or insignificant, in the previously reported mechanical and biodegradation property data. If the changes in suture properties are significant enough, suture manufacturers usually label such changes as the second or third generation of the previous products, e.g., PDSII vs. PDS, Dexon Plus vs. Dexon.

Among all suture materials, stainless steel sutures show the highest tensile breaking strength (113 to 162 kg/mm^2) and moduli of elasticity (8.4×10^3 to 1.17×10^4 N) but the smallest elongation at break (2%).[2,3] Its poor handling characteristics have limited the use of stainless steel despite its strength. Linen sutures behave like steel and are more rigid than most other suture materials. They have a modulus of elasticity of 5.63×10^3 N, 3% elongation at break, and a tensile strength of 65 kg/mm^2. Cotton suture is the weakest suture. It has only a 46 kg/mm^2 tensile breaking strength when tested dry.[3] Of course, slightly higher values would be expected when it is tested wet. Among the absorbable sutures, Holmlund et al.[2] reported that both plain and chromic catgut sutures have almost the same stress–strain properties as polyglycolide (PGA) sutures. But their poor handling properties and intense inflammatory reaction make them less desirable than PGA.

The ultimate solution for choosing suture materials of the right mechanical properties for closing specific wounds might be to select a material whose stress–strain behavior has the best match with the stress–strain curve of the tissue to be sewn. The availability of stress–strain curves of suture materials, like those shown in Figure 6.1, are ideal for such a task. Of course, other properties such as tissue reactions, wound condition (i.e., infection), knot security, handling, and degree of absorption should also be considered, along with the suture's mechanical properties. The final selection will likely be a compromise of these properties for optimum performance.

II. STIFFNESS AND FLEXIBILITY

The stiffness of a suture material determines its performance in terms of handling characteristics and knot strength and security, particularly in closing wounds with small loops.[4,5] It is known that a stiff suture is difficult to tie into a knot, and frequently the knot unties and causes wound disruption. Clinically it is known that the ease of suture bending is important when ligaturing small blood vessels and for closing wounds with small loops. A larger loop is generally required for a stiff suture during wound closure. If a stiff suture is forced into a small loop, particularly in a continuous suturing technique, it has a tendency to spring back, which could make the accurate approximation of the opposite wound edges difficult. It is known in clinical practice that a smaller size of a suture could be used to reduce its stiffness if the larger size of the same suture is too stiff. The ends of a stiff suture could also cause mechanical irritation due to their inability to comply with the topology of the surrounding tissue.[6,7]

Although the stiffness of the commercial suture materials is generally known qualitatively, quantitative stiffness data are not widely available in the literature. The impression of a stiff suture is usually derived from its performance as a knot or by the feel in the surgeon's hands. A more objective means of evaluating stiffness quantitatively is highly desirable. There are three reported methods to obtain stiffness of sutures: bending stiffness, torsional stiffness, and stiffness based upon modulus of elasticity. Although most reported stiffness data of sutures are based upon modulus of elasticity, the stiffness information obtained from a bending test modality may be more appropriate for correlating with suture performance *in vivo*. So far, the most comprehensive reported study of bending stiffness of a large group of commercial sutures was done by Chu and Kizil.[8]

In that study, Chu and Kizil evaluated quantitatively the stiffness of 22 commercial suture materials in terms of their chemical structure, geometrical configuration, coating, and size.[8] The stiffness of suture materials was determined by using the ultrahigh-sensitivity Taber V-5 stiffness tester, model 150B (Teledyne Taber, Tonawanda, New York), an instrument designed to test the bending stiffness of lightweight materials, such as the synthetic and natural fibers, which make up the current commercial sutures. The principle of the test is to bend a specimen of a fixed length (i.e., 1.5 in.) to a predetermined angle (e.g., 7.5 or 15°), and the force required to bend the specimen to this angle is recorded in Taber Stiffness units and used to calculate flexural stiffness, E, according to the formula given in ASTM D747-50:[9]

$$E = 0.006832 \times \{1/(W \times d^3 \times \theta)\} \times T$$

where

E = stiffness in flexure in pounds/inch^2 (convert to kg/cm^2 by multiplying by 0.0703)
W = width of specimen in inches (same as the diameter of a suture)
d = thickness of specimen in inches (diameter of a suture material)
θ = deflection of specimen converted to radian (i.e., 7.5 = 0.1309 radian)
T = measurement in Taber Stiffness units

Three types of stiffness data were obtained. They were initial stiffness, basic stiffness, and resilience. The initial stiffness is the first reading obtained immediately upon bending the suture material to 7.5°, and is generally used for material comparisons. Due to the viscoelastic behavior of polymers, suture materials will creep when held at 7.5° deflection, and this creeping phenomenon will continue within a period of time (usually 1 min) until an equilibrium state is reached with no further measurable change occurring thereafter. Because of this time dependence of stiffness, another stiffness value (1 min after recording the initial stiffness) is measured and is termed the basic stiffness. The elastic quality of the suture materials, called resilience, is then expressed as the ratio of basic stiffness to initial stiffness. Therefore, sutures with higher resilience showed less loss of stiffness over time.

The stiffness data of 22 commercial suture materials are summarized in Tables 6.2 and 6.3. Data in Table 6.2 are the total stiffness values before normalization by the size of the sutures. In terms of total stiffness of suture materials, a decrease in suture size significantly reduces its total stiffness, and the

Table 6.2 Initial and Basic Stiffness in Taber Units of 22 Commercial Suture Materials

Suture	Size	Diameter, in.	Angle of Deflection, degrees, R[a]	Initial Taber Units	Basic Taber Units
Chromic	2-0	0.014	7.5	29	28.5
Dexon®	2-0	0.02	7.5	0.5	0.5
Vicryl®	2-0	0.02	7.5	1.5	1.4
Coated Vicryl	2-0	0.014	7.5	3	3
PDS®	1-0	0.016	7.5	13.5	13.25
PDS	2-0	0.014	7.5	11	10.5
Maxon®	2-0	0.016	7.5	10	8
Silk	2-0	0.02	7.5	1	0.9
Mersilene®	2-0	0.014	7.5	0.9	0.9
Ti-Cron®	2-0	0.015	7.5	0.8	0.7
Ethibond®	2-0	0.013	7.5	3.5	3
Nurolon®	2-0	0.015	7.5	1	1
Surgilon®	2-0	0.016	7.5	0.5	0.5
Ethilon®	2-0	0.019	7.5	3	3
Prolene®	1-0	0.016	7.5	28	26
Prolene	2-0	0.012	7.5	13	11.5
Prolene	5-0	0.0055	7.5	1	1
Prolene	9-0	0.0016	7.5	0.5	0.5
Dermalene®	2-0	0.011	7.5	14.5	13
Gore-Tex®	CV-2	0.025	7.5	1	0.5
Gore-Tex	CV-5	0.014	7.5	0.5	0.25
Gore-Tex	CV-6	0.012	7.5	0.4	0.4

[a] R, deflect to the right

From Chu, C.C. and Kizil, Z., *Surg. Gynecol. Obstet.*, 168, 233, 1989. With permission.

Table 6.3 Flexural Stiffness of 2-0 Commercial Suture Materials

Suture	Initial Stiffness, kg/cm²	Basic Stiffness, kg/cm²	Resilience, Basic/Initial, percent
Chromic catgut	2.77×10^4	2.72×10^4	98
Dexon®	1.15×10^2	1.15×10^2	100
Vicryl®	3.44×10^2	3.21×10^2	93
Vicryl, coated	2.86×10^4	2.86×10^4	100
PDS®	1.05×10^4	1.00×10^4	95
Maxon®	5.60×10^3	4.48×10^3	80
Silk	2.29×10^2	2.06×10^2	90
Mersilene®	8.59×10^2	8.59×10^2	100
Ti-Cron®	5.80×10^2	5.09×10^2	87
Ethibond®	4.50×10^3	3.85×10^3	86
Nurolon®	7.25×10^2	7.25×10^2	100
Surgilon®	2.80×10^2	2.80×10^2	100
Ethilon®	1.69×10^4	1.69×10^4	100
Prolene®	2.30×10^4	2.03×10^4	88
Dermalene®	3.63×10^4	3.25×10^4	89
Gore-Tex®	9.40×10^1	4.70×10^1	50

From Chu, C.C. and Kizil, Z., *Surg. Gynecol. Obstet.*, 168, 233, 1989. With permission.

magnitude of this size dependence of total stiffness varies with the chemical nature of the suture material. For example, 2–0 Prolene had only one half of the total stiffness of 1–0 Prolene. Further reduction in Prolene suture size to 5–0 and 9–0 reduced their total stiffness values to only about 4% and 2% of the

1–0 Prolene, respectively. Similar behavior was also found in Gore-Tex and polydioxanone (PDS) sutures, although the size dependence was less marked.

In order to compare stiffness of suture materials that are chemically and geometrically different from each other, size-normalized stiffness values, flexural stiffness E, can be used and these values are summarized in Table 6.3. A wide range of flexural stiffness values, differing by almost 10^3, was observed for the 22 tested sutures. The newly available synthetic nonabsorbable monofilament suture Gore-Tex showed the lowest flexural stiffness (94 kg/cm^2) among the 11 chemically different types of the same size commercial sutures. This was followed by Dexon, silk, Surgilon, Vicryl, Ti-Cron, Nurolon, Mersilene, Ethibond, Maxon, PDS, Ethilon, Prolene, chromic catgut, coated Vicryl, and finally Dermalene, which had the highest flexural stiffness (3.63×10^4 kg/cm^2). On the basis of this order of flexural stiffness, those suture materials having monofilament form had a higher flexural stiffness than those having a multifilament braided form, except for coated Vicryl suture. This is particularly true when comparing those suture materials having the same chemical structure but different geometrical form. The best example is the comparison between Nurolon and Ethilon. Both sutures are fabricated from nylon 66 but Ethilon, a monofilament nylon 66, had flexural stiffness 23 times that of the braided nylon 66, Nurolon. This demonstrates that geometric form is one of the most important factors in determining a suture's stiffness.

In spite of its monofilament configuration, the Gore-Tex suture is the most flexible suture among all of the tested commercial 2–0 size suture materials. A detailed examination of its surface morphology indicated that in contrast to all other monofilament sutures that are solid, Gore-Tex suture has a porous microstructure with about 50% porous volume.[10] Within this porous structure, there are solid nodules interconnected by tiny but highly oriented fibrils of at least 17 μm length. The large air space created by this unique microporous structure renders Gore-Tex suture extremely flexible under a bending force.

However, the geometrical form of a suture is not the only factor influencing suture stiffness; the chemical constituents also affect its stiffness value, although to a lesser extent. For example, the order of increasing stiffness among the five synthetic solid monofilament sutures was Maxon, PDS, Ethilon, Prolene, and Dermalene. Besides chromic catgut, PDS is the stiffest absorbable suture. A comparison of the basic chemical structures of PDS and Maxon (shown in Chapter 5) clearly indicates that, due to the existence of the trimethylene group in the backbone molecules, Maxon suture would be theoretically expected and, indeed, is observed to be more flexible than PDS, assuming everything else is the same (e.g., physical form, size, orientation, and crystallinity). The recently available PDSII suture, a second generation of PDS, however, appears to change the order of stiffness of monofilament absorbable sutures. Bezwada et al.[11] reported that PDSII is the second most flexible monofilament absorbable suture (next to Monocryl) with a stiffness of 268.9 MPa. The change in fiber morphology found in PDSII from PDS, as described in Chapter 5, is responsible for this significant reduction in stiffness of PDSII sutures.

Although PDS was found to be relatively stiff compared to other synthetic monofilament absorbable sutures, it is more flexible than the same size polypropylene monofilament suture (i.e., Prolene), which has been generally recognized as the stiffest suture. This observation confirms the claim of Ray et al. in their PDS study.[12]

On the basis of chemical structure, polyglycolide (PGA) sutures should be expected to be the stiffest among the four synthetic absorbable sutures. Its high density of ester functional groups, due to the short $-CH_2-$ spacing between two adjacent ester functional groups, results in PGA having high intermolecular hydrogen bond capability. However, in braided form, a PGA suture was the most flexible absorbable suture (1.15×10^2 kg/cm^2) and was only slightly stiffer than the highly flexible Gore-Tex suture among the 16 tested commercial sutures. The low stiffness of Dexon (polyglycolide) suture was solely attributed to its braided geometrical configuration. This observation supports the common belief that any polymer that shows high stiffness in monofilament form due to its chemical constituents can be made, in multifilament braided form, to achieve the desirable flexibility.

Polyolefin-based monofilament sutures (Dermalene suture from polyethylene, and Prolene suture from polypropylene) exhibited the highest flexural stiffness values (3.63×10^4 and 2.3×10^4 kg/cm^2, respectively) of all synthetic absorbable and nonabsorbable sutures, except for coated Vicryl. This must be attributed to their simple chemical structure, which results in their high degree of crystallinity and orientation. Because polyethylene has the simplest and least perturbed chemical structure, it would be expected to have the highest levels of crystallinity and orientation and, in fact, its suture exhibited the highest flexural stiffness of the 11 chemically different sutures studied.

Coating of suture materials is a common practice in manufacture to facilitate suture passage through tissue and, hence, reduce tissue drag. This is particularly true for sutures in braided form. However, coating of suture materials could actually make them stiffer than the corresponding uncoated ones, as shown by Vicryl and polyester sutures. A copolymer-coated Vicryl suture had a flexural stiffness $(2.86 \times 10^4$ kg/cm^2) nearly 100 times greater than the uncoated Vicryl suture (3.44×10^2 kg/cm^2). Similarly, polybutylate-coated polyester suture (Ethibond) was five times stiffer than the uncoated polyester suture (Mersilene). It thus appears true that polymer-coated suture materials become stiffer, primarily because the coating material formed a thin film over the suture that would fill up the interstitial space between fibers and between yarns and bond all the fibers within the yarns together. As a result, the fibers and yarns in a suture were difficult to move or yield under a bending force, which leads to higher stiffness values.

The basic stiffness data followed the same order as the initial stiffness data and were generally less than or equivalent to the latter. This is because the polymers from which these suture materials are made exhibit viscoelastic behavior. Viscoelasticity, a typical characteristic of large molecules, makes plastic materials respond less ideally than those materials with complete elastic characteristics. When these materials are under a constant force, such as the bending force exerted during the stiffness test, the polymeric molecules will rearrange or reorient themselves to reduce or dissipate the externally applied stress. Consequently, the dimension of the material changes, resulting in the loss of its initial stiffness. This phenomenon is called creep in engineering terminology. Therefore, the ratio of basic to initial stiffness would indicate the elastic quality of a material. The higher the ratio, the better the elastic quality and the lower the loss of stiffness due to the viscous behavior of polymers.

Most suture materials with a resilience of less than 90% were those sutures with monofilament form. Examples of these are Maxon, Prolene, Dermalene, and Gore-Tex sutures. Gore-Tex suture showed a resilience of 50%, implying that it lost half of its initial stiffness due to its dimensional change under a constant bending force during a bending stiffness test. Such a large dimensional change was possible only for the Gore-Tex suture because of its high pore density within its porous microstructure, which provided adequate open space for the fibrils and their solid nodules to yield along the direction of bending force. As they yielded under a bending force, the stiffness of the material would decrease. The only exceptions to the low resilience observed in monofilament sutures as a group were sutures made from nylon, such as Ethilon. Nylon sutures were the only suture materials whose resilience was independent of their physical configurational form, and showed no loss of initial stiffness with time (i.e., greater elasticity). This finding is consistent with general experience in using nylon fibers in situations where elasticity is required (e.g., elastic waistbands).

The order of suture stiffness obtained in the study by Chu and Kizil is generally consistent with the semiquantitative results obtained by Holmlund et al.[5] In that study, the stiffness of a suture was evaluated by a torsional method in which one end of a suture specimen was rotated until the other end started to turn. The number of turns the suture took before the other end started to turn was used as an indication of relative stiffness. Among the suture materials tested, Holmlund et al. reported that 2/0 size monofilament nylon, catgut, and Prolene sutures were the stiffest, and that Mersilene, Dexon, and silk were the softest. In Chu and Kizil's study, monofilament nylon, catgut, and Prolene sutures had flexural stiffnesses all above 10^4 kg/cm^2, while Dexon, silk, and Mersilene sutures had flexural stiffness around 10^2 kg/cm^2. Thus, the same conclusion is drawn from the two completely different stiffness testing methods — one with a bending stiffness and the other with a torsional stiffness. However, the stiffness measurement based on bending mode is believed to be a better representation of the conditions that a suture actually experiences *in vivo*. For example, when a loop is made during wound closure, the suture experiences more of a bending force than a torsional force. The bending stiffness measurement also has a greater sensitivity than the torsional stiffness method. For example, the bending stiffness test showed that a monofilament nylon suture (Ethilon) had a lower stiffness value than chromic catgut, while these two sutures exhibited the same degree of torsional stiffness in the study by Holmlund et al.

Young's modulus (the modulus of elasticity) is also used to indicate the stiffness of sutures.[1] Although Young's modulus is a means of indicating the stiffness of a material, it represents flexibility in tensile mode, which may be quite different from the bending stiffness that a suture actually experiences during wound closure. The stiffness derived from Young's modulus may be misleading in evaluating suture materials, as shown by Chu.[1] In that study, silk was found to have the highest Young's modulus (79.0 GPD) among the seven tested commercial sutures, followed by Vicryl, Prolene, Dexon, Mersilene, Nurolon, and Ethilon. Instead of silk being the stiffest on the basis of Young's modulus, Chu and Kizil's[8] study found that silk was one of the most flexible sutures on the basis of the bending stiffness test, and its stiffness is comparable to Surgilon suture.

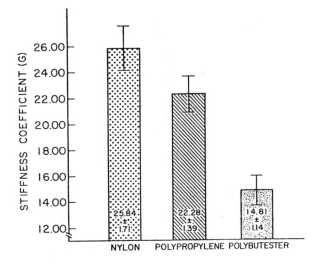

Figure 6.2 Stiffness coefficient (G) of three 3/0 monofilament sutures: polybutester (Novafil®), nylon (Dermalon®), and polypropylene (Surgilene®). See text for the definition of G. (Reproduced from Rodeheaver, G.T. et al., *Surg. Gynecol. Obstet.*, 164, 230, 1987. With permission.)

The recent introduction of several new monofilament sutures like Monocryl[11] and Novafil[13] is intended to improve the handling characteristics by reducing suture stiffness further. Figure 6.2 compares the stiffness coefficient (G) of 3/0 monofilament polybutester (Novafil) with monofilament nylon (Dermalon) and polypropylene (Surgilene) sutures of the same size. Suture stiffness was obtained by bending a fixed length of suture fiber under a constant weight over a pin[13,14] and G was calculated by the following equation:

$$G = \frac{wd^2}{8}$$

where w = weight hung at the each end of the suture, d = the distance between the two ends of a suture after bending over a pin.

The ease of handling Novafil is evident in its relatively low stiffness coefficient, G, which for Novafil is about $^1/_2$ that of Dermalon and $^2/_3$ that of Surgilene sutures. The low stiffness coefficient of Novafil is also reflected in improved knot tying, as described in Section IV, and is attributed to the elastomeric characteristic of the polybutester block copolymer that is not present in either Dermalon or Surgilene. Similarly, monofilament absorbable Monocryl suture has been reported to be the most pliable (in terms of stiffness).[11] Figure 6.3 compares the stiffness (calculated from the product of suture area, moment of inertia, and Young's modulus) of four 2/0 monofilament absorbable sutures. Monocryl has only 24%, 26%, and 72% of the stiffness of Maxon, chromic gut, and PDSII, respectively.

The availability of the present bending stiffness data allows a surgeon's clinical experience of sutures to be quantitatively related to one of the fundamental properties of fibers — stiffness. These data, in addition to many other reported mechanical properties of sutures, can also serve as one of the quantitative bases for surgeons' selection of appropriate suture materials for their particular needs.

III. VISCOELASTIC BEHAVIOR

Synthetic and natural fibers made from semicrystalline polymers exhibit a well-known viscoelastic behavior, namely stress relaxation. When such a fiber is elongated to a fixed strain under a constant temperature and humidity, the resultant stress in the fiber decays with time. The stress may reduce to a limiting value or may disappear completely, depending on many factors, such as the chemical structure of the fiber, the level of strain, and the environmental relative humidity and temperature. Typically, stress relaxation manifests as an initial rapid decay of stress, followed by a near-zero rate of decay at later times on a linear time scale. This viscoelastic behavior has been investigated in the past for many fibers such as nylon, polyesters, polypropylene, wool, viscose rayon, and silk.[15–20] Generally, the rate of stress

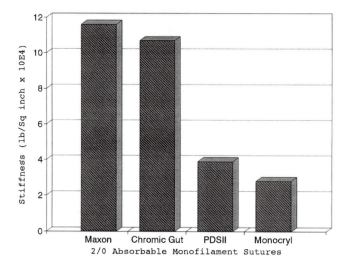

Figure 6.3 A comparison of stiffness value of 2/0 absorbable monofilament sutures, chromic gut, Maxon, PDSII, and Monocryl. (From Bezwada, R.S. et al., *Biomaterials,* 16, 1141, 1995. With permission.)

decay depends on the strain level and this strain-dependent stress decay is probably due to a temperature effect. A rapid extension to a stress level beyond the yield point results in a temperature rise due to a large energy loss (e.g., an increment of 11°C for a 20% extension) and it takes several seconds for the fiber to dissipate the excess heat and thus affects the earlier part of the stress decay curve. This strain level-dependent stress relaxation has been observed in several types of fibers.

Stress relaxation occurs as a result of segmental mobility of the constituent polymeric chains, which enables them to achieve a new equilibrium position. Clearly, factors that affect segmental mobility would also affect stress relaxation and these factors include moisture, temperature, molecular weight, nature of the backbone repeating unit and side-chain substituents, stereoregularity, and orientation. Relative humidity and absorbed moisture affect the stress relaxation of hydrophilic fibers (such as nylon and rayon) to a greater degree than hydrophobic materials (such as polyethylene and polypropylene), presumably due to the plasticizing effect of the absorbed water through disruption of secondary bonds among polymeric chain segments like hydrogen bonding and van der Waals forces. Disruption of the weaker secondary linkages in fibers loosens and increases the mobility of their structure and results in a faster rate of stress decay under a fixed strain. The pH and electrolytes present in water and other immersion media will also affect stress decay, again to a greater degree with absorbable suture materials due to their greater hydrophilicity and pH-dependent degradation.

Stereoregularity of polymer chains affects their stress relaxation and since all fibers exhibit orientation due to their drawing, with not all fibers being drawn to the same degree of orientation, the extent of fiber drawing affects stress relaxation. The rate of stress decay of nylon 66 fibers immersed in distilled water, for example, decreased with increase in the extent of fiber drawing.[21]

These considerations clearly suggest that suture materials, which are drawn fibers, should exhibit stress relaxation effects. However, the propensity for suture materials to undergo stress relaxation[22,23] has received comparatively little attention, although such behavior may have a profound effect on surgical outcome. Typically, relaxation of a ligature could result in leakage from a vessel and consequent delayed hemorrhage; suture relaxation can, however, be beneficial to wound healing, as discussed in Chapter 2. Significant stress relaxation has been demonstrated for certain polymeric suture materials[22] and it was demonstrated, as expected, that the initial rate of stress decay was dependent upon the rate of extension, but the final (steady-state) residual load was independent of strain rate. Stress relaxation of a suture, when held under constant strain, results in a marked reduction in the load required to induce the applied strain. The residual stress levels, shown as percentage retained load, for three sutures subject to stress relaxation are shown in Figure 6.4.[24]

The underlying theory of viscoelasticity is complex, but a brief overview, together with the parallels that can be drawn with elastic behavior, might be useful. With an elastic body, stress is proportional to strain and the elastic modulus is given by the ratio of stress to strain; further, when an elastic body

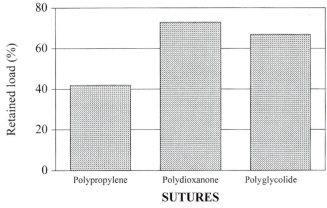

At 45 minutes

Figure 6.4 Residual stress of three sutures, polypropylene, polydioxanone, and polyglycolide under constant strain.

deforms under tensile loading, the axial extension and lateral contraction are related by Poisson's ratio ν. In contrast, for a viscoelastic material, both ν and the elastic modulus exhibit time dependence. It is possible, however, to show that under stress relaxation due to viscoelastic behavior, there is a tensile relaxation modulus, E(t), which may be determined by calculation of the ratio of the residual stress to the applied strain. Sophisticated equations can be derived to account for viscoelastic behavior using a variety of different models and, based on these theories, it is possible to determine relaxation constants for a viscoelastic material. It can be shown that if there is viscous flow under stress relaxation, the stress can decay to zero at sufficiently long times. However, in the absence of viscous flow, stress decays to a finite value and there is an equilibrium or relaxed modulus E_τ at infinite time. The transition time τ characterizes the time scale of viscoelastic behavior and the stress relaxation modulus E(t) will undergo a reduction of about 10^4 $N \cdot m^{-2}$ in the viscoelastic region, the midpoint of which is given by the characteristic time τ. It should be noted that the Boltzmann superposition principle states that strain in a specimen is a function of the entire loading history and that each loading step makes an independent contribution to the final deformation. Thus, the final deformation can be obtained by simple addition of each incremental strain and the total stress at any given time is determined by the sum of the products of the incremental strains and the stress relaxation moduli at each incremental time period. The significance of this in surgical suturing is that each phase of suturing can generate complex stress–strain relationships and, depending upon the characteristics of the suture, correspondingly complex stress relaxation behavior.

It is possible to predict stress relaxation behavior by calculation of the relaxation time spectrum from the measured stress relaxation modulus using Laplace or Fourier transform models. However, a more convenient approach is to perform dynamic mechanical measurements. Dynamic mechanical analysis (DMA), also known as dynamic mechanical spectroscopy (DMS), is now used increasingly for characterizing viscoelastic behavior. The basis of the technique is to subject the specimen to an alternating stress and simultaneously measure the strain. If a sinusoidal, time-carrying tensile force is applied to the test specimen, a small displacement is induced and if the force is applied in the form of a sine wave, the resultant strain is also a sine wave, so that both stress and strain vary sinusoidally.

For a polymeric fiber specimen under DMA, energy dissipation within the sample causes the sample strain to be out of phase with the applied force. Thus, due to the viscoelastic properties of the polymer, the maximum strain does not occur at the same instant as the maximum force. Using this methodology, it is possible to define the stress–strain relationship by a quantity E′ in phase with the stress and quantity E″, which is 90° out of phase with the applied stress,

$$\sigma/\varepsilon = E' - i \cdot E''$$

The real part of the modulus E′, in phase with the stress, is known as the tensile storage modulus and it defines the energy stored in the specimen due to the applied stress. E′ is a measure of the stiffness of the material and is the ratio of the applied stress to strain. The part of the modulus out of phase with the applied stress defines dissipation of energy, and is known as the loss modulus, E''. The loss modulus E'' indicates the ability of a material to dissipate mechanical energy through conversion into heat by molecular motion. Absorption of mechanical energy is often related to movement of molecular segments within the material, e.g., specific groups in the main polymeric chain or polymeric side groups. As the specific groups undergo rotation at a given temperature, a peak occurs in the loss modulus data due to absorption of the energy applied by the mechanical spectrometer. The phase angle, δ, is used to calculate the loss factor, tan δ, which is the ratio of the loss modulus to the elastic modulus (tan $\delta = E''/E'$), and since tan δ is the ratio of the viscous and elastic moduli, it is an index of material viscoelasticity.

DMA is usually performed over a range of temperatures and frequencies. A polymer that exhibits no flow will be rubberlike at low frequencies ($E' \approx 10^5$ Pa, independent of frequency) but is glassy at high frequencies ($E' \approx 10^9$ Pa, also independent of frequency). However, at intermediate frequencies, the polymer exhibits viscoelastic behavior and E' increases with increasing frequency and the rate of change in E' is indicative of the rate of stress relaxation. Complementarily, $E'' = 0$ at low and high frequencies since stress and strain are in phase for the rubbery and glassy states. However, at intermediate frequencies when the polymer is viscoelastic, E'' rises to a peak value at a point close to that at which there are the most rapid changes in E'. The loss factor (tan δ) also passes through a maximum although the tan δ peak is at a slightly lower frequency than the E'' peak since tan $\delta = E''/E'$ and E' is changing rapidly in this frequency range.

DMA allows the rapid and convenient determination of the viscoelastic properties of the sample by providing the major viscoelastic characteristics, namely the tensile storage modulus, E', the phase angle, δ, and the loss modulus, E''.

A recent study characterized the viscoelastic behavior of four suture materials (Prolene, Maxon, Vicryl, and silk) using DMA[23] and showed distinct differences in their viscoelastic constants. Typical DMA curves for Prolene, Maxon, Vicryl, and silk suture are shown in Figures 6.5 to 6.8 and the viscoelastic data for six suture materials are summarized in Table 6.4. The figures show the tensile storage modulus (E'), the loss modulus (E''), and tan δ as a function of the sample temperature. The DMA curve for Prolene (Figure 6.5) shows a number of transitions, namely the β relaxation at 2°C, the α transition (or T_g) at approximately 106°C and melting at 180°C. The β transition, associated with motions occurring within the amorphous regions of the polypropylene, occurs slightly below room temperature and, therefore, this transition should have a major impact on stress relaxation occurring at room or body temperatures. Further, the DMA curve indicates a pronounced change in modulus close to room temperature. The DMA curves for Maxon and Vicryl (Figures 6.6 and 6.7) are similar in appearance but quite different from that of Prolene. The change in modulus occurs at a temperature above room temperature for both materials while the main amorphous phase relaxation event for Vicryl, the T_g, occurs at 74°C although the T_g for Maxon is slightly below body temperature. This T_g value suggests that Maxon should exhibit relaxational behavior at room/body temperature, but such relaxation should not occur with Vicryl because it has a relatively flat modulus response near room temperature. Both materials exhibit subambient relaxation events at approximately –78 and –60°C, respectively. The DMA curve for silk, Figure 6.8, indicates that a change in the storage modulus and the glass transition (T_g at 221°C) only occurs at temperatures close to its decomposition temperature. However, silk has a relatively flat modulus response over a broad temperature range, indicating good handling characteristics.

The dynamic mechanical data obtained for Dexon[24] were similar to that of Vicryl with a β relaxation event at –55°C, the α transition at 72°C and melting at about 202°C (Table 6.4). The DMA data for PDS sutures[24] did not show a β relaxation event and the α transition occurred at 1°C with melting at about 140°C. This suture material has the lowest modulus of the materials tested and might be expected to exhibit "soft" characteristics at room temperature, which is above its T_g.

The relaxation processes occurring at room temperature can be established by performing frequency multiplexing studies in which the modulus data obtained at 25°C ± 50°C is shifted with respect to frequency (or time) to generate a master curve using time–temperature superposition. Figure 6.9 shows the master curves for Prolene, Maxon, Vicryl, and silk. Both Prolene and Maxon show a change in modulus with respect to frequency (or time, since frequency is the inverse of time) at a reference temperature of 25°C, which indicates a propensity for stress relaxation. The stress relaxation observed with Prolene was shown in Figure 6.4. In contrast, the frequency multiplexing data for silk and Vicryl show a very flat modulus response in the vicinity of 25°C, indicating that the modulus of both materials is very stable with respect to time or frequency at 25°C, with both materials having higher moduli than the others. The lower moduli for Prolene and Maxon demonstrated in the frequency multiplexing curves confirms the DMA data in Table 6.4.

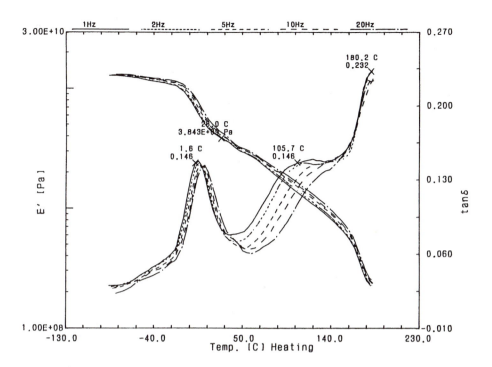

Figure 6.5 Dynamic mechanical analysis (DMA) for the polypropylene monofilament suture, Prolene. The lines correspond to different test frequencies as indicated at the top. (Reproduced from von Fraunhofer, J.A. and Sichina, W.J., *Biomaterials*, 13, 715, 1992. With permission.)

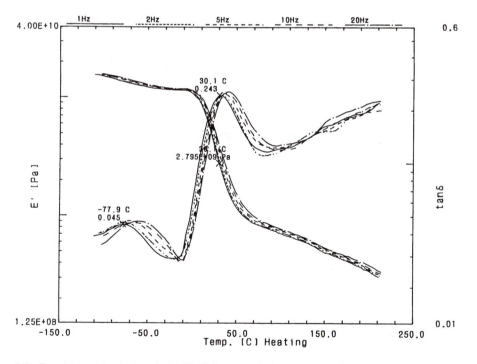

Figure 6.6 Dynamic mechanical analysis (DMA) for the polyglyconate monofilament suture, Maxon. The lines correspond to different test frequencies as indicated at the top. (Reproduced from von Fraunhofer, J.A. and Sichina, W.J., *Biomaterials*, 13, 715, 1992. With permission.)

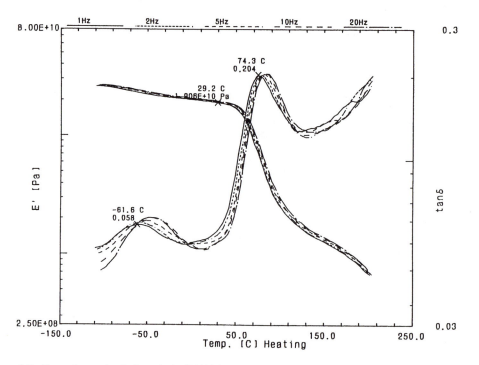

Figure 6.7 Dynamic mechanical analysis (DMA) for the poly(glycolide-L-lactide) multifilament suture, Vicryl. The lines correspond to different test frequencies as indicated at the top. (Reproduced from von Fraunhofer, J.A. and Sichina, W.J., *Biomaterials*, 13, 715, 1992. With permission.)

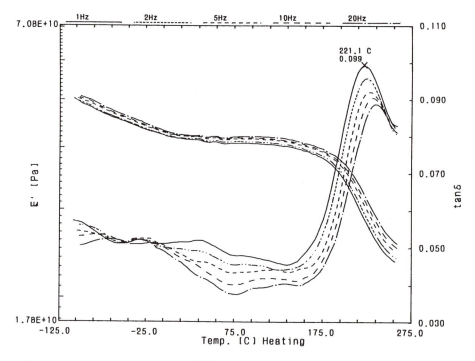

Figure 6.8 Dynamic mechanical analysis (DMA) for the silk multifilament suture. The lines correspond to different test frequencies as indicated at the top. (Reproduced from von Fraunhofer, J.A. and Sichina, W.J., *Biomaterials*, 13, 715, 1992. With permission.)

Table 6.4 Dynamic Mechanical Analysis Data for Sutures at 30°C

Suture	Storage Modulus, E′ (Pa)	Loss Modulus, E″ (MPa)	Tan δ (β transition) (°C)	Tan δ (α transition) (°C)
Dexon	3.9×10^9	3828	−55	72
Maxon	2.8×10^9	3846	−78	30
Prolene	4.4×10^9	1125	2	106
PDS	2.2×10^9	1225		1
Vicryl	2.0×10^{10}	2069	−65	68
Silk	4.0×10^9	3219	—	226

Data from von Fraunhofer, J.A. and Sichina, W.J., *Biomaterials*, 13, 715, 1992. With permission.

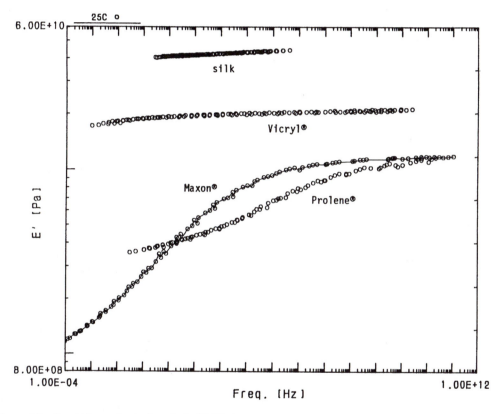

Figure 6.9 Dynamic mechanical analysis (DMA) frequency multiplexing (master) curves for Prolene, Maxon, Vicryl, and silk sutures. (Reproduction from von Fraunhofer, J.A. and Sichina, W.J., *Biomaterials*, 13, 715, 1992. With permission.)

As described in Chapter 4, the cross-sectional stress relaxation vs. time of sutures is closely related to the stability of a suture during knot tie-down and knot security, which depends on the degree of difference between static and dynamic resistance of sutures. Readers should refer to Chapter 4, Section V.B for a detailed description of the issue of cross-sectional stress relaxation.

IV. KNOT STRENGTH AND SECURITY

Sutures are used for two primary purposes, approximation of adjacent cut tissues and ligation (compression) of vessels. Both applications require knots to be tied in the suture so that a secure loop is formed. However, not only must the knot stay tied, i.e., be secure, but the amount of material in the wound must be kept as small as possible to limit foreign body reactions. Clearly then, surgical knots are important aspects of both surgical technique and clinical performance, and a substantial proportion of the total operation time is devoted to knot tying.[25] Nevertheless, it was claimed that many surgeons considered the tying of surgical knots to be more an art form than a science, while the selection of suture materials and suturing technique appeared to be based on tradition, guesswork, or habit.[26] These comments were made even before the introduction and widespread use of synthetic suture materials with their markedly different handling properties compared to those of traditional suture materials. It follows from this that if the selection of suture materials and suturing is based on "tradition, guesswork, or habit," then it is possible that the suture tying technique, particularly the knot construction, employed by many surgeons may not be optimal. For example, one study showed that many surgeons believe that they tie square knots when in fact they tie sliding knots in their sutures.[27]

Irrespective of the knot configuration and the suture material, the weakest link in the surgical suture is the knot and the second weakest point is the portion immediately adjacent to the knot. The strength reduction due to knotting can be as large as 35% to 95%.[27-30] Numerous wound dehiscences are due to either unraveling of the knot with slippage or suture breakage at the knot. This problem becomes more severe with the increasing availability of new, synthetic suture materials and of materials with silicone, poly(tetrafluoroethylene) or PTFE, and similar surface coatings. It has also been found that the tensile failure load of a suture material changes considerably with the suture gauge, knot type, and suturing pattern, particularly for a single loop suture.[31-33] These technique factors can effect up to a 10-times difference in strength.[34] Thus, knot strength and security play an important role in the successful use of sutures in surgery and wound healing.

Surgeons generally cannot use the same knot for every type of suture material. The type of knot used in a given surgical procedure is dictated, in part, by the suture material selected, as well as by the space and access limitations of the surgical site. The tensile properties of any given suture material will change, often markedly, with different knot configurations. Further, in any discussion of suture materials and surgical knots, it well known that a significant variable is the human factor; any given type of knot with a given suture material tied by different individuals, or even by the same person on different occasions, can vary greatly in tensile properties. Accordingly, it is necessary to define and classify surgical knots before the tensile properties of knotted sutures can be discussed.

A. DEFINITION AND CLASSIFICATION

A tied suture has three components, the loop, the knot, and the "tails" or "ears." The loop is created by the knot and performs the function of maintaining the wound edges in apposition or compressing the vessel in ligation. The knot is established by wrapping or twisting together two strands of suture, each wrap or twist being known as a "throw," with the knot being composed of a number of throws snugged against each other. The ears, the third component of the tied surgical suture, are the cut ends of the threads and must be of sufficient length to ensure that there is no loosening or untying of the loop through slippage.[35-37] Commonly, the ears are kept to 2–3 mm in length,[30,38-40] but this varies with the application; the ears might be less than 1 mm in length for buried sutures, but can be 5 to 10 mm in length with sutures that are to be removed subsequently.

A surgical knot, as defined by Taylor,[41] is the fastening made by entangling one or more cords or filaments, so that any tension on the fastening causes an increased contact pressure on the component parts of the knot. A knot stays tied due to the frictional force between the filaments comprising the knot so that both the strength and the security of the knot depend on the coefficient of friction of the suture material as well as on how the knot is tied. The frictional force between the suture threads within the knot is determined by the coefficient of friction of the suture material, the number of crossing points, the contact angle of the threads, as well as the normal forces maintaining contact between the threads.[40,42,43] The contact forces between the threads is determined, at least initially, by the tension applied during knot tying. It was believed that the coefficient of friction was characteristic of each suture material, independent of suture diameter and was linearly related to suture tensile strength and knot security.[40,43] It has been shown, however, that the coefficient of friction is not a material constant for suture materials, a result of their viscoelastic nature (see Section III), and in fact decreases exponentially with increase in applied force, with the rate of change in the coefficient varying with the material.[43] Braided (multifilament) suture materials exhibited higher values of the coefficient of friction and a slower decrease with increasing applied tension than monofilament sutures fabricated from the same material.[43] The significance of these frictional effects can be seen from the observation that multifilament sutures tend to slip less than monofilament sutures,[44] although the suture gauge, the method of tying, and the applied tension all were found to affect knot security.[36,37]

The ideal surgical knot is one that requires the least number of turns or throws to achieve high strength and security. However, as indicated above, small differences in tying technique or the arrangement and sequencing of the throws in a knot can effect a profound change in knot performance, notwithstanding the very wide variety of possible knotting regimens. Surgical knots fall into two categories, symmetric knots and asymmetric knots. Symmetric or flat knots are the familiar square (or reef), granny and surgeons' knots, while asymmetric knots are sliding knots characterized by an unequal distribution of friction between the suture strands within the knot and which are tied by holding one strand under constant tension while the other strand is wrapped around it.[27,35,44-46]

Since knots can vary widely in structure and appearance, it became necessary to establish a systematic classification and nomenclature protocol for describing the different knots for surgical use. The most widely accepted system is that proposed by Tera and Aberg,[28] shown in Figure 6.10. In this system, the Arabic number stands for the number of times the thread ends are twisted about each other, that is, the number of "turns," while the symbols "crossed" (x) or "parallel" (=) indicate how the throws are combined. The "=" symbol indicates that the threads enter and leave on the same side of the other thread, while the "x" symbol indicates that the two threads pass crosswise and are not on the same side, Figure 6.11. Accordingly, a square or reef knot is denoted by 1=1 and the granny knot is designated by 1x1. The surgeon's knot, which has a double turn on the first throw, is designated by 2=1 or 2x1, depending upon which way the threads pass over each other, as in the square (2=1) or granny (2x1) knot, while the double knot, with two turns on each throw, is denoted by 2=2 or 2x2, depending on the relationship between the threads within the knot. Both the number of throws and the throw combination, the "knotting regimen," significantly affect knot strength and stability.

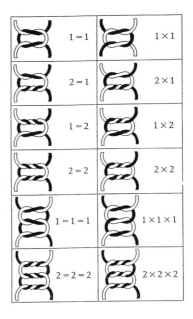

Figure 6.10 Knot classification system by Tera and Aberg. (Data from Tera, H. and Aberg, C., *Acta Chir. Scand.,142(1),* 1, 1976.)

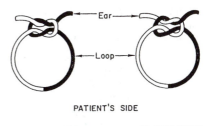

Figure 6.11 Components of tied sutures with either a square (1=1) or granny (1x1) knot configuration. (Reproduced from Batra, E.K. et al., *J. Emerg. Med.,* 10, 309, 1992. With permission.)

PHYSICIAN'S SIDE

Ear

Loop

PATIENT'S SIDE

SQUARE KNOT
l=l

GRANNY KNOT
lxl

124

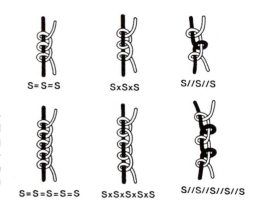

S=S=S   SxSxS   S//S//S

Figure 6.12 Configuration and code of the six different knots. S, sliding throws; =, identical throws around the same suture; X, nonidentical or crossed sliding throws around the same suture; //, sliding throws alternately tied around different sutures. (Reproduced from Trimbos, J.B., *Obstet. Gynecol.*, 64, 274, 1984. With permission.)

S=S=S=S=S   SxSxSxSxS   S//S//S//S//S

The Tera and Aberg classification system had to be modified subsequently to take into account sliding knots, when it became apparent that the clinical use of sliding knots was more common than first thought.[27,30,34,44-46] The conscious or unconscious preference of surgeons for sliding knots stems from the differences in the method of knot construction, notably holding one strand under tension while the second is wrapped around it when tying slip knots. In contrast, when tying a symmetrical knot, the surgeon has to cross either the hands or the suture threads in order to tie the knot. This manipulation has certain disadvantages as far as the surgeon is concerned, including (1) the unavoidable slackening of tension when crossing the hands or suture strands, with its attendant possibility of slippage of the first throw; (2) the loss of time and disruption of smooth hand movements necessitated by the crossing actions; and (3) tying of deep-seated suture loops or ligatures is simpler when one strand is held under tension during knot tying, which leads to the formation of a slip knot.[27,28,40] The designation system for sliding knots is similar to that for a symmetrical knot: S=S designates identical throws around the same suture, SXS indicates nonidentical or crossed throws, while S//S indicates sliding throws alternately tied around different strands.[27,34,45] These sliding knot configurations are shown in Figure 6.12.

B. KNOT EFFICIENCY

The presence of a knot within a thread reduces its tensile strength, a fact well known in textile science and mountaineering. This is clearly demonstrated by Table 6.5, which shows the effect of a simple overhand throw on the tensile failure loads (breaking forces) for several sutures.[33] The data clearly indicate that the presence of even the simplest of knots will reduce the tensile strength by 20% to 50%, a strength reduction found with both mono- and multifilament sutures, although the observed effects vary with the chemical composition, configuration, and gauge of the suture. This strength-reducing effect of knotting has to be taken into account when discussing the clinical use of suture materials since they are always knotted in surgical applications. In order to simplify the discussion of knotted sutures, it is useful to define certain terms.[27,28,34,44,45,47,48]

Knot failure: breakage of the knot or knot slippage that exceeds 2 mm.

Loop-holding capacity (LHC): the force required to break a tied suture loop or provoke slippage of over 2 mm within the knot; this parameter is also known as the knot strength.

Knot holding capacity (KHC): the force required to break the knot or cause it to slip; it is 50% of the loop-holding capacity since in tensile studies of loops, the applied force is divided equally between the two arms of the loop; this parameter may be used to compare loop-holding capacity with the breaking strength of the unknotted thread.

Knot efficiency: the knot-holding capacity of a suture expressed as a percentage of the breaking strength of the unknotted suture thread; this parameter is useful for comparing suture materials of different compositions, structures, and dimensions. A high average knot efficiency for a suture means that the type of knot used is not critical to the knot-holding capacity of the suture and comparable values of knot strength (loop-holding capacity) will be achieved with a wide variety of surgical knots. The corollary to this is that with a suture of low knot efficiency, the surgeon must be more selective in the type of knot that is used because both the strength and security of the suture are highly dependent on the knot type.

Table 6.5 Effect of a Single Knot On Suture Tensile Failure Load (kgf)

Suture/Gauge	USP 1	USP 1/0	USP 2/0
Nylon			
Straight	6.60	5.03	3.79
Knotted	4.06	2.94	2.08
% knotted/straight	61.52	58.45	54.88
Polybutester			
Straight	8.80	6.18	4.35
Knotted	4.93	3.41	2.57
% knotted/straight	56.02	55.18	59.08
Polyglyconate			
Straight	12.97	10.03	7.09
Knotted	7.82	6.96	4.41
% knotted/straight	60.29	69.39	62.20
Polypropylene			
Straight	7.01	4.54	3.37
Knotted	5.56	3.69	2.75
% knotted/straight	79.32	81.28	81.60

Data from von Fraunhofer, J.A., Storey, R.J., and Masterson, B.J., *Biomaterials*, 9, 324, 1988.

Table 6.6 Factors in Suture Knot Efficiency

Intrinsic Factors	Extrinsic Factors
Physical configuration of suture	Surgical knot characteristics
Chemical composition of suture	Suture gauge
Surface treatment/coating on suture	Tension applied during tying
Coefficient of friction of suture material	Number of throws in knot

In fact, there are both intrinsic (suture-dependent) and extrinsic (technique-related) determining factors in the knot holding capacity, i.e., the tensile strength, of a knotted suture and these factors are listed in Table 6.6.

Clearly the physical configuration of the suture (whether it is mono- or multifilament), its chemical composition and coefficient of friction, as well as any surface coating or treatment will affect knot efficiency since these factors are determinants of the frictional force between the suture threads, as discussed earlier. These factors are intrinsic to the suture material while the extrinsic factors, namely those imposed by the surgeon, include the gauge of the suture, the type of surgical knot, the tension applied during knot tying, and the number of throws incorporated into the knot. The effect of the number of throws, suture gauge, and suture material on loop-holding capacity may be seen from Figures 6.13 and 6.14.[49,50] These figures demonstrate that knot security is affected by the suture gauge, the number of throws within the knot, the type of knot, and the physical form of the suture for both monofilament and braided sutures. The effect of the various intrinsic and extrinsic factors on knot security are discussed in the next section.

C. KNOT SECURITY

Clearly it is essential for surgeons to tie knots in sutures that are secure and remain securely tied throughout the duration of the suture loop or ligature placement. The factors involved in obtaining a secure knot are indicated in Table 6.6. Many of these parameters, namely the intrinsic factors, are established by the surgeon when selecting the particular suture to be used, but the extrinsic factors, those related to technique, are established by the surgeon during use. The influence of tying technique, particularly the force applied during knotting, on knot security was clearly established in many studies. Greater knot security, for example, was found with flat knots (square, granny, and surgeon's) and asymmetric (slip) knots when a tension of 1500 g was applied to the suture loop ears than when they were tied loosely with a tension of 500 g.[46] Other studies on the influence of applied tension during knot

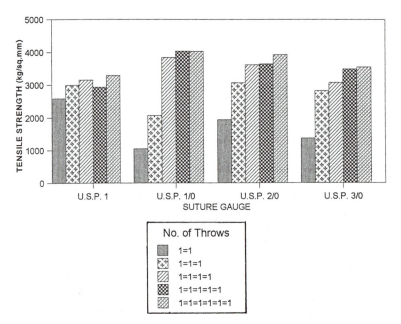

Figure 6.13 Effect of suture gauge and number of throws on tensile strength of coated chromic gut suture loops. (Reproduced from Stone, I.K. et al., *Am. J. Obstet. Gynecol.*, 151, 1087, 1985. With permission.)

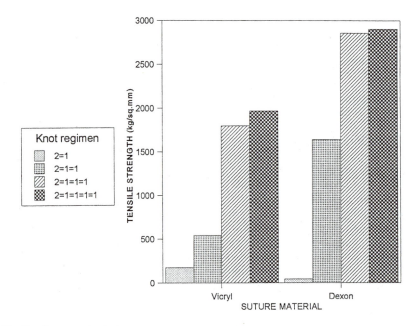

Figure 6.14 Tensile strength of 2/0 Dexon and Vicryl suture loops tied with different knot combinations. (Data from Stone, I.K. et al., *Surface Technol.*, 27, 287, 1986.)

tying have shown similar findings and a tension of 20% of the knot-holding force applied to each throw of the knot provided good knot security.[36,37] These latter studies also demonstrated that faulty technique is easily corrected by didactic information and psychomotor skill training so that in tensile studies, suture loops failed predominantly by breakage rather than slippage. The significance of the applied tension during knot tying follows from considerations of suture material viscoelasticity and the effect of this property on the interstrand friction within a knot which changes with applied tension.[43] The latter study showed that friction decreases with applied load for all types of suture but the decrease was exponential

Table 6.7 Knot Techniques Providing Optimal Knot Security (Knots Fail Predominantly by Breakage, not Slippage)

Suture Material	Form	USP Gauge	Flat Knots	Sliding Knots	Complex Knots	Ref.
Chromic gut	M	2/0, 3/0	1=1=1, 1x1x1, 2=1, 2=1=1, 2x2			31,44,46 50
Dermalon (nylon)	M	1	1=1=1, 2=1=1, 2=2, 2x2			47
Dexon (PGA, polyglycolide)	B	0, 1/0, 2/0, 3/0	1=1, 1=1=1, 2=1, 2=1=1, 2=2, 1x1x1	S=S=S, SxSxS S=S//S	1=1-S, 2=1-S, 1-S//S//S	27,30,34, 44-47,50
Ethilon (nylon)	M	1, 2/0	1=1=1, 2=1=1, 2=1=1=1, 2=2=1			46,47
Maxon (polyglyconate)	M	1, 0, 3/0	1=1=1, 1=1=1=1, 2=1, 2=1=1, 2=1=1=1, 2=2	SxSxSxS, SxSxSxSxS	1-S//S//S	30,44,46, 47
Mersilene (Polyester)	B	3/0	1=1=1, 2=1		1-S//S//S	44
PDS, PDSII (polydioxanone)	M	1, 2/0, 3/0	1=1=1, 1=1=1=1, 2=1=1, 2=2=1	SxSxSxS	SxSxSxS S//S//S	44,45,47 48
PTFE (polytetrafluoroethylene)	M	CV2-CV7	2=1=1=1, 3=1=3=2, 3=1=3=3			53
Prolene (Polypropylene)	M	1, 2/0, 3/0	1=1=1, 1=1=1=1, 2=1, 2=1=1, 2=2, 1x1x1	SxSxSxS	1-S//S//S	44-46,48
Vicryl	B	1, 0, 2/0, 3/0	1=1=1, 2=1, 2=2, 2=1=1, 2=1=1=1	S=S//S	1-S//S//S	44,46,47 51

Note: Form: M: monofilament suture, B: multifilament suture; flat knots: square (1=1), granny (1x1) and surgeon's (2=1); sliding knots: see Figure 6.12; asymmetric/mixed knots.

in form with monofilament and linear with multifilament sutures. Further work is undoubtedly necessary to evaluate the effect of suture throw tension on knot security, but it is clear that technique is one of the most important parameters in knot security.

Knot security appears to be a greater concern with monofilament sutures, which might be anticipated from the higher frictional values observed with multifilament sutures.[43] Accordingly, a variety of knotting techniques are employed to ensure security,[27,30,44-46,47,48] although it is not uncommon for a surgeon to try to improve knot security by selecting a larger gauge of suture material or simply adding extra throws. However, it should be noted that although knot reliability increases with the addition of an extra throw,[27,30,46,47,49,50] the extra throw has the corollary of increasing the knot volume and, consequently, the amount of foreign material in the wound.[51] The use of larger diameter sutures also increases knot security but there is a corresponding increase in knot volume. The increase in knot mass is 36% to 62% for two extra throws with 4/0 suture but the mass increase amounts to 343% to 550% when a 2/0 suture is used in place of a 4/0 size.[51] The greater suture knot mass due to the larger gauge and extra throws will result in a corresponding increase in the size of the inflammatory zone. Although the increase in the size of the inflammatory zone due to two additional throws was 3% to 90%, that arising from the change in suture gauge from 4/0 to 2/0 increased the volume of the tissue reaction sheath by 137% to 255%.[52] Thus, the total knot body is enlarged by a factor of 4 to 6 when suture size increased by a factor of 2, while two extra throws only increases knot mass by a factor of 1.5, with corresponding effects in the tissue reaction sheath. Clearly, adding extra throws to a knot is far preferable to using larger gauge sutures.

The chemical composition and physical conformation of the suture materials have a strong influence on their knot behavior and one knot configuration may provide adequate to good knot security with one suture material but be considered to be unsatisfactory with another material. Unfortunately, the rather limited number of studies on knot security in the literature makes it difficult to present a clear and coherent discussion of the subject. Further, most of these suture studies used different testing regimens so that comparing and contrasting the experimental data is not possible or could be misleading. Nevertheless, certain general statements can be made and these are expanded upon where the information is available.

Catgut (both plain and chromized) and stainless steel (mono- and multifilament) sutures exhibit the highest knot securities of any suture material and rarely exhibit slippage regardless of the knot configuration used. In contrast, coatings such as the silicone or poly(tetrafluoroethylene) used on silk and

Dacron® reduces knot security. Typically, Polydek® and Tevdek® (Teflon®-coated Dacron), Ti-Cron® (silicone-coated silk), and other coated suture materials exhibit lower knot securities than their lightly coated or uncoated counterparts.[52] Likewise, a glycerin-coated chromic gut was found to have a lower knot security than regular chromic gut.[49] These differences are believed to be due, at least in part, to a lower coefficient of friction which allows the knot to slip more easily although the coatings undoubtedly improve handling properties. As previously described in Chapter 4, Section IV, there are several new coating materials for sutures to improve their handling properties without detriment to knot security.

The surface characteristics of the suture material are contributing factors to knot security and materials with a slightly rougher surface, such as catgut and many multifilament sutures, may have superior knot security due to mechanical interlocking of the strands in each turn of the knot. However, even sutures with extremely low friction surfaces, such as the Gore-Tex suture, can be tied into a secure loop with appropriate selection of knotting technique.[53]

A further consideration in knot security is the moisture absorption capability of the suture material; in general, increasing moisture absorption decreases knot security due to the tendency of the sorbed fluid to permeate the suture material and swell the knot loose. This effect appears to outweigh any knot destabilizing effects due to the sorbed fluid reducing frictional forces. Catgut suture is a typical example of this effect since it is known that surface treatments alter the moisture absorption characteristics of the suture material, which in turn changes the knot security.

Numerous studies have demonstrated that knot security, for a given type of knot, increases with increasing numbers of throws in the knot but there is a limiting or maximum knot strength beyond which further throws have little or no effect.[27,30,39,45,46,51] The type of knot and the number of throws that provide maximum knot security vary with both the suture material and the suture gauge; the importance of the suture gauge in knot security was indicated previously.[30,39,51] Notwithstanding the above, projecting laboratory (in vitro) suture strength studies to the surgical (in vivo) arena requires caution, since careful study of surgical procedures indicated that many surgeons tied sliding knots rather than square knots as they thought.[27] Despite this, it is possible to provide some information on the optimal knotting techniques to ensure knot security and these data are summarized in Table 6.7.

It can be seen from this section that a number of factors impinge upon the use of suture materials in surgery and, in particular, the strength and security of surgical knots. Nevertheless, it is possible to achieve knot security with virtually every suture, provided sufficient care is taken with the knotting technique used and the manipulation of the suture threads during knotting. In this regard, it has been shown that knots used to start or end a continuous or running suture pattern are more susceptible to slippage than those used in a simple interrupted pattern, i.e., separate loops are less liable to slip than a running or mattress pattern of loops.[46]

V. SUMMARY

In this chapter the mechanical properties of sutures have been described and discussed. Tensile properties of sutures are discussed and attention is drawn to the differences in the stress-strain curves for the different suture materials. The role of tensile properties in the selection of sutures for surgical use, and the need to match these characteristics to those of the target tissues, has been covered. Comparing the stiffness of different sutures indicates the problems associated with tying small loops in stiff fibers and the limitations on using high modulus sutures as monofilaments. Sutures, being drawn fibers, are subject to stress relaxation and it is shown that marked stress relaxation can occur with these materials. Further, dynamic mechanical analyses of sutures demonstrate the differences in viscoelastic properties of sutures and the significance of these in the stress decay behavior of sutures. Knotting of sutures effects a reduction in the tensile strength but the type of knot and the number of throws will determine the apparent strength of the knotted suture. Although a number of factors determine the security of knotted sutures, it is possible to achieve a secure knot with any suture by selection of the appropriate knotting regimen.

REFERENCES

1. Chu, C.C., Mechanical properties of suture materials: an important characterization, *Ann. Surg.*, 193, 365, 1981.
2. Holmlund, E.W., Physical properties of surgical suture materials: stress-strain relationship, stress relaxation and irreversible elongation, *Ann. Surg.*, 184, 189, 1976.
3. Taylor, T.L., Suture materials: a comprehensive review of the literature, *J. Am. Podiatry Assoc.*, 65, 649, 1975.

4. Chu, C.C., Survey of clinically important wound closure biomaterials, in *Biocompatible Polymers, Metals, and Composites*, Szycher, M., Ed., Technomic Publishing, Lancaster, PA, 1983, 477.

5. Holmlund, D., Tera, H., Wiberg, Y., Zederfeldt, B., and Aberg, C., *Sutures and Techniques for Wound Closure*, Medical and Surgical Publication, New York, 1978.

6. Everett, W.G., Suture materials in general surgery, *Progr. Surg.*, 8, 14, 1970.

7. Edlich, R.F., Panek, P.H., Rodeheaver, G.T. et al., Physical and chemical configuration of sutures in the development of surgical infection, *Ann. Surg.*, 177, 679, 1973.

8. Chu, C.C. and Kizil, Z., Quantitative evaluation of stiffness of commercial suture materials, *Surg. Gynecol. Obstet.*, 168, 233, 1989.

9. Teledyne Taber V-5 Stiffness Tester Instruction Manual, N. Tonawanda, New York, 1979, 13.

10. Leblanc, K.A. and Russo, V.R., Clinical experience with Gore-Tex suture, *J. La. State Med. Soc.*, 138, 39, 1986.

11. Bezwada, R.S., Jamiolkowski, D.D., Erneta, M., Persivale, J., Trenka-Benthin, S., Lee, I.Y., Suryadevara, J., Yang, A., Agarwal, V., and Liu, S., Monocryl suture, a new ultra-pliable absorbable monofilament suture, *Biomaterials*, 16, 1141, 1995.

12. Ray, J.A., Doddi, N., Regula, D. et al., Polydioxanone (PDS), a novel monofilament synthetic absorbable suture, *Surg. Gynecol. Obstet.*, 153, 497, 1981.

13. Rodeheaver, G.T., Borzelleca, D.C., Thacker, J.G., and Edlich, R.F., Unique performance characteristics of Novafil, *Surg. Gynecol. Obstet.*, 164, 230, 1987.

14. Scott, G.V. and Robbin, C.R., Stiffness of human hair fibers, *J. Soc. Cosmet. Chem.*, 29, 469, 1978.

15. Chu, C.C., Stress relaxation of synthetic sutures, in *Advances in Biomaterials*, Vol. 3, Winter, G.D., Gibbons, D.F., and Plenk, H., Eds., John Wiley & Sons, New York, 1982, 655.

16. Morton, W.E. and Hearle, J.W.S., *Physical Properties of Textile Fibres*, John Wiley & Sons, New York, 1975.

17. Feughelman, M., The mechanical properties of fibres and fibre thermodynamics, in *Applied Fibre Science*, Vol. 1, Happey, F., Ed., Academic Press, New York, 1978, 50.

18. Meredith, R. and Hus, B.S., Stress relaxation in Nylon and Terelyene: influence of strain, temperature and humidity, *J. Polym. Sci.*, 61, 253, 1962.

19. Dunell, B.A. and Dillon, J.H., The measurement of dynamic modulus and energy losses in single textile filaments subjected to forced longitudinal vibration, *Textile Res. J.*, 21, 393, 1951.

20. Meredith, R., Relaxation of stress in stretched cellulose fibre, *J. Textile Inst.*, 45, T438, 1954.

21. Lemiszka, T. and Whitwell, J.C., Stress relaxation of fibers as a means of interpreting physical and chemical structure, *Textile Res. J.*, 25, 947, 1955.

22. Metz, S.A., von Fraunhofer, J.A., and Masterson, B.J., Stress relaxation of organic suture materials, *Biomaterials*, 11, 197, 1990.

23. Von Fraunhofer, J.A. and Sichina, W.J., Characterization of surgical suture materials using dynamic mechanical analysis, *Biomaterials*, 13, 715, 1992.

24. Von Fraunhofer, J.A., unpublished data.

25. Tera, H. and Aberg, C., Strengths of knots in surgery in relation to the type of knot, type of suture material and dimension of suture thread, *Acta Chir. Scand.*, 143, 75, 1977.

26. Haxton, H., The influence of suture materials and methods on the healing of abdominal wounds, *Br. J. Surg.*, 52, 372, 1965.

27. Trimbos, J.B., Security of various knots commonly used in surgical practice, *Obstet. Gynecol.*, 64, 274, 1984.

28. Tera, H. and Aberg, C., Tensile strength of 12 types of knot employed in surgery, using different suture materials, *Acta Chir. Scand.*, 142, 1, 1976.

29. Rodeheaver, G.T., Thacker, J.G., and Edlich, R.F., Mechanical performance of polyglycolic acid and polyglactin-910 synthetic absorbable sutures, *Surg. Gynecol. Obstet.*, 153, 835, 1981.

30. Van Rijssel, E.J.C., Trimbos, J.B., and Booster, M.H., Mechanical performance of square knots and sliding knots in surgery: a comparative study, *Am. J. Obstet. Gynecol.*, 162, 93, 1990.

31. Holmlund, D., Tera, H., Wiberg, Y., Zederfeldt, B., and Aberg, C., *Sutures and Techniques for Wound Closure*, Naimark and Barba, New York, 1978.

32. Von Fraunhofer, J.A., Storey, R.J., Stone, I.K., and Masterson, B.J., The tensile strength of suture materials, *J. Biomed. Mater. Res.*, 19, 595, 1985.

33. Von Fraunhofer, J.A., Storey, R.J., and Masterson, B.J., Tensile properties of suture materials, *Biomaterials*, 9, 324, 1988.

34. Trimbos, J.B. and Klopper, P.J., Knot security of synthetic absorbable suture material: a comparison of polyglycolic acid and polyglactin-910, *Eur. J. Obstet. Gynecol. Reprod. Biol.*, 19, 183, 1985.

35. Thacker, J.G., Rodeheaver, G.T., and Moore, J.W., Mechanical performance of surgical sutures, *Am. J. Surg.*, 130, 374, 1975.

36. Batra, E.K., Franz, D.A., Towler, M.A., Rodeheaver, G.T., Thacker, J.G., Zimmer, C.A., and Edlich, R.F., Influence of emergency physician's tying technique on knot security, *J. Emerg. Med.*, 10, 309, 1992.

37. Batra, E.K., Franz, D.A., Towler, M.A., Rodeheaver, G.T., Thacker, J.G., Zimmer, C.A., and Edlich, R.F., Influence of surgeon's tying technique on knot security, *J. Appl. Biomater.*, 4, 241, 1993.

38. Stone, I.K., von Fraunhofer, J.A., and Masterson, B.J., A comparative study of suture materials: chromic gut and chromic gut treated with glycerin, *Am. J. Obstet. Gynecol.*, 151, 1087, 1985.

39. Stone, I.K., von Fraunhofer, J.A., and Masterson, B.J., Knot stability and tensile strength of an absorbable suture material, *Surface Technol.*, 27, 287, 1986.
40. Herrmann, J.B., Tensile strength and knot security of surgical suture materials, *Am. Surg.*, 37, 209, 1971.
41. Taylor, F.W., Surgical knots and sutures, *Surgery*, 107, 498, 1938.
42. Gupta, B.S. and Prosthlethwait, R.W., An analysis of surgical knot security in sutures, in *Biomaterials*, Winter, G.D., Gibbons, D.F., and Plenk, H., Jr., Eds., John Wiley & Sons, New York, 1982, 661.
43. Gupta, B.S., Wolf, K.W., and Prosthlethwait, R.W., Effect of suture material and construction on frictional properties of sutures, *Surg. Gynecol. Obstet.*, 161, 12, 1985.
44. Brouwers, J.E., Oosting, H., de Haas, D., and Klopper, P.J., Dynamic loading of surgical knots, *Surg. Gynecol. Obstet.*, 173, 443, 1991.
45. Trimbos, J.B., van Rijssel, E.J.C., and Klopper, P.J., Performance of sliding knots in monofilament and multifilament suture materials, *Obstet. Gynecol.*, 68, 425, 1986.
46. Rosin, E. and Robinson, G.M., Knot security of suture materials, *Vet. Surg.*, 18, 269, 1989.
47. Brown, R.P., Knotting technique and suture materials, *Br. J. Surg.*, 79, 399, 1992.
48. Trimbos, J.B., Booster, M.H., and Peters, A.A., Mechanical knot performance of a new generation polydioxanone suture (PDS-2), *Acta Obstet. Gynecol. Scand.*, 70, 157, 1991.
49. Stone, I.K., von Fraunhofer, J.A., and Masterson, B.J., A comparative study of suture materials: chromic gut and chromic gut treated with glycerin, *Am. J. Obstet. Gynecol.*, 151, 1087, 1985.
50. Stone, I.K., von Fraunhofer, J.A., and Masterson, B.J., Mechanical properties of coated absorbable multifilament suture materials, *Obstet. Gynecol.*, 67, 737, 1986.
51. Van Rijssel, E.J.C., Brand, A., Admiraal, C., Smit, I., and Trimbos, J.B., Tissue reaction and surgical knots: the effect of suture size, knot configuration, and knot volume, *Obstet. Gynecol.*, 74, 64, 1989.
52. Magilligan, D.J. and DeWeese, J.A., Knot security and synthetic suture materials, *Am. J. Surg.*, 127, 355, 1974.
53. Hertweck, S.P., von Fraunhofer, J.A., and Masterson, B.J., Tensile characteristics of PTFE sutures, *Biomaterials*, 9, 457, 1988.

Chapter 7

Biodegradation Properties

C. C. Chu

CONTENTS

Because suture materials stay either temporarily or permanently inside the body, they are subjected to various types and degrees of biodegradation, particularly in view of the hostile environment of the body. Due to the breakdown of molecules, suture materials often lose their original tensile strength and mass with time. The retention of their tensile strength and the rate of tensile strength loss are vital factors in their usefulness in wound healing. For noncritical surgical conditions, such as small vessel ligature or the coaptation of uncomplicated wounds in rapidly healing tissues, the rate of loss of tensile strength is probably of little importance. For more critical surgical wounds, however, the difference in the rate of loss of tensile strength may be highly significant, particularly in tissues slow to heal, such as tendons and ligaments, and for those with neoplasia, hypoproteinemia, diabetes, etc. In a few situations, suture materials must retain strength for the lifetime of the patient, e.g., an artificial heart valve sutured to the heart. Since the loss of tensile strength of a suture material depends on the animal species, type of tissue, size of suture material, and the testing condition, the reported data vary considerably. In this chapter, the general degradation mechanisms and factors that contribute to the biodegradation of both absorbable and nonabsorbable sutures will be described in detail. In addition, the effect of the recently reported laser assisted fibrinogen bonding techniques on the degradation of suture materials will also be discussed at the end of this chapter.

I. GENERAL BIODEGRADATION PHENOMENA

Although there are many ways in which polymeric materials can be degraded, such as thermal, oxidation, ultraviolet (UV), and mechanical, the degradation of suture materials is mainly through hydrolysis with or without enzymes. However, other modes like UV and oxidation may also play some roles in reported clinical cases of failed sutures in certain physiological environments, like ophthalmology. Whether by hydrolysis or other modes, when a polymer degrades, the backbone macromolecules are broken and their chain length decreases with the duration of degradation. As a result, their physical, mechanical, thermal, and morphological properties change.

There are two basic modes of chain scission: random and terminal (unzipping). The rate of structure and property changes with degradation largely depend on the type of chain scission. Random chain scission indicates that the probability of chain scission at any point of a macromolecule is the same as any other location of the macromolecule. This type of random main-chain scission would usually occur in synthetic polymers with ester or amide linkage and has the most detrimental effect on the physical and mechanical properties of polymers. All synthetic absorbable sutures degrade through this mode of simple hydrolytic random main-chain scission. However, as described later, the morphology of suture materials would also determine the mode of hydrolytic degradation. In the crystalline domains of suture materials, the terminal or unzipping mode of chain scission appears to be more appropriate than random scission. There are no reported data to determine whether absorbable sutures of biological origin, like catgut or reconstituted collagen, degrade through either random or terminal attack of biopolymers by enzymes.

Although degradation of absorbable sutures is their inherent property, the degradation of nonabsorbable sutures is considered undesirable. It is known that silk, nylon, and polypropylene sutures have shown clinically evident degradation in a variety of tissues. It is believed that both random and terminal chain scissions would operate in these nonabsorbable sutures.

There are three most important properties used to describe degradation phenomena of suture materials. They are the loss of tensile strength profile, the loss of mass profile, and the type of degradation products released into surrounding tissues. It is important to recognize that the profile of strength loss always proceeds before the profile of mass or weight loss in sutures because of both the inherent dependence of fiber strength on tie-chain segments in the noncrystalline domains of fibers and the two-stage hydrolytic degradation observed in all semicrystalline fibers. The hydrolytic degradation is known to start in the amorphous regions and then extend to the crystalline domains due to the inability of water molecules to penetrate into the tightly packed crystalline domains. This two-stage hydrolytic degradation mechanism results in distinctive patterns of changes in molecular weight, strength, mass, diameter, level of crystallinity, crystallite size, fiber orientation, and surface and interior morphology. As described later, the hydrolytic scissions of tie-chain segments located in the amorphous regions would be reflected in the observed loss of tensile properties, while the mass loss must come from the destruction of the crystalline domains.

Since most degradation of absorbable sutures is of a hydrolytic nature, the ability of water molecules to penetrate into the sutures determines whether the degradation process proceeds via surface, bulk, or both modes. Bulk hydrolytic degradation would result in a fast loss of tensile strength within a short period of time, while the surface mode of degradation would retain tensile strength for a longer period than the bulk mode. Evidence available so far indicates that absorbable sutures degrade hydrolytically through the bulk mode, while some nonabsorbable sutures, like the polyester- and polyamide-based sutures, degrade through the surface mode.

In this chapter, general information on the mode of chain scission, bulk vs. surface degradation, the reported changes in physical, mechanical, thermal, and chemical properties of sutures upon degradation, and finally those intrinsic and extrinsic factors that have been experimentally determined to affect suture degradation will be described. It is the authors' hope that this chapter will provide readers with the most up-to-date, comprehensive, and systematic understanding of how, what, and why suture materials degrade.

A. RANDOM CHAIN SCISSION VS. DEPOLYMERIZATION

Because hydrolysis of linear polymers results in the cleavage of bonds in the main backbone chains, the mode of bond cleavage certainly influences the changes of chemical, physical, mechanical, and biological properties of the polymers. The two types of bond cleavage in all types of polymer degradations are depolymerization (or unzipping) and random chain scission. The former, essentially the reverse of an addition polymerization, consists of initiation (usually at chain ends), depropagation, and termination stages. The degradation products are essentially the monomers which are repeatedly and consecutively removed from the chain ends during the degradation process. Depolymerization degradation is characterized by a rapid increase in monomer concentration, but the reduction of mechanical and physical properties is not evident at the early stage of degradation. On the contrary, random chain scission occurs purely on a statistical basis and without any preferential site of the chain. Random chain scission is characterized by an early drastic decrease in mechanical properties and molecular weight, but the concentration of end groups increases linearly with time.

Is the hydrolytic degradation of most important synthetic biomedical polymers containing ester or amide linkage of random chain scission or depolymerization nature? Evidence reported in the literature points in favor of random chain scission.[1,2] According to Kuhn's statistic method of random chain scission,[3] the concentration of end groups should be linearly proportional to the duration of degradation as indicated below:

$$N_t - N_o = kt \tag{1}$$

where N_t is the end group concentration at time t; N_o is the end group concentration at time 0; and k is a rate constant.

Equation 1 was derived by assuming all bonds are equally probable toward hydrolysis and are independent of their positions in the chain and the length of the chain. When Equation 1 was applied to both polyesters and polyamides, it was found that both polymers underwent random chain hydrolytic scission.[1] The number of end groups increased linearly with time according to Equation 1. Although the hydrolytic cleavage of amide linkages in linear polyamides is of random nature, it was reported that where the amide groups are located in a cyclic ring, however, they do not appear to hydrolyze randomly.[4] Moiseev et al.[5] and Zaikov[6] found that the hydrolytic cleavage of ester linkages depended on the equilibrium water sorption in the polymer, $C_{H_2O}^o$.

In the case of those biomedical polymers used in thin form (e.g., sutures, tissue adhesives), $C_{H_2O}^o$ can be expected to be reached rapidly and the hydrolysis could occur homogeneously (i.e., within the bulk of the polymer.) Table 7.1 summarizes the diffusion, sorption, and rate constants of some common medical polymers.[5,6] A comparison between polyglycolide (PGA) and poly(ethylene terephthalate) (PET) indicates that, although their diffusion coefficients are in the same order (10^{-9}), their $C_{H_2O}^o$ values are very different from each other (about fivefold difference). On the basis of these parameters, Zaikov et al.[6,7] calculated that there was only a 10^{-3} fraction of hydrolytically sensitive ester bonds in PET cleaved in a 10-year period at 37°C in distilled water. This amount of chain scission is equivalent to 5% loss of molecular weight which, practically, should have no effect on its mechanical properties. On the other hand, the molecular mass of PGA was found to change significantly within a few weeks of immersion in distilled water at 37°C and a much faster loss of tensile strength was observed.

However, Lin et al. have recently postulated that although random chain scissions occur mainly in the amorphous domains of the suture fibers, the scissions of chain segments located in the crystalline regions follow the stepwise manner.[8] This is because the crystalline regions are not permeable to water; hydrolysis of chain segments must occur only at the end of the chain segments located at the end of crystallite (001 and 002 faces that interface with the already hydrolyzed amorphous regions) and propagates sequentially along the crystalline axis into the interior of the crystallites. This one-dimensional stepwise hydrolytic fragmentation (similar to depolymerization) of chain segments in the crystalline regions is thus slower than the three-dimensional random hydrolytic attack of chain segments located in the amorphous regions.

Table 7.1 Diffusion, Sorption, and Hydrolytic Rate Constants of Common Biomedical Polymers at 37°C

Polymer	Level of Crystallinity	D (cm²/s)	$C^\circ_{H_2O}$ (g/C)	$K_{H_2O} C^\circ_{H_2O}$ (m)	$K_{H_2O} C_o$ (min⁻¹ × cm³ × g)	ΔE (kcal/mol)
Polyglycolide	80	$(5 \pm 1) \times 10^{-9}$	0.40 ± 0.03	9×10^{-4}	3.5×10^{-5}	—
Poly(glycolide lactide)	—	—	—	1.5×10^{-3}	1×10^{-4}	—
Polycaproamide	40	$(3 \pm 0.5) \times 10^{-9}$	0.15 ± 0.02	1×10^{-10}	4.0×10^{-10}	20
Polydodecanamide	50	—	0.04	4×10^{-11}	1×10^{-10}	—
Poly(ethylene terephthalate)	40	$(1.5 \pm 0.5) \times 10^{-9}$	0.005	1×10^{-10}	2×10^{-8}	25
Polyethylene	60–70	$(2.3 \pm 0.5) \times 10^{-7}$	2×10^{-4}	—	—	—
Polypropylene	80	$(2.4 \pm 0.5) \times 10^{-7}$	3×10^{-4}	—	—	—
Polycarbonate	Amorphous	$(1.0 \pm 0.2) \times 10^{-7}$	0.004	3.3×10^{-6a}	1×10^{-8}	23
Polydimethyl siloxane	Amorphous	$(7 \pm 1) \times 10^{-9}$	7×10^{-4}	—	—	14

[a] At 70°C. See text for symbols.

From Zaikov, G.E., *J. Macromol. Sci. Rev. Macromol. Chem. Phys.*, 25(4): 551, 1985. With permission.

B. MACROKINETICS OF SURFACE AND BULK HYDROLYSIS

On the basis of the relative magnitudes of equilibrium water sorption and diffusion coefficients, hydrolytic degradation of water-insoluble polymers can be grouped into two broad categories: surface and bulk modes. Their corresponding degradation macrokinetics in the living environment have been proposed by Moiseev et al.[5]

In the surface mode, due to the very low water diffusion coefficient and equilibrium water sorption of the polymer (e.g., PET and polycaproamide), hydrolysis is largely limited to a thin surface layer of the material. The rate of degradation is expressed in Equation 2.

$$dn/dt = K^s(C_p^s \ C_{cat}^s/Z)S \tag{2}$$

where n is the number of scissions of hydrolytically sensitive bonds; t is time; S is the polymer surface area; K^s is the rate constant in hydrolytically sensitive bonds located on the surface of the polymer; C_p^s is the surface concentration of hydrolytically sensitive bonds of the polymer; C_{cat}^s is the concentration of the catalyzing agent on the surface of the polymer; and Z depends on macromolecular packing, cohesive energy of the degradation products in a given medium, and the type of degradation (hydrolysis here).

If the polymer is in a cylindrical fibrous form, as in the case of sutures, the changes of fiber radius (r) and mass (m) with time upon surface hydrolysis with a constant concentration of catalytic agent but without surface roughing, which would increase surface area, could be described by the two equations below:[5]

$$r = r_o - K_{obs}^s \ t/\rho \tag{3}$$

$$m^{1/2} = m_o^{1/2} - K_{obs}^s \ (\pi l/\rho^{1/2})t \tag{4}$$

where $K_{obs}^o = K^s C_p^s \ C_{cat}^s/Z$; r_o is the initial radius; m_o the initial mass; l, fiber length; and ρ, polymer density. As we shall discuss later, the pH of the medium was also found to affect the mode of hydrolysis (i.e., surface vs. bulk).

Because all synthetic absorbable sutures are water-insoluble polymers, water molecules must be able to reach the vicinity of the susceptible ester linkages of the chain molecules for the hydrolysis to occur. This indicates that the role of diffusion becomes an important parameter in determining the rate and extent of hydrolysis. Many investigators have addressed the issue of diffusion and its role as the rate-determining step. Unfortunately, the results were often conflicting.[2] Based on the assumption that water diffusion into a polymer is the rate-determining step, Golike and Lasoski[9] derived a theoretical equation for the kinetics of polymer hydrolysis.

$$kCt = C_o k - (k \ C_o l^2 \ /3) \ (kA/D) \tag{5}$$

where k is the rate constant for chain scission; C_o represents water concentration at the polymer surface; C, effective water concentration [(initial number of water molecules in polymer/moles of polymer) − (number of molecules of ester links hydrolyzed/moles of polymer)]; A is the initial number of ester links per mole of polymer; D, the diffusion coefficient; l is half of a film thickness; t, time. Equation 5 indicates that an increase in thickness, l, would result in a slower rate of hydrolysis. The agreement between Golike and Lasoski's experimental data and the equation led them to conclude that the hydrolysis of PET is diffusion controlled. Their conclusion, however, was challenged by others.[10] In addition to the incorrect mathematic approximation in Golike and Lasoski's study, Davies et al.[10] also pointed out that the diffusion rate of water into PET was found to be 10^3 greater than the hydrolytic reaction. The latter, therefore, should not be diffusion controlled. Thus, Davies et al. attributed the observed slower rate of hydrolysis to other parameters, and the diffusion rate of water into a polymer appears not to be the rate-determining step. The kinetic equations of bulk hydrolysis have been shown to be quite complicated and are not described here.[8]

II. BIODEGRADATION PROPERTIES OF NATURAL ABSORBABLE SUTURES

Numerous studies have demonstrated that the degradation and absorption of catgut sutures is due mainly to the proteolytic enzymes of phagocytes and other cells. Cellular collagenase and proteases eventually degrade and remove catgut and reconstituted collagen sutures. Collagen sutures contain less noncollagenous protein than catgut, but they exhibit mechanisms of degradation and absorption similar to those of catgut sutures. The two most frequent complains about collagen-based absorbable sutures are their characteristic of a very rapid loss of strength during the most critical period of wound healing (i.e., the first week postoperation) and higher than average tissue reactions.

Salthouse et al. used enzyme histochemistry to examine the degradation and absorption of these sutures by implanting the sutures into the gluteal muscles of female Long-Evans rats.[11] It was found that acid hydrolytic activities, as indicated by the acid phosphatase reaction, was present at the suture sites from 1 to 70 d after implantation, with the highest activity found between 4 and 56 d after implantation. Proteolytic activity characterized by the leucine aminopeptidase reaction was barely detectable during the first 4 d, but it increased to a peak of high intensity at 14 d and thereafter. The onset of a loss of tensile strength and the absorption of materials coincided with the activities of these two enzymes, as shown in Figure 7.1. Macrophages at the sites of inflammation were the most enzymatically active cells.

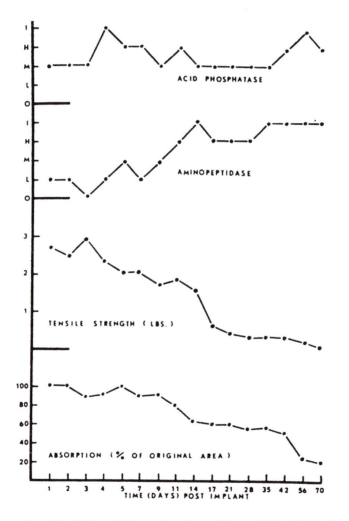

Figure 7.1 A comparison of acid phosphatase and aminopeptidase activity with tensile strength loss and absorption of 3/0 collagen suture. Acid phosphatase activity, denoting the hydrolytic enzyme response, is the highest during the first week of implantation, with a later surge of activity when absorption is nearly complete. Aminopeptidase activity is low during the first week, rises to a peak at 2 weeks, and remains high during absorption. Activity was judged visually to an arbitrary scale: 0, no activity; L, trace; M, moderate; H, increased; and I, intense activity. (From Salthouse, T. N. et al., *Surg. Gynecol. Obstet.*, 129(4), 691, 1969. With permission.)

The acid hydrolytic and proteolytic activities of the macrophages were not restricted to the interiors of the cells. The interstitial fluid exhibited a similar enzymatic activity resulting from a leakage of enzymes from the macrophages during phagocytosis. This extracellular activity, present during the later stages of suture absorption, is believed to be associated with the degradation and digestion of catgut and collagen sutures.

By application of the same enzyme histochemical procedures, Salthouse et al. also examined catgut suture absorption in rabbit cornea, sclera, and ocular muscles. When compared to gluteal muscle, the cornea sites showed predominately alkaline phosphatase activity and more rapid absorption, whereas the scleral sites provided variable results. The findings in ocular muscles were similar to those with gluteal muscle sutures. The study, however, failed to demonstrate a collagenolytic enzyme activity at any point in the degradation process.

Thus, the degradation of these natural absorbable suture materials is a twofold mechanism: (1) the cleavage of the peptide linkage by the acid hydrolytic and collagenolytic activities, evident in a loss of tensile strength; and (2) the absorption and digestion of the cleaved fragments by the proteolytic enzymes during the later stage of degradation.

Jenkins et al. have proposed a similar degradation mechanism at the tissue level for catgut sutures.[12] There are two phases. The first phase, digestion by polymorphonuclear leukocytes, begins about 12 h after implantation and reaches a maximum in 3 d. The second phase, a gradual removal of the suture mass by foreign body giant cells and macrophages, begins at the 7th to 10th day and persists until absorption is complete.

The kinetics of the degradation and absorption of plain and chromic catgut sutures in both *in vitro* enzymatic solutions and *in vivo* were recently reported by Okada et al.[13] They concluded that both plain and chromic catgut sutures exhibited a surface (or heterogeneous) hydrolytic degradation in the presence of *in vitro* enzymatic solutions like collagenase and pepsin due to their large molecular size prohibiting them from entering catgut easily, while the same sutures show bulk (or homogeneous) hydrolytic degradation in the presence of nonenzyme solution. Okada et al., however, reported that both enzymatic and nonenzymatic hydrolyses occurred concurrently in the *in vivo* subcutaneous tissues. Collagenase has a molecular weight of about 109,000 which is big enough not to be diffused into the interior of the catgut suture. The surface-controlled enzymatic hydrolytic degradation of catgut suture is based on a linear relationship between the rate of weight loss and duration of hydrolysis. In other words, the rate of weight loss should be linearly proportional to the total surface area of a suture, as described by Equation 6.[14]

$$(W_t / W_o)^{1/2} = 1 - K(t/r_o d_o) \qquad (6)$$

where W_t = weight of suture at time t; W_o = original weight of suture at time 0; t is the time of hydrolysis; r_o, radius of suture at t = 0; d_o, density of suture at t = 0; and K, rate constant.

Figure 7.2 illustrates such a linear relationship. The initial stage of degradation of both plain and chromic catgut sutures followed the linear relationship with some deviations from the linearity toward the later stage of degradation. The deviation from linearity at the late stage of degradation indicated that catgut sutures lost their weight faster than should result from surface degradation. Chromic catgut retained the linearity longer than plain catgut sutures. It is believed that at the late stage, defects or pores were generated on the surface of catgut sutures, which were large enough to permit the diffusion of enzymes into the interior of the catgut suture to conduct bulk degradation. Thus, a combination of both surface and bulk degradation occurred at the late stage of degradation of catgut sutures; however, the initial stage of degradation was strictly a surface degradation.

Surface degradation of catgut sutures should also lead to a continuous reduction in suture diameter, and theoretically the weight loss profile should coincide with the tensile strength loss profile. However, as shown in Figure 7.3, the profile of tensile strength loss was always faster than the profile of weight loss for both plain and chromic catgut sutures and the difference between the two profiles became larger at longer durations of degradation. One of the possible causes was the generation of molecular defects which had a more profound effect on tensile strength than suture weight. The larger difference between the two profiles observed at a longer duration of degradation must be attributed to a combination of both surface and bulk degradation, since the latter (bulk degradation) has a more detrimental effect on strength loss than the former (surface degradation). As discussed later, therefore, the largest difference between these two profiles would be observed in bulk degradation as found in synthetic absorbable sutures, while the smallest difference should be associated with surface degradation, with a mixed mode (surface + bulk degradation) between the two extreme modes.

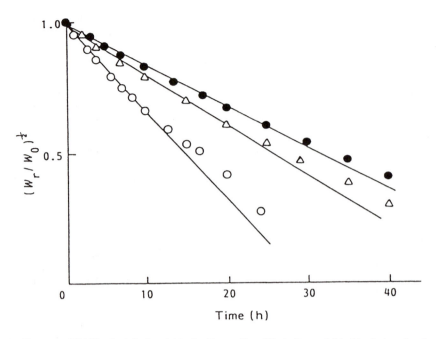

Figure 7.2 The ratio (W_t/W_o) of original weight of collagen fiber, W_o, to the weight of hydrolyzed collagen fiber at time t, W_n as a function of collagenase digestion time. (○) plain 2/0 catgut; (△) 20 plain catgut; (●) 20 chromic catgut. (From Okada, T. et al., *Biomaterials*, 13(7), 448, 1992. With permission.)

The reduction in chromic catgut diameter reported by Okada et al.,[13] however, was contradictory to Walton's reported study of absorbable sutures in joint tissues.[15] Walton observed a significant thickening of 2/0 chromic gut suture (original diameter 0.396 ± 0.008 mm) after 1 week in either the articular cavity (0.513 ± 0.010 mm), muscle (0.509 ± 0.004 mm), or within synovial tissue (0.591 ± 0.026 mm) of ewes, due to absorption of body fluids. A possible cause for the conflicting diameter data is due to the means of measurement of the suture diameter. Walton used an optical microscope, and the chromic catgut sutures were not pretreated by a dehydration process before diameter measurement, which is required for scanning electron microscopic measurement of diameter (used by Okada et al.). The dehydration process under vacuum would reduce swelling of the suture and hence a reduction in suture diameter.

The well-defined surface degradation of catgut sutures *in vitro*, however, became less obvious in *in vivo* rabbit subdermal tissue degradation of catgut sutures. As shown in Figure 7.4, Okada et al. reported that there was a larger difference between weight and strength loss profiles *in vivo* than *in vitro*. The degradation profiles *in vivo* fell between pure *in vitro* degradation without enzyme (bulk degradation mode) and *in vitro* with enzyme (surface degradation mode). In other words, mixed surface (enzymatic) and bulk (nonenzymatic) degradation modes occurred in *in vivo* degradation of catgut sutures. Consequently, Okada et al. suggested that *in vivo* degradation of catgut sutures occurred in three steps: (1) cleavages of secondary bonds like hydrogen bonds and van der Waal's forces through initial hydration, (2) an initial loss of suture mass through further main chain scissions, and (3) subsequent accelerated suture mass loss due to the dissolution of low-molecular-weight fragments and phagocytosis of small fragments.[13] They also determined that the average concentration of enzymes in the subdermal tissue of rabbits was equivalent to 2.5 µg/ml of collagenase.

A linear relationship between suture weight and collagenase concentration was also found in catgut suture degradation. $V_{1/2}$, defined as the reciprocal of the degradation time required for the suture to lose one half of its original weight, increased linearly with collagenase concentration, implying that the rate of degradation of catgut sutures followed first-order kinetics with respect to enzyme concentration as other polypeptides.[16]

The degradation and absorption of collagen-based suture material, according to some authors, appear to be irregular and less predictable.[17,18] Katz and Turner showed that catgut sutures exhibit a varied pattern of absorption in New Zealand rabbits.[18] Irrespective of the size of the suture, however, traces of

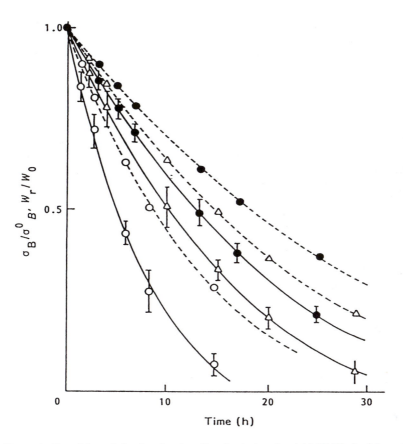

Figure 7.3 The reduction of the relative tensile strength, σ/σ_B (—) and weight, W_r/W_o, (----) for catgut sutures hydrolyzed in phosphate-buffered saline at 37°C and pH 7.4 as a function of collagenase ([E_o] = 250 µg/ml) digestion time. (○) 2/0 plain catgut; (△) 20 plain catgut; (●) 20 chromic catgut. (From Okada, T. et al., *Biomaterials*, 13(7), 448, 1992. With permission.)

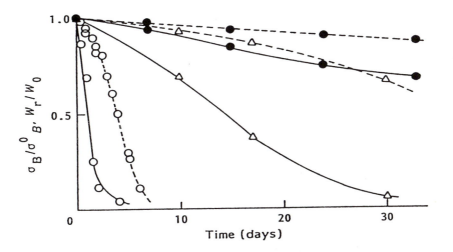

Figure 7.4 Decrease of the relative tensile strength σ/σ_B (—) and weight W_r/W_o (---) for 20 plain catgut suture as a function of incubation time under different conditions. (●) 0.1 *M* PBS at pH 7.4 and 37°C; (△) implanted in the back of rabbit; (○) 0.5% weight NaCl aqueous solution at pH 1.6 and 37°C. (From Okada, T. et al., *Biomaterials*, 13(7), 448, 1992. With permission.)

catgut suture fragments were observed after 75 d of implantation only in isolated instances. Catgut sutures lost most of their strength (70% to 80%) during the first 7 d after implantation.[18]

Since the degradation of catgut and collagen sutures is influenced by proteolytic enzymes, they might be expected to lose strength more rapidly when exposed to organs containing enzymes such as gastrointestinal tract fluids. Evidence of this has been reported by several investigators. Postlethwait et al. showed that 3/0 chromic catgut sutures, when placed within the lumen of the stomach, duodenum, ileum, and colon of rats and dogs, did not retain adequate strength beyond 48 h.[19] In rats, the loss of strength was 12% to 46% of the original value and was most profound in the ileum. Everett implanted chromic catgut in baboons and reported that only about 20% of the original strength of the sutures remained in the colon after 5 d, and nearly no strength was found in the ileum after 2 d.[20] Everett suggested that the rapid degradation of catgut sutures in the colon is due to infection and to the vascularity of the tissue. Howes reported that plain and chromic catgut sutures reached zero strength after 12 and 36 h, respectively, in dogs' stomachs.[21]

These *in vivo* studies of the accelerated degradation of natural absorbable sutures, when exposed to alimentary tract fluids, are consistent with *in vitro* and *in vivo* studies. Jenkins and Hrdina observed that plain catgut sutures were digested in an average time of 11 h, and chromic catgut sutures in excess of 20 h, in HCl and pepsin solution.[22] Okada also found that an accelerated loss of catgut suture mass and strength was found in a pH 1.6 aqueous solution (0.5% by weight NaCl) with a variety of concentrations of pepsin enzyme and the rate of weight loss depended on the concentration of pepsin.[13] Mizuma et al. tested the loop-breaking strength of various sutures in saline, canine serum, bile, and activated and nonactivated pancreatic juice, and found that both plain and chromic catgut sutures disintegrated almost completely within 24 and 48 h, respectively, in enterokinase-activated pancreatic juice (i.e., trypsinogen was activated into trypsin).[23] In an effort to explore the mechanism of degradation of the catgut sutures, the same authors used trypsin inhibitors, such as aprotinin and soybeans, to examine the rate of loss of loop strength of the sutures. It was found that these trypsin inhibitors did not protect the sutures from degradation.[23] This suggests that trypsin may not be the major enzyme responsible for the degradation of catgut sutures.

In addition to the simple presence of proteolytic enzymes, the accelerated degradation of catgut sutures in the gastrointestinal tract can also be attributed to other factors, such as the pH level of the fluid. Chu and Moncrief recently reported the effects of pH on the *in vitro* degradation of both absorbable and nonabsorbable sutures.[24,25] After 7 d, plain 2-0 catgut sutures lost a significant degree of tensile strength in both acidic (37% of strength remained at pH = 3.0) and alkaline (20% remained at pH = 10.0) conditions, while sutures maintained at the physiological pH level retained more strength (61% remained at pH = 7.4). Table 7.2 illustrates these results. In discussing clinical implications, Postlethwait et al.[19] pointed out that the early premature loss of suture strength in the alimentary tract might be disastrous in certain situations, such as the transfixion of a bleeding ulcer.[19] Okada et al.[13] suggested that the accelerated degradation of catgut sutures was a bulk instead of surface phenomenon, as illustrated in Figure 7.5. The difference in the reductions of both weight and strength profiles of both plain and chromic catgut sutures in 0.5% by weight of NaCl aqueous solution of pH 1.6 (without enzymes) became significantly larger than the same sutures with enzymes (Figure 7.4). Surface morphological observations of the lack of change in catgut suture diameter also supported this bulk degradation in the aqueous media without enzyme.

Chromic catgut suture has long been considered as the gold standard for open bladder surgery because of its low morbidity.[26] The function of a suture is to carry physiological force for the wound before the wound gains enough strength to sustain the force. The healing of urinary bladder wounds is essentially complete after 2 weeks and normal bladder strength would be achieved by the third week.[27–29] Thus, the ideal suture for bladder surgery should be able to retain adequate strength during the first week postoperation and should not elicit urinary stone formation. In a comparison with modern synthetic absorbable sutures like polydioxanone (PDS) and Vicryl in rat bladders, Stewart et al. found that there were no significant differences between chromic catgut and PDS and Vicryl sutures in the degree of inflammation, urine pH, and calculogenic potential at the end of 6 months; however, chromic catgut degraded the most. Only 40% of rats had microscopic presence of the suture, while PDS and Vicryl sutures had 80% and 90% of rats with microscopic presence of sutures.[26] Similar findings of very rapid loss of catgut suture strength during the first week postoperation were reported by Cohen et al. in their evaluation of 3/0 chromic surgical catgut in the urinary bladder and subcutaneous tissue of beagle dogs.[30] They reported that chromic catgut lost more than 90% of its original tensile breaking force (0.60 lbs) in bladder at the end of 7 d postoperation. However, catgut sutures appeared not to exhibit this initial rapid loss of strength

Table 7.2 Percent Retention of Tensile Breaking Strength and Elongation at Break of 2/0 Size Suture Materials at Various pH Levels after 7 d and 28 d

	Day	Breaking strength retention (%)			Breaking elongation (%)		
		pH 3.0	pH 7.4	pH 10.0	pH 3.0	pH 7.4	pH 10.0
Plain catgut	7	37	61	20	175	132	42
	28	0	0	0	0	0	0
Dexon®	7	96	91	20	93	91	68
	28	0	0	0	0	0	0
Vicryl®	7	93	95	40	114	106	116
	28	0	0	0	0	0	0
Silk	7	88	87	73	150	164	143
	28	72	81	42	117	146	75
Mersilene®	7	99	101	98	104	103	104
	28	98	99	98	123	115	120
Nurolon®	7	72	77	67	94	99	103
	28	66	72	65	96	102	105
Ethilon®	7	104	102	105	104	100	112
	28	96	96	100	98	98	103
Prolene®	7	97	103	102	95	102	120
	28	103	103	106	111	109	105

From Chu, C.C. and Moncrief, G., *Ann. Surg.*, 198, 223, 1983. With permission.

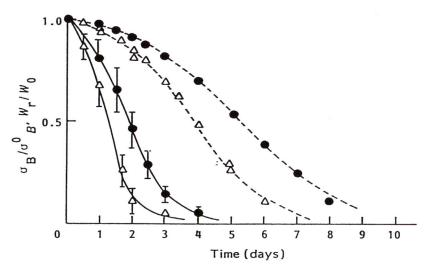

Figure 7.5 Decrease of the relative tensile strength σ/σ_B (—) and weight W_r/W_o (---) for catgut sutures hydrolyzed in 0.5 wt% NaCl aqueous solution at 37°C and pH 1.6 without enzyme as a function of incubation time. (△) 20 plain catgut; (●) 20 chromic catgut. (From Okada, T. et al., *Biomaterials*, 13(7), 448, 1992. With permission.)

after 7 d. Instead, the suture had 22% of its original strength at 14 d and retained 16% of its original strength at 21 d. Cohen et al. also found that the same chromic catgut sutures retained their original strength far better in subcutis (e.g., 41% retention at 7 d) than in bladder (e.g., 10% retention at 7 d) during the first 14 d postoperation.[30] Gorham et al. examined 3/0 plain and chromic catgut sutures in sterile human and rabbit urine with pH ranging from as low as 5.57 to as high as 8.7 *in vitro*.[31] They found that both plain and chromic catgut sutures retained from a low 57% to a high 97% of original tensile breaking strength (TBS) in human urine at the end of 3 weeks *in vitro*, while the same sutures retained slightly lower tensile strength in rabbit urine (69% to 79%) at the end of the same period.

Bartone et al. examined the long-term (130 d) biodegradation and tissue responses to catgut and collagen sutures in a variety of wounded and unwounded organs, including bladder, kidney, liver, and muscle of guinea pigs.[32] They found that both catgut and reconstituted collagen sutures, whether plain

Table 7.3 The Percentage of Each Catgut Suture Type that Remained in the Nonwounded (Series 1) and Wounded (Series 2) Implantation Sites of Various Tissues of Adult Guinea Pigs at Various Periods

| | | 70–85 d | | 100–115 d | | 130 d | | |
| | | Series 1 | Series 2 | Series 1 | Series 2 | Series 1 | Series 2 | Total Retained |
Suture	Tissue							
Plain catgut	Kidney	100	67	100	50	50	50	
	Bladder	100	33	100	50	100	75	71.1
Chromic catgut	Kidney	100	75	75	75	50	50	
	Bladder	100	67	33	100	100	100	78.4
Plain collagen	Kidney	67	83	100	67	100	100	
	Bladder	100	83	100	100	100	100	90.2
Chromic collagen	Kidney	100	100	67	50	100	100	
	Bladder	100	100	100	100	100	100	93.3
Plain catgut	Liver	100	33	50	100	100	67	
	Muscle	67	33	67	75	50	100	72.2
Chromic catgut	Liver	100	100	75	50	100	100	
	Muscle	100	100	75	100	50	50	84.2
Plain collagen	Liver	100	100	100	67	100	100	
	Muscle	100	100	100	100	100	100	97.5
Chromic collagen	Liver	100	100	100	100	100	100	
	Muscle	100	100	100	100	100	100	100.0

From Bartone, F.F. et al., *Invest. Urol.*, 13(6), 390, 1976. With permission.

or chromic, showed a minimal amount of degradation at the end of 130 d with reconstituted collagen sutures showing more resistance to absorption than catgut. As shown in Table 7.3, irrespective of the type of organ, the wounded organs showed faster degradation and absorption of plain catgut and collagen sutures than the same sutures in the corresponding unwounded tissue. Both chromic catgut and collagen sutures, however, showed similar levels of absorption between wounded and unwounded tissues. This indicates that inflammatory reaction is chiefly responsible for the degradation of collagen-based sutures, presumably due to proteolytic enzymic degradation of this class of absorbable sutures. Except in the kidney, there was little difference in the rate of absorption in the tissues examined. Chromic collagen sutures did not show any detectable absorption in muscle and bladder during the whole period of 130 d.

Chromic catgut, however, was found to be unsuitable for fascial closure in rats, in which it lost most of its original tensile strength at the end of 10 d postimplantation (65% loss) and exhibited no measurable strength at 28 d postimplantation.[33] Figure 7.6 illustrates the tensile strength of chromic catgut and other synthetic absorbable sutures used in fascial closure in Sprague Dawley male rats.

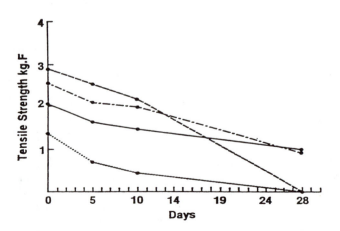

Figure 7.6 Tensile strength at day 0, 5, 10, and 28 for chromic catgut (---), Vicryl (dashed line), Maxon (dot-dashed line), and PDS (solid line) sutures. (From Sanz, L.E. et al., *Obstet. Gynecol.*, 71(3), 418, 1988. With permission.)

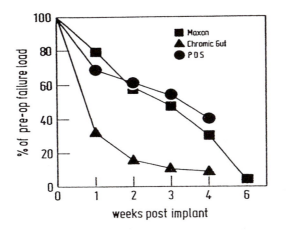

Figure 7.7 Retention of failure load after implantation of three absorbable suture materials in synovial tissue. (▲) Chromic catgut; (●) PDS; (■) Maxon. (From Walton, M., *Clin. Orthop. Relat. Res.*, 242, 303, 1989. With permission.)

The degradation of natural absorbable sutures is also found to be influenced by bacteria. Williams showed that in *in vivo* implantation, plain catgut sutures exhibited a greater degree of degradation (about 14% more) in *Staphylococcus albus* inoculated sites (at $3.8 \times 10^7/0.1$ ml bacterial count) than in noninfected sites in rats.[34] The bacterial effect, however, was insignificant at a lower level of bacterial concentration.

In a series of *in vitro* tests, Sebeseri et al. reported that 3/0 plain catgut sutures dissolved after 1 week of exposure to *Escherichia coli*-infected urine, while about 19% of the suture strength remained in sterile urine solution.[35] Vasselli and Bennett also reported similar findings that catgut lost 50% of its original tensile strength in *E. coli*-infected urine at 7 d.[36] This bacterial effect is consistent with the widespread clinical experience that catgut sutures are degraded more rapidly if a wound is infected.[37] The exact reason for such a rapid degradation is not known. Peacock and Van Winkle attribute this phenomenon to the presence of a large number of inflammatory cells, which increases the concentration of proteolytic enzymes.[37] Conflicting results about the performance of catgut suture in infected urine, however, were reported. El-Mahrouky et al. reported that *E. coli*- and *Proteus*-infected urine resulted in only 8% and 5.8% knot (2=1=1) strength loss of chromic catgut at the end of 10 d *in vitro* incubation.[38] They also found that chromic catgut sutures gained 27% and 4.5% of tensile strength at the end of 10 d immersion in sterile plasma and sterile urine, respectively. It is not clear whether the presence of knots was responsible for the discrepancy between the data from El-Mahrouky et al. and others.

Does the characteristic of a very rapid loss of strength of catgut sutures during the first week postoperation, as observed in other tissues, hold for joint tissues? This issue is important because of the current trend toward early postoperative remobilization after surgery, which imposes physiologic loads upon tissues and hence may accelerate the degradation of catgut sutures. Walton's study of 2/0 chromic catgut sutures in joint tissues of ewes confirms that the same characteristic of degradation of catgut sutures (chromic or plain) observed in other tissues is held in joint tissue, as shown in Figure 7.7.[15] More than 70% of the original tensile breaking force of chromic catgut was lost in synovial tissue during the first week postimplantation. Again, the loss of tensile breaking load slowed down after 2 weeks, with very little further loss observed between 2 and 4 weeks. Walton also found the degradation of chromic catgut in the relatively acellular tissue like synovial fluid was quite different from those highly inflamed adjacent tissues. For example, the portion of chromic catgut suture exposed to the synovial fluid was relatively well preserved, while the same suture embedded in the adjacent cellular tissues had largely disappeared at the end of 4 weeks. This further demonstrates that the previously described mechanism of catgut degradation *in vivo* is through cellular action like phagocytes rather than pure hydrolysis by water as observed in synthetic absorbable sutures.

All the degradation phenomena of catgut sutures described above assume that a normal wound healing process would proceed, i.e., inflammatory reactions occur in wounded tissues. These inflammatory reactions would certainly affect the biodegradation phenomena of absorbable sutures through increasing enzymatic activities associated with inflammatory cells. Will the biodegradation of catgut sutures in nonhealing tissue (hence the lack of inflammatory reaction) be the same as those in normal healing

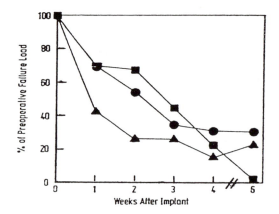

Figure 7.8 Retention of *in vivo* failure load of three absorbable sutures in nonhealing joint tissue. (▲) Chromic catgut; (●) PDS; (■) Maxon. (From Walton, M., *Clin. Orthop. Relat. Res.*, 267, 294, 1991. With permission.)

tissue? Walton recently examined such a scenario by a local application of a steroid like corticosteroid to a synovial incision in the knee of sheep to impede an inflammatory reaction, and hence the normal wound healing.[39] Walton found that although the same characteristic of rapid loss of catgut suture strength during the first week postoperation as reported in normal healing wounds was observed in nonhealing (i.e., noninflammatory) synovial tissue of sheep, the level of strength loss during this initial first week period in the nonhealing synovial tissue was far less than the same suture in the synovial tissue when normal healing was permitted. Figure 7.8 illustrates the percent retention of tensile breaking force of chromic catgut, PDS, and Maxon sutures in nonhealing synovial tissue. In the lack of inflammatory reaction, chromic catgut sutures also retained their strength (above 20%) with insignificant loss from the second to the fifth week postoperation. Gross fragmentation of chromic catgut sutures in corticosteroid-treated wound healing was also far less frequently observed than the comparable healing wound. As a result, the retrieval of chromic catgut sutures in a nonhealing wound was far easier than the same suture in a normal healing wound. Obviously, the lack of macrophage in the corticosteroid-treated wound tissue due to the lack of inflammatory reaction was responsible for the observed better retention of chromic catgut sutures.

In Chapter 5, *Chemical Structure and Manufacturing Processes*, a new type of chromic catgut suture with glycerin coating was mentioned. Does the glycerin coating affect the biodegradation of chromic catgut suture? Stone et al. reported that there was a marked difference in the loss of knot tensile breaking load in the rectus muscle of rats between glycerin-coated and noncoated chromic catgut sutures, as shown in Figure 7.9.[40] The glycerin-treated chromic catgut sutures were initially (nonimplanted) weaker than untreated ones and their strength retentions at 7 and 14 d postimplantation were subsequently lower than the untreated one when a 1=1=1 knot configuration was used for both sutures. The glycerin-treated chromic catgut required 1=1=1=1=1 knot configuration to exhibit the same strength loss pattern as untreated chromic catgut with 1=1=1 knot configuration. The failure of glycerin-treated chromic catgut was by knot slippage, while the untreated chromic catgut failed by breakage at the knot. It thus appeared that glycerin-treated chromic catgut sutures may require additional throws in knotting to provide adequate knot security and knot strength retention *in vivo*. Glycerin-treated chromic catgut sutures, however, elicited the same degree of inflammatory reaction as chromic catgut at 7 d postimplantation.

III. BIODEGRADATION PROPERTIES OF SYNTHETIC ABSORBABLE SUTURES

A. MOLECULAR WEIGHT

The molecular weight of these suture fibers decreased drastically with duration of hydrolysis. Figure 7.10 summarizes the *in vitro* reduction in intrinsic viscosity, [η], in hexafluoroisopropanol of three common synthetic absorbable sutures with time of hydrolysis.[41] The difference in chemical structure on hydrolytic degradation is evident. By 7 d of hydrolysis, about 50% of [η] of Dexon sutures was lost, while Vicryl suture retained 67% of its original [η]. This reported Vicryl data paralleled a study by Fredericks et al. in which they reported 22% of the original inherent viscosity was retained at the end of 35 d of *in vitro*.[42] Maxon sutures show considerable slower reduction in molecular weight than both Dexon and Vicryl.

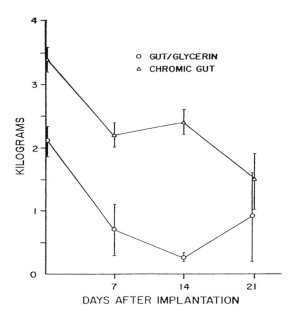

Figure 7.9 Effect of glycerin coating on the implanted fracture load of catgut sutures with 1=1=1 knot configuration. (○) glycerin-coated gut; (△) chromic gut. (From Stone, I.K. et al., *Am. J. Obstet. Gynecol.*, 151 (8), 1087, 1985. With permission.)

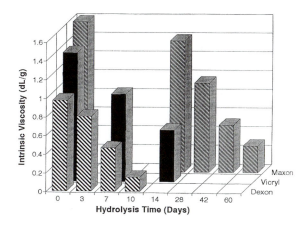

Figure 7.10 Intrinsic viscosity (dl/g) of 2/0 size synthetic absorbable sutures at various durations *in vitro* immersed in phosphate buffers of pH 7.4 at 37°C.

There was no significant reduction in [η] of Maxon before 14 d and it would take more than 28 d of hydrolysis to reach 50% reduction in [η]. The reduction in molecular weight in *in vivo* condition has been reported to be similar to that in an *in vitro* environment. Ray et al. reported that PDS sutures lost about 50% of their original molecular weight at the end of 28 d implantation in the gluteal muscles of rats and these *in vivo* data were parallel to *in vitro* data.[43] Gilding found that *in vivo* degradation of Dexon suture results in a graduate reduction in the high-molecular-weight species and the appearance of low-molecular-weight oligomeric fractions, as demonstrated in the changes in molecular weight distribution (Figure 7.11).[44]

B. MECHANICAL PROPERTIES AND MASS LOSS

Along with the loss of molecular weight, the tensile properties and mass of the absorbable sutures also decrease with hydrolysis time. As shown in Table 7.4, Dexon and Vicryl sutures, in general, have been found to exhibit an insignificant amount of tensile strength after 28 d of implantation or *in vitro*

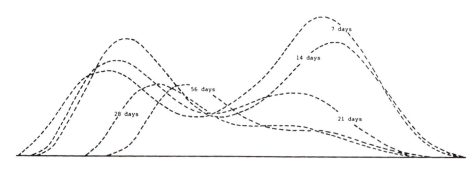

Figure 7.11 Molecular weight distribution of Dexon sutures after various implantation periods in rat. (From Gilding, D.K., in *Biocompatibility of Clinical Implant Materials*, Vol. 2, Williams, D.F., Ed., CRC Press, Boca Raton, FL, 1981, chap. 9. With permission.)

Table 7.4 Absorption Delay of Commercial Synthetic Absorbable Sutures

Suture Materials	Time to Complete Loss of Tensile Strength (d)	Time to Complete Mass Absorption (d)	Absorption Delay (d)	Useful Lifetime[a] (%)
Dexon®	28	50–140	22–112	20–56
Vicryl®	28	90	62	31
PDS®	63	180–240	117–170	26–35
Maxon®	56	210	155	27
Monocryl®	21	90-119	69–98	18–23

[a] The ratio of [the time to complete loss of tensile strength] to [the time to complete mass absorption]. The higher the percentage, the more absorbable the suture.

immersion, while the majority of their mass is still present in tissue for various periods.[45–48] The observed significant delay in mass degradation is a universal phenomenon for all synthetic absorbable sutures. Although the rates of tensile strength and mass loss depend on the hydrolytic environment, such as the type of animals, the site of implantation, the type of buffer, and pH, it appears that more variations in mass loss data than tensile strength loss data have been reported because of the difference in environmental conditions. Craig et al. reported that Dexon sutures were still present in the intramuscular site of rat at 120 d.[45] This is about 45 to 70 d longer than Katz et al. reported.[18] Postlethwait[46] found that Dexon sutures exhibited no tensile strength after 28 d in New Zealand rabbits, while more than 95% to 98% of suture remained at the same period, and close to complete absorption did not occur until about 140 d which is comparable to data from Craig et al.[45]

It appears that *in vitro* conditions promote a faster hydrolytic degradation than the *in vivo* environment. Figures 7.12 and 7.13 summarize the percents of retention of mass and TBS of synthetic absorbable sutures *in vitro* in phosphate buffer of pH 7.4 at 37.5°C.[18,41,48] Dexon sutures exhibited the largest weight loss between 14 and 21 d *in vitro* and reached 50% weight retention at the end of 21 d, while it would take the same suture about 70 d in the intramuscular site of rats to reach 50% weight loss. The same pattern occurs in Vicryl sutures, which, in the *in vitro* environment shows 54% weight loss at 42 d,[41] while in the *in vivo* environment Vicryl sutures exhibit no change in weight at the same duration of hydrolysis.[45] Due to the different types of buffer and pH, there are some discrepancies among different *in vitro* studies. For example, Fredericks et al.[42] reported that almost all of Vicryl suture mass was lost at the end of 42 d (pH = 7.25 sodium phosphate buffer at 37.5°C), while Zhang et al. reported that there was still about 20% weight remaining at the end of 60 d.[41] Reed and Gilding reported that most of Dexon suture strength was lost over the 14- to 28-d period *in vitro* (37°C at pH = 7.0), while the mass of the suture remained unchanged during the same period, and the mass loss began in the fourth week and was completed by 70 to 84 d.[47] The mass loss of Dexon sutures in the *in vivo* environment would not be completed until about 90 d.

One of the most recently commercially available synthetic monofilament sutures, Monocryl, had the shortest retention of tensile breaking strength among the five synthetic absorbable sutures, i.e., a

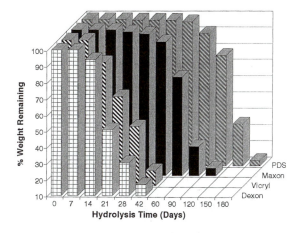

Figure 7.12 Weight loss profiles of four synthetic absorbable sutures *in vitro* in phosphate buffer, pH 7.44, at 37°C.

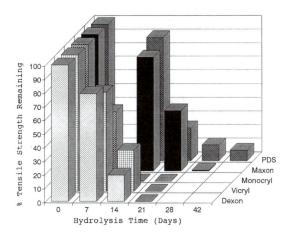

Figure 7.13 Tensile breaking strength remaining of five synthetic absorbable sutures *in vitro* in phosphate buffer, pH 7.44, at 37°C.

negligible amount of strength remained (0.15%) at 21 d. The absorption of Monocryl mass *in vivo* (female Long-Evans rats), however, was not complete until 91 to 119 d postimplantation.[49] The other most recently commercially available synthetic monofilament absorbable suture, Biosyn® from US Surgical,[49a] retains about 82, 66, 37, and 8% of its original tensile breaking strength at 7, 14, 21, and 28 days *in vitro* as shown in Table 7.5.

PDS and Maxon sutures, however, exhibited much longer tensile strength and mass retention than Dexon, Vicryl, Monocryl, and Biosyn sutures. In general, PDS sutures retain their TBS longer than Maxon sutures in both *in vitro* and *in vivo* environments.[33,50,52,53] However, such differences in the rate of TBS retention between PDS and Maxon appear not to be reflected in the healing quality of wound tissue. Foresman et al. reported that there is no significant difference in the wound strength of a variety of tissues (i.e., musculoaponeurotic, gastrotomies and colonic anastomoses) closed with either 7/0 PDS or Maxon sutures over a period of 42 d postoperation.[54]

PDS sutures retained an average of 58% of their original tensile strength at the end of 4 weeks implantation in the subcutis of rats.[33,43,50] However, there was only 20% of the original mass of PDS absorbed at 160 d postimplantation and a complete absorption was not evident until 180 d postimplantation.[33,43,50,51] As long as 240 d for a complete PDS suture absorption have been reported by others.[52,53,55] This prolonged mass absorption was also found in an *in vitro* study.[8] In that *in vitro* study, the rate of tensile strength loss was significantly faster than found by Ray et al. in an *in vivo* study[43] (Figure 7.13).

Table 7.5 *In Vitro* Tensile Breaking Strength Retention of 3/0 Synthetic Absorbable Sutures

Composition (wt%)	Knot (kpsi)	Straight (kpsi)	Modulus (kpsi)	*In Vitro* Strength Retention							
				T_1 %	T_2 %	T_3 %	T_4 %	T_6 %	T_8 %	T_{10} %	T_{12} %
Maxon	61	82	425	88	81	70	69	33	—	—	—
Monocryl	51	97	105	51	21	3	—	—	—	—	—
PDSII	48	77	210	—	—	—	84	—	34	—	10
Vicryl	36	88	844	91	64	35	—	—	—	—	—
Biosyn	50	80	145	82	66	37	8	—	—	—	—

Data from Roby, M.S. et al., US Patent 5,403,347 April 4, 1995.

Table 7.6 Rate Constants for the Hydrolysis of Polyglycolide in Acidic and Basic Media

		Rate Constants (liter mol^{-1} d^{-1}) × 10^3		
pH	**Pellets**	**Fiber (0.0203 cm)**	**Fiber (0.0155 cm)**	**Heat-Treated Fiber (0.0203 cm)**
4.7	13.00 ± 0.24	3.16 ± 0.08	4.16 ± 0.21	5.88 ± 0.26
7.0	17.20 ± 0.93	8.64 ± 0.23	7.00 ± 0.42	n/a[a]
9.2	58.88 ± 3.83	12.84 ± 1.49	n/a[a]	n/a[a]
10.6	148.96 ± 9.02	46.08 ± 1.79	45.08 ± 1.46	53.32 ± 3.99

[a] n/a, data not available. The data are erratic and, hence, the values are not reported.

From Ginde, R.M. and Gupta, R.K., *J. Appl. Polym. Sci.*, 33, 2411, 1987. With permission.

Similar results were also found in Maxon sutures.[33,50,53,56] They retained 30% of their original tensile strength in rat subcutaneous tissues at 42 d; however, it would take 7 months for a complete gross absorption of the same suture. A pharmacokinetic study done by Katz et al. indicates that during the first 6 to 8 weeks postimplantation in rats and dogs, there is negligible loss of radioactivity from the Maxon implant sites, which coincides with the observed negligible suture mass loss.[56] The prolonged suture mass absorption after they have lost all of their function (i.e., tensile strength) results in a typical chronic inflammation with mononuclear macrophages surrounding the sutures.

Monocryl, one of the most recently developed commercial synthetic absorbable monofilament sutures, has the fastest degradation rate among synthetic absorbable sutures, as shown in Figure 7.13. Monocryl suture retains about 50% and 25% of its original TBS at 7 and 14 d postimplantation, respectively, and exhibits no measurable tensile strength at the end of 21 d, while it takes 8 weeks for PDSII to show no measurable tensile strength. The absorption of Monocryl sutures was essentially complete between 90 and 119 d postimplantation.[49]

Does suture size play a role in the rate of hydrolytic degradation? This question, unfortunately, has been controversial because of conflicting reports. Several studies indicate that the retention of TBS and the rate of suture absorption were independent of suture size, i.e., diameter,[18,47,57,58] while other studies showed an effect of suture diameter on suture degradation. It is the author's opinion that the effect of suture diameter on its hydrolytic degradation could occur only in monofilament absorbable sutures but not in multifilament ones. Table 7.6 shows the rate constants for the hydrolysis of polyglycolide (PGA) fibers of two diameter sizes at various pH media.[58] Ginde and Gupta[58] concluded that the reaction rates of hydrolysis of PGA fibers were independent of fiber diameter within the range of experimental errors. This study of monofilament absorbable sutures should shed light on this controversial issue, because all the reported studies used multifilament sutures. These multifilament sutures are made from very fine multifilament fibers and the sizes of the sutures are largely determined by the number of filaments per yarn and strands of yarns used during the braiding process. In other words, variation in suture size of these braided sutures is achieved through the size of yarn strands, which, in turn, is determined by the number of filaments per yarn. The size of each filament remains relatively the same among different sizes of braided sutures. This suggests that even though multifilament sutures have a variety of diameters, the diameter of their constituent fibers are in the same order, which should lead to the same rate of hydrolytic degradation if the degradation is diffusion controlled. If monofilament sutures were used for examining the effect of suture size on hydrolytic degradation, we predict theoretically that there would be a size effect, for the reason that large-diameter monofilament absorbable sutures are expected to have different fiber morphology than small-diameter ones. The cause for this expected difference is due to the crystallization phenomena during melt-spinning. A thick fiber would have a more profound skin-core effect than a thin fiber due to the fact that the dissipation of heat of suture fibers during the cooling stage of a melt-spinning process is more difficult for a thick fiber than a thin one. Therefore, the core of a thick fiber would cool off much more slowly than its skin layer. This gradient of temperature across a fiber cross-sectional area would result in different crystalline morphology, which would subsequently influence its hydrolytic degradation through different rates of diffusion of water molecules.

The significant delay observed in mass degradation of all sutures in both *in vitro* and *in vivo* environments is due to the inherent dependence of fiber strength on fiber morphology that these sutures have. Research on synthetic fibers has given rise to many models of fiber structure and morphology. They are the modified lamellar model proposed by Bonart and Hosemann,[59] the modified fringed micelle

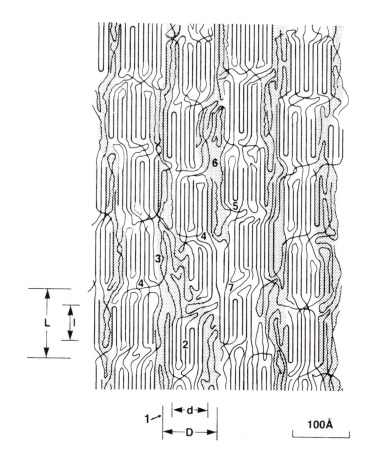

Figure 7.14 Swiss cheese structural model of synthetic fibers. (1) Fibrils, (2) lamellae, (3) partially extended chains in the interfibrillar regions, (4) tie molecules in the interlamellar region, (5) free chain ends, (6) amorphous segments with large free volume and which may give rise to voids, (7) fusion of adjacent microfibrils. Shaded areas represent the interfibrillar amorphous regions. (From Murthy, N.S. et al., *J. Appl. Polym. Sci.*, 40, 249, 1990. With permission.)

model by Hess et al.,[60] the microfibrillar model by Peterlin,[61] and finally the Swiss cheese model by Prevorsek et al.[62] Only the last two models have taken account of the space requirement for the accommodation of chain segments emerged from the 001 crystalline face and the anisotropy of mechanical properties of fibrous structure. In the microfibrillar model of Peterlin,[61] a fiber is composed of dense microfibrils embedded in less dense amorphous matrix. The microfibrils consist of crystalline and amorphous regions alternately arranged in the direction of the fiber axis. These microfibrils are considered to be the strongest element in a fiber and are responsible for the observed physical (e.g., diffusion) and mechanical properties of fibers.[63–66] This microfibrillar model of Peterlin has been found to describe the properties of polyolefin fibers well, but fails to explain the mechanical and dye diffusion data obtained for polyamide and polyester fibers.[67]

Prevorsek et al. suggested that polyamide and polyester fibers could best be described by the Swiss cheese model shown in Figure 7.14.[62,67] The Swiss cheese fibrous model consists of three domains differing in density and molecular orientation: the crystalline part of a microfibril with the highest density and molecular orientation, the amorphous regions within a microfibril with the lowest density and molecular orientation, and the intermicrofibrillar noncrystalline domain that has the density and orientation between the crystalline and amorphous regions of a microfibril. This highly ordered intermicrofibrillar noncrystalline domain was considered by Prevorsek et al.[62,67] to be the most important element of the fiber for controlling fiber properties like strength, modulus, diffusion, and shrinkage tension. Thus, the major difference between the Swiss cheese and microfibrillar models of fiber structure is whether the microfibril or the highly ordered intermicrofibrillar noncrystalline domain determines fiber properties.

In Peterlin's microfibrillar model, microfibrils determine fiber properties, while in the Swiss cheese model, the highly ordered intermicrofibrillar noncrystalline domain determines fiber properties.

Hydrolytic degradation starts in the amorphous regions, as the tie-chain segments, free chain ends, and chain folds in these regions degrade into fragments. The scissions of tie-chain segments would result in the loss of tensile breaking strength. As the degradation proceeds, the size of the fragments reaches the stage where they can be dissolved into the buffer medium. This dissolution removes the fragments from the amorphous regions, and loss of material results. Because the percent of tie-chain segments is relatively low and depends on the molecular weight and fiber spinning conditions, it is not a surprise to observe that these synthetic absorbable sutures lose most of their strength without significant mass loss.

Because alkaline hydrolysis of a fiber like polyethylene terephthalate has been reported to be a surface phenomenon through an initial attack on the surface of the fiber by hydroxyl ions,[68] ester linkages located on the outermost microfibril surface have equal access to the hydrolytic species and should be hydrolyzed regardless of whether the linkages are located in the amorphous or crystalline domains of the outermost microfibril surface. In fact, the ester linkages of the chain molecules located on the crystalline regions of the lateral outermost microfibril surface show remarkable resistance to hydrolytic degradation, compared to the same linkages located in the amorphous regions of the same microfibrils. A possible reason is that, due to crystalline lattice order structure and the lack of chain segmental mobility, it requires two scissions along a chain segment in the lateral crystalline region, separated by a distance smaller than the solubility limit and occurring simultaneously in order for the fragment to detach itself from the backbone chain and to become soluble. If the two scissions are not simultaneous, either of the two chain ends could recombine due to the cage imposed by the crystalline lattice, if it is an acid or neutral hydrolysis (i.e., reversible). The chain segments located in the amorphous domains, however, require only one scission to remove a chain fragment from the remaining chain segment because of the availability of free chain ends and the large free volume which allows water to attack the ester linkages from all different directions. This suggests that it is far less probable to remove a chain fragment from the surface of a crystalline lattice than from the end of a crystalline lattice (e.g., 001 plane). The lack of reduction in the crystallite size along the 110 and 020 planes of Vicryl sutures with hydrolysis as reported by Fredericks et al.[42] also supports this mechanism.

C. LEVEL OF CRYSTALLINITY AND CRYSTALLITE STRUCTURE

In all reported studies of the hydrolytic degradation of synthetic absorbable sutures, the level of crystallinity of the sutures always increases initially with hydrolysis time, reaches to a maximum, and then decreases thereafter. Figure 7.15 illustrates this change in the level of crystallinity in an *in vitro* environment.[8,41,69,70] Due to the lack of theoretical heat of fusion for PDS and Maxon sutures, the experimental heat of fusion was used to indirectly indicate the change in the level of crystallinity with time of hydrolysis. The data in this figure indicate clearly that the time at which the peak level of crystallinity locates varies with the type of suture materials. The location of the peak has been used by Chu as an indicator to predict the rate of hydrolytic degradation of absorbable sutures. For example, the Dexon suture is known to degrade faster than Maxon sutures in terms of tensile strength, mass, and molecular weight loss data, and Dexon sutures have the crystallinity peak appearing at 21 d of hydrolysis, while Maxon sutures peak at 42 d. Among the five synthetic absorbable sutures, PDS sutures show the least apparent maximum pattern of their level of crystallinity with hydrolysis time. Their maximum heat of fusion occurs at about 120 d. This would suggest that PDS would degrade the slowest among the five synthetic absorbable sutures. This prediction agrees with the data in Table 7.4 that PDS sutures show the longest absorption delay among the five absorbable sutures.

The maximum pattern of the level of crystallinity as a function of hydrolysis time was also reported by Ginde and Gupta in their *in vitro* study of the effect of pH on PGA fibers.[58] The peak level of crystallinity appeared between 3 and 4 weeks of hydrolysis in the medium of pH 4.7, which coincided with an earlier study reported by Chu et al.[69,72] The hydrolysis of the same PGA fibers in a highly alkaline medium (pH 10.6) was distinguished from that in acidic medium by a marked and sharp peak level of crystallinity instead of a broad peak found in acidic medium at 3 weeks *in vitro* immersion.

Secondary crystallization was suggested to be the cause for the maximum pattern of crystallinity with hydrolysis time.[69] With the hydrolytic degradation in the amorphous regions during the early stage of hydrolysis, main-chain scissions result in a lesser degree of entanglement of long-chain molecules located in these regions, as well as lower axial elastic moduli and tensile strength. Therefore, the remaining undegraded chain segments in the amorphous regions acquire better chain mobility; they can move and reorganize themselves from a disordered to an ordered state. Further crystallization is induced

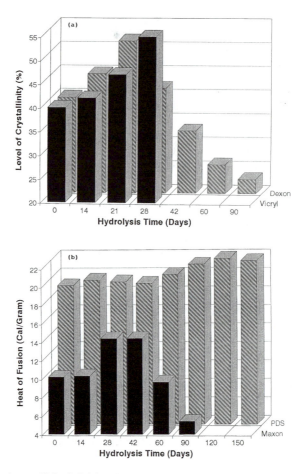

Figure 7.15 The level of crystallinity (%) (a) or heat of fusion (b) of synthetic absorbable sutures upon *in vitro* hydrolysis in phosphate buffer.

and an increase in crystallinity is expected and was indeed observed. The degree of crystallinity reaches a maximum at the end of the first stage of degradation, and starts to decrease as hydrolysis proceeds to the second stage and destroys the crystalline lattice. During the first stage, the loss of tensile strength is also the greatest due to the scission of tie-chain segments, while the second-stage degradation is chiefly responsible for the mass loss.

Upon hydrolysis, the prolonged retention of suture mass along with the retention of most of their fiber morphology indicate that there must be little change in crystal structure of the crystallites after the sutures lose their tensile strength completely. There were two studies reported to confirm this conclusion.[8,42] The wide angle X-ray diffraction flat films of partially hydrolyzed PDS suture fibers are shown in Figure 7.16. The d spacing along the fiber axis of these partially hydrolyzed PDS sutures was found to be 6.38 Å. This d spacing was independent of hydrolysis time up to 90 d (no data were obtained beyond 90 d due to loss of physical integrity of the fiber). This finding indicates that hydrolysis had no significant effect on the crystal structure of PDS fiber up to 90 d. This result was consistent with the observed lack of change in birefringence. This lack of significant change in average molecular orientation (described in the next section) and crystal lattice structure at the end of 90 d hydrolysis coupled with only 8.60% of PDS suture mass lost at the same hydrolysis interval are consistent with the hydrolytic mechanism proposed by Chu et al.[69,71]

Similar findings were reported by Fredericks et al.[42] in their study of Vicryl sutures. Table 7.7 summarizes the changes in crystallite size, orientation, and long period due to *in vitro* hydrolysis.[42] There is no change in crystal structure of the Vicryl crystallites remaining at 42 d. The orientation of the crystallites remains high throughout the study period (42 d). The Vicryl crystallite size in the direction perpendicular to the fiber axis, [110] and [020] planes, exhibits very little change within the study period. The crystallite size along the fiber axis, [002] plane, however, shows a significant reduction (15%

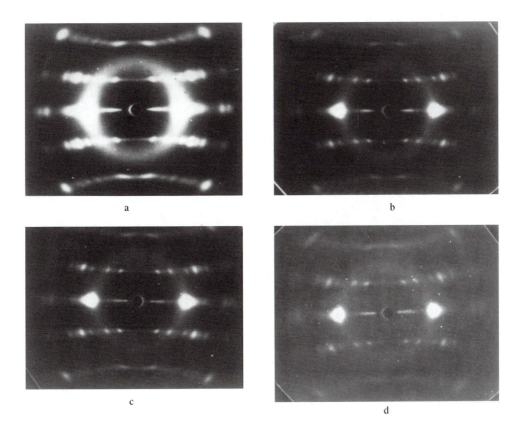

Figure 7.16 Wide-angle X-ray diffraction patterns of PDS sutures as a function of *in vitro* hydrolysis time (a) control; (b) 28 d; (c) 60 d; (d) 90 d. (From Lin, H. L. et al., *J. Biomed. Mater. Res.*, 27(2), 153, 1993. With permission.)

reduction) during the first 28 d of hydrolysis. This reduction in the crystallite size along the fiber axis agrees with the above-mentioned one-dimensional stepwise hydrolytic fragmentation occurring only at the ends of the chain segments located at the end of the crystallite. This reduction in crystallite size along the fiber axis would also be reflected in the reduction in the long period of Vicryl crystallite (from 87Å at 0 day to 66Å at 28 d).

D. ORIENTATION

The observed tensile strength and weight loss profiles described above and surface morphology described in the next section indicate that the loss of suture function (i.e., tensile strength) occurred with virtually no mass loss and no visible morphological changes. This suggests that the average molecular orientation (a combination of crystalline and amorphous orientation) inside a fiber should not change either within the same time interval. In a study of the relationship between birefringence and hydrolysis time of 2/0 PDS sutures,[8] there was no significant effect of hydrolysis time (up to 60 d) on average molecular orientation of PDS sutures. Therefore, although virtually no TBS could be found at the end of 60 d hydrolysis, there was no disruption of the overall fiber structure, particularly the crystalline regions. Most of the hydrolytic activity during the first 60 d was believed to occur in the noncrystalline regions, i.e., scission of tie-chain segments. This lack of birefringence change with hydrolysis time up to 60 d coincided with the lack of significant change in crystal lattice parameters found from X-ray diffraction flat-film patterns described above.

One of the unique aspects of these absorbable sutures is their fiber orientation that does not exist in nonfibrous, biodegradable materials. This characteristic anisotropy implies that the hydrolytic degradation process along the fiber axis (i.e., parallel to fiber molecules) should be different from the direction perpendicular to the fiber axis because different ways of molecular packing and arrangement would result in different rates of water diffusion through the materials, i.e., different rates of hydrolysis. Up to

Table 7.7 Change of Physical Properties of Vicryl Suture as a Function of *In vitro* Hydrolysis

Time (d)	Inherent Viscosity (dl/g)	Crystallinity (%)	Density (g/cm³)	Orientation f (φ)	Orientation Qualitative	Crystallite size (Å) (110)	(020)	(002)	Diameter (mm)	Tensile Strength Remaining (%)	Weight Loss (%)	Long Period SAXS (Å)
0	1.373	40	1.537	0.966	High	69	40	82	21.9	100	0	87
7	1.063	39	1.537		High	72	40	78	21.5	89.6	0.6	87
14	0.722	42	1.540		High	75	41	77	21.8	73.7	1.1	81
21	0.562	47	1.544		High	76	45	73	22.5	33.9	1.7	77
28	0.310	55			High	74	42	70	21.4		9.6	66
35	0.302				High				21.1		76.7	
42					High				21.3		98.3	

From Fredericks, R.J. et al., *J. Polym. Sci. Phys. Ed.*, 22, 57, 1984. With permission.

the present time, there is only one reported study examining different rates of hydrolysis due to orientation of suture fibers.[8]

In that study, Lin et al.[8] used a dye diffusion approach to examine the dye diffusion phenomena along both the lateral (perpendicular to the fiber axis) and the longitudinal (parallel to the fiber axis) directions of partially hydrolyzed 2/0 PDS suture fibers. The dye diffusion coefficients, D, at both lateral ($D_\perp$) and longitudinal ($D_\parallel$) directions were calculated from the following equation:[73]

$$D = X^2/2t \tag{7}$$

where X is the distance of dye diffusion and t the time of dyeing. A plot of X against $t^{1/2}$ would yield a straight line with a slope of $(2D)^{1/2}$. The isotropy index, ϕ, defined as the ratio of $D_\perp$ to $D_\parallel$, was thus calculated. The activation energy of dye diffusion, ΔE in kilocalories per mole, was obtained from the following equation:

$$Ln\ D = Ln\ D_o - \Delta E/RT \tag{8}$$

where T is the absolute temperature of the dye bath in degrees Kelvin and R is a gas constant (0.002 kcal/K/mol).

Table 7.8 summarizes the $D_\perp$ and $D_\parallel$ at various dyeing temperatures and hydrolysis times. There was a significant effect of hydrolysis time and dyeing temperature on dye diffusion coefficients. The data in the table illustrate that both the $D_\perp$ and $D_\parallel$ increase with an increase in dyeing temperature and hydrolysis time (Figure 7.17). The $D_\parallel$ was always much greater than the $D_\perp$. For example, $D_\parallel$ of an unhydrolyzed PDS suture was about 1300 times greater than the $D_\perp$ at 30°C dyeing temperature, and about 220 times greater than the $D_\perp$ at 60°C dyeing temperature. This significant dependence of dye diffusion coefficient on the relative direction of dye diffusion to the fiber axis must be closely related to the characteristic of anisotropic morphology of PDS fibers and will be discussed later.

As PDS suture fibers were hydrolyzed, their corresponding dye diffusion coefficients increased with the duration of hydrolysis, and the magnitude of increase depended on the dyeing temperature. The process of hydrolysis had more significant effect on $D_\perp$ than on $D_\parallel$. This significant difference in the dependence of dye diffusion coefficient along and perpendicular to the fiber axis on hydrolysis time indicated that the hydrolytic degradation of absorbable fibers is highly anisotropic. The change of fiber morphology due to the hydrolysis was more profound in the lateral than longitudinal direction.

An isotropy index, ϕ, and its dependence on hydrolysis time and dyeing temperature are given in Figure 7.18. This definition of the isotropy index implies that an increase in the index as a result of hydrolysis should show an increase in the isotropic characteristic of a fiber. When the index equals 1.0, $D_\perp$ becomes identical with $D_\parallel$. Thus, the difference in morphological characteristic of a fiber between the longitudinal and lateral directions of the fiber disappears as far as dye diffusion behavior is concerned. The data in Figure 7.18 show that ϕ increased with increasing hydrolysis time; however, the magnitude of increase depended on dyeing temperature. The duration of hydrolysis had no significant effect on the isotropy index of PDS fibers at the lowest and highest dyeing temperatures. A further analysis of the isotropy indices indicated that the process of hydrolysis lowered the dyeing temperature required for exhibiting more isotropic dye diffusion phenomena.

The activation energy of dyeing at different durations of hydrolysis showed that $\Delta E_\perp$ was much greater (about 6 to 12 times) than $\Delta E_\parallel$. $\Delta E_\parallel$ showed a continuous decrease with increasing hydrolysis time, while $\Delta E_\perp$ showed a maximum pattern with hydrolysis time. The much greater $\Delta E_\perp$ observed was consistent with the observed lower $D_\perp$. The observed continuous decrease in $\Delta E_\parallel$ is expected from hydrolysis which would result in the dissolution of chain fragments. Consequently, the fiber structure becomes more porous, and dye molecules are thus expected to have less obstacle or energy barrier to overcome when they diffuse into the interior of a partially hydrolyzed fiber. The $\Delta E_\parallel$ was reduced to half of its original value at the end of 42 d of hydrolysis. The $\Delta E_\perp$, however, did not show its continuous reduction with hydrolysis time. $\Delta E_\perp$ reached a maximum value at 28 d of hydrolysis and then decreased thereafter.

This difference in activation energy revealed the amorphous morphological structural difference between the lateral and longitudinal directions of a fiber. Obviously, the arrangement of amorphous chain segments along the fiber axis (in the intermicrofibrillar noncrystalline domain) provided less energy barrier for dye molecules to overcome than perpendicular to the fiber axis (amorphous regions within individual microfibrils). A detailed correlation of this observation to fiber morphology will be given later.

Table 7.8 Dye Diffusion Coefficient and Isotropy Index of Partially Hydrolyzed PDS 2/0 Suture at Different Dyeing Temperatures

Dyeing Temperature (°C)	Hydrolysis Time (d)	Lateral $D \times 10^{-8}$ (mm²/s)	Longitudinal $D \times 10^{-5}$ (mm²/s)[a]	Isotropy[a] Index ($\times 10^{-4}$)
30	0	1.75	2.33	7.51
	14	2.17	2.56	8.48
	28	2.27	2.71	8.38
	42	2.32	2.92	7.95
40	0	2.38	2.42	9.83
	14	2.62	2.65	9.89
	28	2.95	2.90	10.17
	42	3.81	2.98	12.78
50	0	2.51	2.73	9.19
	14	5.51	2.91	18.93
	28	7.26	2.99	24.28
	42	8.57	3.03	28.28
60	0	14.42	3.16	45.63
	14	16.19	3.27	49.51
	28	16.36	3.42	47.83
	42	16.65	3.47	47.98

[a] Isotropy index is defined as the ratio of lateral dye diffusion coefficient to longitudinal dye diffusion coefficient.

From Lin, H.L. et al., *J. Biomed. Mater. Res.*, 27(2), 153, 1993. With permission.

It was also found that the hydrolytic process of PDS suture altered the structure of the fiber to such an extent that the lowest temperature at which a particular dye could significantly diffuse into the fiber, T_D, became a function of hydrolysis time. Figure 7.19 illustrates the dependence of T_D on hydrolysis time at lateral and longitudinal directions of the fiber. The data indicate that T_D decreased with increasing hydrolysis time in both lateral and longitudinal directions, and lateral T_D was much higher than longitudinal one. Because T_D relates to the flexibility of chain segments in the amorphous regions, a lower T_D implies that the chain segments are flexible enough to allow dye to diffuse into fibers at a lower dyeing temperature. The initial (0 day) lateral T_D was twice greater than the longitudinal T_D. This indicates that chain segments in the amorphous regions located along the longitudinal direction of the fiber had a greater mobility and yield easier from the advancement of dye molecules than the ones in the lateral direction. This finding was consistent with the dye diffusion coefficient and activation energy data previously observed: that a lower longitudinal T_D associated with a higher dye $D_\parallel$ and lower dye diffusion $\Delta E_\parallel$.

From the dye diffusion data obtained in PDS suture fibers, the Swiss cheese model appears to be a better representative of PDS fiber structure. Since the crystalline blocks in the microfibrils are impermeable to dye molecules, the only way for dye to diffuse into PDS suture fibers is through the amorphous domains of the microfibrils (lateral dye diffusion) and the intermicrofibrillar noncrystalline regions (longitudinal dye diffusion). Obviously, the relative position of the impermeable crystalline blocks between two adjacent microfibrils would only influence lateral dye diffusion. There are two possible arrangements of these macrolattices as proposed by Prevorsek et al.[62] These are shown in Figure 7.20. The dye diffusion data obtained in this study indicate that the B type of macrolattice arrangement is more appropriate for PDS fiber to explain the significant difference between $D_\perp$ and $D_\parallel$. Because dye molecules must go through the amorphous channels between macrolattices, lateral dye diffusion must encounter the tortuosity of the diffusion channels, while the longitudinal dye diffusion does not. As a result, $D_\perp$ is expected to be, and was found to be, much smaller than $D_\parallel$ in the study by Lin et al.[8]

In addition to this tortuosity of diffusion channels, the level of void volume, the extent of chain segmental mobility, and the free volume in the amorphous domains also contribute to dye diffusion.[74–77] Whether these parameters affect the dye diffusion of PDS suture fiber depended on the extent of hydrolysis, and the relative magnitude of glass transition temperature of PDS to the dyeing temperature. If the dyeing temperatures (30 to 60°C) were above the T_g of PDS (about −10°C), then both the free volume (arising from chain segmental mobility) as well as voids (arising from the dissolution of hydrolytically fragmented chain segments) could contribute to the dye diffusion. This suggests that as hydrolytic scissions of PDS amorphous chain segments proceeds, both more void contents (due to the

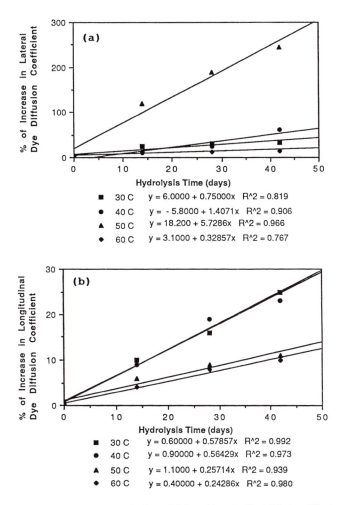

Figure 7.17 The percentage of increase in the lateral (a) and longitudinal (b) dye diffusion coefficients of 2/0 size PDS sutures as a function of *in vitro* hydrolysis time at different dyeing temperatures. (■) 30°C, (●) 40°C, (▲) 50°C, (♦) 60°C. (From Lin, H. L. et al., *J. Biomed. Mater. Res.*, 27(2), 153, 1993. With permission.)

dissolution of fragmented chain segments) and higher chain segmental mobility (due to less chain entanglement) could result. This provides an easier dye diffusion path as reflected in an increase in both $D_\perp$ and $D_\parallel$ with increasing hydrolysis time. The observed continuous decrease of T_D with hydrolysis time supported the argument that an increase in chain segmental mobility resulted from increasing extent of hydrolysis. However, due to the difference in detailed amorphous morphological structure located in the intermicrofibrillar domains and within a microfibril, the level of impact of hydrolysis on the dye diffusion coefficient, T_D, and activation energy were expected, and found, to be different at different directions of dye diffusion (i.e., lateral vs. longitudinal). The data showed that the longitudinal dye diffusion was characterized by a higher $D_\parallel$ and lower T_D and activation energy than the lateral one. Thus, we could conclude that in the PDS system the chain segments in intermicrofibrillar noncrystalline domains have a higher segmental mobility, and their spacial arrangement provides a more void volume, and less tortuous path than the chain segments located in the noncrystalline regions of microfibrils.

Because the kinetics of diffusion of water along the two perpendicular directions of a suture fiber have been found to be significantly different, suture fibers with different levels of orientation must affect their hydrolytic degradation rate. There are only two reported studies that indirectly confirm this theoretical prediction.[58,70,78] In these two reported studies, Chu and Browning[70,78] and Ginde and Gupta[58] found that heat- or annealing-treated suture fibers without strain applied to them would increase the rate of tensile strength loss upon *in vitro* hydrolysis when compared with unannealed ones. The most probable cause is the reduction in fiber orientation upon unstrained annealing, which facilitates the diffusion of

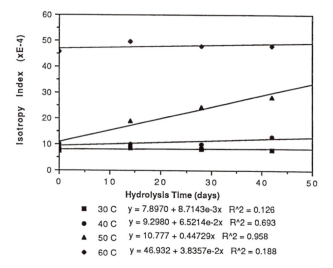

30 C   y = 7.8970 + 8.7143e-3x   R^2 = 0.126
40 C   y = 9.2980 + 6.5214e-2x   R^2 = 0.693
50 C   y = 10.777 + 0.44729x   R^2 = 0.958
60 C   y = 46.932 + 3.8357e-2x   R^2 = 0.188

Figure 7.18 Isotropy index of 2/0 size PDS suture fiber as a function of *in vitro* hydrolysis time at different dyeing temperatures. (■) 30°C, (●) 40°C, (▲) 50°C, (♦) 60°C. (From Lin, H. L. et al., *J. Biomed. Mater. Res.*, 27(2), 153, 1993. With permission.)

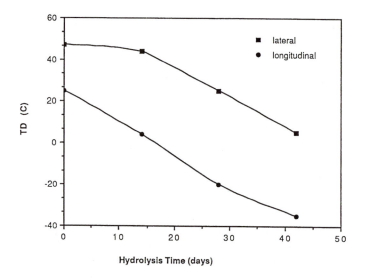

Figure 7.19 The change of both the lateral and longitudinal dye diffusion T_d of 2/0 PDS sutures *in vitro* hydrolysis time. (From Lin, H. L. et al., *J. Biomed. Mater. Res.*, 27(2), 153, 1993. With permission.)

water molecules into suture fibers. The faster loss of TBS in less oriented suture fibers is also consistent with the observed higher rate constant of hydrolysis associated with heat-treated PGA fibers shown in Table 7.6. The details of the effect of fiber morphology on the hydrolytic degradation of absorbable sutures are given in Section III.F.1 of this chapter.

E. SURFACE MORPHOLOGY

Any degradation process results in mass loss. Unlike nonfibrous polymers, which exhibit relatively nonmorphological interest due to mass loss, the synthetic absorbable suture fibers exhibit unique change in surface morphology upon hydrolysis. Based on the existing available data, multifilament Dexon and Vicryl sutures show distinctive different hydrolysis-induced morphological changes from monofilament PDS, Maxon, Monocryl, and Biosyn sutures. However, there is a universal observation among synthetic absorbable sutures. Most of the loss of tensile properties of an absorbable suture occurs without any

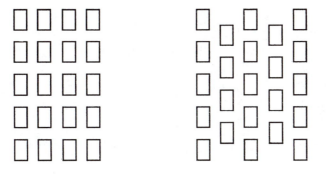

Figure 7.20 Macrolattice structure models of synthetic fibers. (From Prevorsek, D.C. et al., *J. Macromol. Sci. Phys. B*, 8(1-2), 127, 1973. With permission.)

apparent surface morphological change of the suture, and the onset of apparent surface morphological changes is frequently associated with the onset of suture mass loss.

Both Dexon and Vicryl multifilament sutures exhibit no visible surface morphological changes up to 14 d *in vitro*. As hydrolysis progresses to 28 d, the surface of the filament becomes rough and fragmentation of constituent filaments (perpendicular to the fiber axis) appear by day 40, as shown in Figure 7.21.[41,71] As hydrolysis proceeds to the late stage, the size of the fragments becomes smaller (e.g., 90 d sample). It is interesting to know that the loss of suture mass becomes evident when the fragmentation of constituent filaments appears. The cross-sectional surface of the fragment ends appears very smooth. Due to the coating material, Vicryl sutures, however, do not exhibit profound surface cracks as Dexon sutures do. The detachment of surface coating materials from the braided multifilaments was observed at 28 d. All braided multifilaments were degraded to many microfibrils and the braided structure was totally lost. The diameter of the Vicryl braided sutures remains relatively constant during the entire period of hydrolysis (i.e., 42 d) even though less than 20% of the suture mass remains. This is consistent with the study by Fredericks et al., in which they reported that there was virtually no change in Vicryl suture diameter at the end of 42 d *in vitro*.[42] They suggested that the remaining polymer mass forms a type of skeleton throughout the suture to preserve its external shape and dimensions.

The observed smooth ends of Dexon suture fragments prompted Chu and Campbell to suggest that the amorphous domains of the adjacent microfibrils are located at a common cross-sectional plane normal to the fiber axis.[71] As a microcrack forms at one point of the filament surface on the outermost microfibrils, it will propagate circumferentially around the fiber and deeply into the fiber along this common cross-sectional plane, where the amorphus domains of adjacent microfibrils are located. As hydrolysis proceeds further, the microcracks cut through the fiber along this common plane and result in relatively smooth and sharp scissions along various parts of the fiber. Experimentally, no cracks propagating along the fiber axis (c axis) have been observed in these multifilament Dexon and Vicryl sutures. This is because once a microcrack forms, it would meet stronger hydrolytic resistance in the crystalline regions and would be less likely to grow along the fiber axis. It will continue to hydrolyze along the a-b plane, where the more open and less resistant amorphous regions are located. Figure 7.22 is a schematic drawing of the propagation of a crack.

In a more recent study by Chu et al. on the use of PGA fibers as one of the components for bicomponent woven vascular fabrics, they observed a very unusual and informative morphological change of the fibers with hydrolysis.[79–81] These PGA fibers have the same chemical structure as Dexon sutures and are all multifilaments. Different fiber processing conditions appear to be responsible for this difference in surface morphology of the same type of fibers. As shown in Figure 7.23, circumferential surface microcracks was observed and the appearance of the surface microcracks were much more regular along the fiber axis than Dexon sutures, which do not show such regular arrangement of surface microcracks. A detailed examination of the regions where the surface microcracks were formed indicated that not all materials located in the microcrack regions were equally susceptible to hydrolysis. There were many microfibrils remaining in the microcrack regions, while the materials surrounding these microfibrils were hydrolyzed and removed. These microfibrils appeared to hold the fiber together by connecting the two adjacent, more hydrolytically resistant, portions (i.e., the portions without microcracks) of the fiber together before complete fragmentations of the fiber occurred. The dimension of these microfibrils was about 0.5 μm.

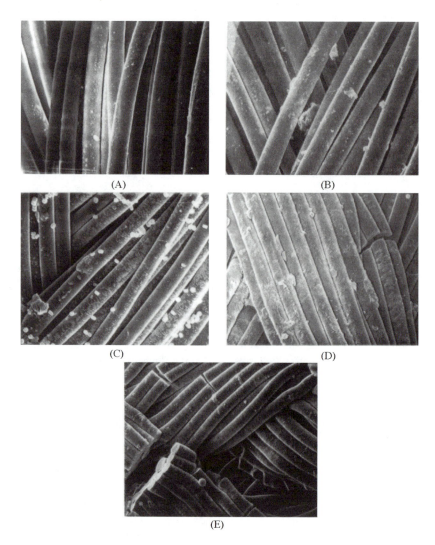

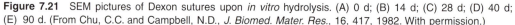

(A) (B) (C) (D) (E)

Figure 7.21 SEM pictures of Dexon sutures upon *in vitro* hydrolysis. (A) 0 d; (B) 14 d; (C) 28 d; (D) 40 d; (E) 90 d. (From Chu, C.C. and Campbell, N.D., *J. Biomed. Mater. Res.*, 16, 417, 1982. With permission.)

This observed PGA fiber morphology suggests that the fiber itself has a composite structure of microfibrils impregnated within amorphous domains. A recent study by Chu of the bulk birefringence of these microfibrils and fibers indicated that the microfibrils had a birefringence of 0.240, which was significantly higher than the fiber (0.0019). These birefringence data suggest that the observed microfibrils are far more oriented than the PGA fiber where these microfibrils reside. Due to its highly oriented and crystalline nature, microfibrils are more resistant to hydrolysis than the surrounding amorphous domains. As the surrounding amorphous matrix is first hydrolyzed and removed, it reveals the remaining microfibrils, as shown in Figure 7.23. Such a unique arrangement of surface microcracks on PGA fibers was also observed by Chu et al. in a study of knitted bicomponent vascular fabrics.[80,81] In that study, PGA and Dacron fibers were knitted into jersey tubular fabrics and examined after *in vitro* hydrolytic degradation. After dyeing the partially hydrolyzed bicomponent fabric with a blue dye, a series of circumferential blue bands alternatively arranged along the length of PGA fiber were observed. The widths of the dyed and undyed bands, however, were not uniform. This suggests that not every part of the PGA fiber along its axis exhibits the same level of hydrolytic sensitivity; thus, there are some domains that are more susceptible to hydrolysis than the remaining portions of the fiber. These domains are arranged in such a way that they regularly alternate with the more hydrolytic-resistant portion of the fiber. This arrangement of blue bands in the knitted bicomponent fabrics was very similar to the above-mentioned circumferential surface microcracks observed in PGA fibers in bicomponent woven fabrics.

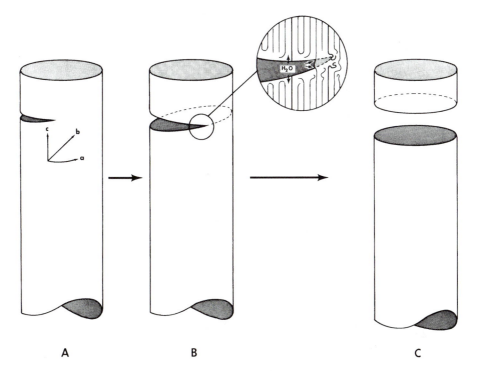

Figure 7.22   A schematic drawing of the circumferential propagation of a crack on a fiber surface. (A) Initiation of a microcrack. (B) This microcrack propagates circumferentially around the fiber and deeply into the fiber along the amorphous regions of each microfibril. The insertion illustrates that water molecules hydrolyze more chain segments located in the amorphous regions than those located in the crystalline regions. (C) As the crack completely propagates through the fiber, fragmentation of fibers results. (From Chu, C.C. and Campbell, N.D., *J. Biomed. Mater. Res.*, 16, 417, 1982. With permission.)

It is still puzzling why the hydrolytically sensitive domains randomly distribute along the PGA fiber axis. What are the origin and factors that dictate their distribution? Why do the hydrolytically sensitive and resistant domains alternately arrange along the fiber axis? Similar patterns of crack formation have been found from undrawn and drawn nylon 66 filaments treated in oxygen-water systems.[82] Stress concentration due to crystallization of smaller molecules produced during the oxidative degradation was suggested as a possible cause for the crack formation in nylon 66.

The monofilament PDS, Maxon, Monocryl, and Biosyn suture fibers, however, exhibit surface morphological changes with hydrolysis time completely different from the multifilament Dexon and Vicryl sutures, and hence may suggest different types of hydrolytic mechanism. PDS sutures do not show any apparent surface morphological change until after 90 d (corresponding to less than 9% weight loss) *in vitro*.[8,83] However, circumferential cracks start to appear in a regular manner at 120 d and are followed by subsequent detachment of surface layers from the underneath fiber at 150 d, as illustrated in Figure 7.24.[8] Obviously this detachment of large surface layers contributed to the massive weight loss observed in Figure 7.12. Similar morphological changes in the hydrolytically degraded polycaproamide fibers were also reported.[5] As we describe later in this chapter, this pattern of PDS surface morphology changes under the influence of various extrinsic factors like enzymes and γ-irradiation.

The monofilament Maxon suture fibers show somewhat different surface morphological changes than PDS, as shown in Figure 7.25.[41] There are no visible surface morphological changes before 42 d *in vitro* in phosphate buffer of pH 7.44. Longitudinal cracks start to appear on the 2/0 Maxon suture surface at 42 d and the diameter of the suture is reduced to 94%. The appearance of these longitudinal surface cracks is also reflected in the loss of almost all TBS (0.6% retention) at this period of hydrolysis. These longitudinal surface cracks, straight and parallel to the fiber axis, are not observed in either Dexon or Vicryl multifilament sutures over the complete period of their degradation. Nonparallel longitudinal cracks start to appear at 60 d and the diameter of the Maxon suture is reduced to 90% of its original value. Circumferential surface cracks perpendicular to the fiber axis start to appear at 90 d and its

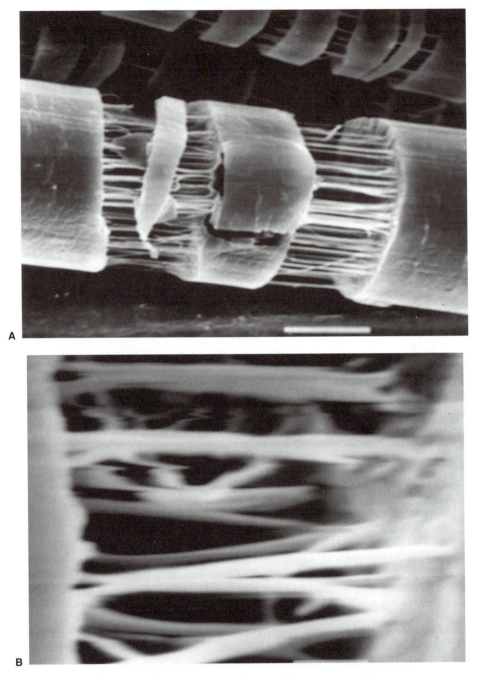

Figure 7.23 Surface morphology of partially hydrolyzed PGA fiber as one of the yarn components of a bicomponent vascular fabric. (A) Surface microcracks on PGA warp yarns of a bicomponent woven fabric; (B) a close-up view (×10,000) of the surface microcrack region. Note the microfibrils connected between two adjacent blocks of PGA fiber. (From Yu, T.J. and Chu, C.C., *J. Biomed. Mater. Res.*, 27, 1329, 1993. With permission.)

diameter is reduced by 22% (from 400 to 315 μm). These sequences of surface morphological changes with hydrolysis time indicate that the Maxon monofilament suture degrades through the concentric removal of the outermost surface layer by the hydrolytic dissolution of the surface molecular chain fragments. As a result, the diameter of the suture continuously decreases with hydrolysis time. It is believed that the thickness of a Maxon monofilament suture fiber is mainly responsible for this observed unique pattern of surface morphology with hydrolysis time. For example, a 2/0 size Maxon monofilament suture has an initial diameter of about 400 μm, while the constituent fibers of the same size Dexon

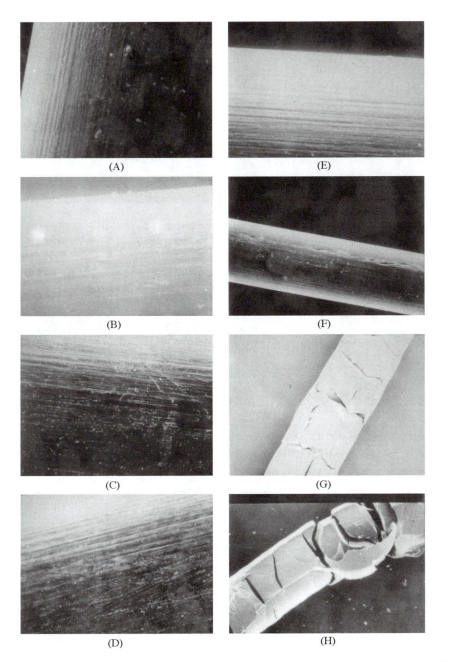

Figure 7.24 SEM micrographs of 2/0 PDS sutures undergoing *in vitro* hydrolysis. (A) 0 d; (B) 14 d; (C) 28 d; (D) 42 d; (E) 60 d; (F) 90 d; (G) 120 d, (H) 150 d. (From Lin, H. L. MS thesis, Cornell University, May 1990.)

multifilament braided suture has about 10 to 15 μm diameter. Due to the very small diameter of the individual fiber in Dexon or Vicryl sutures, the formation of surface cracks on these individual fibers would be able to cut though the whole fibers much faster than the significantly thicker monofilament Maxon or PDS sutures. This leads to the observed fragmented Dexon or Vicryl filaments with smooth fragment ends. Like other synthetic absorbable sutures, this pattern of surface morphology with hydrolysis time changes with different extrinsic factors, as we describe later.

F. INTRINSIC AND EXTRINSIC FACTORS AFFECTING BIODEGRADATION

The general biodegradation phenomena described above in terms of the changes in chemical, physical, mechanical, thermal, and morphological properties are under common *in vitro* (various buffers of pH

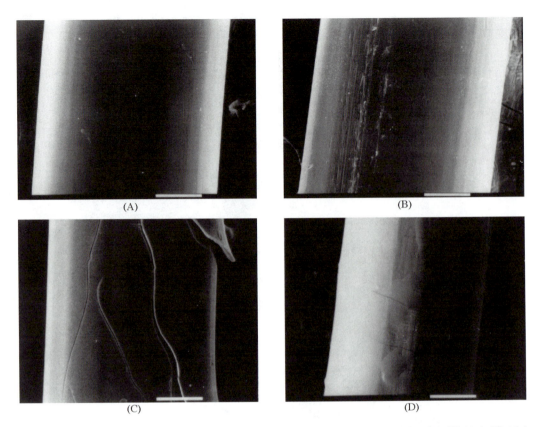

Figure 7.25 SEM micrographs of 2/0 Maxon sutures undergoing *in vitro* hydrolysis. (A) 0 d; (B) 28 d; (C) 60 d; (D) 90 d. (From Zhang, L. et al., *J. Biomed. Mater. Res.*, 27, 1425, 1993. With permission.)

from 7.2 to 7.44 at 37°C) or *in vivo* (subcutis or intramuscular sites of rat or rabbit model) environments. When other environmental factors like acidic pH, electrolytes, temperature, γ-irradiation or intrinsic parameters like chemical variation of glycolide and lactide are imposed, different biodegradation phenomena are expected to occur.

Up to the present time, several intrinsic and extrinsic factors have been identified either experimentally or theoretically to influence the biodegradation of synthetic absorbable sutures. They include substituents of various sizes α, β, or γ to the carbonyl function group (steric effect), substituents of various electron withdrawing or releasing capability (inductive effect), annealing treatment, pH, electrolytes, temperature, external strain or stress applied, γ-irradiation, plasma coating, enzymes, lipids, synovial fluids, bacteria, and a unique surface chemical reaction which could accelerate surface hydrolytic degradation of PGA without altering its bulk properties. The effects of these intrinsic and extrinsic factors on the chemical, physical, mechanical, thermal, and morphological properties of synthetic absorbable sutures are described individually in the remainder of this chapter.

1. Intrinsic Factors
a. Substituent Effect

Intrinsic factors are those that relate to the chemical and physical structure of the synthetic absorbable sutures, such as substituents, orientation, level of crystallinity, and molecular weight. Their effects on the biodegradation of synthetic absorbable sutures are due to the changes in material characteristics which subsequently reflect in their biodegradation properties. Due to the requirements of enormous resources to examine the effect of intrinsic factors, very few studies are available in the literature. Recent reported theoretical research work in Chu's laboratory appears to provide a better means to examine the effects of intrinsic factors than the traditional experimental approach. Pratt and Chu were the first to use semiempirical computational chemistry to examine a wide range of parameters (steric hindrance, hydrophobicity, electron inductive effect) on the hydrolytic degradation of synthetic linear aliphatic polyesters.[84,85] The findings from these theoretical calculations allow investigators not only to better understand

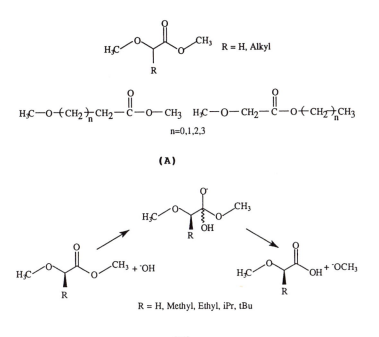

Figure 7.26 (A) Chemical structure of glycolic ester model compounds for steric hindrance effect. (B) Chemical reaction of two-step hydrolysis of glycolic ester model compounds. (From Pratt, L. and Chu, C.C., *J. Comput. Chem.*, 14(7), 809, 1993. With permission.)

the degradation mechanism and the effect of several chemical parameters at the molecular level but also to be able to intelligently predict the possible hydrolytic degradation properties of biodegradable polymers even before they are synthesized. This could considerably reduce the time and cost of research and development of new biodegradable polymers for both biological and environmental uses.

Steric Hindrance Effect The hydrolysis of α substituted (2-methoxy) methyl acetate was used as a model for examining the effect of different substituents on the hydrolysis of substituted PGA. In addition, homologues of the glycolic ester containing up to three additional methylene groups, as well as the ethyl, *n*-propyl, and *n*-butyl esters of 2-methoxy acetic acid, were modeled in order to examine the effects of chain length on the alkyl and acyl portions of the molecule on hydrolysis, since a longer chain will act as an electron donor. The chemical structure of these model compounds is given in Figure 7.26(A). Although the polyester hydrolysis could be catalyzed by either acid or base, the slightly alkaline pH (7.44) was chosen for this theoretical calculation because it is the physiological pH and most reported experimental studies use this pH. The two-step hydrolysis of these model compounds in pH 7.44 consists of an attack of the hydroxide ion on the carbonyl carbon, followed by methoxide elimination from this tetrahedral intermediate. This tetrahedral species shown in Figure 7.26(B) was chosen as the starting structure and preoptimized by molecular mechanics, as it was more convenient to perform the calculations on the reverse reaction. Four water molecules were placed about the hydroxyl group in an approximately symmetrical manner and optimized to the most stable structure by MNDO.[86] Four waters of solvation provides the best compromise between chemical accuracy and the time (i.e., cost) of supercomputer use. All MNDO calculations were performed with the MOPAC[87] package of programs. For comparison, duplicate AM1[88] calculations were run on selected molecules.

The second step of hydrolysis, i.e., the elimination of methoxide from the tetrahedral intermediate, is the rate-determining step and hence is the most important for determining the substituent effect. Table 7.9 summarizes the reaction enthalpies for both the unsolvated and solvated hydroxide attack and methoxide elimination steps of α substituted glycolic acid methylesters. In the solvated case, the hydroxide ion attack becomes progressively less exothermic with increasing substituent size. The most dramatic effect is the rate-determining elimination step, where the methoxide elimination is favored by the larger substituents in both the unsolvated and tetrasolvated cases, and actually becomes exothermic for the tetrasolvated *R-t*-butyl substituted intermediate. Thus, although the equilibrium is less favorable

Table 7.9 Reaction Enthalpies for (ΔH) the Two-Step Hydrolysis of Alpha-Substituted Glycolic Acid Methyl Esters

Substituent	ΔH Hydroxide Attack	ΔΔH*	ΔH Methoxide Elimination	ΔΔH*
H	−48.214 kcal/mol	0.000	10.189 kcal/mol	0.000
Methyl (re)	−49.092	−0.878	9.363	−0.826
Methyl (si)	−47.969	0.245	9.168	−1.021
Ethyl (re)	−51.375	−3.161	8.545	−1.644
Ethyl (si)	−51.175	−2.961	11.209	1.020
iPr (re)	−47.772	0.442	7.756	−2.433
iPr (si)	−46.501	1.713	8.539	−1.650
t-Butyl (re)	−46.396	1.818	5.127	−5.062
t-Butyl (si)	−45.861	2.353	8.537	−1.652
H·4H$_2$O	−44.109	0.000	8.287	0.000
Methyl (re)·4H$_2$O	−40.649	3.460	7.228	−1.059
Methyl (si)·4H$_2$O	−42.487	1.622	9.265	0.978
Ethyl (re)·4H$_2$O	−45.090	−0.981	8.188	−0.099
Ethyl (si)·4H$_2$O	−42.387	1.722	9.048	0.761
iPr (re)·4H$_2$O	−43.045	1.064	7.442	−0.845
iPr (si)·4H$_2$O	−38.641	5.468	5.248	−3.039
t-Butyl (re)·4H$_2$O	−33.916	10.193	−1.269	9.556
t-Butyl (si)·4H$_2$O	−34.703	9.406	0.556	−7.731

* ΔΔH = (ΔH of α-substituted) − (ΔH of unsubstituted).

From Pratt, L. and Chu, C.C., *J. Comput. Chem.*, 14(7), 809, 1993. With permission.

toward the formation of the tetrahedral intermediate, the rate of hydrolysis would be expected to be faster with very large α substituents due to the added driving force toward methoxide elimination.

Similar calculations were performed on the unsolvated hydroxide attack on, and methoxide elimination from, glycolic ester homologues. The data show little effect of the number of methylene groups in the acyl portion of the molecule on the reaction enthalpies. However, it appears that an increase in the number of methylene groups in the alkyl portion of the ester had a more profound effect on the rate-determining step than it did on the acyl fragment. The largest effect of the carbon chain length on the reaction enthalpy is seen in the alkoxide elimination step, where a longer chain in the alcohol fragment appears to destabilize the tetrahedral intermediate more than the product alkoxide ion, thereby lowering the reaction enthalpy by as much as 3.5 kcal/mol. Overall, the effect of chain length was relatively small compared to the effect of substituents α to the carbonyl group. It, therefore, appears that the effects of alkyl substituents are largely steric in nature, since the electron releasing effect of additional methylene groups in the repeat unit is relatively small. Figure 7.27 summarizes the relative rate constants, K_{rel} = exp($ΔΔH^*$/RT) where $ΔΔH^*$ is the activation enthalpy of the rate-determining methoxide elimination step, of the various α substituted glycolic esters. The data in this figure show a decrease in the rate of hydrolysis by about a factor of 10^6 with isopropyl substituents, but nearly a sixfold increase with t-butyl substituents.

The calculations described above were performed on small molecules in both gas and solution phases, where rotational energy barriers are relatively low. Actual hydrolysis of synthetic biodegradable fibers, however, is far more complicated than the assumptions imposed in the calculation, due to the complex fiber structure and morphology. Research on synthetic fibers has given rise to many models of fiber structure and morphology, all of which describe the fiber consisting of alternating crystalline and amorphous regions. The amorphous regions consist largely of tie-chain segments which connect the highly crystalline regions. Most of the initial loss of fiber tensile strength takes place by random chain scissioning of tie-chain segments. Unlike small molecules in solution, the polymer chains are partially oriented in the amorphous regions and therefore have a higher energy barrier to bond rotation, decreasing the ability of the tetrahedral intermediates to adopt the most stable conformation. Therefore, the calculated results should be taken as a lower limit to the enthalpies of hydrolysis of synthetic biodegradable fibers.

Pratt and Chu[84] found that alkyl substituents on the glycolic esters cause an increase in activation enthalpies, and a corresponding decrease in reaction rate, up to about three carbons, while alkyl substituents bulkier than isopropyl make the rate-determining elimination step more facile. It, therefore, appears that polymers containing α-isopropyl groups, or slightly larger linear alkyl groups, such as n-butyl, n-pentyl, etc., will show a longer strength retention, given the same fiber morphology. The quantitative

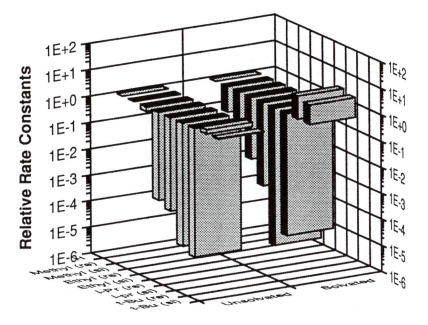

Figure 7.27   Calculated relative rate constants for the hydrolysis of α-substituted esters of glycolic acids. (From Pratt, L. and Chu, C.C., *J. Comput. Chem.*, 14(7), 809, 1993. With permission.)

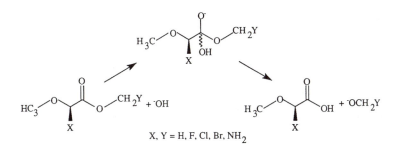

X, Y = H, F, Cl, Br, NH₂

Figure 7.28   Chemical reaction of two-step hydrolysis of either halogen- or amino-substituted glycolic ester model compounds. (From Pratt, L. and Chu, C.C., *J. Mol. Struct.*, 304, 213, 1994. With permission.)

study of the effects of the chemical structure on fiber morphology is currently beyond the capability of semiempirical methods. These effects should also play a significant role in the rate of fiber degradation.

Inductive Effect   The substituent effects reported above are largely steric in nature, as alkyl substituents are relatively weak electron donors. As shown in Figure 7.28, electron withdrawing substituents α to the carbonyl group would be expected to stabilize the tetrahedral intermediate resulting from hydroxide attack, which would favor hydroxide attack but disfavor alkoxide elimination. Electron releasing groups would be expected to show the opposite effect.[85] Similarly, electronegative substituents on the alkyl portion of the ester would stabilize the formation of alkoxide ion and thus favor the elimination step. This theoretical prediction was recently confirmed by Pratt and Chu in a study of the effect of electron donating and electron withdrawing groups on the rate of hydrolytic degradation of linear aliphatic polyesters.[85] It is difficult, however, to make a quantitative prediction of substituent effects based on electronegativity alone, since steric and conformational effects will also influence the calculated reaction and activation enthalpies. In particular, the small size of fluorine, compared to the other halogens, may cause significant deviations from the predicted patterns of reactivity.

In the study by Pratt and Chu,[85] halo- and amino-methyl (2-methoxy) acetate, and its acyl and alkyl homologues, were chosen as model compounds. The location of the halo or amino substitution ranged from α, ß, to γ substitutions. The halogenated carbon was assigned the R absolute configuration and reactions were modeled corresponding to attack by the hydroxide ion on both the re and si faces, followed by alkoxide elimination from the two diastereomeric tetrahedral intermediates. The amine carbons were chosen with the same absolute configuration, in this case, the S isomer, due to the lower priority of the amine group. All MNDO calculations were performed with the MOPAC package of programs and run on an IBM 3090 supercomputer. Molecular geometries were optimized using the PRECISE keyword, which increases the self consistent field (SCF) convergence criteria by a factor of 100. Starting geometries of the unsolvated esters were obtained by molecular mechanics, using the MMX force field of PC Model.[89]

For the attack of hydroxide ions on α-halogen substituted glycolic esters, the reaction enthalpy (ΔH_{rxn}) was more exothermic than the unsubstituted ester, with the largest effects found with chloro substitution. The attack on the fluoro ester from the si face was nearly 7 kcal/mol more exothermic than from the re face. The smallest substituent effects were seen in the aminoesters, making the re attack slightly less exothermic and the si attack more exothermic by about the same amount.

These α-halogen substituents decreased the activation enthalpy (ΔH_{act}) of the hydroxide ion attack from the re face, and no activation barrier could be found with a Br substituent. Attack from the si face showed no discernable pattern in activation enthalpies, although Br and amino substituents raised the barrier above that of the unsubstituted ester.

More dramatic differences in reaction enthalpies were observed in the rate-determining alkoxide elimination step, as reported in Table 7.10. Similar values were observed for elimination following attack on the re and si faces, with the R intermediate being more stable by about 1 kcal/mol, except the *R*-fluoro intermediate, which is less stable than the S isomer by about 2 kcal/mol. As in the case of hydroxide attack, the aminoesters showed the smallest substituent effects. As with the halogen substituents, the *R*-amino intermediate was more stable than the S isomer by about 1 kcal/mol.

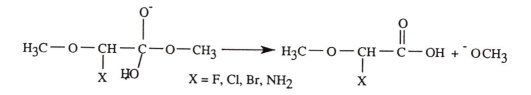

Table 7.10 Reaction and Activation Enthalpies of Methoxide Elimination from Alpha-Substituted Glycolic Esters

	R Intermediate					S Intermediate			
X	**ΔHrxn**	**ΔΔH**	**ΔHact**	**ΔΔH**	**X**	**ΔHrxn**	**ΔΔH**	**ΔHact**	**ΔΔH**
H	10.189	0.000	18.618	0.000	H	10.189	0.000	18.618	0.000
F	16.055	5.866	30.325	11.707	F	18.593	8.404	26.854	8.236
Cl	19.148	8.959	23.774	5.156	Cl	18.368	8.179	23.877	5.259
Br	18.454	8.265	23.665	5.047	Br	17.435	7.246	23.728	5.110
NH₂	12.124	1.935	20.655	2.037	NH₂	11.143	0.954	19.415	0.797

From Pratt, L. and Chu, C.C., *J. Mol. Struct.*, 304, 213, 1994. With permission.

The activation enthalpy of methoxide elimination from the R-tetrahedral intermediate of the fluoro ester was 3.3 kcal/mol higher than from the S isomer, indicating a greater stabilization of the ground state relative to the transition state. A similar but smaller effect was observed for elimination from the *R*-amino intermediate.

Halogen and amine substitution at the alkyl fragment of the ester showed the same pattern as α substitution on the attack by hydroxide ion on the carbonyl group, but with much smaller reaction enthalpy differences. The largest effects were observed with chlorine and bromine substitution. Activation enthalpies were lower than that of the unsubstituted methyl ester by as much as 1.3 kcal/mol.

However, significant substituent effects are seen in the substituted methoxide elimination step, where large differences are seen in both the reaction and activation enthalpies. Chlorine and bromine substitutions cause the elimination step to become exothermic, and lower the activation barrier to about 5 kcal/mol, as shown in Table 7.11. Similar but smaller effects are observed with fluorine substitution, and little effect is seen with amine substitution.

$$H_3C-O-CH_2-\underset{\underset{HO}{|}}{\overset{\overset{O^-}{|}}{C}}-O-CH_2X \longrightarrow H_3C-O-CH_2-\overset{\overset{O}{\|}}{C}-OH + {}^-OCH_2X$$

$$X = F, Cl, Br, NH_2$$

Table 7.11 Reaction and Activation Enthalpies of Alkoxide Elimination from Glycolic Halomethyl and Aminomethyl Esters

X	$\Delta Hrxn$	$\Delta\Delta H$	$\Delta Hact$	$\Delta\Delta H$
H	10.189	0.000	18.618	0.000
F	3.634	–6.555	14.053	–4.565
Cl	–20.872	–31.061	3.919	–14.699
Br	–16.008	–26.197	4.032	–14.586
NH$_2$	9.161	–1.028	18.341	–0.277

From Pratt, L. and Chu, C.C., *J. Mol. Struct.*, 304, 213, 1994. With permission.

Figure 7.29 illustrates the effects of electron donor (or withdrawing) substituents and their location from the carbonyl carbon position on the relative rate constant, $K_{rel} = \exp(\Delta\Delta H^*/RT)$ where $\Delta\Delta H^*$ is the activation enthalpy of the rate-determining methoxide elimination step. The data suggest that the magnitude of the inductive effect on the hydrolysis of glycolic esters decreases significantly as the location of the substituent is further away from the α carbon. This is not a surprise because the inductive effect is very distance sensitive. In all three locations of substitutions (α, β, and γ), Cl and Br substituents exhibit larger inductive effects than other elements. This is particularly true in the α position. The difference among various elements becomes much smaller in the β and γ positions. It is quite surprising, however, that the effect of F was smaller than that of Cl or Br, where the elimination step actually became exothermic when the α position was substituted with either Cl or Br. Although F is the most electronegative of the group (4.0 electronegativity), the larger size of the Cl and Br atoms may more effectively delocalize the negative charge. These larger atoms are also more sterically hindered in the tetrahedral intermediate and this may contribute an additional driving force toward the alkoxide elimination. A substantial lowering of the activation barriers of this rate-determining step is reflected in the very large relative rate constants, especially with Cl and Br substitution, as shown in Figure 7.29. Only a slight decrease in reaction and activation enthalpies was observed with the aminomethyl ester, indicating a slight charge delocalization by nitrogen.

In conclusion, Pratt and Chu[85] found that the rate of ester hydrolysis has been found to be greatly affected by halogen substituents due primarily to charge delocalization. α substituents on the acyl portion of the ester favor the formation of the tetrahedral intermediate but retard the rate-determining alkoxide elimination step. Interpretation of the β and γ substituent effects is less straightforward, as differences apparently arise from a combination of relatively small inductive, steric, and conformational effects. Halogen substituents on the alkyl fragment have only a slight effect on the enthalpy of hydroxide attack, but greatly accelerate the elimination step by stabilization of the forming alkoxide ion. This effect falls off rather slowly with distance from the carbonyl group, and is still significant in the γ position. Therefore, the polymer degradation rate can be modified by altering both the number of methylene groups in the repeat unit, and the position of the heteroatoms. Rapid degradation could be achieved with chlorine substitution in the alkyl portion of the ester, adjacent to the carbonyl group, while α fluorine substitution in the acyl fragment would slow the rate-determining step, if the number of methylene groups was sufficiently large to avoid the inductive effects in the alkyl portion of the polyester.

b. Morphological Effect

The wide range of application of synthetic biodegradable polymers requires different polymer processing conditions. As a result, different morphology of polymers is obtained. This morphological difference in synthetic biodegradable polymers must influence their subsequent degradation in a biological environment,

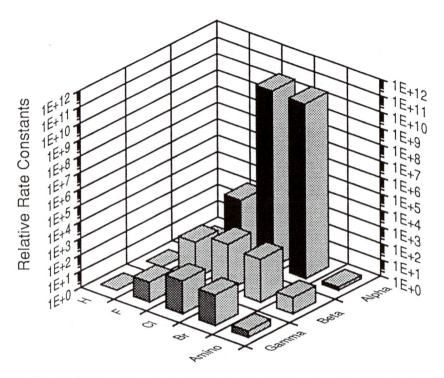

Figure 7.29 Calculated relative rate constants for the hydrolysis of electron donor (or withdrawing) α-substituted esters of glycolic acids. (From Pratt, L. and Chu, C.C., *J. Mol. Struct.*, 304, 213, 1994. With permission.)

and would reflect in their different rates of hydrolysis even though the polymers have the same chemical constituents. This is because the hydrolytic degradation of synthetic biodegradable polymers, particularly those in fibrous form, has been found to be closely related to the accessibility of amorphous regions of the polymers to water, the relative portions of amorphous to crystalline regions, and the chain orientation in the amorphous regions.[42,72,78,90] Thus, a synthetic biodegradable polymer in fibrous form, like PGA suture, would be expected to degrade differently from a bone plate or drug delivery device made of PGA.

Chu et al. recently examined the effect of polymer morphology on the hydrolytic degradation of PGA suture fibers.[79,90] Three types of PGA samples differing in physical form were used: (1) multifilament-braided Dexon suture of 2/0 size from Davis & Geck, (2) PGA polymer chips of molecular weight (M_w) about 60,000 from Polyscience, and (3) capillary-rheometer extruded PGA monofilament fiber from the same PGA chips as in (2). It was found that the levels of crystallinity of these three types of PGA samples exhibited a different relationship with the duration of hydrolysis (Figure 7.30). An unoriented PGA rheometer fiber showed a rapid increase in the level of crystallinity during the very early stage of hydrolysis (i.e., 7 d) and its crystallinity remained at a constant level thereafter for a long period of hydrolysis (about 40 d). Dexon sutures, however, showed a characteristic maximum pattern in crystallinity with a peak at 30 d of hydrolysis. PGA chips showed a similar characteristic in crystallinity vs. hydrolysis time as Dexon suture, but the onset of the crystallinity level occurred about 5 d earlier than Dexon sutures and the width of the maximum peak was much broader than for Dexon sutures. These findings suggest that the orientation of molecules is an important factor in influencing the rate of hydrolysis. The difference in crystallinity onset time indicated that unoriented PGA degraded faster than oriented PGA. Subsequent weight loss study of these three PGA samples also confirmed this observation. Morphologically, the typical circumferential surface cracks observed in oriented PGA sutures, however, were not found in unoriented PGA samples. Instead, micropores were found in unoriented PGA samples and these pores increased in number and size as hydrolysis proceeded.

A similar morphological effect of PGA on its hydrolytic degradation has also been reported by Ginde and Gupta.[58] They examined the *in vitro* hydrolytic degradation of PGA pellets and fibers at a variety of pH media. They found that PGA pellets degraded faster than PGA fibers in terms of mass and strength losses and surface morphology, even though PGA pellets had an initial higher level of crystallinity than the PGA fibers. PGA pellets showed circumferential and longitudinal surface cracks as early as 7 d in

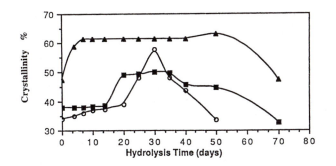

Figure 7.30 The change of the crystallinity level of three PGA samples differing in morphology as a function of *in vitro* hydrolysis time. (○) Dexon suture fiber; (■) PGA chip; (▲) rheometer PGA fiber. (From Chu, C.C. and Kizil, Z., *3rd International ITV Conference on Biomaterials — Medical Textiles*, Stuttgart, W. Germany, 1989, p.24. With permission.)

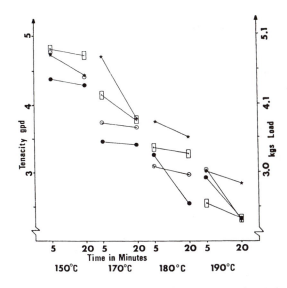

Figure 7.31 The effects of annealing temperature, time, and percent extension on tenacity of 2/0 PGA sutures through a three-factor analysis. Percent extensions during annealing were (●) freely hung; (○) 0%; (□) 1%; (★) 10%. (From Browning, A. and Chu, C.C., *J. Biomed. Mater. Res.*, 20, 613, 1986. With permission.)

water media and became more severe and frequent at longer periods of hydrolysis. On the contrary, PGA fibers did not show any surface crack up to 28 d.

c. Annealing Effect

On the basis of the proposed hydrolytic degradation mechanism of synthetic absorbable sutures described earlier in this chapter, any alteration of the ratio of crystalline to amorphous regions of these materials is expected to result in a different degree of degradation rate. Chu and Browning[70,78] examined such an approach by using the annealing method to alter the hydrolysis rate of 2/0 size PGA sutures *in vitro* in phosphate buffer of pH 7.4 at 37°C.

The sutures were annealed under selected axial strain (freely hung, 0%, 1%, and 10%) at four temperatures (150, 170, 180, and 190°C) and two durations (5 and 20 min). It was found that annealing treatments, in general, did alter the mechanical properties of PGA sutures, as well as their degradation properties. Figure 7.31 demonstrates the synergistic relationships among annealing temperature, time, and percent of axial extension and their effects on tensile strength of PGA sutures. Most of the annealing treatments (i.e., temperature, time) resulted in lower tenacity and breaking elongation when compared with the control samples. PGA sutures that have been exposed to any level of axial tension during annealing, however, exhibited more resistance toward hydrolytic degradation than the freely hung specimens. Before hydrolysis, freely hung specimens had the same strength as the strained ones, but the former showed a faster loss of strength than the latter as degradation proceeded.

Such a difference in hydrolytic degradation may indicate that a different morphologic rearrangement of the amorphous and crystalline regions within microfibrils occurred, due to the different conditions of annealing (i.e., freely hung vs. strained). Under a freely hung annealing condition, the tie-chain segments located in amorphous domains can acquire less constrained conformations, which subsequently could bring the crystal blocks they connect back to the original arrangement before drawing. As a consequence, the characteristics of fiber structure are lost gradually and this is reflected in the observed shrinkage. The amount of shrinkage (an indication of loss of fiber structure) depends on the severity of the annealing treatments, particularly temperature treatment. At annealing temperatures below the melting point of the fiber the memory effect of the tie-chain molecules succeeds only partially, thus producing incomplete shrinkage. Annealing at a temperature slightly above its melting point may achieve nearly complete shrinkage and loss of fiber characteristics as reported by Prevorsek and Tobolsky.[91] This tendency of annealed polymers to return to the stage of less oriented conformation was also demonstrated by Siegmann and Geil[92] in an electron microscopy and X-ray scattering study of the neck region of polyoxymethylene.

The loss of fiber characteristics and a return to a more disoriented packing of parallel lamellae with much less material connection in the fiber direction are particularly profound in the freely hung PGA specimens and are believed to be responsible for the observed hydrolytic resistance. According to the hydrolytic degradation mechanism of PGA proposed by Chu,[69] the reduction in orientation of the lamellae in the freely hung annealed specimens will orient the end faces of the crystallites away from the fiber axis which could expose the end faces more directly to the surrounding water to facilitate so-called preferential end attack.

The rearrangement of the tie-chain molecules to the less constrained (amorphous) conformations in the freely hung annealed PGA suture also results in the observed higher breaking elongation through uncoiling of the amorphous conformations. In the clamped and strained samples, however, breaking elongation decreased with more severe strain treatment. This is due to the fact that stress applied during annealing will uncoil and disentangle the molecules in the amorphous regions, and as a result, the fewer entanglements will present the material with fewer opportunities to extend before break. This would lead to a reduction in elongation which involves the uncoiling of molecules.

The anneal effect on suture hydrolysis mentioned above was also confirmed by Ginde and Gupta[58] in their study of the effect of heat treatment of the hydrolysis of PGA fibers. As shown in Table 7.5, the rate constant of hydrolysis for the heat-treated PGA fiber was 86% greater than the untreated one of the same suture diameter over a wide range of pH of the degradation media.[58]

2. Extrinsic Factors

a. Effect of pH of Media

Since all commercial synthetic absorbable sutures have ester linkages, they are subject to hydrolysis as simple organic esters. However, is the hydrolytic degradation of these absorbable sutures affected by the pH of the medium in the same way that it is affected in the simple organic esters? Are the reversibility and irreversibility of hydrolysis in simple organic esters applicable to polymeric systems? How does the tensile strength of the suture material change with pH of a medium? Furthermore, it is important to understand the pH-dependent degradation of these suture materials, because surgical suture materials should be able to retain adequate strength under all possible physiologic and pathologic conditions. It is known that the pH of gastric juice in the stomach can reach as low as 0.9 to 1.5, while pancreatic juice in the duodenum ranges from 7.5 to 8.2.[93,94] The urinary pH often ranges from 4.5 to 8.0.[95] In the latter case, although the reported data are in conflict, absorbable sutures should be used. Nonabsorbable sutures should not be used in the urinary tract because their presence incites the formation of urinary calculi.[96] This peculiar requirement in urologic surgery further indicates the importance of studying the pH-dependent degradation of synthetic absorbable sutures. To answer these questions, a series of studies have been reported.[24,25,97,98]

Plain catgut sutures showed the widest range of change of breaking elongation within the pH levels studied. Breaking elongations were the highest at the acidic medium (175%) and the lowest at the high-alkaline medium (42%) in plain catgut sutures.

In Figure 7.32, the percentage retention of tensile strength of Vicryl sutures was plotted against the pH levels at different periods of immersion. This plot not only illustrates the pH dependence of the

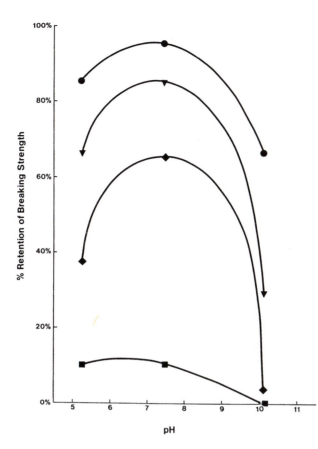

Figure 7.32 The percentage retention of breaking strength of 2/0 poly (glycolide-lactide) copolymer absorbable sutures at various pH levels. (●) Day 7; (▼) day 14; (♦) day 21; (■) day 28. (From Chu, C.C., *Ann. Surg.*, 195(1), 55, 1982. With permission.)

hydrolytic degradation of these synthetic absorbable sutures but also shows how this pH dependence changes with the duration of immersion.

In Vicryl sutures, all the curves have one common character — a convex shape. The maximum retention of tensile strength occurred around the pH level of 7.0, whereas smaller percentages of retention of tensile strength were observed at both acidic and strong alkaline solutions. The shape of the convex curves depended on the duration of immersion. The curves became sharper as the duration of immersion increased from 7 to 21 d, and then became broad at 28 d.

In Dexon sutures, a continuous decrease in the percentage retention of tensile strength was observed with an increase in the pH level from 5.25 to 10.09 at day 7. Therefore, Dexon sutures retained the highest amount of tensile strength at a pH level of 5.25 at day 7. The data indicate a change, however, at day 14 when sutures from the physiologic pH (7.44) exhibited better retention of tensile strength than Dexon sutures from the acidic and high alkaline buffers. Thus, a similar convex curve shape as for Vicryl sutures is found in Dexon sutures at day 14. As degradation proceeded to day 21, no measurable strength could be detected at the pH level of 10.09 and Dexon sutures retained better strength in acidic conditions than in slight and strong alkaline conditions. This tendency was also observed at day 28.

The reasons for the significant difference in the degradation behavior between the acidic and slightly alkaline buffers (pH = 5.25 and 7.44) and the highly alkaline buffer (pH = 10.09) are not clear. It could be attributed to two factors: the cage effect in the crystalline regions, and the pH effect on the hydrogen bond. They are elucidated as follows.

The hydrolysis of simple organic esters in a neutral or an acidic medium generally has the characteristic of reversibility of the reaction, which alkaline hydrolysis does not have. Whether this unique characteristic (reversibility) still exists in polymeric substances is not known. It is believed, however, that the probability of two fragmentary chain ends located in the amorphous region recombining (i.e., reversing) is too small to be significant.[99] But due to the far more restricted mobility of chain segments located in the crystalline lattice, the two chain ends resulting from a hydrolytic cleavage in this lattice might have a better chance to recombine. This so-called "cage effect," a concept which involves the recombination of reactive species, has been demonstrated in the acid hydrolysis of cellulose and other types of chain scission degradations.[100–102] If this cage effect indeed exists, it could slow down the degradation of PGA sutures in both acidic and neutral buffer media. The cage effect may not be restricted to the crystalline phase only. A high viscosity in the amorphous regions, due to either high molecular weight or low crystallinity, might create such a cage. It is believed, however, that the cage effect in the crystalline regions would be more pronounced and important than the same effect in the amorphous region.

The significantly faster degradation of PGA in the highly alkaline buffer (pH = 10.09) than in the acidic one could be attributed to the irreversible nature of hydrolytic degradation. The cage effect is thought to be inapplicable to alkaline hydrolysis because of the irreversible nature of the hydrolysis. After 21 d in pH = 10.09 buffer, no trace of suture materials could be detected. The crystalline part of the suture material was completely degraded. This is in contrast to acidic and neutral degradations. Thus, the existence and the extent of crystalline regions in PGA would have a stronger effect on degradation in a neutral or an acidic buffer than in a highly alkaline buffer.

The other possible cause for the difference in degradation behavior at different pH levels might be related to the hydrogen bond. It is a well-established fact that in macromolecules the capability of hydrogen bonding between two adjacent chain segments is lost at a higher pH level.[103] Strong hydrogen bonds exist, due to stereoregularity and the ester groups of PGA. Hydrogen bonds are not destroyed in acidic and neutral media. Consequently, they stabilize the chain segments in the amorphous and crystalline regions, and result in a "relatively" more rigid and compact amorphous structure than that of the polymer without hydrogen bonds. Conversely, the amorphous structure of PGA in a higher pH medium is relatively open, due to its lack of capability in forming hydrogen bonds. Due to different pH conditions, varying degrees of openness in the amorphous structure result in different levels of accessibility of the hydrolytic species to the PGA chain segments located in the amorphous structure. A more open amorphous structure of PGA in an alkaline buffer would degrade the sutures faster than the specimens in a buffer of lower pH level, because of the better accessibility of the hydrolytic species in the former.

It is highly possible that both mechanisms, the cage effect and pH-dependent hydrogen bonding, operate in PGA hydrolytic degradation. The former, however, will function predominantly in the crystalline region, while the latter will occur mainly in the amorphous region.

The observed pH dependence of Dexon and Vicryl sutures was also confirmed by Gorham et al.[31] and Ginde and Gupta.[58] Gorham et al. examined in vitro Vicryl sutures and mesh incubated in rabbit and human urine of various pH.[31] As shown in Figure 7.33, 3/0 Vicryl sutures lost their tensile breaking force much faster at pH 8.2 normal human and rabbit urine than at lower pH. For example, about 59% of the original Vicryl tensile breaking force was lost at pH 8.2 urine at 7 d, while those same sutures at pH 7, 6.1, and 5.8 retained more than 80% of their original tensile breaking force at the same period of incubation. However, the data at pH <7.0 indicated that Vicryl sutures in acidic urine hydrolytically degraded more slowly than neutral pH. This is quite different from Chu's data described previously (Figure 7.32). It is difficult to explain why the data from Gorham et al. do not follow the well-known fact that acids should catalyze the hydrolysis of organic esters, as shown in Chu's data.

Ginde and Gupta[58] conducted a thorough study of the effect of pH on the hydrolysis of PGA fibers and pellets. They concluded that the rate of hydrolysis was an order of magnitude faster in alkaline vs. acidic media. The faster hydrolytic degradation at a highly alkaline medium was also evident in mass loss, level of crystallinity, rate constants, and surface morphology. The rate constant at pH 10.6 medium ($46.08 \pm 1.79 \times 10^3$ liter/mol/d) was six times the rate constant at the neutral pH ($8.64 \pm 0.23 \times 10^3$ liter/mol/d) as shown in Table 7.5. PGA fibers retained more than 80% of their mass at the end of 6 weeks in vitro, if the pH of the medium was ≤ 9.2. But no measurable PGA fiber mass could be found at the same period in pH 10.6 medium. The dramatic rapid reduction in the level of crystallinity after peaking at the end of 3 weeks in vitro in pH 10.6 medium agreed with the mass loss profiles.

Reed and Gilding[47] and Holm-Jensen and Agner[104] also reported the effect of pH on absorbable suture degradation. Holm-Jensen and Agner concluded that the degradation of Dexon sutures was not significantly affected within the pH range of 2 to 11. Reed and Gilding reported that there is no significant difference in the degradation rate of PGA and poly (glycolide-lactide) copolymers of compositions of 50/50 and 70/30 mol% within the pH levels of 5.0 and 9.0. This discrepancy between the data from Chu et al. and others was surprising, as these absorbable sutures are of linear aliphatic polyesters whose hydrolytic degradation should be pH dependent.

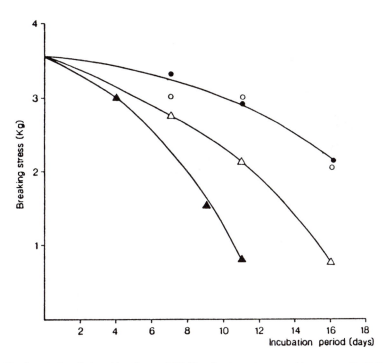

Figure 7.33 The loss in tensile breaking force of 3/0 Vicryl sutures in normal human and rabbit urine at 37°C. (●) pH 5.8; (○) pH 6.1; (△) pH 7.0; (▲) pH 8.2 (rabbit urine). (From Gorham, S.D. et al., *Urol. Res.*, 15, 53, 1987. With permission.)

The accelerated hydrolysis of synthetic absorbable sutures at pH other than 7.44 is particularly noticeable in certain pathologic conditions. Milroy reported that the presence of infection within the bladder enhanced the dissolution of Dexon sutures.[105] This early dissolution was tentatively attributed to an increase in bladder pH level to as high as 8.39 as a result of a urea splitting microorganism (e.g., *Proteus*) degrading the urine to ammonia. Milroy's speculation on the pH dependence of the hydrolysis of these synthetic absorbable sutures is consistent with Chu's reported studies of the effect of pH on the degradation of synthetic absorbable sutures.

The reported pH-dependent hydrolysis of absorbable sutures like Dexon and Vicryl sutures deserves the attention of surgeons in their selection of these suture materials for their particular needs. In the case of an acidic environment such as the stomach, there is very little difference in hydrolysis rate between Dexon and Vicryl sutures; the latter is only slightly better than the former. In the case of an alkaline environment, such as physiologic pH, or a *Proteus*-infected urinary track, Vicryl sutures appear to retain much better tensile strength than Dexon sutures, and hence are the better choice in that circumstance. This difference in strength retention should be considered along with the capability of the suture materials to elicit the formation of urinary calculi in the selection of proper suture materials for urologic surgery.

b. Effect of Electrolytes

The human body consists of a high percentage of electrolyte fluid containing Na, Ca, Mg, and K ions. The presence of these electrolytes is expected to alter the solvation sphere surrounding biodegradable materials. If the presence of these electrolytes makes the environment unfavorable for water molecules to diffuse into biodegradable polymers, it should be reflected subsequently in degradation properties. For example, a change of ionic strength of a fluid due to the presence of electrolytes will alter the behavior of water molecules in the fluid. That, in turn, should alter the hydrolytic degradation of synthetic absorbable polymers. Such an electrolyte effect on the biodegradation properties of absorbable sutures was recently reported by Pratt et al.[106] They examined the effect of electrolytes on tensile and thermo-dynamic properties of Dexon and Vicryl sutures. They also used a theoretical molecular modeling of the solvation sphere to gain a basic understanding of the mechanism behind the observed electrolyte effect.

Both PGA and Vicryl sutures showed a considerably higher retention in tensile breaking strength (TBS) (and hence a slower rate of hydrolytic degradation) when hydrolyzed in NaCl and MgCl$_2$ solutions

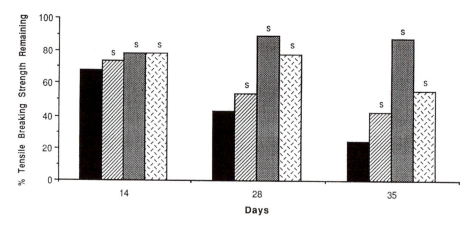

Figure 7.34 The effect of electrolytes on the tensile strength retention of 2-0 Dexon sutures; left to right in each group of four bars, the shaded columns indicate deionized water; 20% magnesium chloride; 54% magnesium chloride; 25% sodium chloride. S, statistically significant; N, not statistically significant; *t*-test at 95% level, deionized water as control. (From Pratt, L. et al., *J. Polym. Sci. Chem. Ed.*, 31, 1759, 1993. With permission.)

than in the deionized water control. As shown in Figure 7.34, the highest TBS was retained in 54% $MgCl_2$ solution, while the control showed the lowest retention of TBS over the entire period of study. The extent of retention of TBS was also dependent on the concentration of electrolyte. Better retention of TBS was observed in a more concentrated electrolyte solution than in a less concentrated solution. A comparison between 20% and 54% $MgCl_2$ solutions demonstrated this point of view. It was also found that the electrolyte effect became more profound at a later stage of hydrolysis. For example, both Dexon and Vicryl fibers showed about 10% loss of the original TBS at the end of 14 d in the $MgCl_2$ solution and no further loss of tensile strength thereafter (till the end of the study at 35 d), while the control exhibited consistently lower retention of TBS over the same period and reached 13.5% retention of TBS at the end of 35 d. Although the NaCl solution showed electrolyte effects similar to the $MgCl_2$ solution, the effects were less dramatic.

This observed electrolyte effect on the retention of TBS of synthetic absorbable sutures was closely related to the observed surface morphology, water uptake data, calculated chemical potential difference ($\Delta\mu$), and molecular modeling describing below.

The significantly better retention of TBS found in the electrolyte solutions was consistent with the observed surface morphology of these biodegradable suture fibers. Figure 7.35 illustrates the observed different surface morphology of Dexon and Vicryl suture fibers due to different media. Both Dexon and Vicryl suture fibers in 54% $MgCl_2$ solution showed surface morphology not much different from the corresponding unhydrolyzed ones after 35 d, while the same fibers in the control media (deionized water) exhibited either many fiber fragmentations (in Dexon) or distinctive circumferential cracks (in Vicryl). Such circumferential cracks were also found in previous studies by Chu and coworkers[71] of γ-irradiated biodegradable suture fibers and were closely related to the accelerated loss of TBS. Thus, the observed much better retention of fiber surface morphology of Dexon and Vicryl sutures in electrolyte solutions agrees with their significantly better retention of TBS.

Hydrolytic degradation of these biodegradable polymers cannot begin until water molecules reach chain segments located in the noncrystalline domains to initiate chain scission reactions. Thus, a measure of water uptake and its rate would provide needed information to explain the observed electrolyte effect. The largest amount and fastest rate of water uptake of PGA disks (and hence the fastest degradation in terms of the loss of TBS) were associated with the deionized water, followed by the NaCl solution. The water uptakes in $MgCl_2$, LiCl, and $ZnCl_2$ solutions were the smallest and of comparable magnitude. Thus, both the amount and rate of water uptake data agree well with the aforementioned TBS data. It should be pointed out that the decrease in water uptake after the maximum was attributed to PGA mass loss resulting from hydrolytic degradation.

The calculated chemical potential differences of water ($\Delta\mu$) between electrolyte solutions and pure water at 37°C are summarized in Table 7.12. The data are in good agreement with the observed water uptake and the retention of TBS. In electrolyte solutions, the chemical potential of water is always smaller than the chemical potential of pure liquid water. Thus, $\Delta\mu$ is negative. The magnitude of this

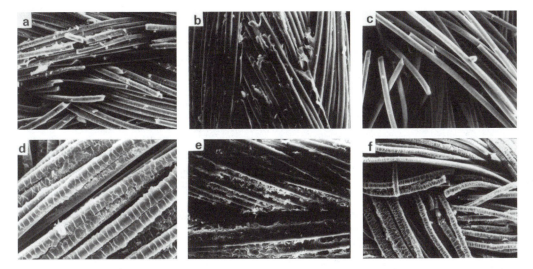

Figure 7.35 SEM of partially hydrolyzed Dexon (a-c) and Vicryl (d-f) sutures for 35 days. (a,d) In deionized water, (b, e) in 54% MgCl$_2$, (c,f) in phosphate buffer. (From Pratt, L. et al., *J. Polym. Sci. Chem. Ed.*, 31, 1759, 1993. With permission.)

Table 7.12 Chemical Potential Difference ($\Delta\mu$) of Different Electrolyte Solutions at 37°C

Solution (by Weight)	γ	$\Delta\mu$ (kJ)
25% NaCl	0.8574	–0.6488
20% MgCl$_2$·6H$_2$O	0.7883	–0.6634
54% MgCl$_2$·6H$_2$O	0.3588	–2.8029

From Pratt, L. et al., *J. Polym. Sci. Chem. Ed.*, 31, 1759, 1993. With permission.

chemical potential difference is also related to the concentration of electrolytes, as evident in the MgCl$_2$ solution. Since activity coefficient, γ, tends to decrease with increasing electrolyte concentration, a higher concentration of electrolyte in a solution results in a larger negative value of $\Delta\mu$. The largest negative value of $\Delta\mu$ is associated with the 54% MgCl$_2$ solution. This also agrees with the observed slowest hydrolytic degradation rate of PGA in this electrolyte solution in terms of water uptake and loss of TBS.

Our understanding of the effect of lowered water chemical potential in solution on water uptake, and hence loss of TBS, is that the polymer initially contains little water, so the chemical potential of water there is very low. Diffusion of water into the polymer is driven by the chemical potential difference between the polymer and the solution outside, so lowered water chemical potential in the solution slows the diffusion process, resulting in both slower uptake and reduced water concentration in the polymer when equilibrium with respect to mass transfer is reached. This effect is illustrated schematically in Figure 7.36.

The electrolyte effect on the hydrolytic degradation of absorbable sutures was further understood by a molecular modeling of a solvation sphere. MNDO/H calculations showed water molecules distributed rather evenly about the polymer segment in the absence of coordinated metal ions (i.e., in the absence of electrolytes).[106] The presence of electrolytes, however, resulted in a greatly perturbed solvation sphere. Metal ions from electrolytes coordinated rather strongly to the carbonyl oxygen atoms with minimum metal–oxygen distances of 1.78, 2.08, and 2.07 Å for beryllium, lithium, and zinc, respectively. The bonding between the carbonyl oxygens and the coordinated metals appears to have a considerable degree of covalent character, as indicated by the calculated charges on the atoms. Far from being fully ionized, the beryllium, lithium, and zinc atoms carry respective average charges of +0.39, +0.32, and +0.57. Likewise, the chloride counterions are much less than fully ionized with average charges of –0.40 and –0.42 for zinc and beryllium chlorides, and the coordinated water molecules were nearly neutral in charge. The stronger coordination of the metal ions to the carbonyl oxygens as opposed to the sp^3 oxygens

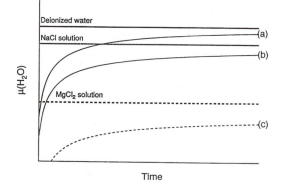

Figure 7.36 Schematic illustration of the changes of chemical potential of water, μ, as a function of electrolytes and hydrolysis time. (a) Deionized water; (b) NaCl solution; (c) MgCl$_2$ solution. (From Pratt, L. et al., *J. Polym. Sci. Chem. Ed.*, 31, 1759, 1993. With permission.)

was further supported by MMX force field calculations.[89] Although obviously a very crude approximation to the structure of the solvation sphere, the force field calculation consistently gave a shorter metal–oxygen distance when bound to the carbonyl oxygen.

Besides metal ion–water coordination, the chloride counterions were also coordinated to the metals in the inner solvation sphere. This coordination of the metal ions to the polymer leads to a disruption of the solvation sphere and subsequently retards the absorption of water into the fiber as reflected in the observed slower water uptake and lower rate of TBS loss.

In conclusion, Chu et al. demonstrated that the presence of ionic salts could retard the hydrolytic degradation of PGA and Vicryl sutures. The decrease in water uptake of the polymer can be explained by a decrease in the chemical potential of the water in the presence of electrolytes, as opposed to that of pure water. On a molecular level, a disruption of the polymer solvation sphere due to the presence of electrolytes was observed by molecular orbital calculations.

c. Effect of External Stress Applied

The effect of external stress or strain on the biodegradation of synthetic absorbable sutures was recently studied by Chu[107] and Miller and Williams.[108] The purpose was to determine whether strained absorbable sutures would degrade differently from unstrained ones. It has been known in studies of polymer degradation that mechanical stress imposed on polymers during degradation could accelerate the degradation process. Examples include the faster hydrolysis of polyamide,[109] and the accelerated autoxidation of polyethylene.[110] Biomedical materials like synthetic absorbable sutures may also be subjected to the same stress-accelerated hydrolytic degradation as other nonbiomedical polymers because of the residual stress, surgical techniques, and clinical conditions. The residual stress of suture fibers may result from the highly drawn process (orientation) during fiber spinning. This orientation process assumes the molecules away from the most stable random conformation and leads to residual stress. In any surgical practice of wound closure by sutures, the sutures could be subjected to various degrees of external stress and strain when surgeons pull them taut during tying knots. In certain clinical conditions, such as a patient's cough, or when wounds develop severe edema, sutures could experience stress. The combination of external stress/strain with body fluid environment could result in a synergic effect on the hydrolytic degradation of absorbable sutures.

Both studies indicate that absorbable sutures indeed degraded faster than unstrained ones and the level of accelerated degradation depended on the percent of strain (or elongation) applied to the sutures. Increasing the level of elongation would accelerate the hydrolytic degradation, and the effect of elongation was more pronounced as the duration of immersion increased. Figure 7.37 illustrates the effect of strain on *in vitro* loss of TBS of 2/0 PGA sutures. Beyond 14 d, no TBS could be detected with 5% strained Dexon sutures, while there was about 84% retention of original tensile strength of unstrained PGA sutures. This accelerated hydrolytic degradation of strained PGA sutures was also evidenced in changes of the level of crystallinity with hydrolysis time. The onset of an accelerated increase in the level of crystallinity of 5% strained PGA sutures occurred as early as 7 d, while the onset time for the unstrained PGA controls was 20 d. This suggests that the rate of hydrolytic chain scission in the amorphous regions

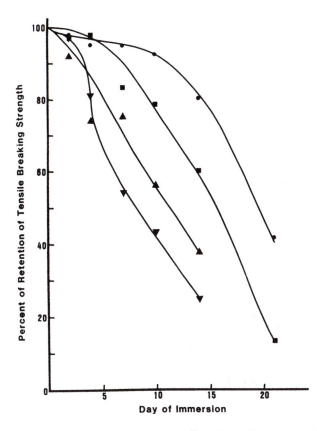

Figure 7.37 Effect of external stress/strain on the retention of tensile breaking strength of 2/0 size PGA sutures under *in vitro* hydrolysis at 37°C. (●) unstrained control; (■) 1% strained; (▲) 2.5% strained; (▼) 5.0% strained. (From Chu, C.C., in *Surgical Research -— Recent Developments*, Hall, C.W., Ed., Pergamon Press, New York, 1985, pp. 111–113. With permission.)

of strained PGA suture fibers is faster than unstrained ones. This observed acceleration *in vitro* hydrolytic degradation of strained PGA sutures was also reported *in vivo* by Miller and Williams.[108] PGA sutures at 25% and 50% of the breaking strain were subcutaneously implanted in the dorsal surface of Half-Lop rabbits for up to 28 d. The strained PGA sutures hydrolyzed more rapidly after 1 week implantation. The most elongated PGA sutures (50%) lost all of their tensile breaking load at about the 17th day of postimplantation, while the 25% elongated and unstained PGA sutures retained 50% and 85% of their original tensile breaking loads, respectively.

The effect of external stress or strain on suture hydrolysis rate has also been confirmed in Vicryl sutures. Zhong et al. recently examined the effect of applied external stain on mechanical and thermal properties of 2/0 Vicryl sutures in hydrogen peroxide (H_2O_2).[111] Their results support data described above from Chu[107] and Miller and Williams.[108] Figure 7.38 illustrates the stress-strain curves of 14 d *in vitro* hydrolysis in four different media: in deionized water without strain, in deionized water with 4% strain applied, in 6% H_2O_2 without strain, and in 6% H_2O_2 with 4% strain applied. The level of 4% strain is slightly beyond the yield point (3%) of Vicryl suture. The prestrained Vicryl sutures lost about 59% of their unhydrolyzed TBS in deionized water, while the unstrained sutures lost only about 43%. Irrespective of whether they were strained or unstrained, the presence of 6% H_2O_2 in media accelerated the strength loss significantly more than the deionized water medium alone. The effect of H_2O_2 on the strength loss of Vicryl sutures appeared to be independent of the concentration of H_2O_2. Figure 7.39 summarizes the retention of the ultimate TBS of 2/0 Vicryl sutures in various media. The accelerated effect of applied strain in various media was also confirmed in the change of crystallinity level. As described in Section III.C, the change in the level of crystallinity could be used as an indicator to measure the rate of hydrolysis of absorbable sutures. Zhong et al.[111] reported that Vicryl sutures in H_2O_2 media

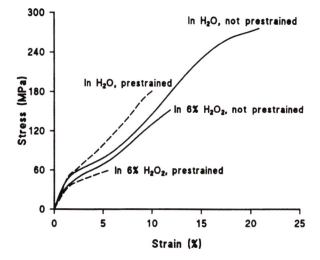

Figure 7.38   The effect of prestrain and H_2O_2 on the stress and strain of undyed 2/0 Vicryl suture. (From Zhong, S.P. et al., *Clin. Mater.*, 14, 183, 1993. With permission.)

exhibited a maximum level of crystallinity as early as 7 d *in vitro*, irrespective of applied strain or not; while the level of crystallinity of the same sutures in deionized water media had not reached a maximum at the end of 14 d *in vitro*. However, readers should be aware that the observed difference in the rate of strength loss between water and H_2O_2 media could be due to pH difference between the two media.

There are several possible reasons behind the observed stress/strain induced accelerated hydrolytic degradation of absorbable sutures. They are (1) stress-induced chemical reaction, (2) stress-induced alteration of morphological structure, and (3) stress-induced accelerated diffusion of small molecular species. It is known that when an external stress is applied to semicrystalline polymers, stress-induced chemical reactions controlled by the level of stress/strain, chemical constituents of chain molecules and chain conformation, and/or alteration of morphological structure could occur. The former (stress-induced reaction) would occur in high-molecular-weight materials like polymers and has been documented by Porter and Casale[112] and Silberberg and Henenberg.[113] This is because molecules would flow or slip under external stress/strain to release the imposed mechanical energy. When molecular weight is high, the high degree of entanglement among chain molecules would retard their slippage which, in turn, would store the imposed mechanical energy within segments of molecules. This would increase the energy level of molecules and may lead to either the distortion of chemical bonds and eventually their breakage, with the production of macroradicals, or the reduction in the activation energy for other chemical reactions. Some examples of stress-induced chemical reactions are the photodegradation of polyolefins[114] and oxidation of nylon 66.[115]

The alteration of molecular and gross morphological structure upon external stress/strain was reported by Rapoport and Zaikov in their study of stress-induced oxidation of polymers.[116] The applied external stress would change the molecular dynamics and molecular conformation which closely relate to the formation of a transition complex required for any chemical reaction to occur. Carter and Wilkes reported that uniaxial tension of an absorbable copolyester of glycolide and L-lactide (the same polymer used to make Vicryl suture) resulted in a distinctive gross morphological change in spherulites.[117] Using a standard chemical etching technique, they reported that a circular spherulite was transformed into an ellipsoidal shape upon uniaxial deformation. Different regions of a spherulite deformed differently, depending on the direction of the applied stress relative to the fibril axis within a spherulite and the related interstitial amorphous materials. For example, in the equatorial region of the spherulite, where the crystalline fibrils and interstitial amorphous materials are perpendicular to the principal applied stress, these two types of materials (fibrils and amorphous sandwiched between two adjacent fibrils) mechanically behaved like they are connected in "series" upon external stress. In other words, the least resistant material (i.e., interstitial amorphous) would pick up the external stress, yield and deform first, while the more resistant material (i.e., crystalline fibrils) would resist the deformation imposed by the external stress. As a result, a splaying of the crystalline fibrils would form and lead to more accessible amorphous

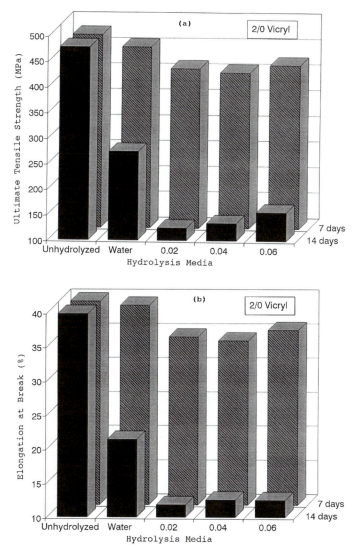

Figure 7.39 The mechanical properties of undyed 2/0 Vicryl suture treated in different concentrations of H_2O_2 at 7 and 14 d *in vitro*. (Data from Zhong, S.P. et al., *Clin. Mater.*, 14, 183, 1993. With permission.)

materials to low molecular species like water or H_2O_2 for hydrolysis. An accelerated loss of mechanical strength could thus result from this increased exposure of amorphous domains.

The third factor is the stress-induced accelerated diffusion of low-molecular-weight species. Peterlin reported that the sorption of low-molecular-weight species into semicrystalline polymers increased with increasing external stress applied below the yield point of polymers.[118] This is because the random coiled chain segments within the amorphous domains are extended upon the application of initial stress which subsequently reduce the volume occupied by chain segments and facilitate the accommodation of low-molecular-weight permeants. The accelerated diffusion of low-molecular-weight species upon external stress could also be attributed to the generation of submicrocracks in microfibril structure as reported by Peterlin.[61] He found that external stress applied to fibers could induce the retraction of the ends of microfibrils which were the origin of submicrocracks.[61] The submicrocracks of the microfibrils located on the outer surface of a fiber are believed to have a more important influence on the hydrolytic degradation of the fiber, because alkaline hydrolysis of a fiber has been reported to be a surface phenomenon and water molecules will have better access to enter the submicrocracks on the outer surface of a fiber.

Which of the three factors contribute to the observed accelerated loss of tensile strength in absorbable sutures? Based on data by Zhong et al,.[111] they hypothesized that the stress-induced chemical reaction is unlikely to be responsible for the observed faster loss of tensile strength in both water and H_2O_2 media, since the extent of external stress was near the yield point, and the Vicryl suture that was strained for 14 d in vacuum (for the purpose of eliminating stress-induced oxidation) had the same TBS as the unstrained and unhydrolyzed Vicryl sutures. Therefore, Zhong et al. suggested that the second (morphology) and third (diffusion) factors were the most probable causes. When semicrystalline fibers like PGA or Vicryl sutures are subject to a low level of external force (i.e., less than yield stress), the tie-chain segments located in the amorphous regions will be uncoiled and become taut. This would create additional free space within the amorphous domains to facilitate the diffusion of small-molecular-weight species like water or H_2O_2. As the level of stress/strain increases to a level slightly above yield point, main-chain bonds will be ruptured initially almost exclusively in the tie-chain segments connecting the two crystalline blocks. The shortest tie-chain segments will be broken first. This rupture of main-chain bonds in the amorphous regions would create new void space in the regions and hence allow more water molecules to penetrate into the suture fibers for a faster hydrolytic degradation. The possible formation of submicrocracks in microfibrils would also facilitate the diffusion of water and/or H_2O_2 into these sutures.

d. Effect of Temperature

Although all *in vitro* and *in vivo* hydrolytic degradation studies of synthetic absorbable sutures have been conducted at 37°C, it is theoretically predicted that other temperatures should result in different rates of hydrolysis. This is because the diffusion rate of water molecules through absorbable sutures depends on the relative magnitude of T_g of the suture materials to degradation temperature. In theory, water diffusion into a polymer could either not happen or happen at a very slow rate at a temperature lower than T_g of the polymer, due to the inability of chain segments to yield to the advancement of water molecules. Because hydrolytic degradation must require the diffusion of water molecules into the interior of a material, a hydrolytic degradation at a temperature lower than T_g of a suture material would occur either very slowly and be restricted to the surface, or not at all. The five commercial synthetic absorbable sutures have a wide range of T_g, some below 37°C (e.g., Maxon and PDS), while others are near or above body temperature (e.g., Dexon and Vicryl). Thus, it is expected that these absorbable sutures would degrade significantly differently at temperatures above or below their T_g. An example is given in Figure 7.40 for Vicryl sutures and Figure 7.41 for Maxon sutures.

As shown in Figure 7.40, the effect of hydrolytic degradation temperature on the loss of tensile strength and mass of Vicryl is very dramatic. A highly significant reduction in the hydrolytic degradation rate (in terms of tensile strength and weight loss) of Vicryl sutures was found when the hydrolysis was conducted at a temperature (room temperature) less than T_g. For example, at the end of 28 d, a 4.0 Mrad irradiated Vicryl that was hydrolyzed at room temperature retains 53.9% of its original tensile breaking load, while the unirradiated Vicryl exhibits no measurable tensile breaking load at 37°C hydrolysis. It is known, from studies by Chu et al. on the effect of γ-irradiation (described later) on the hydrolytic degradation of various synthetic absorbable sutures,[41,71,83] that γ-irradiation would significantly accelerate the loss of both tensile strength and suture mass. For example, 2 Mrad irradiated Vicryl exhibited no TBS at the end of 14 d *in vitro* hydrolysis at 37°C, while the same dosage irradiated Vicryl retained 74% of its original tensile breaking load at the end of 28 d hydrolysis at room temperature. Similar findings were also found in the weight loss of sutures during *in vitro* hydrolysis, as shown in Figure 7.40b. There is virtually no change in irradiated suture mass (98% retention) during the 60 d of *in vitro* hydrolysis at a temperature lower than T_g of the suture, while those irradiated sutures hydrolyzed at 37°C exhibited no measurable suture mass at the end of 14 d for 2.0 Mrad and 60 d for 0.1 Mrad. Similar observations were found in Maxon sutures, as shown in Figure 7.41. Thus, the temperature of hydrolysis lower than T_g could reduce the hydrolysis rate of absorbable sutures to such an extent that a highly γ-irradiated absorbable suture would exhibit a far better retention of tensile breaking load and suture mass than an unirradiated one hydrolyzed at $T > T_g$.

Similar temperature effects on the hydrolytic degradation of 1/0 Dexon sutures were also reported by Reed and Gilding.[47] As shown in Figure 7.42, there was a significant temperature effect on both tensile strength and mass loss below and above T_g of Dexon (36°C). Dexon sutures hydrolyzed at 25°C retained more than 60% of their original tensile breaking force at the end of 12 weeks, while the same sutures hydrolyzed at 50°C exhibited no strength at about 10 d. Both the rates of tensile strength and

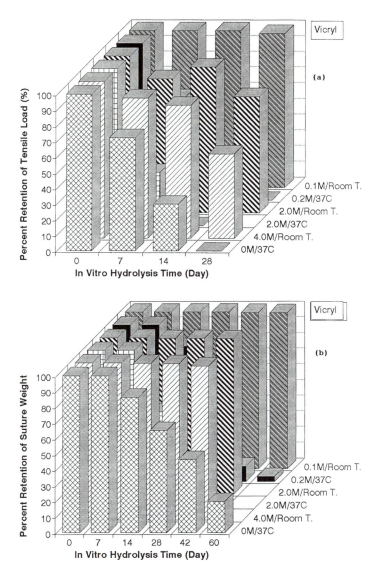

Figure 7.40 Effect of hydrolysis temperature on the hydrolytic degradation of Vicryl sutures. (a) Retention of tensile breaking load; (b) retention of suture mass.

mass losses showed discontinuity at T_g. The temperature coefficient (i.e., the slope of the plot of rate of tensile or mass loss vs. temperature) above T_g was about seven times greater than that below T_g.

e. Effect of γ-Irradiation

Gamma-irradiation of fiber-forming polymers can result in simultaneous chain scission and crosslinking. Whether the reaction will be characterized by predominant scission or by crosslinking depends on several factors, including the chemical structure of materials to be irradiated, the amount of dosage, the rate of dosage, the environment of the material during irradiation, and the heat of polymerization.[119,120] The orientation of long-chain molecules has also been reported to have some influence on the direction of the overall radiation reaction, and was due to the differences in chain mobility.[121] In the linear saturated polyesters, such as PGA and PGL, D'Alelio et al.[102] reported that the crosslinking reaction would occur if the radicals formed on the carbon atoms of the methylene group in the main chains combine together, whereas the scission process would be expected to occur within the ester moiety.

In general, the effect of γ-irradiation on synthetic absorbable sutures is undesirable because it leads to an accelerated loss of TBS upon biodegradation. Consequently, all existing synthetic absorbable sutures cannot be sterilized by a conventional ^{60}Co γ-irradiation process. This well-known adverse effect

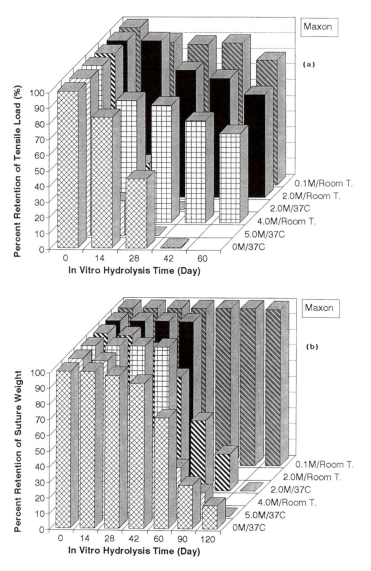

Figure 7.41 Effect of hydrolysis temperature on the hydrolytic degradation of Maxon sutures. (a) Retention of tensile breaking load; (b) retention of suture mass.

of γ-irradiation on the biodegradation properties of synthetic absorbable sutures, however, has recently been overcome by Chu and Lee.[122] In that study, Chu and Lee suggested the incorporation of extremely low temperature and vacuum during γ-irradiation would result in biodegradation properties of γ-irradiated synthetic absorbable sutures similar to the corresponding ethylene oxide sterilized absorbable sutures. The details of the research are given toward the end of this section.

Polyglycolide Sutures In the case of PGA, Figure 7.43 summarizes the possible routes of chain crosslinking and scission. The predominant effect of γ-irradiation on PGA sutures is thought to be scission across the dosage range studied, based on the reported reduction in mechanical properties of PGA upon γ-irradiation.[41,48,123–125] In the Chu et al. study, a steady and progressive decline in the mechanical properties of PGA sutures with increasing irradiation dosage was observed.[123] There was a sharp drop in breaking strength between the dosage levels of 0 and 2.5 Mrad (6.03 to 4.82 gpd), but the decrease was smaller between the 2.5 and 5.0 Mrad dosage (4.82 to 4.50 gpd). The tensile properties then showed another significant decrease between 20 and 40 Mrad.

The loss of molecular weight of Dexon sutures due to γ-irradiation was also reported by Reed and Gilding.[125] As shown in Figure 7.44, the loss of both M_w and M_n of a Dexon suture with γ-irradiation dosage is significant, particularly at the sterilization dosage of 2.5 Mrad. The faster loss of M_n than M_w

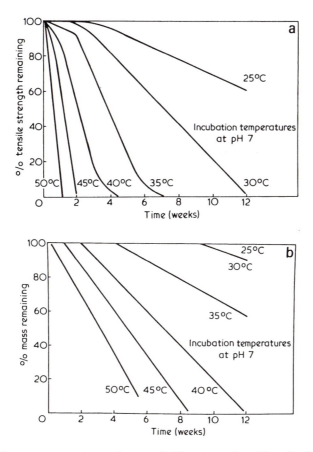

Figure 7.42 Effect of temperature on the tensile strength (a) and mass loss (b) profiles for 0 size PGA sutures. (From Reed, A.M. and Gilding, D.K., *Polymer*, 22(4), 494, 1981. With permission.)

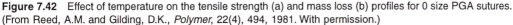

Figure 7.43 Possible routes of chain crosslinking and chain scission of γ-irradiated PGA sutures. (From Chu, C.C. and Campbell, N.D., *J. Biomed. Mater. Res.*, 16, 417, 1982. With permission.)

also suggests that γ-irradiation leads to the unzipping of PGA molecules rather than random chain scissions. The even faster loss of M_{n-1} than M_n at a dosage as low as 1 Mrad supports this unzipping mechanism because M_{n-1} is more sensitive to the low-molecular-weight portion of the molecular weight distribution curve.

The observed γ-irradiation effect on PGA sutures (chain scission) is consistent with the results of a study by D'Alelio et al.,[102] on a series of saturated polyesters. They concluded that the primary factor

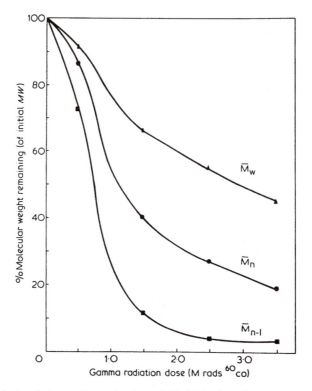

Figure 7.44 Effect of γ-irradiation on the molecular weight distribution of Dexon suture (PGA). (From Reed, A.M. and Gilding, D.K., *Polymer*, 20, 1459, 1979. With permission.)

responsible for the direction of overall radiation effect in the saturated linear polyester is the chemical structure of the diol segment of the main chain. As the number of –CH$_2$– groups in the diol segment increases from 2 to 10, the major observable effect of irradiation changes from chain scission to chain crosslinking. In the PGA system, there is only one –CH$_2$– group in each ester segment. Thus, degradation would be more favorable to occur than crosslinking in the γ-irradiated PGA specimens. This chemical structure effect on the direction of γ-irradiation reaction of saturated linear polyesters is attributed to the weakened bond between alkyl group and acyl oxygen resulting from the ester bond resonance as shown below.[102]

Chain scissions would occur in these already partially weakened bonds when irradiated. As the number of –CH$_2$– groups increases, the distance between two adjacent electron-withdrawing ester groups also increases. This makes any weakening of main chain bonds through ester resonance ineffective. Consequently, it would decrease the scission reaction and relatively increase the crosslinking effect.

The scission of polymer chains is also expected to be more pronounced in the amorphous regions than in the crystalline regions. This might be due to the so-called "cage effect," a concept which involves the recombination of initial radicals before they can diffuse out of an active cage and undergo reactions other than recombination elsewhere. The crystalline regions of the microfibrillar model act as effect cages because of the dense and compact packing of immobile chain segments. The trapped free radicals can recombine and reduce the number of effective scissions. Therefore, γ-irradiation would result in more chain scissions in the amorphous regions than in the crystalline domains. This additional degradation (due to γ-irradiation) of the chain segments located in the amorphous regions would reduce their

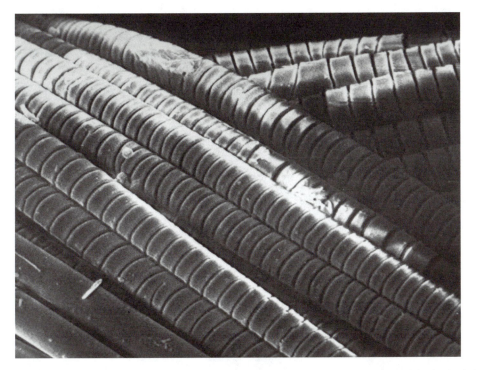

Figure 7.45 Scanning electron micrographs of 20 Mrad irradiated 2/0 PGA sutures after 40 d *in vitro* hydrolysis in pH 7.4 phosphate buffers at 37°C. (From Chu, C.C. and Campbell, N.D., *J. Biomed. Mater. Res.*, 16, 417, 1982. With permission.)

degree of long-chain entanglement before hydrolysis and result in a more open amorphous structure than in unirradiated specimens. This effect would make the chain segments in these regions more accessible to hydrolytic species and hence faster biodegradation as reported by Chu et al.[41,48,71,72,83]

Besides the faster biodegradation upon γ-irradiation, Chu et al. found that γ-irradiated absorbable sutures like PGA exhibited unusual and unique surface morphology upon hydrolysis. Figure 7.45 shows such a unique surface morphology of PGA sutures. A comparison between Figure 7.45 (irradiated) and Figure 7.21 (unirradiated) PGA sutures indicated that γ-irradiation results in far more severe surface cracks on absorbable sutures than unirradiated ones. The severity of the surface cracks depends on the dosage of γ-irradiation and the extent of hydrolysis. Higher dosages of γ-irradiation, or longer immersion in buffer solutions, or both, resulted in more severe and regular surface cracking. The cracks always propagated circumferentially and in a direction perpendicular to the fiber axis. No cracks propagating along the c axis (fiber axis) have been observed in PGA sutures. This is because once a microcrack forms, it would meet stronger hydrolytic resistance along the c axis due to the presence of the crystalline regions and would be less likely to grow along this direction. It will continue to hydrolyze along the a–b directions (cross-sectional plane), where the more open and less resistant amorphous regions are located.

Vicryl, PDS, and Maxon Sutures Similar γ-irradiation effect on the accelerated loss of tensile properties, mass loss, and intrinsic viscosity, and changes in heat of fusion and wettability were also found in Vicryl, PDS, and Maxon sutures.[41,84] However, the magnitude of γ-irradiation effects varied with the type of absorbable sutures. Figure 7.46 is the representative data on Vicryl and Maxon sutures.

Before hydrolysis, γ-irradiation alone significantly affected the tensile breaking force of both Vicryl and Maxon sutures, as shown in Figure 7.46.[41] As the irradiation dosage reached to 2.0 Mrad, only 79% of the original Vicryl tensile breaking force remained. A further increase in irradiation dosage slightly reduced the tensile breaking force further from 79% (2.0 Mrad) to 70.1% (5.0 Mrad). Maxon monofilament sutures, however, appeared to be more resistant to γ-irradiation than PGA and Vicryl sutures. For example, 89.8% and 82.9% of the original tensile breaking force remained for 2.0 and 5.0 Mrad unhydrolyzed Maxon, respectively. The degree of γ-irradiation degradation in the unhydrolyzed PDS sutures in terms of the retention of tensile breaking force (RTBF) is not proportional to the dosage of radiation. For example, the losses of about 7%, 25%, and 64% of RTBF at 5, 10, and 20 Mrad,

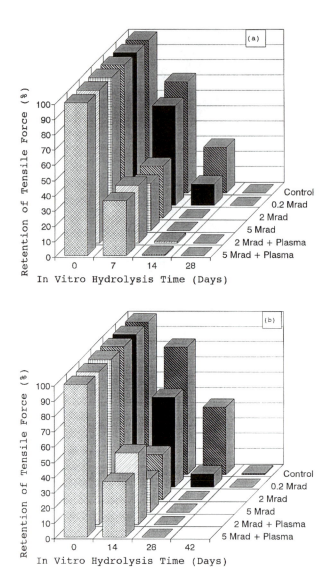

Figure 7.46 Percentage of retention of tensile breaking force of Vicryl and Maxon sutures as a function of *in vitro* hydrolysis time in phosphate buffer solution of pH 7.44 at 37°C. (a) Vicryl, (b) Maxon. (From Zhang, L. et al., *J. Biomed. Mater. Res.*, 27, 1425, 1993. With permission.)

respectively, were observed. Thus, the greatest loss of tensile strength of unhydrolyzed PDS sutures was observed between 10 and 20 Mrad.

Upon hydrolysis, γ-irradiation effects on RTBF became more pronounced for Vicryl, Maxon, and PDS sutures. Seventy percent of original tensile breaking force of 2.0 Mrad treated Vicryl was lost within 7 d of immersion. At 14 d, no tensile breaking force remained. The unirradiated control Vicryl sutures lost most of their tensile breaking force between 7 and 14 d of hydrolysis (from 72.4% to 29.8%), and no tensile breaking force could be measured at the end of 28 d. For the irradiated and hydrolyzed Maxon sutures, only less than 30% of its original tensile breaking force remained at the end of 14 d with 2.0 Mrad irradiation. A further increase in irradiation dosage to 5.0 Mrad reduced the original TBS further to 21.8% at 14 d. Both 2.0 Mrad and 5.0 Mrad treated Maxon exhibited no measurable tensile strength at 28 d. Unirradiated Maxon controls lost most of their tensile breaking force between 14 and 42 d. At the end of 42 d, the breaking force of Maxon sutures was negligible (0.6% retention). γ-Irradiation at the level as low as 5 Mrad was sufficient to significantly increase the susceptibility of PDS fibers to hydrolysis and less than 10% RTBF of 5 Mrad treated PDS sutures was observed at 28 d *in vitro* in buffer, while the unirradiated PDS control retained more than 75% RTBF at the same period of hydrolysis.

Table 7.13 $[\eta]_D/[\eta]_0$ of Vicryl and Maxon Sutures vs. γ-Irradiation Dosage Before Hydrolysis

$[\eta]_D/[\eta]_0$	0 Mrad	0.2 Mrad	2.0 Mrad	5.0 Mrad
Vicryl	1.00	0.95	0.89	0.56
Maxon	1.00	0.92	0.89	0.84

From Zhang, L et al., *J. Biomed. Mater. Res.*, 27, 1425, 1993. With permission.

γ-Irradiation also accelerated the weight loss of Vicryl, PDS, and Maxon sutures. For example, both 2.0 and 5.0 Mrad irradiated Vicryl lost their weight completely at the end of 42 d, while the unirradiated control still retained 46.5% of its initial weight at the same hydrolysis period. Similar observations were also found for Maxon and PDS sutures. Unirradiated Maxon sutures retained 14.6% of their original weight at the end of 120 d *in vitro* in buffer, while the 5.0 Mrad γ-irradiation treated Maxon exhibited significant weight loss as early as 28 d and the weight was unmeasurable at the end of 120 d.

Along with the mass loss, molecular weight of these absorbable sutures is also significantly affected by γ-irradiation as demonstrated by the loss of the intrinsic viscosity, $[\eta]$, of these absorbable sutures. Table 7.13 shows the ratio of $[\eta]_D$ (of irradiated samples) to $[\eta]_0$ (of unirradiated control samples) of both Vicryl and Maxon sutures in HFIP solvent at 18°C.[41] The data indicated that γ-irradiation alone reduced the $[\eta]$ of Vicryl and Maxon, and the magnitude of reduction depended on γ-irradiation dosage. The decrease of $[\eta]$ of irradiated Maxon was less than that of irradiated Vicryl sutures. This indicates that Vicryl sutures are more sensitive to the γ-irradiation-induced degradation than Maxon sutures, and the tensile property data also support this finding.

The $[\eta]$ data of absorbable sutures could be used to determine whether the predominant effect of γ-irradiation is main-chain scission or crosslinking via the following formula derived by Zhang et al.[41]

$$[\eta]_D/[\eta]_0 = (1 + KD)^{-a} \tag{9}$$

$$\text{where } K = [G(s)/2 - 2G(x)] \, (\mu m/100N_A) \tag{10}$$

G(s), defined as radiation chemical yields caused by chain scission, is the number of molecules or atoms produced or decomposed per 100 eV of absorbed energy; G(x) is the corresponding G value for crosslinking; D is the irradiation dosage in eVg^{-1}. If G(s)>4G(x), γ-irradiation effect will be mainly chain scissions.[126] Under the condition of G(s)<4G(x), the structure of the polymer will be converted into a three-dimensional network through cross-linking. Based on the assumption that a is equal to 0.6 because of the fact that, for most polymeric materials, a varies from 0.5 to 1.0 and a for poly-D,L-lactide was reported to be from 0.64 to 0.67,[127] the constant K (relates to molecular weight) could be calculated by the nonlinear regression program (NLIN).[128]

$$K_V = 0.2337 \qquad a = 0.6 \text{ for Vicryl}$$

$$K_M = 0.0778 \qquad a = 0.6 \text{ for Maxon}$$

Both K_V and K_M are positive, which means G(s)/2 – 2G(X)>0 or G(s)>4G(x) from Equation 10. Therefore, Zhang et al. concluded the effect of γ-irradiation on Vicryl and Maxon sutures was mainly chain scissions.

The thermal properties, such as heat of fusion and melting point, of Vicryl and Maxon sutures were also changed as a function of γ-irradiation conditions and hydrolysis time. After γ-irradiation, not only the position of the maximum ΔH appeared at an earlier time, but also the magnitude of the maximum ΔH decreased, depending on the dosage level. These observed changes in ΔH and T_m were related to the two-stage degradation mechanism proposed by Chu[69,72] and were described previously in Section I.

Will the observed accelerated hydrolytic degradation of γ-irradiated synthetic absorbable sutures be due to any change in their surface wettability upon irradiation? Wettability studies of γ-irradiated Maxon monofilament sutures indicate that the accelerated hydrolytic degradation observed in γ-irradiated synthetic absorbable sutures is not due to change in surface wettability of the sutures.[41] Both the surface contact angle and work of adhesion of irradiated Maxon and its control do not change with γ-irradiation up to 5 Mrads. For example, 5 Mrad irradiated but unhydrolyzed Maxon and its corresponding control have 72.9 and 72.4 dynes/cm of W_{SL} (work of adhesion), respectively. The effect of γ-irradiation on

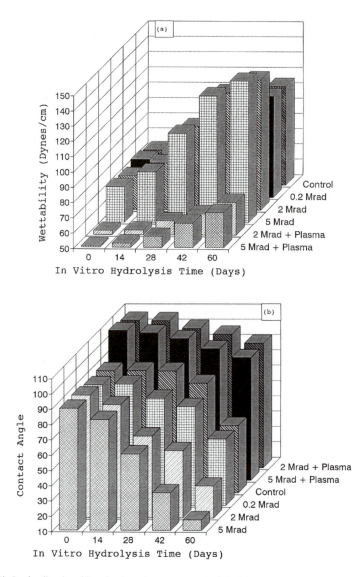

Figure 7.47 Work of adhesion (dyne/cm) and contact angle (θ) of Maxon as a function of *in vitro* hydrolysis time in phosphate buffer solution of pH 7.44 at 37°C. (a) Work of adhesion (dyne/cm); (b) contact angle (θ). (From Zhang, L. et al., *J. Biomed. Mater. Res.*, 27, 1425, 1993. With permission.)

surface wettability, however, becomes significant as hydrolysis proceeds, as illustrated in Figure 7.47. The change in W_{SL} and θ of Maxon control is not observed until after 42 d of hydrolysis. At the end of 60 d, W_{SL} increased significantly to 158% of the 0 d Maxon control. Correspondingly, at this critical period (42 d), the weight loss of Maxon became visible, the ΔH reached a maximum, and the tensile strength was completely lost. After γ-irradiation, this critical period appeared at an earlier time (14 d for both 2.0 Mrad and 5.0 Mrad). Up to 60 d of hydrolysis, the W_{SL} of irradiated Maxon samples increased to 200% of the unhydrolyzed controls, as compared to 158% for the unirradiated Maxon. The observed increase in W_{SL} with hydrolysis in both control and irradiated Maxon was attributed to the fact that hydrolysis of this class of polymers would create more polar hydrophilic groups, such as –OH and –COOH, on the surface, which makes the suture surface more hydrophilic and is subsequently reflected in the observed increasing W_{SL} with hydrolysis time.

Surface morphological study by scanning electron microscope revealed that, before hydrolysis, γ-irradiation did not result in any apparent change in surface appearance of Vicryl, Maxon, and PDS sutures. However, subsequent *in vitro* hydrolysis showed vast difference in the change of fiber surface morphology, depending on hydrolysis time, dosage, and type of sutures.

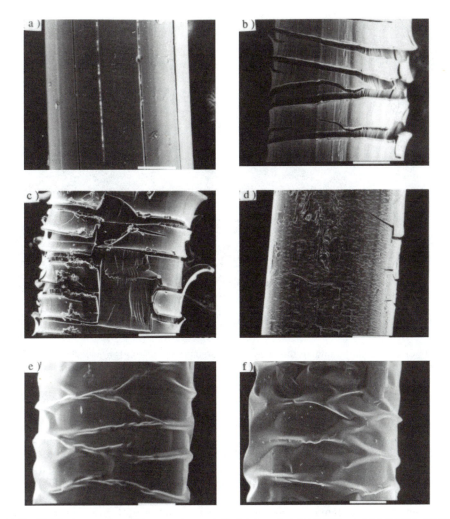

Figure 7.48 SEM micrographs of Maxon sutures at 42 d: (a) control; (b) 0.2 Mrad; (c) 2.0 Mrad; (d) 5.0 Mrad; (e) 2 Mrad + Parylene Plasma; (f) 5 Mrad + Parylene Plasma. (From Zhang, L. et al., *J. Biomed. Mater. Res.*, 27, 1425, 1993. With permission.)

In Vicryl sutures, the filament cleavage was observed as early as 7 d hydrolysis at 2.0 Mrad dosage. This cleavage became more severe as the dosage increased to 5.0 Mrad; however, Vicryl sutures did not show the same unique surface morphology of irradiated Dexon sutures. The time for the disintegration of the braid structure of Vicryl was reduced to 28 d for the 2.0 Mrad and 5.0 Mrad irradiated Vicryl from the 42 d unirradiated Vicryl control. These observed morphological changes of hydrolyzed control and irradiated Vicryl sutures were consistent with the observed tensile strength and mass loss profiles. For example, control Vicryl lost about 30% of its original tensile breaking force at 7 d, while up to 70% of their original tensile strength was lost for 2.0 Mrad and 5.0 Mrad irradiated samples.

Upon hydrolysis, the change in surface morphology of monofilament synthetic absorbable sutures like Maxon and PDS due to γ-irradiation is very different from the multifilament Dexon and Vicryl sutures described above. Figures 7.48 and 7.49 illustrate the surface morphological changes of Maxon and PDS sutures at various times of hydrolysis and γ-irradiation dosage levels. Figure 7.48 illustrates the surface morphologic changes of Maxon sutures as a result of γ-irradiation at 42 d of hydrolysis. In general, all control and irradiated Maxon sutures exhibited three common features along hydrolysis time: (1) formation of surface cracks without a significant dimensional change at an earlier period; (2) subsequent removal of the outermost skin layer, which leads to a reduction in suture diameter; (3) the degradation of the interior core with a wrinkle surface appearance at the late period. For example, longitudinal cracks of control Maxon started to appear at 42 d. As hydrolysis proceeded to 60 d, circumferential cracks appeared and the diameter of the suture decreased to 91%. At 90 d of hydrolysis, the surface cracks became deeper, followed by the removal of the outer skin layer and a further reduction

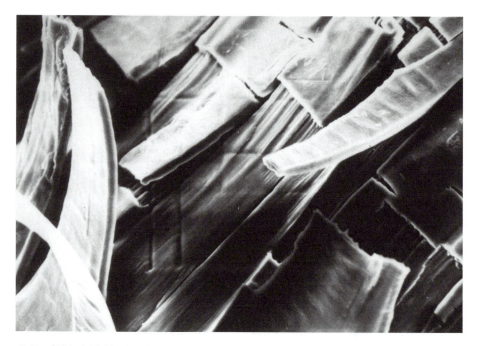

Figure 7.49 SEM of 20 Mrad and 14 d hydrolyzed PDS suture in buffers. The microfibrils beneath the skin layer are evident. (From Williams, D.F. et al., *J. Appl. Polym. Sci.*, 29, 1865, 1984. With permission.)

of suture diameter by 22% (from originally 400 to 315 μm) through the hydrolytic dissolution of the fragments on the surface and interior of Maxon sutures. In the case of γ-irradiated Maxon sutures, each of the three common features mentioned above appeared at an earlier hydrolysis time. At the late periods of hydrolysis (42 d), the control and irradiated Maxon showed quite drastic morphological differences. A comparison of Figure 7.48, (a) to (d) indicates that γ-irradiation resulted in more severe surface cracks which is also reflected in the faster tensile strength and mass loss as described earlier. It is interesting to know that the reduction in Maxon fiber diameter was not as fast as its mass loss. For example, the diameter of 2.0 Mrad Maxon was about 400 μm at 0 d and 342 μm at 60 d (85% of the original diameter). Within the same period, the removal of surface skin should result in 30% of mass loss (because $\Delta m \propto 2\Delta r$, Δm is the change in mass, Δr is the change in diameter); however, the actual mass loss was 56%. This suggests that the mass loss of sutures must also occur simultaneously in the interior of the suture.

PDS sutures exhibit similar γ-irradiation-induced surface morphology as Maxon sutures. Figure 7.49 illustrates the surface morphology of 20 Mrad irradiated PDS upon 14 d hydrolysis in buffer. The concept that a macrofibril consists of a number of microfibrils can be seen in this figure. Beneath the peeling layers, an array of microfibrils of size ranging from several hundreds to thousands of angstroms were evident. This microfibrillar structure was not apparent on the peeling layer, which is the outermost skin of the fiber. This difference in morphological appearance seems to be attributed to the so-called skin-core effect. Since the polymer chains on the skin layer are exposed to the ambient environment first during the melt spinning of the fiber, they crystallize faster than the internal polymer molecules. They experience less shear stress in the molten stage, and the formation of microfibrils is thus less apparent than the inner polymer molecules.

The susceptibility of PDS to γ-irradiation-induced accelerated hydrolysis must be attributed to its chemical structure. As shown in Chapter 5, PDS has the same chemical structure as PGA suture, except it has an additional ether functional group that PGA does not have. It is well known that the incorporation of oxygen atoms into the main chains leads to a significant increase in the probability for main chain scissions.[121] This susceptibility toward chain scission is also influenced by the number of CH_2 groups in the ether linkage or the relative concentration of the oxygen. For example, poly(methylene oxide) undergoes exclusive chain scission,[129] while poly(tetramethylene oxide) undergoes chain scission and crosslinking.[130] This lower ratio of chain scission to crosslinking in the poly(tetramethylene oxide) was attributed to the fact that the C–O to C–C ratio is lower in this polymer than in polymethylene oxide.[101] The ethylene oxide portion of the PDS repeating unit has the content of ether linkage falling between methylene and tetramethylene oxides. Thus, PDS would be expected to undergo mainly but not exclusively chain scission. In the absence of oxygen, however, poly(ethylene oxide) will gel when irradiated at a dosage of 4.5 to 7.5×10^4 rad.[131]

γ-Irradiation has been found to result in chain scissions on synthetic absorbable sutures. Will such an alteration of their structure affect their susceptibility toward enzymatic degradation? Since the chain scission process would result in more chain ends, and it was previously mentioned that enzymatic degradation of synthetic polymers proceeds through terminal (i.e., chain ends) attack, therefore, γ-irradiation on synthetic absorbable sutures may promote their susceptibility toward enzymatic attack. This issue has been addressed by Chu and Williams,[124] and is reviewed in Section III.F.2.g below.

Factors Affecting γ-Irradiation Efficiency Besides the chemical structures of suture materials which influence the effects of γ-irradiation, there are other factors that could affect their irradiation efficiency. These factors include oxygen, dose rate, linear energy transfer, and irradiation temperature (T_{irr}).[126]

The effects of varying the irradiation temperature, especially with respect to the glass transition temperature of suture materials, T_g, have probably been examined less than any of the other factors. In theory, a pair of macromolecular radicals formed as a result of γ-irradiation-induced main chain scissions have certain probabilities to recombine. The extent of recombination depends on molecular chain mobility. Chain segments with restricted segmental mobility due to crystalline structure, orientation, or being at a temperature below their T_g would be expected to facilitate the recombination of a pair of macromolecular radicals and hence would show less γ-irradiation-induced degradation. This theoretical prediction was experimentally confirmed in the UV irradiation of nonsuture materials.[126,132] It was found that the quantum yields of main chain scission, $\phi(s)$, depend on the relative magnitude of the temperature during UV irradiation (T_{irr}) to the glass transition temperature of polymers.[126,132] $\phi(s)$ increased very slowly with temperature when $T_{irr} < T_g$. In the vicinity of T_g, $\phi(s)$ increased dramatically and approached a limiting value. Recently, Chu et al. extended this theoretical concept to synthetic absorbable sutures and found that the absorbable suture materials also followed the theoretical prediction as other polymers.[48].

In that study of both Dexon and Maxon sutures by Chu et al.,[48] they found that T_{irr} indeed had an effect on the rate of tensile strength loss with hydrolysis time. The benefit of γ-irradiation at $T_{irr} < T_g$ was found with hydrolyzed Dexon and Maxon sutures. With a few exceptions, both Dexon and Maxon sutures consistently exhibited higher retention of tensile breaking force over the specified hydrolysis periods when T_{irr} was less than T_g. Similar benefits were also found in the unhydrolyzed sutures. For example, Dexon sutures irradiated at 55°C ($>T_g$ of Dexon) lost 17% (2 Mrad) and 34% (10 Mrad) of the TBS of their unirradiated controls, while the same sutures irradiated at –78°C ($<T_g$ of Dexon) lost only 6% (2 Mrad) and 24% (10 Mrad) of their unirradiated controls. A similar pattern was observed in Maxon sutures.

Chu et al. attributed the observed T_{irr} effect of irradiated absorbable suture fibers to cage reaction. It is known that fiber strength depends on the tie-chain segments located in the amorphous domains of microfibrils. When γ-irradiation of suture materials was done at –78°C (i.e., $T_{irr} < T_g$), the resulting Norrish type I macromolecular radicals due to chain scissions of the tie-chain segments have a better opportunity to recombine than the same radicals produced upon γ-irradiation at $T_{irr} > T_g$. This higher probability of macromolecular radical recombination was further enhanced by the orientation effect of fibers and thus resulted in a better retention of tensile breaking force as observed in this study. Cage reaction could also be enhanced by viscosity of the medium, namely molecular weight.[133] It is generally observed that the higher the viscosity of the medium, the more important cage reaction becomes. This is because the radicals generated from γ-irradiation become less mobile when viscosity is high and the geminate radicals produced in close proximity have a better chance to recombine before they diffuse apart. Accordingly, the efficiency of radical production in the initiation step decreases when viscosity increases. In the study by Chu et al., the original intrinsic viscosity of Maxon was higher than that of Vicryl sutures before hydrolysis. Based on the viscosity effect on cage reaction, a smaller level of γ-irradiation-induced chain scission on the Maxon sutures than that on the Vicryl sutures should be expected. This means Maxon sutures should be more resistant to γ-irradiation degradation than Vicryl, as evident in the observed physical and mechanical properties by Chu et al.[41,48]

However, it appeared that the benefit of irradiation at $T_{irr} < T_g$ became less obvious at a longer duration of hydrolysis or a higher irradiation dosage applied. This suggested that an overwhelmingly high dosage of γ-irradiation must overpower the propensity for cage recombination of pairs of macromolecular radicals at a $T_{irr} < T_g$ of the material because the rate of radical generation became much faster than the rate of cage recombination.

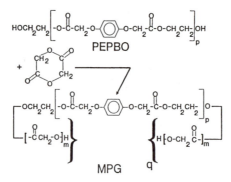

Figure 7.50 Chemical structure of modified PGA (MPG) which is a copolymer of glycolide and poly(ethylene 1,4-phenylene-bis-oxyacetate) PEPBO. (Source: Jamiolkowski, D.D. and Shalaby, S.W., in *Radiation Effect of Polymers*, Clough, R.L. and Shalaby, S.W., Eds., ACS Symp. Ser. 475, American Chemical Society, Washington, D.C., 1991, 300. With permission.)

Potential Application of γ-Irradiated Absorbable Sutures Although the accelerated hydrolytic degradation of γ-irradiated synthetic absorbable sutures is largely undesirable in most wound closure, Duprez et al. have used this change in degradation properties to their advantage in skin closure of small children.[134] Absorbable sutures, in general, are not used for skin closure, due to the fact that the sutures are removed before they are biodegraded. Anesthesia is usually applied before the removal of sutures to eliminate pain and discomfort, particularly when dealing with patients who are young children. It is psychologically desirable for young patients and their parents. In order to eliminate the practice of using general anesthesia in children during the removal of sutures (such practice also saves cost), Duprez et al. used fast absorption Vicryl (Vicryl Rapide®) that had been previously treated by γ-irradiation on 27 children (18 months to 8 years) with a congenital or traumatic defect of their limbs requiring reconstructive surgery. They found that Vicryl Rapide could be easily and completely removed without either local or general anesthesia and pain or discomfort, simply by wiping the wound area with a dressing between 12 and 16 d postoperation. There was no complication of wound rupture, nor any inflammation or infection in patients with grafts and flaps for syndactylia. The long-term (11.3 months) results of wound healing using Vicryl Rapide were similar to those obtained with nonabsorbable sutures. Duprez et al. also examined the time required for a complete absorption of fast absorption Vicryl in mice grafted with human skin. Total absorption occurred within 35 d, whereas normal Vicryl sutures required about 90 d for complete absorption (See Table 7.4). A recent study of this fast absorption Vicryl on the cytokinetics of crypt cells in colonic anastomoses of rats indicated that there was no statistically significant difference in the crypt cell production rate (CCPR) of an anastomosis closed with Vicryl Rapide when compared with controls (without anastomosis), while a nonabsorbable stainless steel suture resulted in a statistically significant increase in CCPR.[135] The details of this study are described in Chapter 8.

Making Synthetic Absorbable Sutures Sterilizable by γ-Irradiation Because of the adverse effect of γ-irradiation on the mechanical properties of synthetic absorbable sutures, they are sterilized by ethylene oxide. There is a great desire to develop γ-irradiation-sterilizable synthetic absorbable sutures in medical industry to take advantage of this highly convenient and reliable method of sterilization.

Shalaby et al.[136,137] have reported that the incorporation of about 10 mol% of a polymeric radiostabilizer like poly(ethylene 1,4-phenylene-bis-oxyacetate) (PEPBO) into PGA would make the PGA copolymer sterilizable by γ-irradiation without significant accelerated loss of mechanical properties upon hydrolysis when compared with the unirradiated PGA copolymer control (MPG). The chemical structure of this MPG is shown in Figure 7.50. Table 7.14 shows the changes in tensile breaking force of both MPG and PGA sutures implanted intramuscularly and subcutaneously in rats for various periods. MPG fibers γ-irradiated at 2.89 Mrads did not show any loss in tensile breaking force during the first 14 d postimplantation when compared with unimplanted samples. On the contrary, PGA sutures γ-irradiated at 2.75 Mrads lost 62% of the tensile breaking force of unimplanted samples. The absolute tensile breaking force of the 2.89 Mrad irradiated MPG at the end of 14 d postimplantation was higher than the unirradiated PGA sutures at the same period, even though the latter had a higher initial (0 d) tensile breaking force than the former. There was no tensile breaking force remaining for the irradiated PGA at the end of 21 d, while both 2.89 and 5 Mrads irradiated MPG retained 72% and 55% of their corresponding 0 d controls, respectively. The absorption profile in terms of the cross-sectional area

Table 7.14 *In Vivo* Breaking Strength Retention Data of Modified Polyglycolide (MPG) and Polyglycolide (PGA) Braids

	Days Postimplantaiton			
	0	7	14	21
MPG braid, nonirradiated				
Pounds	9.51	11.63	9.96	9.23
Percent Retention	100	122	105	97
MPG braid, irradiated 2.89 Mrads				
Pounds	9.43	10.63	9.82	6.76
Percent Retention	100	113	88	72
MPG braid, irradiated 5 Mrads				
Pounds	8.58	9.44	7.80	4.71
Percent Retention	100	110	92	55
PGA braid, nonirradiated				
Pounds	13.41	15.05	9.90	6.85
Percent Retention	100	112	74	51
PGA braid, irradiated 2.75 Mrads				
Pounds	12.76	11.06	4.91	0.00
Percent Retention	100	87	38	0
PGA braid, irradiated 5.33 Mrads				
Pounds	12.91	9.70	2.04	0.00
Percent Retention	100	75	16	0

From Jamiolkowski, D.D. and Shalaby, S.W., in *Radiation Effect of Polymers*, Clough, R.L. and Shalaby, S.W., (Eds.), ACS Symp. Ser. 475, American Chemical Society, Washington, D.C., 1991, 300. With permission.

remaining followed the same pattern as tensile breaking force profiles, namely irradiated MPG retained higher cross-sectional area remaining than irradiated PGA fibers *in vivo*. For example, MPG retained about 49% cross-sectional area at the end of 91 d postimplantation, while the unmodified PGA suture had only 19.5% cross-sectional area remaining.

The inherently more hydrolytic resistance of MPG must be attributed to the presence of aromatic groups in the backbone chain. This aromatic polyester component is also responsible for the observed γ-irradiation stability. It is not known at this time whether the new γ-irradiation-resistant MPG is biocompatible with biologic tissues, due to the lack of published histologic data. Based on the chemical structure of MPG, it is expected to be less biocompatible than PGA due to the aromatic ring.

A recent patent awarded to Chu and Lee suggests that the well-known adverse effect of γ-irradiation on the mechanical and biodegradation properties of synthetic absorbable polymers like sutures could be drastically minimized by modifying the process of irradiation sterilization procedures.[122] Their modification of existing ^{60}Co γ-irradiation sterilization methods included pretreating the biomaterials/devices with high vacuum (about 10^{-5} torr) and low temperature (about –196°C or –77°K) prior to and during γ-irradiation. Figures 7.40 and 7.41 show the effects of irradiation temperature below (–78°C) and above (55°C) T_g on the tensile breaking force of 2/0 PGA suture at 7 d *in vitro* hydrolysis. Chu speculated that a better retention of mechanical properties of synthetic absorbable biomaterials upon hydrolysis would be expected if an even lower irradiation temperature than –78°C was used, such as the liquid nitrogen temperature (–196°C), along with a high vacuum environment during γ-irradiation sterilization. Such a prediction was confirmed by the recently awarded patent.[122]

The purpose of pretreating absorbable biomaterials and devices with an extremely low temperature (below T_g of all existing absorbable biomaterials) is to drastically reduce chain mobility of those tie-chain segments (mainly responsible for mechanical property and its loss with hydrolytic degradation) located in the amorphous domains of the suture materials. Such a reduction in chain mobility would permit more opportunity for the recombination of chain ends (i.e., cage effect) broken by γ-irradiation and hence would reduce the premature loss of mechanical properties of irradiated absorbable biomaterials and devices. The purpose of pretreating absorbable sutures with high vacuum before and during ^{60}Co γ-irradiation is to eliminate or reduce irradiation-induced oxidation so that the benefit of "cage effect" (i.e., recombination of broken chain ends) could be realized. Thus, a combination of extremely low temperature and vacuum should provide the maximum protection of absorbable sutures from the adverse effect of γ-irradiation sterilization described earlier. The lack of ESR signal of the synthetic absorbable sutures upon Chu et al.'s modified γ-irradiation sterilization method, i.e., no free radicals present, further supports the findings of the lack of adverse effect of this new sterilization method on the mechanical properties of these absorbable sutures.[122a]

Figure 7.51 summarizes the effect of such a combined pretreatment of 2/0 PGA and Vicryl sutures on the retention of tensile breaking force upon *in vitro* hydrolytic degradation. The strength loss profile of ^{60}Co γ-irradiation sterilization under conventional conditions (no vacuum and room temperature) is also included as the controls to demonstrate the merits of Chu et al.'s sterilization method. The absorbable sutures sterilized by Chu et al.'s modified sterilization method retained a better tensile breaking force over the entire period of hydrolysis (0 to 21 d) and the difference between the two force loss profiles became even bigger at longer duration of hydrolysis. For example, there was no measurable tensile breaking force for the conventionally ^{60}Co γ-irradiated Dexon sutures at 17 d, while the same sutures irradiated by Chu et al.'s method still retained 40% of their original tensile breaking force at the same duration of hydrolysis. Similar findings were observed in Vicryl sutures. A study of viscosity average molecular weight of these irradiated absorbable sutures indicated that those absorbable sutures sterilized by Chu et al.'s method also support their findings in mechanical properties. There was no change in viscosity average molecular weight of PGA and Vicryl sutures sterilized by Chu et al.'s proposed method, while the same sutures sterilized by conventional ^{60}Co γ-irradiation exhibited a significant loss of molecular weight.

Therefore, the study by Chu et al. indicates that the proposed modified ^{60}Co γ-irradiation sterilization (high vacuum and extremely low temperature during irradiation) could completely eliminate the well-known adverse effect of conventional ^{60}Co γ-irradiation sterilization on synthetic absorbable biomaterials and devices. The Chu et al.'s modified γ-irradiation sterilization could not only revitalize the use of ^{60}Co as a better source for sterilization of synthetic absorbable biomaterials and devices without the fear of deteriorated mechanical and biodegradation properties, but also eliminate the toxicity concern of ethylene oxide sterilization.

f. Effect of Free Radicals

Matlaga and Salthouse demonstrated that the biodegradation of synthetic absorbable sutures is closely related to macrophage activity through the close adhesion of macrophage onto the surface of the absorbable sutures.[138] It is also known that inflammatory cells, particularly leukocytes and macrophages, are able to produce highly reactive oxygen species like superoxide ($\cdot O_2^-$) and hydrogen peroxide during inflammatory reactions toward foreign materials.[139,140] These highly reactive oxygen species participate in the biochemical reaction, frequently referred to as respiratory burst, which is characterized by the one electron reduction of O_2 into superoxide via either NADPH or NADH oxidase, as shown below. The reduction of O_2 results in an increase in O_2 uptake and the consumption of glucose.

$$2O_2 + NADPH \xrightarrow{\text{(NADPH Oxidase)}} 2 \cdot O_2^- + NADP^+ + H^+ \tag{11}$$

The resulting superoxide radicals are then neutralized to H_2O_2 via the cytoplasmic enzyme superoxide dismutase (SOD).

$$2 \cdot O_2^- + 2H^+ \xrightarrow{\text{(SOD)}} H_2O_2 + O_2 \tag{12}$$

Williams et al. suggested that these reactive oxygen species may be harmful to polymeric implant surfaces through their production of highly reactive, potent, and harmful hydroxyl radicals $\cdot OH$ in the presence of metals like iron, as shown in the following series of redox reactions.[141-143]

$$\cdot O_2^- + M^{n+} \rightarrow O_2 + M^{(n-1)+} \tag{13}$$

$$H_2O_2 + M^{(n-1)+} \rightarrow \cdot OH + HO^- + M^{n+} \tag{14}$$

The net reaction will be:

$$\cdot O_2^- + H_2O_2 \rightarrow \cdot OH + HO^- + O_2 \tag{15}$$

and is often referred to as the metal-catalyzed Haber-Weiss reaction.[144]

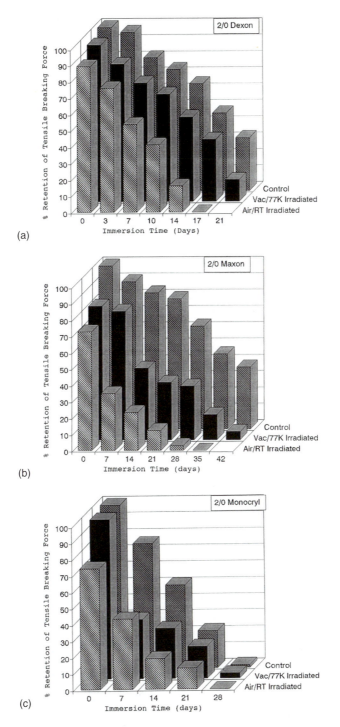

Figure 7.51 The retentions of tensile breaking force (kg) of 2/0 Dexon (a), Maxon (b), and Monocryl (c) sutures in PBS of pH 7.44 at 37°C after a modified 2 Mrad γ-irradiation sterilization (Vac/77°K), room temperature/air (air/RT) γ-irradiation sterilization, and ethylene oxide sterilization (control). The percent is based on the 0 d control. (From Chu, C.C. and Lee, K.H., U.S. Patent 5,485,496, January 16, 1996).

Although the role of free radicals in the hydrolytic degradation of synthetic absorbable sutures is largely unknown, a preliminary study of Vicryl suture in the presence of aqueous free radical solution prepared from H_2O_2 and ferrous sulfate, $FeSO_4$, raised the possibility of the role of free radicals in the biodegradation of synthetic absorbable sutures. As shown below, both ·OH radicals and OH^- are formed

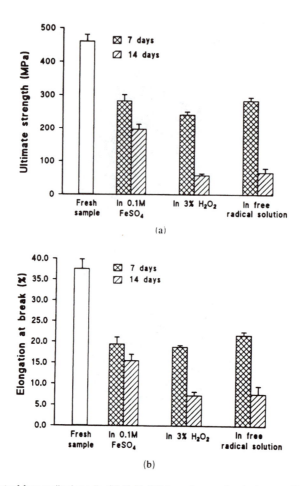

Figure 7.52 The effect of free radical media (H$_2$O$_2$/FeSO$_4$) on the mechanical properties of 2/0 Vicryl sutures. (a) Ultimate strength (MPa); (b) elongaton at break (%). FeSO$_4$ and H$_2$O$_2$ served as the control media. (From Zhong, S.P. et al., *Plast. Rubber Composites Processing Appl.*, 21, 89, 1994. With permission.)

in the process of oxidation of Fe^{2+} by H$_2$O$_2$ and could exert some influence on the subsequent hydrolytic degradation of Vicryl sutures.

$$Fe^{2+} + H_2O_2 \rightarrow Fe^{3+} + \cdot OH + OH^-$$

Scanning electron microscopy results indicated that Vicryl sutures in the presence of free radical solutions exhibit many irregular surface cracks at both 7 and 14 d *in vitro*, while the two controls (H$_2$O$_2$ or FeSO$_4$ solutions) did not have these surface cracks. However, Vicryl sutures treated in one of the two controls (FeSO$_4$) exhibited rough surface, but the other control (H$_2$O$_2$) still retained the same smooth surface appearance as the unhydrolyzed one.

Surprisingly, the presence of surface cracks on Vicryl suture treated in the free radical solutions did not accelerate the tensile breaking strength loss as would be expected, as shown in Figure 7.52. At 7 d *in vitro*, the 3% H$_2$O$_2$ control media resulted in the lowest tensile breaking strength, while both the free radical and the control FeSO$_4$ media had the same tensile breaking strength. The pattern changed at 14 d in that the free radical and the control 3% H$_2$O$_2$ media had the same tensile breaking strength, while the FeSO$_4$ media resulted in the highest retention of tensile breaking strength.

Thermal properties of Vicryl sutures under these three different media indicated that the different rates of degradation occurred due to different media (Table 7.15). Both the free radical and 3% H$_2$O$_2$ media showed the classical maximum pattern of the change of the level of crystallinity with hydrolysis time, as described earlier in this chapter (Section III.C). The level of crystallinity of Vicryl sutures peaked at 7 d in both media (free radical and 3% H$_2$O$_2$). The time for peak appearance in these two media was

Table 7.15 Thermal Properties of Vicryl Sutures Upon *In Vitro* Hydrolysis in Free Radical, H_2O_2, and $FeSO_4$ Solutions

	$\Delta H/\Delta D$[a]	T_m
Fresh	0·869	469·1, 474·6[b]
In 0·1 M $FeSO_4$ 7 d	0·870	472·6
In 3% H_2O_2 7 d	2·324	469·56, 473·28[b]
In free radical solution 7 d	1·590	473·28, 474·99[b]
In 0·1 M $FeSO_4$ 14 d	1·610	470·39, 473·02[b]
In 3% H_2O_2 14 d	0·908	470·39
In free radical solution 14 d	0·878	472·32

[a] $\Delta H/\Delta D$: half peak height/half peak width.
[b] The main peak position.

From Zhong, P.J. et al., *Plast. Rubber Composites Processing Appl.*,, 21(2), 1994. With permission.

considerably earlier than Vicryl sutures in conventional physiological buffer media. Based on Chu's suggestion of using the time for the appearance of crystallinity peak as an indicator of degradation rate, it appears that these two media accelerated the degradation of Vicryl sutures when compared with regular physiological buffer solution. The $FeSO_4$ media did not show the maximum crystallinity during the period of *in vitro* study (14 d), indicating no accelerated degradation of Vicryl sutures in this medium. The highest retention of tensile breaking strength at 14 d observed in $FeSO_4$ medium agreed with the thermal data.

Based on their preliminary data, Williams et al. proposed the possible routes of the role of ·OH radicals in the hydrolytic degradation of Vicryl sutures shown in Figure 7.53. Unfortunately, the possible role of OH^-, one of the by-products from Fenton reagents ($H_2O_2/FeSO_4$), was not considered in the interpretation of their findings. OH^- species could be more potent than ·OH toward hydrolytic degradation of synthetic absorbable sutures. This is because hydroxyl anions are the sole species which attack carbonyl carbon of the ester linkages during alkaline hydrolysis, as described earlier in this chapter (Section III.F.2.a). Since equal amounts of ·OH and OH^- are generated in Fenton reagents, the observed changes in morphological, mechanical, and thermal properties could be partially attributed to OH^- ions as well as ·OH radicals. Because no pH value was given in the study by Williams et al., it is difficult to assess the role of OH^- ions in their data.

Chu et al. recently reported that superoxide ions could have a significant effect on the hydrolytic degradation of synthetic absorbable sutures.[144a] They found that there was a significant reduction in molecular weight, mechanical and thermal properties of these sutures over a wide range of superoxide ion concentration, particularly during the first few hours of contact with superoxide ions. For example, PGA suture lost almost all of its mass at the end of 24 hours' (25°C) contact with superoxide ions, while the same suture would take at least 50 days in *in vitro* buffer for a complete mass loss. The surface morphology of these sutures was also altered drastically. The exact mechanism behind these findings is not fully known; however, the possibility of simultaneous occurrence of several main-chain scissions by three different nucleophilic species was suggested by Chu et al.

Chu et al. have also recently reported that the addition of Fenton agent or hydrogen peroxide to the degradation medium would retard the well-known adverse effect of the conventional γ-irradiation sterilization of synthetic absorbable sutures.[144b] They found that these γ-irradiated sutures retained better tensile breaking strength in the Fenton medium than in the regular buffer media. Chu et al. postulated that the γ-irradiation-induced α-carbon radicals in these sutures react with the hydroxyl radicals from the Fenton agent medium and hence neutralize the adverse effect of α-carbon radicals on the backbone chain scission. This suggested mechanism is supported by the observed gradual loss of ESR signal of the sutures in the presence of Fenton agent in the medium.

g. Effect of Enzymes

Enzymes, proteins with a molecular weight ranging from 10^3 to 10^6, are major chemical species in the living system and catalyze a variety of chemical reactions. They are usually soluble in water because of their hydrophilic groups, such as $-NH_2$, $-OH$, or $-COOH$. Enzymes are synthesized for various purposes; they can be used to catalyze the hydrolysis of a chemical bond (a hydrolase) or to oxidize a molecule (an oxidase).

Polyglycolide:

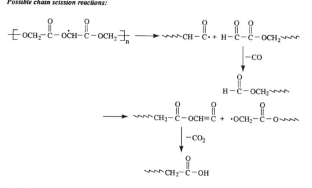

Possible chain scission reactions:

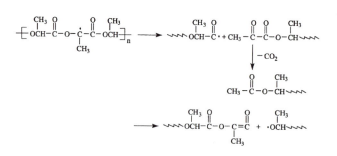

Cross-linking or termination of the reactions:

$$R\cdot + R'\cdot \longrightarrow R-R'$$

Polylactide:

Possible chain scission reactions:

Figure 7.53 Schematic illustration of possible routes for the attack of HO· on Vicryl sutures. (From Zhong, S.P. et al., *Plast. Rubber Composites Processing Appl.*, 21, 89, 1994. With permission.)

Enzyme-aided degradation of either natural or synthetic polymers could proceed in a random or terminal mode as described previously. For example, α-amylase randomly hydrolyze C_1-C_4 linkages of the amylose chain and hence α-maltose and glucose are the end products.[132] ß-amylases hydrolyze the same C_1-C_4 linkage but at the nonreducing end of the chain, so that maltose molecules are removed successively. Not all proteases hydrolyze proteins in the same way. Trypsin degrades the carbonyl groups of arginine and lysine only, while pepsin and chymotrypsin randomly attack the peptide linkages. In the case of synthetic polymers, enzymes are believed to attack at the chain ends of polymers and will be discussed later.

Regardless of their purposes, all enzymes are substrate specific and their catalytic activities relate to their chain conformation. Any change in their chain conformation due to pH or temperature of the medium will result in a loss of their catalytic function. The importance of the substrate chain conformation in the ease of formation of enzyme-substrate complex is demonstrated in the faster enzymatic degradation of denatured vs. native proteins.[145] This occurs because a denatured protein assumes a statistically favorable random coil conformation which can form the enzyme-substrate complex more easily. Because enzymes were originally designed for biopolymers or processed biopolymers (e.g., catgut or reconstituted collagen sutures) which have existed for thousands of years, it is still not known how nature would react to synthetic polymers which have only been available for less than 100 years. It is believed that the creation of a new enzyme for a new synthetic substrate would take months, years, or decades to develop, depending on the species. Usually, microorganisms are capable of adapting to new synthetic substrates better than highly organized species like human beings.[132] For example, *Pseudomonas aeruginosa* that was placed in contact with a polyamide-6 and began to proliferate after only 56 d of contact, will immediately grow on a new polyamide-6 substrate.[132] This demonstrates the ability of microorganisms to adapt to new sources of nutrition via the development of new enzymes within a relatively short period.

It has often been argued that *in vivo* synthetic polymer degradation may be aided by enzymes. This was based on the histological observation of the presence of macrophage immediately adjacent to degradable polymers, the principal producer of a series of lysosomal enzymes including hydrolases. As pointed out by Kopecek and Ulbrich,[145] high-molecular-weight substrates may be degraded upon lysosomal enzymatic action in three ways:

1. Endocytosis after the substrate has been captured into the cell
2. Release of the lysosomal enzymes into both the extracellular and intracellular spaces during inflammation
3. The process of autophagy

Because the size of the surgical implants is always significantly larger than biological cells, and because most polymers are insoluble in body fluids, the two broad processes of endocytosis, (1) the ingestion of particulate matters (phagocytosis) and (2) the engulfment of small droplets of extracellular fluid (pinocytosis), and the process of autophagy appear to be inapplicable to the initial stage of biodegradation of biodegradable surgical devices and materials. Thus, the release of lysosomal enzymes into the extracellular space is the most probable process in response to the presence of biodegradable surgical implants. Such a process is especially common with older macrophage populations (chronic inflammation)[146] and in the surrounding sites of toxic substances.[147] It is important to recognize that such enzymatic activities of macrophage are mainly responsible for the degradation and absorption of natural absorbable sutures, such as catgut and reconstituted collagen. This is evident in the comparison of acid phosphatase and aminopeptidase activities with tensile strength loss and absorption of 3-0 collagen suture shown in Figure 7.1 earlier in this chapter.[148] Whether or not such release of lysosomal enzymes from macrophage will aid in the degradation and absorption of synthetic biodegradable wound closure biomaterials is inconclusive and controversial.

It has been previously mentioned that degradation of biopolymers with the assistance of enzymes proceeds either in a random or terminal scission mode. Schnabel postulated that,[132] contrary to biopolymers, synthetic polymers, except polyvinyl alcohol and poly-ε-caprolactone, are usually attacked only at the chain ends and thus degradation is affected by molecular weight of the polymers. The higher the molecular weight, the smaller the number of chain ends available for enzymatic attack. These fewer chain ends in high-molecular-weight polymers may not be readily accessible to enzymes because they are often lost in the mass of entangled polymer matrix. Consequently, the rate of degradation should be low as the molecular weight of polymers increases. Potts et al.[148] demonstrated such a molecular weight effect on the microbial degradation of hydrocarbons. A study of the effect of γ-irradiation on the *in vitro* enzymatic degradation of PGA absorbable sutures, by Chu and Williams, also suggested that the hypothesis of preferential terminal attack of absorbable polymers by enzymes may be the route for the eventual enzymate-aided absorption of absorbable sutures *in vivo*.[124] In addition to the effect of molecular weight of substrates described above, the morphology of absorbable sutures (i.e., crystallinity and orientation) must also bear a relationship to the enzymatic degradation of synthetic absorbable sutures because crystalline domains are not accessible by enzymes which are significantly larger than water molecules. Because of their large molecular size, enzymes are too large to be able to diffuse into the interior of a synthetic biodegradable polymers. Therefore, enzymes must limit their activity to the surface or a thin surface layer of the implants, unless microcracks initially existed or resulted from other types of degradation.[6]

It is known that one of the conditions to facilitate enzyme-aided hydrolysis is the hydrophilicity of the polymer substrate. A hydrophobic polymer such as PET, although it contains hydrolytically sensitive bonds, may have a very limited degree of hydrolytic degradation due to the difficult accessibility of the extracellular fluids to the hydrolyzable bonds. It is thus expected that enzymes may not be able to catalyze the hydrolysis of synthetic hydrophobic polymers consisting of hydrolyzable bonds. This general belief, however, has been challenged by Smith et al., who studied *in vitro* enzymatic degradation of three relatively hydrophobic polymers, namely, PET, nylon 66, and poly(methylmethacrylate).[149] They found that PET degraded significantly faster in the esterase solution than in the buffer control.[149] This faster rate of PET degradation in esterase was most significant at the beginning of the immersion and the

Table 7.16 Comparison of Enzyme Activity, Methylene Blue Binding, and Absorption at Polyglactin 910 Suture in Rats

| Days | | | Acid Phosphatase[a] | Dehydrogenase[a] | Oxidase[a] | Methylene Blue[b] | Suture Remaining[c] (%) |
A	B	C					
	7	7	±	+	+	±	100
	14	14	+	+	+	±	100
7	7	14	±	+	+	±	100
	21	21	+	+	+	±	100
7	14	21	+	+	+	±	100
14	7	21	±	+	+	±	100
	28	28	++	++	++	+++	100
7	21	28	++	++	++	+++	100
14	14	28	+	++	++	+++	100
21	7	28	±	++	++	+++	100
	35	35	++	+++	+++	+++	100
7	28	35	++	+++	+++	+++	100
14	21	35	+	+++	+++	+++	100
21	14	35	+	+++	+++	+++	100
	42	42	+	+++	+++	++	90
7	35	42	+	+++	+++	++	90
14	28	42	++	+++	+++	++	90
21	21	42	+	+++	+++	++	90
	56	56	+	+	+	+	40
7	49	56	+	+	+	+	40
14	42	56	+	+	+	+	40
21	35	56	+	+	+	+	40

Note: A, *in vitro* incubation 38°C, pH 7.3; B, *in vivo* implantation; C, total time in aqueous environment, hydrolysis, *in vitro* plus *in vivo*.

[a] Enzyme activity grading: ±, trace activity; +, moderate activity, normal level; ++, increased activity; +++, intense activity. Acid phosphatase activity in macrophages at implant site. Dehydrogenase and cytochrome oxidase activity in cells adjacent to suture filaments.

[b] Methylene blue grading; ±, faint blue staining; + pale blue staining; ++, blue staining; +++, deep blue staining. Methylene blue dye binding at pH 2.5 by suture filaments in cross section.

[c] Suture absorption measured as percentage of cross-sectional area remaining, estimated to nearest 10%.

From Salthouse, T.N. and Matlaga, B.F., *Surg. Gynecol. Obstet.*, 142(4), 544, 1976. With permission.

difference in rate would gradually be narrowed with time, suggesting that the enzymatic catalytic effect was somehow gradually retarded as degradation proceeded. There was virtually no difference in the hydrolysis rate between esterase and the buffer control systems after 15 d. Papain was found to influence PET hydrolysis, but in a different way. Trypsin and chymotrypsin, however, did not affect the hydrolytic degradation of PET. This difference in enzymatic effect may suggest that different mechanisms of hydrolysis are involved, depending on the enzyme type and the interaction between the enzyme and the substrate. Contrary to PET, the hydrolytic degradation of nylon 66 was not influenced by esterase but by papain, trypsin, and chymotrypsin. These three enzymatic effects on nylon 66 had one common characteristic — the effect did not start until about 4 d of immersion and lasted for the duration of the testing period (15 to 16 d). Poly(methylmethacrylate), however, was not affected by any of four enzymes tested.

Synthetic absorbable sutures are expected to behave differently from nonabsorbable polymers in the presence of enzyme. This is because of the relatively high hydrophilicity of the absorbable sutures and their capability to produce lower-molecular-weight species with hydrolysis. These low-molecular-weight degradation products could provoke additional tissue reactions (i.e., more enzymes would be released by inflammatory cells). In addition, the biologic system must be able to metabolize these low-molecular-weight degradation products by enzymes. Salthouse and Matlaga[150] used histochemical procedures to study the mechanism of suture absorption. As shown in Table 7.16, they identified several important enzymes presented in tissues immediately adjacent to Vicryl absorbable sutures. These enzymes are (1) alkaline phosphatase leucine, generally associated with neutrophils and confined to the 7-d suture implant only; (2) acid phosphatase aminopeptidase and β-glucuronidase, associated with macrophages

Table 7.17 Effects of Various Enzymes on the Breaking Tensile Strength of Polyglycolide

Enzyme	Time	Control Breaking Strength (kg) ± S.D.	Buffer Treated Breaking Strength (kg) ± S.D.	% Loss	Enzyme Treated Breaking Strength (kg) ± S.D.	% Loss
In Preparation Without Ammonium Sulfate						
Carboxypeptidase A	2 weeks	4.45 ± 0.06	3.26 ± 0.12	26.7	2.57 ± 0.04	42.2
α-Chymotrypsin	2 weeks	4.78 ± 0.05	3.58 ± 0.05	25.1	2.97 ± 0.11	41.6
Clostridiopeptidase A	3 weeks	4.70 ± 0.01	2.36 ± 0.13	49.8	0.98 ± 0.08	79.1
	4½ weeks	4.76 ± 0.02	0.33 ± 0.12	93.1	0.07 ± 0.03	98.5
Ficin	3 weeks	4.70 ± 0.01	2.29 ± 0.06	51.3	1.60 ± 0.10	66.0
In Solutions Containing Ammonium Sulfate						
Bromelain	2 weeks	4.40 ± 0.07	3.96 ± 0.09	10.9	2.34 ± 0.10	46.9
	3 weeks	4.97 ± 0.14	3.98 ± 0.07	19.9	1.31 ± 0.13	73.6
Esterase	2 weeks	4.21 ± 0.15	3.51 ± 0.11	15.2	1.75 ± 0.20	58.4
	3 weeks	3.99 ± 0.10	1.59 ± 0.13	60.2	0.00 ± 0.00	100
Leucine aminopeptidase	5 days	5.07 ± 0.07	4.44 ± 0.07	12.4	0.50 ± 0.15	90.1
	7 days	4.82 ± 0.08	4.18 ± 0.04	13.3	0.00 ± 0.00	100

From Williams, D.F. and Mort, E., *J. Bioeng.*, 1(3), 231, 1977. With permission.

and giant cells at suture sites and the exhibited higher activity between 28 and 35 d postimplantation with β-glucuronidase exhibiting a lower level of intensity; (3) nonspecific esterase, frequently associated with giant cells and with activity lower than other hydrolases like acid phosphatase, β-glucuronidase, and aminopeptidase; (4) adenosine triphosphatase occurred from 28 to 42 d postimplantation and in areas close to suture fibers; (5) succinic dehydrogenase and lactic, isocitric, and malic dehydrogenases, with their highest activity in Vicryl suture between 28 and 42 d and in cells adjacent to suture fibers undergoing hydrolysis; (6) cytochrome oxidase, with its activity more conspicuous in cells bordering the Vicryl fibers, with a minimal activity at a distance remote from the suture site.

The experimental evidence from Salthouse and Matlaga's study demonstrates that the primary breakdown of Vicryl sutures is independent of cellular or enzyme activity and that the only requirement for these sutures to degrade is an aqueous environment. Oxidoreductase enzymes, however, appear to be associated with the metabolism of the degradation products of these sutures. This high activity associated with oxidative enzymes was not found in cells removed from the suture implantation sites. Salthouse et al. suggested that the increase in oxidative enzymes associated with the citric acid cycle indicates the glycolic and lactic acid degradation products are being actively metabolized by those cells in contact with the suture filaments. Salthouse and Matlaga concluded their enzymatic study by suggested the following *in vivo* scheme:

Vicryl suture + water
↓
glycolic and lactic acids
↓
macrophage oxidoreductase enzymes
↓
carbon dioxide and water

In contrast, Williams and Mort[151,152] demonstrated that certain enzymes, under some conditions, are able to influence the degradation of PGA and polylactides. Williams and Mort[151] found that certain enzymes, under some *in vitro* conditions, were able to influence the degradation of 2/0 PGA sutures as shown in Table 7.17. Acid phosphates, papain, pepsin, peptidase, pronase, proteinase K, and trypsin had no apparent effect on PGA sutures. Ficin, carboxypeptidase A, chymotrypsin, and clostridiopeptidase A all produced significantly greater amounts of degradation, often increasing the rate of hydrolysis by a factor of two. Bromelain, esterase, and leucine amino peptidase-treated PGA sutures lost all of their tensile strength after 3 weeks, while the untreated ones lost only 13.3% of their original value within

Table 7.18 Effects of γ-Irradiation on *In Vitro* Enzymatic Degradation of 2/0 Polyglycolide Absorbable Sutures

Time (d)		Dosage			
		0 Mrad	5 Mrad	10 Mrad	20 Mrad
0		5.40 ± 0.51 kg	3.95 ± 0.40 kg	3.66 ± 0.29 kg	3.11 ± 0.32 kg
3	E	3.88 ± 0.54	2.20 ± 0.31	2.24 ± 0.29	1.33 ± 0.72
		(3.94 ± 1.45)	(3.25 ± 0.28)	(2.74 ± 0.31)	(1.53 ± 0.44)
	α	4.92 ± 0.25	3.53 ± 0.33	2.55 ± 0.40	1.90 ± 0.48
		(4.43 ± 0.12)	(3.34 ± 0.15)	(2.41 ± 0.58)	(1.78 ± 0.35)
	T	4.75 ± 0.53)	3.04 ± 0.49	2.48 ± 0.41	1.35 ± 0.37
		(4.46 ± 0.36)	(2.93 ± 0.33)	(2.58 ± 0.30)	(2.05 ± 0.21)
7	E	2.77 ± 0.18	1.43 ± 0.36	1.06 ± 0.13	0.29 ± 0.14
		(3.99 ± 0.88)	(2.15 ± 0.43)	(1.64 ± 0.38)	(0.74 ± 0.22)
	α	4.28 ± 0.33	2.21 ± 0.20	1.57 ± 0.19	0.89 ± 0.05
		(3.74 ± 0.31)	(2.20 ± 0.17)	(1.69 ± 0.12)	(1.06 ± 0.13)
	T	4.67 ± 0.18	2.14 ± 0.33	1.76 ± 0.13	1.14 ± 0.12
		(4.17 ± 0.52)	(1.75 ± 0.26)	(1.80 ± 0.17)	(0.85 ± 0.06)
14	E	0.45 ± 0.12	0	0	0
		(3.56 ± 0.76)	(0.85 ± 0.22)	(0.52 ± 0.18)	(0.16 ± 0.07)
	α	2.76 ± 0.34	0.06 ± 0.03	0	0
		(2.71 ± 0.51)	(0.57 ± 0.17)	(0.74 ± 0.06)	(0.19 ± 0.09)
	T	3.81 ± 0.47	0.64 ± 0.26	0.30 ± 0.07	0
		(4.06 ± 0.24)	(0.62 ± 0.11)	(0.50 ± 0.19)	(0.08 ± 0.03)

Note: E, esterase; α, α-chymotrypsin; T, trypsin. Data in parentheses from the corresponding buffer solutions at 95% confidence limit. Values are mean breaking load.

From Chu, C.C. and Williams, D.F., *J. Biomed. Mater. Res.*, 17(6), 1029, 1983. With permission.

the same period. It was, however, difficult to take into account quantitatively the effect of ammonium sulfate whose presence in the media was required to stabilize the enzymes on the observed accelerated hydrolysis. The enzymes that did influence the hydrolysis were mainly (although not exclusively) of the type (esterases) that might be expected to attack an aliphatic polyester on the basis of its molecular structure.

As mentioned earlier, the alteration of the structure of polymer chains by γ-irradiation may change the susceptibility of the polymer toward enzymatic degradation. Thus, those enzymes like trypsin which show no effect on PGA initially may influence its degradation after the alteration of its physical and chemical structures by γ-irradiation. This possibility was recently examined by Chu and Williams[124] in the *in vitro* study of the effect of γ-irradiation on the role of enzymes in PGA suture hydrolysis.

Of the three enzymes studied (esterase, α-chymotrypsin, and trypsin), esterase showed the greatest enzymatic effect on the degradation of the unirradiated and irradiated PGA sutures as shown in Table 7.18. Irradiation made the suture more susceptible to esterase attack than was the case with an unirradiated sample, as evidenced by the lower percentage of retention of tensile breaking strength in enzymatic solutions. The effect of trypsin on PGA sutures was not observed until 20 Mrads of radiation were applied. Trypsin-treated, 20 Mrad-irradiated PGA sutures lost 13% more than their corresponding buffer control group after 3 d of immersion. The findings for trypsin demonstrated the hypothesis that synthetic high-molecular-weight polymers, which are initially resistant to enzymatic degradation, can become prone to enzymatic attack after the alteration of their physical and chemical structures.

Mizuma et al.[23] also concluded that trypsin does not accelerate the hydrolytic degradation of PGA sutures *in vitro* after they compared the percent of loss of tensile strength of PGA sutures exposed to nonactivated canine pancreatic and enterokinase activated pancreatic juices. By the end of 14 d, PGA sutures lost about 60% of their original tensile strength in the former, while they lost only 30% in the latter.

Holbrook used urine as a model to examine the enzymatic effect on PGA degradation.[153] He found that amylase, hyaluronidase, and urokinase failed to show enzymatic catalytic degradation, but the addition of porcine esterase into a control urine did accelerate the breakdown of PGA sutures. The suture in the esterase-treated urine had only 15% of the tensile strength (0.09 kg) of the urine control (0.61 kg) after 3 d. This esterase-accelerated degradation of PGA was further confirmed by competitive inhibition

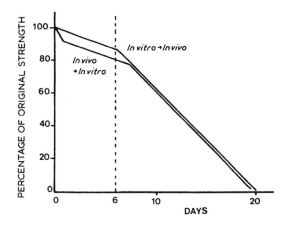

Figure 7.54 Degradation profiles of polyglycolide sutures with transfer between *in vivo* and *in vitro* conditions at 6 d.

with another ester (glyceryl triacetate-triacetin). Thus, Holbrook concluded that the destruction and fracturing of PGA sutures is more than the result of pure hydrolysis.

By effecting a transfer between *in vitro* and *in vivo* conditions, Williams also showed that there is something specific about the immediate environment in bodily implantation that influences the hydrolytic degradation of PGA sutures.[152] As shown in Figure 7.54, there was a rapid initial loss of strength of about 10% during the first 2 d postimplantation which was not observed under *in vitro* conditions. Those sutures that were transferred from an *in vitro* to an *in vivo* environment at day 6 exhibited this rapid loss of strength immediately after the transfer.

In an attempt to identify which enzymes were responsible, those released by polymorphonuclear leukocytes during the acute inflammatory response, or those released by the macrophages of the chronic response, Williams used a novel approach involving repeated implantation, removal, and reimplantation of PGA sutures for short periods of time.[154] It was found that the reimplanted PGA sutures, which experienced a series of acute responses, had slightly higher degradation rates than the control group, which only experienced acute response once followed by chronic response (55.8% strength remaining in repeated implantation, removal, and reimplantation compared to 59.9% in control group at $p<0.005$). The difference, however, was hardly conclusive enough to prove the hypothesis that the enzymes released from cells in response to the trauma of implantation are responsible for the initial rapid loss of strength during the first few days after implantation.

The possible role of enzymes in the hydrolytic degradation of synthetic absorbable sutures was further demonstrated by Persson et al.[155] in their study of the effect of the enzymatic wound cleaning surgical practice on 3/0 PGA sutures. Varidase, an enzymatic solution consisting of streptokinase and streptodornase, has been used as a wound cleanser in infected wounds to remove necrotic tissues, fibrin, pus, and coagulated blood.[156] Because the cleaning procedures involve the soaking of the wound with Varidase solution, the sutures in the wound are in close contact with the enzymatic solution. Persson et al.[155] found that a statistically significant difference ($p<.05$) in tensile breaking strength, elongation at break, and toughness (area under stress-strain curve) of the PGA sutures was observed between saline- and Varidase-incubated 3/0 PGA sutures. For example, the percentage of retention of original tensile breaking strength, elongation at break, and toughness at day 15 were 59%, 52%, and 29% for the Varidase-incubated PGA group, while the saline-incubated PGA sutures retained 71%, 65%, and 47%, respectively. Similar differences in the change of mechanical properties of 3/0 PGA sutures were observed in artificially created abdominal wounds in male Wistar rats. The authors thus concluded that there is a potential risk of wound rupture with the continuous use of Varidase in PGA-sutured wounds for a long postoperation period. However, it seems to be safe to use Varidase in PGA-sutured wounds for a short postoperation period (less than 10 d).

All the *in vivo* biodegradation properties of synthetic absorbable sutures reported in the literature include the involvement of direct contact of inflammatory cells to these sutures. As described earlier, Salthouse and Matlaga[150] suggested that the close adhesion of macrophages onto the Vicryl suture surface must bear a direct relationship to the observed *in vivo* biodegradation properties. In order to isolate the

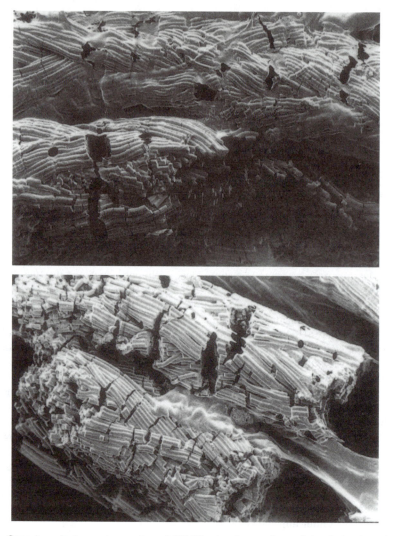

Figure 7.55 Scanning electron micrographs of 2/0 Vicryl sutures after poly(methylmethacrylate) (PMMA) chamber implantation subcutaneously in rats for 14 d. (From Zhong S.P. et al., *Clin. Mater.*, 14, 145, 1993. With permission.)

effect of these biological cells from the general *in vivo* environment, Zhong et al. have reported a study of the biodegradation properties of Vicryl sutures in a controlled acellular *in vivo* environment.[157] Vicryl sutures were confined with a poly(methylmethacrylate) chamber which had a pore size <0.45 μm and the chamber was implanted subcutaneously in Lister rats. Because of the pore size, no biological cells were expected to penetrate into the chambers; however, biochemicals like enzymes could still diffuse into the chamber. Their SEM observations indicated that Vicryl sutures under this controlled *in vivo* environment degraded faster than *in vitro* phosphate-buffered saline (PBS) medium. A comparison between the *in vivo* chamber environment (Figure 7.55) and *in vitro* PBS medium (Figure 7.56) indicated that the *in vivo* chamber environment induced a faster degradation, as evident in the earlier appearance of multiple surface cracks. Far more severe fragmentations were observed in the chamber environment at 14 d, while the same suture in PBS showed far sparser fragments and fewer surface cracks. This study, however, did not determine whether these two environments would alter the tensile strength loss profiles.

In terms of the kinetics of enzymate-catalyzed hydrolysis of PGA, Zaikov suggested the addition of the term $0.8(1 - K_{enz}^s \, C_{enz}^{-s} \, t/N\gamma\rho)^2$ to the general kinetic Equation 16 shown below.[6] K_{enz}^s, the rate constant of enzyme-accelerated degradation, is $1.0 \times 10^{-2} \, d^{-1}$.

$$\alpha = m/m_o = [1 - 0.2 \, (1 - e^{-Ka \, Ca \, t})^2] + [0.8 \, (1 - K_c C_c \, t/N\gamma\rho)^2]$$

$$\text{Amorphous term} \qquad \text{Crystalline term} \qquad (16)$$

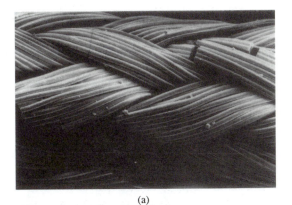

(a)

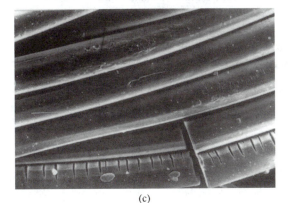

(b)

(c)

Figure 7.56 Scanning electron micrographs of 2/0 Vicryl sutures after *in vitro* degradation in PBS medium for 14 d. (a) ×150; (b) ×480; (c) ×1000. (From Zhong S.P. et al., *Clin. Mater.*, 14, 145, 1993. With permission.)

where K_a is the effective rate constant, which includes the rate constant of random scission of ester linkages in the amorphous regions and the rate constant of unzipping the ester bonds located at the ends of crystallites. Its value is 5×10^{-2} cm^3 × d^{-1} × g^{-1} in water at 37°C.

K_c, effective rate constant in the crystalline regions; 1.3×10^{-2} × d^{-1} in water at 37°C

C_a, average water content in the amorphous regions

C_c, average water content at the side face of crystallites

N, number of crystallites in a cross-sectional area of a fiber

γ, average radius of the crystallite (¹/₂ of the minor axis of the ellipsoid density of crystallites)

ρ, density of crystallites

0.2 and 0.8, the volume proportions of amorphous and crystalline regions, respectively

Table 7.19 Tensile Breaking Loads of Sutures After Incubation in Broths and Bacterial Cultures

Suture	Bacteria	Broth	Breaking Strength (kg)		
			Control	In Broth	In Culture
Catgut	*Strep. mites*	Tryptone soya	3.41	2.34	2.25
	E. coli	Peptone-glucose	2.19	1.70	1.81
	E. coli	Brain-heart	3.38	2.67	2.37
	Staph. albus	Brain-heart	2.85	1.65	2.09
PGA	*Strep. mites*	Tryptone soya	4.77	1.31	2.79
	E. coli	Peptone-glucose	4.20	2.06	3.01
	E. coli	Brain-heart	4.55	2.74	3.27
	Staph. albus	Brain-heart	4.63	0.59	0.96

From Williams, D.G., *J. Biomed. Mater. Res.,* 14, 329, 1980. With permission.

The first term relates to the kinetics of hydrolysis in the amorphous phase, while the second term relates to that in the crystalline phase. This is consistent with the two-stage hydrolytic degradation mechanism of synthetic absorbable sutures proposed by Chu.[69] On the basis of the above equation, the effects of fiber structure and water content in PGA suture fibers on the rate of hydrolysis are readily illustrated. Increasing both C_a and C_c or either one of them will decrease the ratio of m/m_o, i.e., faster rate of hydrolysis.

In conclusion, at the beginning of implantation, enzymes may have difficulty in degrading synthetic absorbable suture materials because of their high molecular weight and enzyme-substrate specificity. Hydrolysis by water molecules alone is believed to be the major mechanism causing these sutures to degrade during the initial stage. Once the long chain molecules of these sutures are broken into short chain fragments by this initial pure water hydrolysis, lysosomal enzymes such as esterase could start to function efficiently through the so-called preferential terminal attack. Any chemical or physical means which could increase the number of chain ends of a polymer will make initially enzymatically resistant synthetic biodegradable polymers more prone to enzymatic degradation.

h. Effect of Bacteria

Since bacteria are also a source of enzymes, it is speculated that bacteria in an infected wound can also influence the degradation of synthetic absorbable sutures. Williams tested three types of bacteria (*E. coli, S. albus,* and *Streptococcus mites*) and found that PGA sutures degraded less rapidly in the presence of bacteria than they did in a control broth, as shown in Table 7.19.[34] PGA sutures in the broth degraded 20% to 13% faster than the same suture in the same broth with bacteria included. The same results were observed in the subsequent *in vivo* experiment in rats. PGA sutures of size 2/0 implanted subcutaneously in the *S. albus*-infected sites of the white hooded Lister rat of the Liverpool strain exhibited 38% loss of tensile breaking strength, while the same suture in the noninfected sites showed 40.7% loss of strength. The difference was statistically significant at the $p < .05$ level.

Williams' data clearly indicate that the enzymes from the tested bacteria do not catalyze the degradation of PGA sutures. One of the possible causes for the observed slower rate of degradation in the presence of bacteria is that the bacteria adhere onto the suture surface and may act as a physical barrier to isolate the suture from the surrounding medium. This slower rate of degradation of PGA sutures in the presence of bacteria was consistent with Bucknall's study in which 2/0 PGA sutures were used to close *S. aureus*-infected abdominal fascia.[158] As shown in Table 7.20, after 10 d, there was only a 24% loss of initial tensile strength in the infected wound, while the same sutures lost 65% of their original tensile strength in the noninfected rats. Infection, however, did not accelerate or slow the degradation of PGA sutures at a later period of postoperation. Bucknall attributed this slower degradation rate of PGA during the early period of postimplantation to the fact that the vigorous polymorphonuclear cell reaction around the suture strands in the infected wound may slow the invasion of foreign-body giant cells and macrophages which are chiefly responsible for the absorption of PGA sutures *in vivo*.[158,159] Other factors, such as pH change due to bacterial metabolism, may inhibit the enzymatic esterase absorption process *in vivo* and hence slow down the degradation process of PGA. Bucknall also pointed out that the bacteriocidal nature of the degradation product of PGA sutures would clear the bacteria in the wound rapidly, and the normal rate of degradation would progress. The same rate of degradation observed at the late period in both infected and noninfected wounds supported this point of view.

Table 7.20 *In Vivo* Tensile Breaking Strength of Sutures in *Staphylococcus aureus*-Infected Abdominal Wounds of Rats

Suture	Period (d)	Unused (new) Strength (kg)	Unused (new) Elongation (%)	Noninfected Strength (kg)	Noninfected % loss	Infected Strength (kg)	Infected % loss
Silk	0	3.88	18				
	10			2.73	29	3.34	14
	30			1.04	73	2.91	25
	70			0.65	83	1.46	62
	200			0.16	96	—	—
Monofilament nylon	0	3.33	79				
	10			3.22	3	2.62	21
	30			3.09	7	3.19	4
	70			2.79	16	3.10	7
	200			2.67	20	—	—
Polyglycolide	0	6.65	36.3				
	10			2.30	65	5.02	24
	30			0.51	92	0.27	96
	70			0.08	99	0.08	99
Multifilament nylon	0	3.83	36				
	10			3.21	16	3.67	4
	30			3.10	19	3.44	10
	70			2.98	22	2.22	42

From Bucknall, T.E., *J. R. Soc. Med.*, 74, 580, 1981. With permission.

Table 7.21 *In Vitro* Tensile Breaking Force (kg) of 3/0 Polyglycolide Suture Material Incubated in Bacterial-Infected Human Urine at 37°C

	Sterile	Infected with 10^9 Organisms of E. coli	Strep. faecalis	Proteus	Pseudomonas
Broth	1.91	1.83	1.77*	1.80*	1.73*
Human urine	2.19	2.28	2.22	0.00[†]	2.03*

Note: Comparison with sterile * $P < .05$; [†] $P < .001$.

From Holbrook, M.C., *Br. J. Urol.*, 54(3), 313, 1982. With permission.

In a study of PGA suture degradation in infected human urine, Holbrook,[153] however, found that there was no tensile strength after 3 d incubation of 3/0 PGA sutures in *Proteus mirabilia*-infected human urine, while other microorganisms, such as *E. coli*, *Streptococcus faecalis*, and *Pseudomonas*, had little effect on PGA degradation in infected human urine. Table 7.21 summarizes his results. Multiple circumferential surface cracks, like those observed by Chu in γ-irradiated PGA sutures, were also observed on Holbrook's PGA sutures after 3 d incubation in the *Proteus mirabilia*-infected urine.

The accelerated degradation of PGA sutures in infected human urine was also reported by Sebeseri et al.[35] They reported that 3/0 PGA sutures dissolved completely on the third day of immersion in *E. coli*-infected urine, while it took 6 d for the same suture to be completely degraded in noninfected urine at 36°C. The same PGA sutures in physiologic saline solution still retained 50% of their original tensile breaking strength at the same duration of immersion. Hovendal and Schwartz,[160] using the same suture materials and methods, observed statistically less significant difference between sterile and *E. coli*-infected urine ($p < .05$), but significant difference between physiological saline and *E. coli*-infected urine ($p < .01$) over a 10-d period.

Schiller et al.[161] confirmed the effect of bacteria on the degradation of five 3/0 absorbable sutures in sterile and both *E. coli*- and *P. mirabilia*-infected canine urine. Their most significant finding is that *P. mirabilia*-inoculated urine promoted the tensile property loss significantly faster than either *E. coli*-infected or sterile urine in all five absorbable sutures (chromic catgut, PGA, Vicryl, PDSII, and Maxon). For example, PGA and Vicryl were too weak to be tested after 24 h incubation in *P. mirabilia*, while

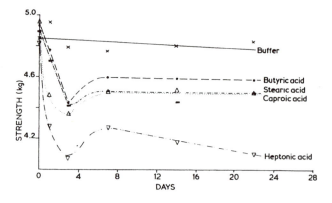

Figure 7.57 Tensile breaking strength of PGA sutures as a function of *in vitro* period of immersion in various lipid solutions. (From Sharma, C.P. and Williams, D.F., *Eng. Med.*, 10, 8, 1981. With permission.)

the same sutures exhibited little or no loss of tensile properties in sterile or *E. coli*-infected urine at the end of the same period (24 h). PDSII and Maxon sutures were too weak to test at the end of 7 and 10 d incubation in *P. mirabilia*-infected urine, respectively. The same PDSII suture, however, exhibited no loss of tensile properties at the end of 7 d in both sterile and *E. coli*-infected urine. Chromic catgut was the only absorbable suture in the group which retained its tensile properties for the longest period of immersion, i.e., 21 d. One of the possible causes for the profound effect of *P. mirabilia* was the alkalinity of the medium. *P. mirabilia*-infected urine had a pH of 8.8, while the sterile and *E. coli*-infected urine had pH of 6.1 and 6.8, respectively. It is known from Chu's published work[25,97,98] that an alkaline pH had a significant adverse effect on the hydrolytic degradation of synthetic absorbable sutures. Because of the small difference in pH between the sterile and *E. coli*-infected urine, no significant effect would be expected between these two media, as observed in the study by Schiller et al.[161]

Sharma and Kumar examined the effect of *S. aureus*-inoculated wounds (5.38×10^8/ml) in buffaloes on tensile strength retention of Dexon, catgut, linen, and Prolene sutures.[162] They found that Dexon sutures in *S. aureus*-infected wounds lost their tensile strength significantly ($p<.05$) faster than clean or infected but antibiotic (penicillin)-treated wounds at 3, 9, and 15 d postimplantation. Dexon sutures in clean wounds retained the highest strength, followed by infected but antibiotic-treated wounds. Catgut sutures showed similar behavior as Dexon sutures, but there was no statistically significant difference ($p<.05$) in catgut strength retention between clean and infected but antibiotic-treated wounds. All linen sutures whether in clean, infected, or infected but treated wounds exhibited a gradual loss of tensile strength with time. For example, a loss of 23% to 30% of the day 3 strength was found at 90 d postimplantation in clean, infected, and infected but treated wounds. Infection, however, did not lead to a faster loss of linen sutures.

i. Effect of Lipids

It is well known from several studies by various investigators that lipids can affect the structure of biomedical polymers, particularly silicone rubber, used as the ball component of artificial heart valves or as a joint component.[163–165] The absorption of lipids onto silicone rubber is believed to be mainly responsible for the observed fracture and its subsequent malfunction.

Whether or not lipids in tissues are able to influence the degradation of PGA sutures is not conclusive. There is only one reported study.[166] Sharma and Williams examined the role of various lipids, such as butyric, caproic, heptonic, and stearic acids, in PGA degradation, as shown in Figure 7.57,[166] 2/0 PGA sutures in phosphate buffer solutions containing lipids degraded significantly faster than the buffer control, particularly within the first 3 d of immersion. There was, however, a slight increase in strength thereafter before the strength of the suture decreased again. The magnitude and rapidity of tensile breaking strength loss depended on the concentration of the lipid. The concentration effect occurred at the very early stage of immersion (e.g., 2 h of immersion), and an increase in concentration of lipids accelerated the degradation of the sutures. It is speculated that the large molecular size of the lipid molecules could open up the amorphous regions of the fiber to facilitate subsequent hydrolytic degradation.

Andriano et al. reported that lipids like cholesterol may have some effect on the *in vitro* degradation of absorbable poly(*ortho*-ester) (POE) films.[167] They found that, although there was no apparent difference in the rate of loss of mechanical properties and mass when compared to deionized water, there was a 28% reduction in inherent viscosity of a 65:35 poly(*ortho*-ester) with original $M_w = 59,000$, in a cholesterol emulsion, while the deionized control lost only 6% inherent viscosity after 5 weeks immersion. However, the effect of lipid was the most pronounced in cloudy POE films having microscopic bubbles and there were only minor changes in the loss of mass and mechanical properties of uniform and clear POE films. It appears that studies of the effect of cholesterol on POE films were inconclusive because of inconsistent film quality.

j. Effect of Synovial Fluid

The use of absorbable suture materials in orthopedic surgery requires special precaution because the rate of loss of strength of absorbable sutures may accelerate under clinical conditions, particularly the high physiologic force imposed on sutures during early mobilization after orthopedic surgery, a practice that is frequently used, and the presence of synovial fluid that has different biochemical compositions than subcutaneous tissues. Based on the effect of external stress applied on suture degradation described earlier, it is reasonable to predict that absorbable sutures used in orthopedic surgery would degrade faster than the standard *in vivo* condition in which sutures are not stressed and minimal tissue trauma in subcutaneous environment are observed. In addition, torn meniscus is frequently associated with an inflammatory synovitis through anterior-cruciate-deficient knees. This inflammatory condition may accelerate the biodegradation of the absorbable sutures used for meniscal repair.

The very few published studies of the effect of synovial fluid or the physiological force imposed by synovium on absorbable suture strength were reported by Barber and Gurwitz[168,169] and Walton.[15] Because the meniscus repair by suture is considered to have the greatest promise for retaining the normal knee mechanism, Barber and Gurwitz suggest that the preservation of meniscus is very important during the treatment of knee pathology and holds the best long-term prognosis. However, the choice of sutures for a proper repair of torn meniscus is not easy because of the lack of clear understanding of the healing process of torn meniscus. It is known that meniscus requires a longer time to heal than other tissues, as reported by Arnoczky and Warren.[170] They found that as long as 8 months were required to completely heal a longitudinal tear of dog meniscus. This slow healing process in torn meniscus demands a longer retention of tensile strength on sutures. This requirement is further confirmed by Barber and Gurwitz that synthetic absorbable sutures lose their strength faster when exposed to synovial fluid than normal subcutaneous implantation.[168] Figure 7.58 demonstrates the effect of synovial fluid on the biodegradation of PDS and Vicryl sutures. PDS exposed to synovial fluid consistently exhibited better retention of tensile breaking force than those exposed to subcutaneous tissue. However, Vicryl sutures showed a faster loss of tensile breaking force when exposed to synovial fluid than in subcutaneous tissue. Readers should be aware that there was a difference in suture size. Those sutures used by Barber and Gurwitz (exposed to synovial fluid) were 1/0 size in rabbit, while the same type of sutures exposed to rat subcutaneous tissue were 2/0 size. Thus, the difference observed in Figure 7.58 may be attributed to differences in animal species and suture size.

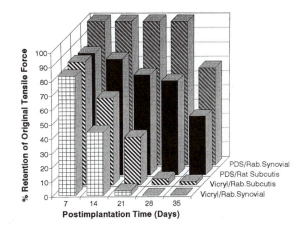

Figure 7.58 Effect of synovial fluid of rabbits on the tensile breaking force retention of Vicryl and PDS sutures when compared with the same sutures subcutis. (Replotted from data of Barber, F.A. and Gurwitz, G.S., *Am J. Knee Surg.*, 1, 189, 1988.)

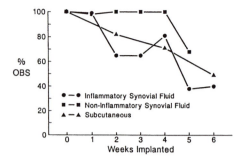

Figure 7.59 The changes in original tensile breaking strength (OBS) of 1/0 PDS sutures in various environments. (■) Noninflammatory synovial fluid in rabbits; (●) inflammatory rabbit synovial fluid; (▲) subcutaneous in rat. (From Barber, F.A. and Gurwitz, G.S., *Arthroscopy*, 4, 272, 1988. With permission.)

Because repairable longitudinal peripheral meniscal tears are likely associated with arthritis or inflammatory synovitis, Barber and Gurwitz also examined the effect of inflammatory synovial fluid on the biodegradation properties of absorbable sutures in New Zealand rabbits.[169] PDS sutures of 1/0 size in inflammatory synovial fluid consistently exhibited lower retentions of original tensile breaking force than the same sutures in noninflammatory synovial fluid, as shown Figure 7.59. The presence of exudates like neutrophils and serum proteins, as well as the breakdown products from torn articular cartilage, should be responsible for the observed accelerated loss of strength of PDS sutures. Both Howell et al.[171] and Mainardi[172] reported that inflammatory and/or arthritic rabbit or human knees have significantly higher elevation of enzymes and activities like neutral metalloproteoglycan-degrading enzymes and serine protease.[171,172] These biochemicals resulting from inflammatory response are believed to be responsible for the observed faster tensile strength loss of PDS in inflammatory synovial fluid.

Walton took a different approach to examine the combined effect of physiological force imposed by orthopedic tissues (e.g., synovium) and inflammation from surgical trauma on the biodegradation properties of absorbable sutures.[15] He demonstrated that the inflammatory postoperative synovial tissue and the mechanically stressed nature of the wound could degrade absorbable sutures faster than the commonly used *in vivo* testing condition. Both 2/0 PDS and Maxon sutures exhibited a faster loss of tensile breaking force when these sutures were used for a mattress closure of sheep synovial tissue (i.e., sutures were subject to force imposed by the synovial tissue) than the same sutures that were simply implanted into the medial parapatellar synovial pouch (i.e., no physiological force experienced by the implanted sutures) over 4 weeks postoperation. Walton thus questioned the validity of the commonly used implantation procedures (i.e., no stress applied to sutures in subcutaneous tissue with minimal tissue trauma) in the evaluation of suture performance in orthopedic surgery.

k. Effect of Plasma Surface Modification

The degradation of absorbable sutures could well be controlled by the rate of water permeation into the sutures. From the hydrolytic degradation studies of absorbable sutures, it is expected that any modification which could retard the diffusion (D) and solubility (S) of H_2O and/or enzyme molecules into the suture should be able to slow down their hydrolytic degradation process. Although there are many ways to retard the diffusion and solubility of water molecules in absorbable sutures, the use of plasma surface deposition to regulate the rate of tensile strength loss was recently reported by Loh et al.[173] The advantages of using plasma surface modification are that it could:

1. Change the water wettability, W, and solubility parameter, S, of the substrate by creating a hydrophobic surface
2. Crosslink the outermost layers of the polymers, thereby decreasing the diffusivity, D, of water molecules in this region
3. Retain those useful bulk properties like stiffness because the modification was limited to less than 1000 Å
4. Increase convenience in conducting the surface modification

The plasma surface treatment conditions are summarized in Table 7.22. Figure 7.60 summarizes the percentages of tensile breaking strength of the plasma surface-treated absorbable sutures. The percentage above (or below) the 100% mark in the bar graph indicates the amount better (or worse) than the corresponding untreated control at a particular hydrolysis time. Statistical analysis of these data indicate

Table 7.22 Plasma Surface Modification Parameters
for Four Synthetic Absorbable Sutures

Code	Types of Plasma Gas	Treatment Thickness
A1	Parylene N	400 Å
A3	Parylene N	1000 Å
C0	Methane	200 Å
C1	Methane	400 Å
C2	Methane	600 Å
C3	Methane	1000 Å
D1	Trimethylsilane	400 Å
D3	Trimethylsilane	1000 Å
E1	Tetrafluoroethene	400 Å
E2	Tetrafluoroethene	600 Å
E3	Tetrafluoroethene	1000 Å

From Loh, I.H. et al., *J. Appl. Biomater.*, 3(2), 131, 1992. With
permission.

that some of the plasma surface treatments resulted in significant statistical advantage over controls
($p<.05$). For example, all the four plasma surface treatment conditions for PDSII sutures (C0, C1, E1,
and E3) exhibited significant advantage over the corresponding untreated PDSII sutures at the later stages
of hydrolytic degradation (i.e., at 28 and 42 d). The improvement ranged from about 60% to 180% better
than the controls. Most of the plasma surface treatments for Vicryl sutures also showed better tensile
strength retention than the control (e.g., A3, C1, C3, E3). The range of improvement was from 20% to
80% better than the controls. In the Dexon sutures, the range of improvement on tensile breaking strength
retention was from 10% to 80% better than the control with E1-treated Dexon sutures exhibiting the
best result (80% better at 28 d). The results from Maxon sutures, however, were not as good as the other
absorbable sutures.

The improved tensile breaking strength retention of the plasma surface-treated absorbable sutures
observed was also consistent with the wettability data shown in Figure 7.61. All the plasma surface-
treated absorbable sutures exhibited higher hydrophobicity than the corresponding controls, as evidenced
in contact angle (θ), specific wettability (SW), and work of adhesion (W) data. For example, both
untreated PDSII and Maxon sutures had contact angles of about 71°, while the contact angle of all the
treated PDSII and Maxon sutures increased to 90° and above. In addition, all the treated PDSII and
Maxon sutures showed negative SW, while the corresponding controls exhibited positive SW, as expected
from our hypothesis that the creation of a more hydrophobic surface on the absorbable sutures by the
plasma surface treatments would certainly improve the retention of tensile breaking strength of absorbable
sutures.

It is known that water molecules must be able to permeate into these materials before hydrolysis can
occur. This water permeability depends on three factors: the adsorption of water onto the surface of the
material, the diffusion of surface-adsorbed water into the interior of the material due to the chemical
potential gradient of water, and subsequent dissolution of diffused water inside the material. The
wettability controls the first step of water permeation (adsorption of water on the surface of material).
Obviously, a more hydrophobic surface would reduce the amount of water adsorption on the material
surface which should reduce the subsequent permeation of water into the material. The second step of
permeation (water diffusion) is mainly controlled by macromolecular interaction, namely large-scale
segmental mobility. Macromolecules with more rigid chain characteristics either due to aromatic groups,
unsaturated bonds in the backbone, or crosslinking between backbone chains would reduce this diffusion
step. The last step of permeation (water dissolution) is determined by polymer-permeant interaction. A
stronger interaction would result in a larger solubility of the permeant in the material matrix.

In the case of hydrolysis, both the diffusivity and the solubility of water are found to be largely
affected by the polarity (i.e., cohesive energy density) of materials.[174] However, due to crosslinking and
hence the lack of large-scale segmental mobility resulting from plasma treatment, the permeability
characteristic of plasma-treated polymers must deviate from this diffusion-dissolution mechanism
described above. Yasuda suggested the permeability of plasma-treated polymers exhibits the characteristics of both the diffusion-dissolution mechanism and the molecular-level sieve mechanism. The latter
is controlled by the size of the permeant.[175]

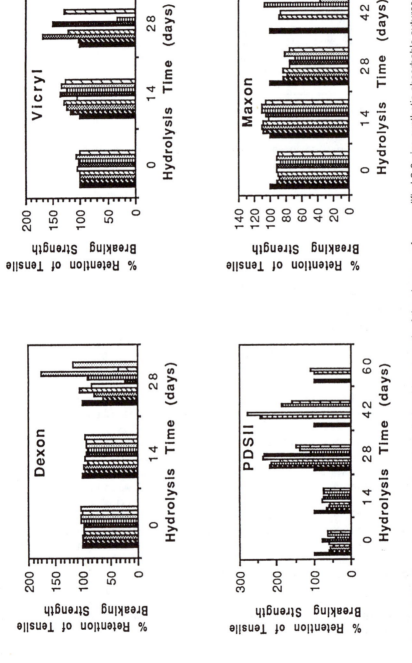

Figure 7.60 Percentage of retention of tensile breaking strength of the plasma surface modified 2-0 size synthetic absorbable sutures as a function of *in vitro* hydrolysis time in phosphate buffer of pH 7.44 at 37°C. The corresponding untreated sutures at the corresponding hydrolysis time serve as the controls. *Dexon suture:* control, A1, B3, C1, C2, C3, D1, E1, E2, E3. *Vicryl suture:* control, A1, B3, C1, C2, C3, D1, E2, E3. *PDSII suture:* control, A1, B3, C0, C1, C3, D1, E1, E3. *Maxon suture:* Control, A1, B3, C0, C1, C3, D1, D3, E3.

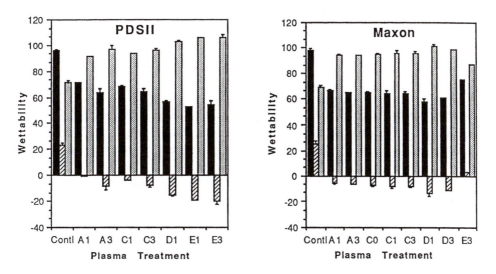

Figure 7.61 Wettability of unhydrolyzed plasma surface treated 2-0 size synthetic absorbable sutures (SAS). Contact angle (θ), specific wettability (Dynes/cm), and work of adhesion (Dynes/cm). The corresponding untreated SAS serve as the controls. (From Loh, I.H. et al., *J. Appl. Biomater.*, 3(2), 131, 1992. With permission.)

A comparison between tensile strength data and wettability findings in the study by Loh et al.[173] indicates that a hybrid mechanism controls the hydrolysis of plasma surface-treated synthetic absorbable sutures. For example, although a considerable improvement in hydrophobicity was found in plasma-treated Maxon sutures, there was no significant improvement in their retention of tensile breaking strength. A close examination of the earlier periods of hydrolysis (i.e., 14 d, Figure 7.60) of Maxon sutures showed that the two plasma-treated Maxon sutures (methane and trimethylsilane) revealed better tensile breaking strength retention (83% to 93%) than the control (80%). The advantage observed at the earlier period of hydrolysis must be attributed to the increase in initial hydrophobicity of the plasma-treated Maxon sutures found in the wettability study. But this advantage disappeared at longer periods of hydrolysis, probably due to the eventual permeation of water into the Maxon suture through the molecular sieve mechanism. Thus, it appears that the barrier for small permeants like water should largely depend on the degree of crosslinking or the sieve size. The hydrophobic surface generated by the plasma treatment delays the time of water diffusion rather than retards its diffusion. This points out that the future direction for optimizing the plasma treatment to maximize its advantage is to control the sieve size through the degree of crosslinking and type of plasma gases.

Plasma surface treatment also accelerated the mass loss of synthetic absorbable sutures upon hydrolysis and the degree of accelerated weight loss depended on the types of absorbable suture and plasma treatment conditions. For example, C0- and C1-treated Maxon sutures exhibited twice the rate of weight loss as the control at 42 d, while most of the plasma-treated PDSII sutures showed about three to four times faster weight loss than the untreated PDSII sutures at the same interval. Similar observation was also found in the plasma-treated Dexon sutures. Vicryl sutures were the only ones which did not show consistently higher rate of weight loss over the periods of study. This observed accelerated weight loss without the expenses of faster tensile strength loss could have one major advantage in wound closure. As given in Table 7.4, the absorption delay of the four synthetic absorbable suture fibers in both *in vitro* and *in vivo* conditions is very high for all four commercial synthetic absorbable sutures. There is a need for a faster loss of suture mass after the suture becomes useless (i.e., no tensile strength left) because it could reduce the extent of undesirable chronic foreign body reactions.

Surface morphological study by SEM revealed that the plasma surface treatments did not alter the appearance of fiber morphology of unhydrolyzed sutures; but subsequent hydrolysis revealed vast differences in the change of surface morphology of monofilament absorbable sutures with hydrolysis time. However, the multifilament braided Dexon and Vicryl exhibited little morphological difference between the plasma-treated sutures and their corresponding controls. The lack of any visible surface morphological difference from their corresponding untreated controls among all four types of absorbable suture before hydrolysis proceeded is due to the extremely thin plasma surface (in the order of 1000 Å). Figure 7.62 illustrates some of the unique surface morphological changes of plasma-treated absorbable

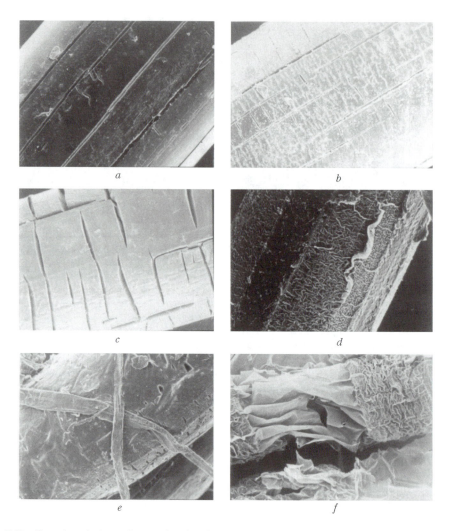

Figure 7.62 Scanning electron micrographs of surface morphology of methane plasma surface treated Maxon sutures after various periods of *in vitro* hydrolysis in phosphate buffer at 37°C. (a) 42 d hydrolyzed control; (b) 42 d hydrolyzed C1 plasma treated; (c) 90 d hydrolyzed control; (d) 90 d hydrolyzed C1 plasma treated; (e) 120 d hydrolyzed control; (f) 120 d hydrolyzed C1 plasma treated. (From Loh, I.H. et al., *J. Appl. Biomater.*, 3(2), 131, 1992. With permission.)

sutures as a result of hydrolysis. During the late periods of hydrolysis (greater than 60 d), the two monofilament absorbable sutures (PDSII and Maxon) showed quite drastic morphological differences between plasma-treated and untreated controls and between PDSII and Maxon sutures. There was no visible difference between plasma-treated and untreated PDSII sutures up to 60 d. However, major differences started to emerge thereafter. In both plasma-treated and untreated Maxon suture fibers, the surface cracks appeared earlier (as early as 42 d) and were more severe than for PDSII sutures. The untreated Maxon exhibited mainly longitudinal cracks, while the plasma-treated one showed equal appearance of longitudinal and circumferential cracks.

Another unique aspect of surface morphological change with hydrolysis was that the plasma-treated Maxon suture fibers was the very thin, paper-like material (<1 μm) with a lot of void space between the thin layers in the interior of the core suture fiber at 120 d *in vitro* hydrolysis. This suggests that very little Maxon suture mass remained at 120 d. This observation was consistent with the weight loss data (i.e., 98% weight loss). Since most of the weight loss occurred between 42 and 90 d (about 62% of the original weight was lost), while the diameter of the treated Maxon suture fiber was only reduced by 15% and the integrity of the suture core outline was still intact, this high degree of suture mass loss must occur in the interior of the core. The exposed very thin paper-like material with a lot of empty space at 120 d (Figure 7.62f) illustrates this point of view. The untreated Maxon controls, however, did not show this unique morphological change, and its diameter at 120 d of hydrolysis (i.e., 270 µm) was significantly larger than the plasma-treated Maxon sutures (i.e., 160 µm).

It is a general belief that a highly crosslinked plasma surface, in which segmental mobility is severely restricted, should behave similarly to rigid sieves. If this is true, uniaxial or biaxial deformation of the surface could occur only through bond strain and subsequent bond breakage. This may predispose to premature failure due to the formation of surface cracks during actual clinical use of sutures (e.g., tying knots). SEM data from the study by Loh et al.[173] showed no apparent surface crack in both uniaxial and knotting deformation of PDSII and Maxon sutures. Their surface morphology was identical to the untreated and deformed controls. It appears that the concern of possible premature failure due to strained plasma-treated surface layer does not apply in the conditions employed here. The lack of adverse effect of the plasma modification on absorbable suture was also found in the bending stiffness data. In general, the plasma treatments used either slightly lowered the bending stiffness of absorbable suture which is advantageous (e.g., C3 in Maxon, Vicryl, and C2 in Dexon) or showed no statistical difference from the controls. PDSII sutures, however, were the only ones which showed slight increase in bending stiffness.

The only major adverse effect of the plasma surface treatment of absorbable sutures was the reduction of tensile breaking force before hydrolysis, particularly with PDS sutures. A comparison of the tensile breaking strength of 0 d plasma-treated absorbable sutures with their corresponding controls indicates that PDSII sutures had the largest reduction in initial tensile breaking strength due to plasma surface treatment, followed by Maxon sutures. Dexon and Vicryl sutures did not show any adverse effect from the plasma surface treatment as evident in their initial (0 d) tensile breaking strength. The percentage of tensile strength loss of plasma-treated PDSII ranged from 23% to 50% of the untreated control. D1 treatment showed the worst reduction in initial tensile strength, while C3 exhibited the least initial tensile strength loss. This initial (0 d) lower tensile strength found in the plasma-treated PDSII and some Maxon sutures might be attributed to the photodegradation of the fibers during plasma surface treatment. Since plasma treatment involves excited gas species like free radicals, ions generated by radio frequency power, the resulting photons discharged from these excited gas species could generate UV radiation, which may cause photochemical degradation of the treated sutures. This finding also suggests the need to redesign the plasma reactor to minimize UV-originated photodegradation.

In conclusion, data on plasma surface modification of absorbable sutures obtained by Loh et al.[173] are encouraging and may indicate a convenient and less expensive alternative for changing the biodegradation properties of synthetic absorbable sutures with minimal adverse side effects.

I. Effect of Dialkyltitaneous Surface Modification

Several linear synthetic absorbable sutures have been used experimentally as synthetic vascular grafts and the data obtained indicate that these biodegradable polyesters have the capability to regenerate arterial tissues through hydrolytic degradation.[176–182] This regeneration of arterial tissues was attributed to the activation of macrophages by the degradable graft materials.[180,183,184] This macrophage activation subsequently induces a transinterstitial migration and proliferation of primitive mesenchymal cells, which then differentiate into cells with the ultrastructural and functional characteristics of smooth muscle-like myofibroblasts and endothelial-like cells.[180]

Yu et al. recently postulated that the degradation products of biodegradable polyesters and their rate of release into the surrounding environment must bear a relationship to the experimentally observed arterial tissue regeneration capability.[181] This hypothesis suggests that an ideal biodegradable polymer for arterial tissue regeneration should be able to release enough degradation products for activating macrophages to produce the required growth factors for accelerated wound healing, without the expense of premature loss of strength of the material during the early stage of hydrolytic degradation. However, none of the existing synthetic biodegradable fibers could achieve the degradation properties required by an ideal vascular graft. A faster degradation of a biodegradable fiber is always accompanied by a rapid loss of its mechanical properties. This inherent structure-property relationship in fibers makes any conventional chemical modification of synthetic absorbable suture fibers for meeting the goal of ideal biodegradable vascular grafts impossible. However, a recent report by Pratt and Chu appears to overcome this inherent difficulty.[185] They selectively altered the rate of degradation on this class of polymer surface without adversely affecting bulk properties by way of surface functional group transformation, where the surface ester linkages of PGA were converted to more hydrolytically sensitive vinyl ether functionalities with dimethyltitanocene, using the method of Petasis and Bzowej.[186] Because the conversion was

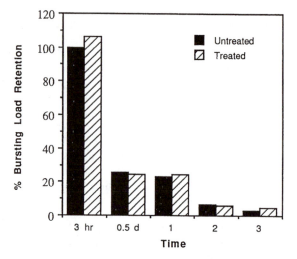

Figure 7.63 Bursting strength loss of treated and untreated PGA disks as a function of hydrolysis time. (From Pratt, L.M. and Chu, C.C., *J. Polym. Sci. Chem. Ed.*, 32, 949, 1994. With permission.)

limited to the surface layer of biodegradable polyesters, a faster degradation was achieved without premature accelerated loss of strength of the materials.

Figure 7.63 illustrates the effect of selective surface degradation on the mechanical properties of partially hydrolyzed PGA disks. For each hydrolysis period, a student *t*-test showed no statistically significant difference in bursting force between the treated and untreated PGA disks at the 95% confidence level. They, therefore, conclude that the chemical surface modification had no significant effect on either the initial strength of the material or its strength loss profile upon hydrolysis. The restriction of the chemical reaction to the surface of PGA was further demonstrated by the results of the intrinsic viscosity data. Those intrinsic viscosity data suggest that only the first few millimeters beneath the polymer surface were subject to the titanocene reaction and the reaction results in a lower-molecular-weight species.

The limitation of the titanocene reaction to the surface of biodegradable polyesters was further confirmed by a laser confocal microscopic evaluation. Figure 7.64 summarizes the maximum dye penetration as a function of the duration of chemical treatment (hours) and hydrolysis time (days). It appears that either longer duration of chemical treatment or hydrolysis time, in general, increased the maximum depth of dye penetration (MDDP) in both treated and untreated PGA disks with some variations for the treated samples at longer durations of both titanocene reaction and hydrolysis. For example, the MDDP of the unhydrolyzed disks increased from 12 mm in the untreated disk to 25 mm in the 10 h chemically treated disk, a 108% increase in MDDP due to chemical treatment alone. The MDDP of untreated control disks continuously increased from about 12 mm at 0 d hydrolysis to about 22 mm at the end of the 4-d hydrolysis period, an 83% increase in the depth of dye penetration due to hydrolysis alone. It is understandable that hydrolysis of PGA disks results in more microporous space which allowed dye to penetrate deeper into the interior of the disk. The titanocene-treated PGA disks, however, behaved differently than the untreated ones, particularly at the later stages of hydrolysis. The MDDP of the 4-h treated disks reached a peak of 32 mm at the end of 2 d of hydrolysis and then decreased thereafter. Compared to the longer treatment times, the 4-h treatment time generated fewer low-molecular-weight species, and so the removal of the surface layer by hydrolysis was much slower than with longer treatment times. No apparent difference in surface morphology was observed between the untreated and 4-h treated samples. Longer chemical treatment times, however, generated more and lower-molecular-weight species on the surface. They were more easily removed by hydrolysis to expose the underlying core material, and hence a reduction in MDDP would be expected and was observed at a shorter hydrolysis time.

The exact mechanism of this metathesis reaction is still not known, but it is believed to involve a polar intermediate since the reaction is fastest in aprotic polar solvents such as THF. Figure 7.65 illustrates the scheme of the dimethyltitanocene-induced surface chemical degradation on PGA. Enol ethers are easily hydrolyzed in dilute aqueous acid. It appears that fortuitous moisture in the THF solution and/or the protons from the polymer end groups were sufficiently acidic to cause cleavage of the vinyl ether

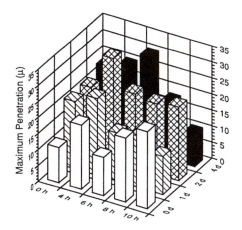

Figure 7.64 Maximum depth of dye penetration as a function of titanocene treatment time (hours) and duration of hydrolysis (days). (From Pratt, L.M. and Chu, C.C., *J. Polym. Sci. Chem. Ed.*, 32, 949, 1994. With permission.)

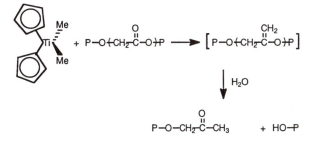

Figure 7.65 Reaction mechanism of titanocene chemical modification of polyglycolide and its subsequent hydrolysis. (From Pratt, L.M. and Chu, C.C., *J. Polym. Sci. Chem. Ed.*, 32, 949, 1994. With permission.)

group formed from the PGA metathesis reaction. To find out the reason for this unusual acid sensitivity, semiempirical molecular orbital calculations were used. The observed unusual instability of the vinyl ether resulting from the metathesis reaction of PGA was caused by a stabilization of the cationic intermediate which results from the rate-determining protonation of the vinyl ether.

IV. BIODEGRADATION PROPERTIES OF NONABSORBABLE SUTURES

A. NATURAL NONABSORBABLE SUTURES

Among nonabsorbable sutures, the ones which are most susceptible to degradation are silk and cotton. Postlethwait conducted a long-term comparative study of nonabsorbable sutures.[187] Figure 7.66 summarizes his results. It is clear that silk sutures lost all their strength after 2 years of implantation; this loss of strength is more severe during the first 12 weeks, when there was a loss of about 80% of original strength.[187] This loss of strength of silk sutures has also been reported by Greenwald et al.,[188] Van Winkle and Salthouse,[189] and Sato et al.[190] Greenwald et al. reported that 2/0 silk lost a significant amount of its mechanical properties at 6 weeks postimplantation in male adult Sprague-Dawley rats, such as the loss of 56% of its original tensile breaking strength, as shown in Figure 7.67. However, Van Winkle and Salthouse[189] reported that silk sutures reached zero strength much earlier, i.e., in 390 d. The discrepancy may be due to the difference in coating materials, the site of implantation, or to the differences in the species of animal. Does the property of strength loss of nonabsorbable silk suture pose any clinical problem? There are very few reported cases in the literature about such a concern. Sato et al. reported that the biodegradation of silk sutures was responsible for 11 noninfected aortic pseudoaneurysms at the suture line of patients with 1.8 to 26.8 years postimplantation of synthetic vascular grafts.[190] In one

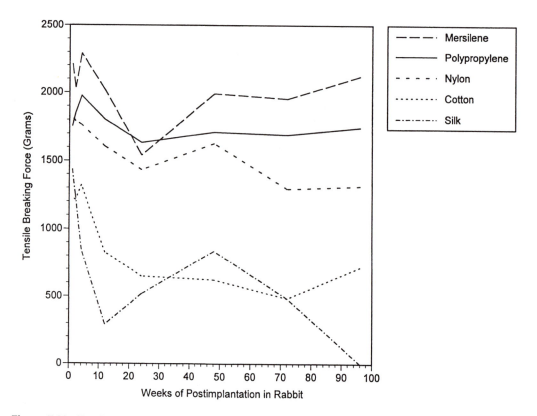

Figure 7.66 Tensile strength of five nonabsorbable sutures after implantation in rabbits for 2 years. (From Postlethwait, R.W., *Ann. Surg.,*171(6), 892, 1970. With permission.)

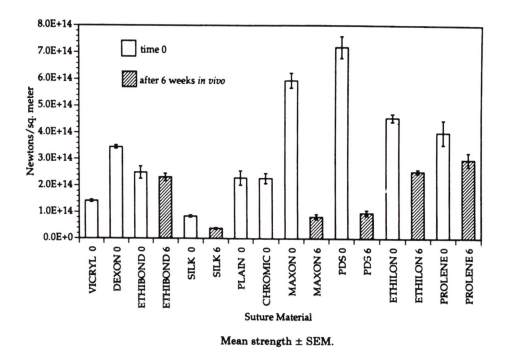

Figure 7.67 Tensile breaking strength (N/m²) of 10 suture materials before and after 6 weeks *in vivo* in rats. (From Greenwald, D. et al., *J. Surg. Res.,* 56, 372, 1994. With permission.)

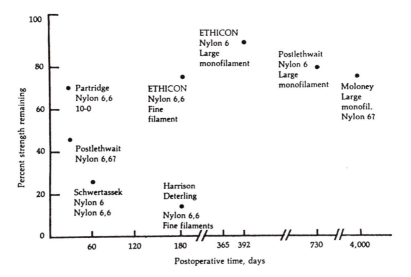

Figure 7.68 Tensile strength loss of nylon 6 and nylon 66 sutures. (From Kronenthal, R.L., *Am. Intra-Ocular Implant Soc. J.*, 3, 222, 1977. With permission.)

patient 19 years postimplantation of a Teflon graft, silk sutures were completely disintegrated into powder-like fragments on the grafts.

The effect of coating materials on silk degradation was studied by Postlethwait et al.[191] and the data were somewhat erratic. Irrespective of the surface treatment — dyed, waxed, or Teflon-coated — no significant differences in tensile strength could be found after 42 postoperative d in rabbits.

Similar to PGA sutures, silk sutures lost their strength slower in the infected than noninfected wound, as demonstrated in Bucknall's study.[158] He reported that there was only 25% loss of initial tensile strength in *S. aureus*-infected abdominal wounds in rats, while there was 27% tensile strength remaining in the noninfected abdominal wound 30 d postoperation. The silk sutures in infected wounds still remained stronger (38% of the original strength) than in noninfected wounds (17% of original strength). The delay in giant cell appearance due to infection was postulated to explain such a slower degradation in the presence of infection.

Postlethwait reported cotton sutures degraded to a lesser degree and lost approximately half their tensile strength by the end of the first year. Tensile strength remained more or less constant during the second year.[187]

B. SYNTHETIC NONABSORBABLE SUTURES

1. Nylon Sutures

Among the synthetic nonabsorbable sutures, nylon is probably the one most susceptible to degradation. The degradation of nylon *in vivo* was reported as early as 1958, when nylon fabrics were found to lose 80% of their strength during a 3-year implantation.[192] A great deal has appeared in the literature about the degradation of nylon sutures, and it is often conflicting. Figure 7.68 summarizes some of the important findings.[193] It is obvious that nylon 66 and nylon 6 degrade to a different degree; the percent strength remaining ranged from as low as 20% to as high as 75% in nylon 66 and from 75% to 90% in nylon 6. This wide range of degradation data is attributed to variations in test methods, such as animal species and location of suture, and to variations in materials like monofilament types, braiding, and size. Two things, however, were in common. First, most of the data indicated that once the initial loss in strength had occurred, the remaining strength did not change significantly during the remainder of the period of implantation. Second, nylon 6, in general, is slightly more resistant than nylon 66 to hydrolytic degradation, but the small difference is clinically insignificant. Recently, Greenwald et al. reported that 2/0 nylon suture (Ethilon) showed the second worst loss of mechanical properties (e.g., about 45% of its original tensile breaking strength) among four nonabsorbable sutures tested (silk, Ethilon, Prolene, and Ethibond) at 6 weeks postimplantation in rats (Figure 7.67).[188]

The initial loss of strength of nylon sutures was suggested by Kronenthal to be due to the hydration of the nylon sutures by body fluids immediately after implantation.[193] Nylon is able to absorb 12% water.

The absorbed water would act as a plasticizer and could disrupt the existing hydrogen bonds between nylon molecules, and hence reduce the strength of the suture. As suggested by Williams, there are many chemicals other than water, such as lipids and enzymes, which might contribute to this initial decrease in the strength of sutures.[152] The role of lipids and enzymes in PGA suture degradation was discussed earlier, but their effect on nylon sutures is unknown. Schwertassek and Dvorak used pepsin to examine the vulnerability of nylon fibers to enzymatic attack *in vitro* and concluded that enzymes, possibly lysozymes, may contribute to the *in vivo* degradation of nylon fibers through amide linkage.[194] Mehta found clinically detectable degradation of nylon sutures in second iris clip or iridocapsular implants inserted after aspiration of cataracts in children and speculated that macrophages and their enzymes may be responsible for the degradation of nylon sutures.[195] A further indication of the possible role of enzymes in nylon degradation was reported by Williams.[196] He found that nylon 66 degrades faster in the tissues of an acute inflammatory response than in the more quiescent chronic phase of tissue response.

The morphological change in intraocular nylon sutures as a result of degradation was reported by Blanksma and Siertsema.[197] The nylon sutures broke off where they made a sharp bend to pull through the hole in the pseudophakos. Transverse surface cracks were found in the sharply bent portion of the knot and in the two long broken extremities. These observed surface cracks were also reported in the SEM study by Jongebloed et al. of mechanical and biochemical effects of nylon (Perlon and Supramid) sutures in human eyes.[198] Based on their SEM data, severe degradation occurred at the ends (in contact with the tissue) of the Perlon suture retrieved from a patient after 6.5 years of implantation. The middle part of the Perlon suture, which was not in contact with tissue, however, did not show visible surface degradation. As shown in Figure 7.69, a segment of a Supramid loop of a retrieved Fedorov-type intraocular lens exhibited a similar surface crack pattern of degradation as Perlon sutures. A reduction of Supramid diameter was found in this severely biodegraded segment. This unique pattern of surface cracks on biodegraded nylon sutures is also similar to those observed on absorbable PGA sutures. Blanksma and Siertsema[197] suggested that the suture thread under tension would be more susceptible to degradation, because the so-called internal surface was enlarged and the possibility of hydrolysis increased. Drew et al.[200] also suggested that nylon may fatigue or break if it is tied under tension when anchoring Worst medallion lens.

Several other investigators also reported the tapered-end appearance of degraded nylon sutures.[199,200] Among them, Cohan et al. observed three configurations of suture ends at the point of break: fracture, erosion, and smoothed, as shown in Figure 7.70.[199] Cohan et al. also calculated the probabilities in percent of finding a broken nylon suture. Their results are 1 ± 1 at 12 months, 10 ± 3 at 24 months, 24 ± 5 at 36 months, and 36 ± 6 at 48 months.[199] Contrary to data from Blanksma and Siertsema, Cohan et al. suggested that knots, bends, and other areas of stress were never the areas most susceptible to degradation.[199] The area of most pronounced nylon suture degradation always occurred behind the iris. They thus concluded that nylon sutures are contraindicated for fixation of Worst lens because they are susceptible to degradation. Kronenthal, in a review of nylon sutures in the anterior chamber of the eye, suggested the use of more stable sutures in eye surgery, because it seems that the eye is not homogeneous in its promotion of nylon degradation.[201] The difference between the environments anterior and posterior to the iris, in pH, cell type, and distribution and mechanical stress factors remains to be determined.

Anderson et al. examined the effect of pH and morphological factors on the rate of *in vitro* hydrolytic degradation of nylon 6 multifilament and monofilament sutures.[202] They reported that hydrolysis of nylon 6 sutures and films is a bulk phenomenon and not restricted to their surface. The calculated first-order rate constants for multifilament and monofilament nylon 6 sutures at 37°C and pH 7.4 were very similar, 6.19 and 6.12×10^{-5}/d, respectively. The rate constants increased by at least 34% as pH of the solution decreased from 7.4 to 6.0. As observed and described for synthetic absorbable sutures, an increase in the level of crystallinity of nylon 6 upon hydrolysis was also found in the study by Anderson et al.[202] Many other workers, such as Troutman,[203] Taylor,[204] and Boruchoff and Donshik,[205] have also reported the degradation of nylon sutures after several years *in vivo* as indicated by visual observation.

2. Polyester Sutures

Polyethylene terephthalate (PET) sutures contain ester bonds which should be hydrolyzed readily. Clinically, no PET sutures have been reported to degrade to any significant level. Greenwald et al. found that there was no change in mechanical properties of Ethibond sutures for 6 weeks implantation in rats.[188] In a long-term study of nonabsorbable sutures, Postlethwait found that multifilament PET and Teflon-coated PET sutures showed virtually no change in tensile strength in the abdominal wall muscles of rabbits over a period of 2 years.[187] Similarly, Cook et al. reported that all three types of PET sutures

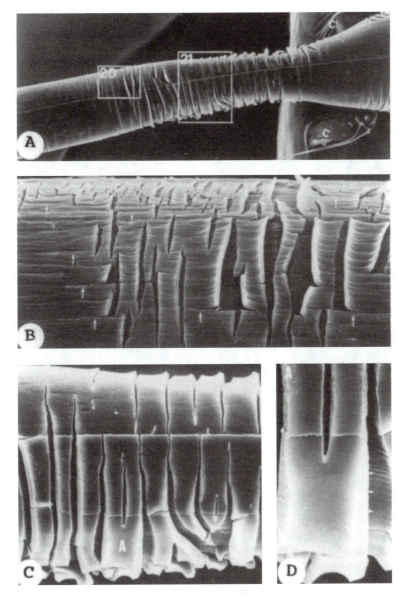

Figure 7.69 The Supramid loop close to a Fedorov-type intraocular lens retrieved from a patient after 10 yrs. (A) ×75; c, cell deposit; (B) ×455 of the portion marked 20 in (A); (C) ×275 of the portion marked 21 in (A); (D) ×610 of (C). (From Jongebloed, W.L. et al., *Doc. Ophthalmol.*, 61, 303, 1986. With permission.)

(Mersilene, Ethibond, and Biolite® carbon-coated Mersilene) of sizes 1/0, 2/0, and 1, which were used to repair incised medial collateral ligaments, retained more than 98% of their tensile strength after 48 weeks in dogs.[206]

Other types of polyester sutures like polybutester (Novafil), however, have been reported to exhibit long-term *in vivo* degradation.[207] Because a proper corneosclearal wound healing after cataract surgery is known to be longer than 12 months in human, McClellan et al. examined the stability of Novafil sutures in the eyes of rabbits for a period of 23 months. They reported that after 23 months 9/0 Novafil sutures used to close corneosclearal wound in the eyes of female Castle Hill pigmented rabbits exhibited distinctive surface degradation characterized by multiple small transverse cracks and/or longitudinal cracks. Some small transverse cracks led to the development of severe and deep transverse clefts in the knot regions, presumably because high stress regions of the knot caused the enlargement of the small transverse cracks deep into the interior of the suture.

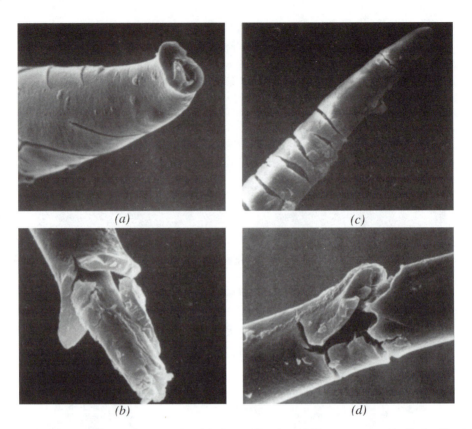

(a)

(c)

(b)

(d)

Figure 7.70 Scanning electron micrographs of broken 10/0 nylon 66 iris sutures used to fix the Worst lens. (a) Fractured tip and longitudinal cracking, ×2000; (b) eroded tip with peeling, ×5000; (c) smooth tip with circumferential crack, ×2000; (d) peeling and longitudinal cracking in section from behind iris, away from site of break, ×3000. (From Cohan, B. E. et al., *Am. J. Ophthalmol.,* 88, 982, 1979. With permission.)

3. Polypropylene Sutures

Due to the lack of hydrolyzable bonds, polyolefin sutures, such as polyethylene and polypropylene (PP), are not subjected to hydrolytic degradation. Thus, they retain their original strength very well for a long time in most *in vivo* environments. Postlethwait showed no loss of strength of PP sutures during the 2-year implantation in rabbit.[187]

Although the class of polyolefins is resistant to hydrolysis, it is susceptible to degradation by catalytic active carbon, oxidation, free radicals, and biodegradation. In many published studies of the recycling of plastic wastes like PP, it was found that PP can be degraded into aromatic hydrocarbons over metal-containing (e.g., Fe and Pt) activated carbon catalyst.[208–210] PP oxidation is not as well known as hydrolysis in biomedical polymers. The human body, due to the presence of O_2 in various forms, is a potentially powerful oxidizer. Liebert et al. examined the rate of oxidation of polypropylene fibers with and without antioxidant implanted subcutaneously in hamsters.[211] They found that the pure fiber (without antioxidant) degraded by an oxidation mechanism similar to high-temperature autoxidation. The degradation began to occur after only about 10 d and this initiation period lasted about 108 d. The degradation product, $>C=O$ group, was observed after 99 d of implantation. Whether this observation is applicable to polypropylene suture materials *in vivo* is not known and needs further study.

However, Cacciari et al. recently reported that pure isotactic PP films without any prior chemical or physical treatment underwent biodegradation after incubation with four microaerophilic microbial communities in limited O_2 environment.[212] Evidence of PP biodegradation included weight loss and CH_3Cl-extracted degradation products which were hydrocarbons. The findings of enzymatic attack of PP films by Cacciari et al. agree with other reported studies of biodegradation of other types of polyolefins like polyethylene.[213,214] The adaptability and metabolic flexibility of microorganisms are believed to be the reasons for the reported biodegradation of polyolefins, which have been thought to be highly resistant to biodegradation. These biodegradation studies of PP were originated from environmental recycling of plastic wastes. Whether the human body would provide a similar environment to those reported for the biodegradation of PP sutures is not fully understood. There are a few studies that indicate that PP sutures may not be recalcitrant to biodegradation and may be subject to biodegradation in the human environment.[188,198,215]

The reports of PP biodegradation in the human body environment, particularly in intraocular surgery where the transmission of UV light through the cornea may cause UV-induced degradation, have been controversial. Drews,[216] Lerman,[217] and Fechner et al.[218] reported that PP intracameral sutures or intraocular lens (IOL) haptics did not cause clinically significant degradation, particularly in elderly patients who spend most of their time indoors and have a shorter life span, and human cornea could act as a filter to remove any UV light <300 nm. On the other hand, Jongebloed et al.,[198, 220] Altman et al.,[215] and Apple et al.[219] have found that PP sutures or PP haptics of IOLs exhibited unique surface cracks after various periods of implantation in human eyes. Jongebloed et al. reported that Prolene loops of an open J-lens retrieved from a patient after 1 year exhibited severe surface degradation, as evident by the appearance of very regular circumferential striations, shown in Figure 7.71.[198] However, no surface biodegradation on the parts of the Prolene loop that were not in contact with tissue was observed. These characteristic circumferential surface cracks of PP sutures were also found in a study by Altman et al. of a 10/0 PP iris fixation suture after 5 years and 3 months implantation.[215] Although the surface circumferential cracks were limited in depth, their effect on the extent of embrittlement of PP should not be underestimated. This is because photooxidation-induced surface microcracks of PP fibers may lead to further crack propagation under stress, which would lead to premature failure.[221] However, the 4/0 PP IOL haptic retrieved from the same patient did not show any visible surface degradation. Altman et al. attributed the difference to the extent of orientation of fibers. 10/0 PP sutures were drawn about up to four times after melt-spinning which is significantly smaller than the theoretical draw ratio of 20. Because highly oriented fibers would be least affected by UV irradiation, a partially oriented PP suture is thus less resistant to UV-induced degradation.

Most reported biodegradation of PP sutures or PP IOL haptics is based on surface morphological observation by SEM. There is only one reported study of loss of mechanical properties of PP sutures due to implantation. Greenwald et al. found that Prolene suture lost about 26% of its original tensile breaking strength 6 weeks postimplantation in rats, as shown in Figure 7.67.[188] It is difficult to understand why the Prolene suture lost one quarter of its strength within such a short period of implantation.

V. LASER-INDUCED DEGRADATION OF SUTURE MATERIALS

Although much laser welding of tissues for wound closure does not involve suture materials, a recently reported technique of wound closure, laser-assisted fibrinogen bonding (LAFB), involves the use of sutures with laser. LAFB is used to reinforce sutured closure in a variety of tissues like vascular, gastrointestinal, urinary, and skin.[222–228] Because of the presence of sutures during LAFB procedures, it has been a concern whether the laser applied during LAFB procedures would damage the underlying sutures. Unfortunately, there are virtually no reports of studies that examine such a concern, except the work by Ashton et al.[229]

In that study, Ashton et al. examined the effect of LAFB procedures on 10 absorbable and nonabsorbable suture materials of both 3/0 and 6/0 sizes. Their results are summarized in Table 7.23. They used both the LAFB procedures with (group 3) and without (group 2) the presence of indocyanine green dye (approved by the Food and Drug Administration) which has a maximum absorption at 805 nm. The purpose of the dye is to enhance laser absorption because the diode laser with a peak emission at 808 nm is poorly absorbed by water presence in tissues. As shown in Table 7.23, 3/0 black silk from Ethicon is the only one in group 2 which showed the most significant laser-induced degradation without the presence of dye, a 75% reduction in its original tensile breaking force. White silk sutures from Ethicon, however, showed a relatively smaller adverse laser effect than its black counterpart, a 22% reduction of its original tensile breaking force. The difference between these two silk sutures is their color. Black absorbs energy far more than white and hence black silk suture would be expected to show more adverse effect than the white one. The other four nonabsorbable sutures (green Polydek II from Deknatel, white Gore-Tex from Gore and Associates, blue Prolene from Ethicon, and clear Novafil from Davis & Geck) showed negligible laser-induced degradation (97.7% to 100.7% retention of tensile breaking force), irrespective of size and color of the sutures. Among the four 3/0 absorbable sutures (beige Dexon, violet-dyed and undyed Vicryl, and chromic catgut) in group 2, only Dexon showed no laser-induced degradation, while the other three had about 13% to 15% loss of their original tensile breaking force. Contrary to silk

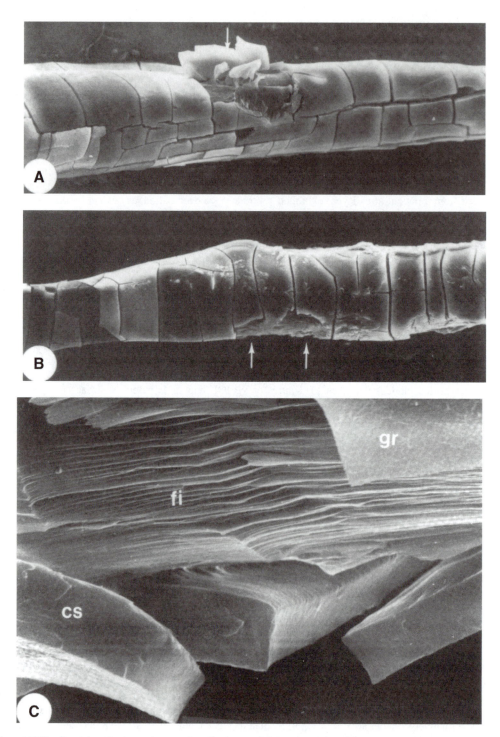

Figure 7.71 Scanning electron micrographs of polypropylene retrieved from human eyes. (A) Part of a polypropylene suture that remained in a human eye for 6.5 years as a fixation suture for an intraocular lens. Note the distinctive regular pattern of circumferential striations, ×325. (B) Part of the left side of the same suture at ×225. Note the circumferential cracks in the surface layer and some missing parts of the surface layer. (C) Subsurface layer of the same polypropylene suture at ×2500. fi — fibrillar character; gr — granular character. Note the exposed subsurface fibrillar character. (From Jongebloed, W.L. et al., *Doc. Ophthalmol.*, 61, 303, 1986; Jongebloed, W.L. and Worst, J.F.G., *Doc. Ophthalmol.*, 64, 143, 1986. With permission.)

Table 7.23 Effects of Laser-Assisted Fibrinogen Bonding Procedures on Tensile Breaking Force of Suture Materials

Suture Material	N	Strength[a] (lbs)	Retention[b]	Suture Material	N	Strength[a] (lbs)	Retention[b]
3-0 Polyester				**3-0 Silk (white)**			
Group 1	6	8.93 ± 0.38	—	Group 1	5	6.36 ± 0.30	—
Group 2	4	8.75 ± 0.31	98.0%	Group 2	5	5.00 ± 0.06*	78.6%
Group 3:				Group 3:			
10 s	5	8.38 ± 0.39	93.8%	10 s	4	4.34 ± 1.78	68.2%
15 s	6	7.09 ± 2.14	79.4%	15 s	2	4.50 ± 0.77	70.8%
30 s	6	5.82 ± 3.50	65.2%	30 s	4	5.11 ± 0.42	80.3%
60 s	7	5.74 ± 2.65*	64.3%	60 s	6	5.13 ± 0.67	80.7%
3-0 Polyglactin (violet-dyed)				**3-0 Silk (black)**			
Group 1	5	9.82 ± 0.54	—	Group 1	5	6.36 ± 0.30	—
Group 2	5	8.34 ± 0.37*	84.9%	Group 2	5	1.60 ± 0.71*	25.2%
Group 3:				Group 3:			
10 s	4	7.96 ± 1.62	81.1%	10 s	4	6.09 ± 0.08	95.8%
15 s	6	2.58 ± 2.69*	26.3%	15 s	6	6.04 ± 0.10	95.0%
30 s	5	0.29 ± 0.28*	3.0%	30 s	5	5.56 ± 0.87	87.2%
60 s	5	0.09 ± 0.05*	0.1%	60 s	6	0.42 ± 0.43*	6.6%
3-0 Polyglactin (undyed)				**6-0 Polypropylene (blue)**			
Group 1	5	10.86 ± 0.82	—	Group 1	6	1.30 ± 0.12	—
Group 2	5	9.52 ± 0.49*	87.7%	Group 2	5	1.27 ± 0.08	97.7%
Group 3:				Group 3:			
10 s	4	7.29 ± 3.04*	67.1%	10 s	12	0.64 ± 0.78	49.2%
15 s	6	1.29 ± 1.39*	11.9%	15 s	10	0.72 ± 0.73	55.4%
30 s	5	0.89 ± 1.49*	8.2%				
60 s	5	0.14 ± 0.04*	1.3%				
3-0 Polyglycolide				**6-0 Polybutester (clear)**			
Group 1	5	12.09 ± 0.71	—	Group 1	3	1.46 ± 0.24	—
Group 2	5	11.97 ± 0.52	99.0%	Group 2	3	1.47 ± 0.11	100.7%
Group 3:				Group 3:			
10 s	6	8.38 ± 3.08	77.6%	10 s	3	1.25 ± 0.49	85.6%
15 s	5	5.37 ± 3.26*	44.4%	30 s	3	1.06 ± 0.87	72.6%
30 s	5	0.64 ± 0.30*	5.4%	60 s	3	0.62 ± 0.90	42.5%
60 s	5	0.09 ± 0.05*	0.7%				
3-0 Chromic gut				**6-0 Polytetra-fluoroethylene**			
Group 1	9	9.03 ± 1.25	—	Group 1	4	4.45 ± 0.09	—
Group 2	5	7.69 ± 0.87*	85.2%	Group 2	5	4.31 ± 0.23	93.6%
Group 3:				Group 3:			
10 s	7	5.42 ± 1.67*	60.0%	20 s	4	4.45 ± 0.11	100.0%
15 s	5	3.24 ± 0.25*	35.9%	30 s	4	4.60 ± 0.35	103.4%
30 s	7	2.78 ± 1.13*	30.8%	60 s	4	4.59 ± 0.07	103.1%
60 s	5	0.0*	0.0%				

Note: *N*, number; Group 1, no exposure to laser or dye-enhanced solder; Group 2, exposed to laser only; Group 3, exposed to laser with addition of dye-enhanced solder.

* Significant at $P < .05$ as compared with Group 1.

[a] Percentage of original suture strength.

[b] Pound force at break.

From Ashton, R.C. et al., *J. Surg. Res.*, 53, 39, 1992. With permission.

sutures, it appeared that color of a suture did not contribute to the level of laser-induced degradation in the absorbable sutures (violet-dyed Vicryl vs. undyed Vicryl).

The presence of indocyanine dye in LAFB procedures (group 3), however, led to significant degradation in strength of all suture materials, except Gore-Tex suture, which retained its strength irrespective of time (up to 60 s). Many absorbable and nonabsorbable sutures were degraded to such an extent that they only retained their original tensile breaking force in single digits after 60 s LAFB exposure (e.g., dyed or undyed Vicryl, Dexon, black silk) or not at all (chromic gut). Absorbable sutures as a group were affected by LAFB procedures more than the nonabsorbable sutures. For example, all four absorbable sutures showed <1.3% retention of their original tensile breaking force at the end of 60 s of LAFB procedures, while most nonabsorbable sutures tested retained >42% of their original tensile breaking force, except black silk and Prolene sutures, which were very prone to LAFB-induced degradation.

The level of degradation of suture materials in the presence of laser-enhanced dye also depended on the duration of LAFB procedures. Duration of laser exposure greater than 10 s (e.g., 15 s) resulted in the largest degradation in tensile breaking force of all four absorbable sutures tested. It is important to know that normal LAFB procedures rarely involve more than 10 s laser exposure. The effect of the color of a suture on its susceptibility toward the laser-induced degradation was most evident between white and black silk sutures. After 60 s, the white silk suture retained 80.7% of its original tensile breaking force, while the black one had only 6.6% retention.

Finally, Ashton et al. pointed out that the size of the dye-enhanced solder drop had a significant effect on the extent of suture degradation, particularly at shorter time of laser exposure. This is because the outer surface of the solder drop is exposed to the thermal energy of the laser first. If the suture subsequently passes through the solder drop in such a way that the suture is closer to the outer surface, the suture would experience more thermal energy from the laser than the same suture that passes through the center of the solder drop.

The difference in the susceptibility of the sutures toward the laser-induced degradation in LAFB procedures must be attributed to the thermal and chemical properties of the suture materials. Among the synthetic suture materials, Gore-Tex suture has the highest melting temperature and hence was not affected by the LAFB procedures. Prolene suture has the lowest melting temperature among the tested synthetic sutures and hence showed the least tolerance toward laser. Ashton et al. attributed the laser sensitivity of the two natural suture materials (chromic catgut and silk) to the protein nature of these suture materials. They turn into pyrolytic products upon heating, via a dehydration process.

REFERENCES

1. Ravens, D.A.S., The chemical reactivity of poly(ethylene terephthalate): heterogeneous hydrolysis by hydrochloric acid, *Polymer*, 1, 375, 1960.
2. Ravens, D.A.S. and Sisley, J.E., Cleavage reactions, in *Chemical Reactions of Polymers*, Fettes, E.M., Ed., Interscience, New York, 1964, chap. 8.
3. Kuhn, W., Uber die Kinetik des Abbaues hochmolekularer kettin, *Berichte*, 63, 1503, 1930.
4. Heiken, D., Hermans, P.H., and Veldhoven, H.A., Kinetics of the acid hydrolysis of cyclic oligomers from nylon 6 and nylon 66, *Makromol. Chem.*, 30, 154, 1959.
5. Moiseev, Y.V., Daurova, T.T., Voronkova, O.S., Gumargalieva, K.Z., and Privalora, L.G., The specificity of polymer degradation in the living body, *J. Polym. Sci. Polym. Symp.*, 66, 269, 1979.
6. Zaikov, G.E., Quantitative aspects of polymer degradation in the living body, *J. Macromol. Sci. Rev. Macromol. Chem. Phys.*, C25, 551, 1985.
7. Moiseev, Y.V. and Zaikov, G.E., *Chemical Resistance of Polymers in Reactive Media*, Plenum, London, 1985, 426.
8. Lin, H.L., Chu, C.C., and Grubb, D., Hydrolytic degradation and morphologic study of Poly-p-dioxanone, *J. Biomed. Mater. Res.*, 27, 153, 1993.
9. Golike, R.C. and Lasoski, S.W., Kinetics of hydrolysis of polyethylene terephthalate films, *J. Phys. Chem.*, 64, 895, 1960.
10. Davies, T., Goldsmith, P.L., Ravens, D.A.S., and Ward, I.M., The kinetics of the hydrolysis of polyethylene terephthalate film, *J. Phys. Chem.*, 66, 175, 1962.
11. Salthouse, T.N., Williams, J.A., and Willigan, D.A., Relationship of cellular enzyme activity to catgut and collagen suture absorption, *Surg. Gynecol. Obstet.*, 129, 691, 1969.
12. Jenkins, H.P., Hrdina, L.S., Owens, F.M. et al., Absorption of surgical gut (catgut): duration in tissues after loss of tensile strength, *Arch. Surg.*, 45, 74, 1942.
13. Okada, T., Hayashi, T., and Ikada, Y., Degradation of collagen suture *in vitro* and *in vivo*, *Biomaterials*, 13, 448, 1992.
14. Hayashi, T. and Ikada, Y., Enzymatic hydrolysis of copoly(N-hydroxyalkyl L-glutamine/γ-methyl L-glutamate) fibres, *Biomaterials*, 11, 409, 1990.

15. Walton, M., Strength retention of chromic gut and monofilament synthetic absorbable suture materials in joint tissues, *Clin. Orthop. Rel. Res.*, 242, 303, 1989.

16. Hayashi, T., Tabata, Y., and Nakajima, A., Biodegradation of poly(amino acid) *in vitro*, *Polym. J.*, 17, 463, 1985.

17. Rhoads, J.E., Hotenstein, H.F., and Hudson, I.F., The decline in strength of catgut after exposure to living tissues, *Arch. Surg.*, 34, 209, 1937.

18. Katz, A.R. and Turner, R.J., Evaluation of tensile and absorption properties of polyglycolic acid sutures, *Surg. Gynecol. Obstet.*, 131, 701, 1970.

19. Postlethwait, R.W., Ulin, A.W., Skarin, R.M. et al., Breaking strength loss of intraluminal suture materials in gastrointestinal tract, *Chir. Gastroenterol.*, 8, 18, 1974.

20. Everett, W.G., Suture materials in general surgery, *Prog. Surg.*, 8, 14, 1970.

21. Howes, E.L., Factors determining the loss of strength of catgut when embedded in tissue, *JAMA*, 90, 530, 1928.

22. Jenkins, H.P. and Hrdina, L.S., Absorption of surgical gut (catgut). 11. Pepsin digestion tests for evaluation of duration of tensile strength in the tissues, *Arch. Surg.*, 44, 984, 1942.

23. Mizuma, K., Lee, P.C., and Howard, J.M., The disintegration of surgical sutures in exposure to pancreatic juice, *Ann. Surg.*, 186, 718, 1977.

24. Chu, C.C. and Moncrief, G., An in-vitro evaluation of the stability of mechanical properties of surgical suture materials in various pH conditions, *Ann. Surg.*, 198, 223, 1983.

25. Chu, C.C., A comparison of the effect of pH on the biodegradation of two synthetic absorbable sutures, *Ann. Surg.*, 195, 55, 1982.

26. Stewart, D.W., Buffington, P.J., and Wacksman, J., Suture material in bladder surgery: a comparison of polydioxanone, polyglactin, and chromic catgut, *J. Urol.*, 143, 1261, 1990.

27. Rasmussen, F., Healing of urinary bladder wounds. Morphologic and biochemical studies, *Proc. Soc. Exp. Biol. Med.*, 123, 470, 1966.

28. Rasmussen, F., Biochemical analysis of wound healing in the urinary bladder, *Surg. Gynecol. Obstet.*, 124, 553, 1967.

29. Hasting, J.C. and Van Winkle, W., Jr., Organ differences in post-operative healing, *Surg. Forum.*, 23, 29, 1972.

30. Cohen, E.L., Kirschenbaum, A., and Glenn, J.F., Preclinical evaluation of PDS (polydioxanone) synthetic absorbable suture vs. chromic surgical gut in urologic surgery, *Invest. Urol.*, 30, 369, 1987.

31. Gorham, S.D., Monsour, M.J., and Scott, R., The in vitro assessment of a collagen/Vicryl (Polyglactin) composite film together with candidate suture materials for use in urinary tract surgery, *Urol. Res.*, 15, 53, 1987.

32. Bartone, F.F., Shervey, P.D., and Gardner, P.J., Long term tissue responses to catgut and collagen sutures, *Invest. Urol.*, 13, 390, 1976.

33. Sanz, L.E., Patterson, J.A., Kamath, R., Willett, G., Ahmed, S.W., and Butterfield, A.B., Comparison of Maxon suture with Vicryl, chromic catgut, and PDS sutures in fascial closure in rats, *Obstet. Gynecol.*, 71, 418, 1988.

34. Williams, D.G., The effect of bacteria on absorbable sutures, *J. Biomed. Mater. Res.*, 14, 329, 1980.

35. Sebeseri, O., Keller, U., Spreng, P. et al., The physical properties of polyglycolic acid sutures (Dexon) in sterile and infected urine, *Invest. Urol.*, 12, 490, 1975.

36. Vasselli, A.J. and Bennett, A.H., Suture material in urologic and gynecologic surgery, *Infect. Surg.*, 2, 522, 1983.

37. Peacock, E.E., Jr. and Van Winkle, W., Jr., *Wound Repair*, 2nd ed., W.B. Saunders, Philadelphia, 1976, 218.

38. El-Mahrouky, A., McElhaney, J., Bartone, F.F., and King, L., In vitro comparison of the properties of polydioxanone, polyglycolic acid and catgut sutures in sterile and infected urine, *J. Urol.*, 138, 913, 1987.

39. Walton, M., Strength retention of chromic gut and synthetic absorbable sutures in a nonhealing synovial wound, *Clin. Orthop. Relat. Res.*, 267, 294, 1991.

40. Stone, I.K., von Fraunhofer, J.A., and Masterson, B.J., A comparative study of suture materials: chromic gut and chromic gut treated with glycerin, *Am. J. Obstet. Gynecol.*, 151, 1087, 1985.

41. Zhang, L., Loh, I.H., and Chu, C.C., A combined γ irradiation and plasma deposition treatment to achieve the ideal degradation properties of synthetic absorbable polymers, *J. Biomed. Mater. Res.*, 27, 1425, 1993.

42. Fredericks, R.J., Melveger, A.J., and Dolegiewitz, L.J., Morphological and structural changes in a copolymer of glycolide and lactide occurring as a result of hydrolysis, *J. Polym. Sci. Phys. Ed.*, 22, 57, 1984.

43. Ray, J.A., Doddi, N., Regula, D., Williams, J.A., and Melveger, A., Polydioxanone (PDS), a novel monofilament synthetic absorbable suture, *Surg. Gynecol. Obstet.*, 153, 497, 1981.

44. Gilding, D.K., Biodegradable polymers, in *Biocompatibility of Clinical Implant Materials*, Vol. 2, Williams, D.F., Ed., CRC Press, Boca Raton, FL, 1981, chap. 9.

45. Craig, P.H., Williams, J.A., Davis, K.W. et al., A biologic comparison of polyglactin 910 and polyglycolic acid synthetic absorbable sutures, *Surg. Gynecol. Obstet.*, 141, 1, 1975.

46. Postlethwait, R.W., Polyglycolic acid surgical suture, *Arch. Surg.*, 101, 489, 1970.

47. Reed, A.M. and Gilding, D.K., Biodegradable polymers for use in surgery: poly (glycolic)/poly (lactic acid) homo and copolymers. II. *In vitro* degradation, *Polymer*, 22, 494, 1981.

48. Chu, C.C., Zhang L., and Coyne, L., Effect of irradiation temperature on hydrolytic degradation properties of synthetic absorbable sutures and polymers, *J. Appl. Polym. Sci.*, 56, 1275, 1995.

49. Bezwada, R.S., Jamiolkowski, D.D., Erneta, M., Persivale, J., Trenka-Benthin, S., Lee, I.Y., Suryadevara, J., Yang, A., Agarwal, V., and Liu, S., Monocryl suture, a new ultra-pliable absorbable monofilament suture, *Biomaterials*, 16, 1141, 1995.

49a. Roby, M.S., Bennett, S.L., and Liu, C.K., Absorbable block copolymers and surgical articles fabricated therefrom, U.S. Patent, 5,403,347, April 4, 1995.

50. Bourne, R.B., Bitar, H., Andreae, P.R. et al., *In vivo* comparison of four absorbable sutures: Vicryl, Dexon plus, Maxon and PDS, *Can. J. Surg.*, 31, 43, 1988.

51. Friberg, L.G., Mellgren, G.W., Eriksson, B.D. et al., Subclavian flap angioplasty with absorbable suture polydioxanone (PDS). An experimental study in growing piglets, *Scand. J. Thorac. Cardiovasc. Surg.*, 21, 9, 1987.

52. Knoop, M., Lunstedt, B., and Thiede, A., Maxon and PDS — evaluation and physical and biologic properties of monofilament absorbable suture materials, *Langenbecks Arch. Chir.*, 371, 13, 1987.

53. Metz, S.A., Chegini, N., and Masterson, B.J., In vivo and in vitro degradation of monofilament absorbable sutures, PDS and Maxon, *Biomaterials*, 11, 41, 1990.

54. Foresman, P.A., Edlich, R.F., and Rodeheaver, G.T., The effect of new monofilament absorbable sutures on the healing of musculoaponeurotic incisions, gastrotomies, and colonic anastomoses, *Arch. Surg.*, 124, 708, 1989.

55. Marti, R., Burgues, L., Gabarro, I. et al., Synthetic absorbable PDS explant for the treatment of retinal detachment, *J. French Ophthalmol.*, 9, 373, 1986.

56. Katz, A., Mukherjee, D.P., Kaganov, A.L., and Gordon, S., A new synthetic monofilament absorbable suture made from polytrimethylene carbonate, *Surg. Gynecol. Obstet.*, 161, 213, 1985.

57. Pavan, A., Bosio, M., and Longo, T., A comparative study of poly(glycolic acid) and catgut as suture materials. Histomorphology and mechanical properties, *J. Biomed. Mater. Res.*, 13, 477, 1979.

58. Ginde, R.M. and Gupta, R.K., In vitro chemical degradation of poly(glycolic acid) pellets and fibers, *J. Appl. Polym. Sci.*, 33, 2411, 1987.

59. Bonart, R. and Hoseman, R., Fibrillar strukauren in Kaltverstecktem linearen polyyathylen, *Kolloid Z. Z. Polym.*, 186, 16, 1962.

60. Hess, K., Mahl, H., and Guter, E., Elektronenmikroskopishe Darstellung Grober Langsperioden in Zellulosefasern und ihr Vergleich mit den perioden anderer Faserarten, *Kolloid Z. Z. Polym.*, 155, 1, 1957.

61. Peterlin, A., Morphology and properties of crystalline polymers with fiber structure, *Text. Res. J.*, 42,20, 1972.

62. Prevorsek, D.C., Harget, P.J., Sharma, R.K., and Reimschuessel, A.C., Nylon 6 fibers: changes in structure between moderate and high draw ratios, *J. Macromol. Sci. Phys.*, 8, 127, 1973.

63. Peterlin, A., Radical formation and fracture of highly drawn crystalline polymers, *J. Macromol. Sci.*, B6, 583, 1972.

64. Williams, J.L. and Peterlin, A., Transport properties of methylene chloride in drawn polyethylene as a function of the draw ratio, *J. Polym. Sci. A*, 2(9), 1483, 1971.

65. Peterlin, A., Molecular model of drawing polyethylene and polypropylene, *J. Mater. Sci.*, 6, 490, 1971.

66. Peterlin, A., Mechanical properties of polymeric solids, *Annu. Rev. Mater. Sci.*, 2, 349, 1972.

67. Prevorsek, D.C., Structure of semicrystalline fibers from interpretation of anelastic effects, *J. Polym Sci. C*, 32, 343, 1971.

68. Waters, E., The dyeing of Terylene polyester fiber, *J. Soc. Dyers Colour*, 66, 609, 1950.

69. Chu, C.C., Hydrolytic degradation of polyglycolic acid: tensile strength and crystallinity study, *J. Appl. Polym. Sci.*, 26, 1727, 1981.

70. Chu, C.C. and Browning, A., The study of thermal and gross morphologic properties of polyglycolic acid upon annealing and degradation treatments, *J. Biomed. Mater. Res.*, 22, 699, 1988.

71. Chu, C.C. and Campbell, N.D., Scanning electron microscopic study of the hydrolytic degradation of poly(glycolic acid) suture, *J. Biomed. Mater. Res.*, 16, 417, 1982.

72. Chu, C.C. and Louie, M., A chemical means to examine the degradation phenomena of polyglycolic acid fibers, *J. Appl. Polym. Sci.*, 30, 3133, 1985.

73. Takagi, Y. and Hattori, H., Studies on the drawing of polyamide fibers. III. Change of dye-diffusion behavior into polyamide fibers with drawing, *J. Appl. Polym. Sci.*, 9, 2167, 1965.

74. Subramanian, D.R., Venkatamam, A., and Bhat, N.V., Studies on dyeing and mechanical properties of nylon 6 filaments subjected to swelling treatments, *J. Appl. Polym. Sci.*, 27, 4149, 1982.

75. Moore, R.A.F. and Weigmann, H.D., Dyeability of Nomex aramid yarn, *Text. Res. J.*, 56, 180, 1986.

76. Murthy, N.S., Reimschuessel, A.C., and Kramer, V., Changes in void content and free volume in fibers during heat setting and their influence on dye diffusion and mechanical properties, *J. Appl. Polym. Sci.*, 40, 249, 1990.

77. Rohner, R.M. and Zollinger, H., Porosity versus segmental mobility in dye diffusion kinetics — a differential treatment: dyeing of acrylic fibers, *Text. Res. J.*, 56, 13, 1986.

78. Browning, A. and Chu, C.C., The effect of annealing treatments on the tensile properties and hydrolytic degradative properties of polyglycolic acid sutures, *J. Biomed. Mater. Res.*, 20, 613, 1986.

79. Chu, C.C., Recent advancements in suture fibers for wound closure, in *Hi-Tech Fibrous Materials*, Vigo, T.R. and Turbak, A.F., Eds., American Chemical Society Symp. Ser. 457, American Chemical Book, Washington, D.C., 1991, 167.

80. Yu, T.J. and Chu, C.C., Bicomponent vascular grafts consisting of synthetic biodegradable fibers. I. *In vitro* study, *J. Biomed. Mater. Res.*, 27, 1329, 1993.

81. Chu, C.C. and Lecaroz, L.E., Design and *in vitro* testing of newly-made bicomponent knitted fabrics, in *Advances in Biomedical Polymers*, Gebelein, C.G., Ed., Plenum Press, New York, 1987, 185.

82. Vachon, R.N., Rebenfeld, L., and Taylor, H.S., Oxidative degradation of nylon 66 filament, *Text. Res. J.*, 38, 716, 1968.

83. Williams, D.F., Chu, C.C., and Dwyer, J., The effects of enzymes and gamma irradiation on the tensile strength and morphology of poly(p-dioxanone) fibers, *J. Appl. Polym. Sci.*, 29, 1865, 1984.

84. Pratt, L. and Chu, C.C., Hydrolytic degradation of γ substituted polyglycolic acids: a semi-empirical computational study, *J. Comput. Chem.*, 14, 809, 1993.

85. Pratt, L. and Chu, C.C., The effect of electron donating and electron withdrawing substituents on the degradation rate of bioabsorbable polymers: a semi-empirical computational study, *J. Mol. Struct.*, 304, 213, 1994.

86. Dewar, M.J.S. and Thiel, W.J., Ground states of molecules. 39. MNDO results for molecules containing hydrogen, carbon, nitrogen, and oxygen, *J. Am. Chem. Soc.*, 99, 4907, 1977.

87. Stewart, J.J.P. QCPE 581.

88. Dewar, M.J.S., Zoebisch, E.G., Healy, E.F., and Stewart, J.J.P., Development and use of quantum mechanical molecular models. 76.AM1 — A new general purpose quantum mechanical molecular model, *J. Am. Chem. Soc.*, 107, 3902, 1985.

89. PC Model Serena Software, Box 3076, Bloomington, IN 47402-3076.

90. Chu, C.C. and Kizil, Z., *3rd International ITV Conference on Biomaterials –Medical Textiles*, Stuttgart, W. Germany, 1989, 24.

91. Prevorsek, D.C. and Tobolsky, A.V., Determination of nonflow shrinkage ratio in oriented fibers, *Text. Res. J.*, 33, 795, 1963.

92. Siegmann, A. and Geil, P.H., Heat relaxation of drawn polyoxymethylene, *J. Macromol. Sci.*, B4, 557, 1970.

93. Houssay, B.A., *Human Physiology*, McGraw-Hill, New York, 1951.

94. Cantarow, A. and Schepartz, B., *Biochemistry*, 4th ed., W.B. Saunders, Philadelphia, 1967, 262.

95. Guyton, A.C., *Textbook of Medical Physiology*, W.B. Saunders, Philadelphia, 1976, 496.

96. Kaminski, J.M., Katz, A.R., and Woodward, S.C., Urinary bladder calculus formation on sutures in rabbits, cats and dogs, *Surg. Gynecol. Obstet.*, 146, 353, 1978.

97. Chu, C.C., In-vitro degradation of polyglycolic acid sutures: effect of pH, *J. Biomed. Mater. Res.*, 15, 7954, 1981.

98. Chu, C.C., The effect of pH on the in vitro degradation of poly(glycolide-lactide) co-polymer absorbable sutures, *J. Biomed. Mater. Res.*, 16, 117, 1982.

99. Chu, C.C., An *in vitro* study of the effect of buffer on the degradation of poly(glycolic acid) sutures, *J. Biomed. Mater. Res.*, 15, 19, 1981.

100. Sharples, A., The hydrolysis of cellulose and its relation to structure, *Trans. Faraday Soc.*, 53, 1003, 1957.

101. Franck, J. and Rabinowitch, E., Some remarks about free radicals and the photochemistry of solutions, *Trans. Faraday Soc.*, 30, 120, 1934.

102. D'Alelio, G.F., Haberli, R., and Pezdirtz, G.F., Effect of ionizing radiation on a series of saturated polyester, *J. Macromol. Sci. Chem.*, 2, 501, 1968.

103. Bovey, F.A. and Winslow, F.H., *Macromolecules: An Introduction to Polymer Science,* Academic Press, New York, 1979.

104. Holm-Jensen, S. and Agner, E., Syntetisk absorberbart suturmateriale (PGA) sammenlignet med catgut, *Ugeskrift Laeger*, 136, 1785, 1974.

105. Milroy, E., An experimental study of the calcification and absorption of polyglycolic acid and catgut sutures with the urinary track, *Invest. Urol.*, 14, 141, 1976.

106. Pratt, L., Chu, C., Auer, J., Chu, A., Kim, J., Zollweg, J.A., and Chu, C.C., The effect of ionic electrolytes on hydrolytic degradation of biodegradable polymers: mechanical properties, thermodynamics and molecular modeling, *J. Polym. Sci. Chem. Ed.*, 31, 1759, 1993.

107. Chu, C.C., Strain-accelerated hydrolytic degradation of synthetic absorbable sutures, in *Surgical Research — Recent Developments*, Hall, C.W., Ed., Pergamon Press, New York, 1985, 111.

108. Miller, N.D. and Williams, D.F., The *in vivo* and *in vitro* degradation of poly(glycolic acid) suture material as a function of applied strain, *Biomaterials*, 5, 365, 1984.

109. Bershtein, V.A. and Egorova, L.M., Hydrolysis of oriented polyamide in a field of mechanical stresses, *Vysokomol. Soedin. Ser. A*, 19, 1260, 1977.

110. Kaufman, F.S., Jr., A new technique for evaluating outdoor weathering properties of high density polyethylene, *Appl. Polym. Symp.*, Weatherability of Plastics, issue 4, Kamal, M.R., Ed., New York, 1967, 131.

111. Zhong, S.P., Doherty, P.J., and Williams, D.F., The effect of applied strain on the degradation of absorbable suture *in vitro*, *Clin. Mater.*, 14, 183, 1993.

112. Porter, R.S. and Casale, A., Recent studies of polymer reactions caused by stress, *Polym. Eng. Sci.*, 25, 129, 1985.

113. Silberberg, A. and Henenberg, M., Relaxation of stored mechanical stress along chemical reaction pathways, *Nature*, 312, 746, 1984.

114. Nguyen, T.L. and Rogers, C.E., Effect of uniaxial deformation on the photodegradation of polyolefines, *Polym. Sci. Eng. Conf.*, 53, 292, 1985.

115. George, G.A., Egglestone, G.T., and Riddell, S.Z., Stress-induced chemiluminescence from nylon 66 fibers, *J. Appl. Polym. Sci.*, 27, 3999, 1982.

116. Rapoport, N.Y. and Zaikov, G.E., Kinetics and mechanism of the oxidation of stressed polymer, in *Developments in Polymer Degradation,* Grassie, N., Ed., Elsevier, London, 1985, 207.

117. Carter, B.K. and Wilkes, L., Some morphological investigations on an absorbable copolyester biomaterial based on glycolic and lactic acid, in *Polymers as Biomaterials*, Shalaby, S.W., Hoffman, A.S., Ratner, B.D., and Harbett, J.A., Eds., Plenum Press, New York, 1984, 67.

118. Peterlin, A., Depedence of diffusive transport on morphology of crystalline polymers, *J. Macromol. Sci. Phys.*, 11, 57, 1975.

119. Shalaby, S.W., *Irradiation of Polymeric Materials*, Vol. 527, ACS Symp. Ser., Reichmanis, E., Frank, C.W., and O'Donnell, J.H., Eds., American Chemical Society, Washington, D.C., 1993, 315.

120. Charlesby, A., *Atomic Radiation and Polymers*, Pergamon, Oxford, England, 1960.

121. Sehnabel, W., *Aspects of Degradation and Stabilization of Polymers,* Jellinek, H.H.G., Ed., Elsevier, New York, 1978, chap. 4.

122. Chu, C.C. and Lee, K.H., γ-irradiation sterilization of biomaterial medical devices or products with improved degradation and mechanical properties, U.S. Patent 5,485,496, January 16, 1996.

122a. Lee, K.H. and Chu, C.C., Electron spin resonance study of free radical properties of polyglycolic acid upon γ-irradiation sterilization, 5th World Biomaterials Congress, Toronto, Canada, May 29–June 2, 1996.

123. Campbell, N.D. and Chu, C.C., The effect of γ-irradiation on the biodegradation of polyglycolic acid synthetic sutures — tensile strength study, in *27th International Symposium on Macromolecules*, Vol. II, Strasbourg, France, July 6-9, 1981.

124. Chu, C.C. and Williams, D.F., The effect of γ-irradiation on the enzymatic degradation of polyglycolic acid absorbable sutures, *J. Biomed. Mater. Res.*, 17, 1029, 1983.

125. Reed, A.M. and Gilding, D.K., Biodegradable polymers for use in surgery — poly(glycolic)/poly(lactic acid) homo and copolymers. I. *Polymer*, 20, 1459, 1979.

126. Jellinek, H.H.J., *Aspects of Degradation and Stabilization of Polymers*, Elsevier, New York, 1983, 153.

127. Birkinshaw, C., Buggy, M., and Henn, G.G., Irradiation of poly-D,L-lactide, *Polym. Degradation Stability*, 38, 249, 1992.

128. Cary, N.C., *SAS User's Guide — Statistics*, SAS Institute, Raleigh, N.C., 1982.

129. Fischer, V.H. and Langbein, W., Radiation-induced reactions in poly(oxmethylene), *Kolloid Z. Z. Polym.*, 217, 329, 1967.

130. Golden, J.H., Degradation of poly(tetramethylene oxide). II. Ionising radiation, *Makromol. Chem.*, 81, 51, 1965.

131. Van Brederode, R.A., Rodriguez, F., and Cocks, G.G., Crosslinking poly(ethylene oxide) in dilute solutions by gamma rays, *J. Appl. Polym. Sci.*, 12, 2097, 1968.

132. Schnabel, W., *Polymer Degradation: Principles and Practical Applications*, Hanser International, Wein, 1981, 112.

133. Koenig, T., Fischer, H., and Kochi, M.J.K., *Free Radicals,* Vol. 1, John Wiley & Sons, New York, 1973, chap. 4.

134. Duprez, K., Bilweis, J., Dupre, A., and Merle, M., Experimental and clinical study of fast absorption cutaneous suture material, *Ann. Chir. Main,* 7, 91, 1988.

135. Hubens, G., Totte, E., Van Marck, E., and Hubens, A., Effects of nonabsorbable and rapidly absorbable suture material on the cytokinetics of crypt cells in colonic anastomoses in the rat, *Eur. Surg. Res.*, 24, 97, 1992.

136. Jamiolkowski, D.D. and Shalaby, S.W., A polymeric radiostabilizer for absorbable polyesters, in *Radiation Effect of Polymers*, ACS Symp. Ser. 475, Clough, R.L. and Shalaby, S.W., Eds., American Chemical Society, Washington, D.C., 1991, 300.

137. Shalaby, S.W. and Johnson, R.A., Synthetic absorbable polyesters, in *Biomedical Polymers: Designed-to-Degrade System,* Shalaby, S.W., Ed., Hanser Publisher, New York, 1994, chap. 1.

138. Matlaga, V.F. and Salthouse, T.N., Electron microscopic observations of polyglactin 910 suture sites, in *First World Biomaterials Congress,* Abstr., Baden, Austria, April 8-12, 1980, 2.

139. Devereux, D.F., O'Connell, S.M., Liesch, J.B., Weinstein, M., and Robertson, F.M., Induction of leukocyte activation by meshes surgically implanted in the peritoneal cavity, *Am. J. Surg.*, 162, 243, 1991.

140. Badwey, J.A. and Kamovsky, M.L., Active oxygen species and the functions of phagocytic leucocytes, *Annu. Rev. Biochem.*, 49, 695, 1980.

141. Ali, S.A.M., Zhong, S.P., Doherty, P.J., and Williams, D.F., Mechanisms of polymer degradation in implantable devices. I. Poly(caprolactone), *Biomaterials*, 14, 648, 1993.

142. Zhong, S.P., Doherty, P.J., and Williams, D.F., A preliminary study on the free radical degradation of glycolic acid/lactic acid copolymer, *Plast., Rubber Composites Processing Application*, 21, 89, 1994.

143. William, D.F. and Zhong, S.P., Are free radicals involved in the biodegradation of implanted polymers? *Adv. Mater.*, 3, 623, 1991.

144. Haber, F. and Weiss, J., The catalytic decomposition of hydrogen peroxide by iron salts, *Proc. R. Soc. Lond. Ser. A*, 147, 332, 1934.

144a. Lee, K.H., Won, C.Y., and Chu, C.C., Hydrolysis of absorbable polymeric biomaterials by superoxide, 5th World Biomaterials Congress, Toronto, Canada, May 29–June 2, 1996, p. 91.

144b. Lee, K.H. and Chu, C.C., The role of free radicals in hydrolytic degradation of absorbable polymeric biomaterials, 5th World Biomaterials Congress, Toronto, Canada, May 29–June 2, 1996, p. 811.

145. Kopecek, J. and Ulbrich, K., Biodegradation of biomedical polymers, *Prog. Polym. Sci.*, 9, 1, 1983.

146. Niemi, M. and Sylven, B., On the chemical pathology of interstitial fluid, *Acta Pathol. Microbiol. Scand.*, 72, 205, 1968.

147. Salthouse, T., Cellular enzyme activity at the polymer-tissue interface: a review, *J. Biomed. Mater. Res.*, 10, 197, 1976.

148. Potts, J.E., Biodegradation, in *Aspects of Degradation and Stabilization of Polymers*, Jellinek, H.H.G., Ed., Elsevier, Amsterdam, 1978, 617–657.

149. Smith, R., Oliver, C., and Williams, D.F., The enzymatic degradation of polymers *in vitro, J. Biomed. Mater. Res.*, 21, 991, 1987.

150. Salthouse, T.N. and Matlaga, B.F., Polyglactin 910 suture absorption and the role of cellular enzymes, *Surg. Gynecol. Obstet.*, 142, 544, 1976.

151. Williams, D.F. and Mort, E., Enzyme-accelerated hydrolysis of polyglycolic acid, *J. Bioeng.*, 1, 231, 1977.

152. Williams, D.F., Some observations on the role of cellular enzymes in the *in vivo* degradation of polymers, in *Corrosion of Implant Materials*, Syre, H.B. and Achyara, A., Eds., ASTM Special Technical Publication, American Society for Testing and Materials, Philadelphia, 684, 61, 1979.

153. Holbrook, M.C., The resistance of polyglycolic acid sutures to attack by infected human urine, *Br. J. Urol.*, 54, 313, 1982.

154. Williams, D.F., Biodegradation of surgical polymers, *J. Mater. Sci.*, 17, 1233, 1982.

155. Persson, M., Bilgrav, K., Jensen, L., and Gottrap, F., Enzymatic wound cleaning and absorbable sutures: an experimental study on Varidase and Dexon sutures, *Eur. Surg. Res.*, 18, 122, 1986.

156. Poulsen, J., Kristensen, Y.N., Brygger, H.E., and Delikaris, P., Treatment of infected surgical wounds with Varidase, *Acta Chir. Scand.*, 149, 245, 1983.

157. Zhong, S.P., Doherty, P.J., and Williams, D.F., The degradation of glycolic acid/lactic acid copolymer *in vivo, Clin. Mater.*, 14, 145, 1993.

158. Bucknall, T.E., Abdominal wound closure: choice of sutures, *J.R. Soc. Med.*, 74, 580, 1981.

159. Bucknall, T.E., Factors influencing wound complications: a clinical and experimental study, *Ann. R. Coll. Surg. Engl.*, 65, 71, 1983.

160. Hovendal, C.P. and Schwartz, W., Polyglycolic acid (Dexon) sutures in *Escherichia coli* infected urine, *Scand. J. Urol. Nephrol.*, 13, 105, 1979.

161. Schiller, T.D., Stone, E.A., and Gupta, B.S., *In vitro* loss of tensile strength and elasticity of five absorbable suture materials in sterile and infected canine urine, *Vet. Surg.*, 22, 208, 1993.

162. Sharma, A.K. and Kumar, A., Strength of suture materials after implantation in clean and infected wounds in buffaloes, *Indian Vet. J.*, 69, 435, 1992.

163. Meester, W.D. and Swanson, A.B., In vivo testing of silicone rubber joint implants for lipid absorption, *J. Biomed. Mater. Res.*, 1, 193, 1972.

164. Carmen, R. and Mutha, S.C., Lipid absorption by silicone rubber heart valve poppets: *in vivo* and *in vitro* results, *J. Biomed. Mater. Res.*, 6, 327, 1972.

165. Moacanin, J., Lawson, D.D., Chin, H.P., Harrison, E.P., and Blankenhoon, D.H., Prediction of lipid uptake by prosthetic heart valve poppets from solubility parameter, *Biomat., Med. Devices Artif. Org.*, 1, 183, 1973.

166. Sharma, C.P. and Williams, D.F., Effects of lipids on the mechanical properties of PGA sutures, *Eng. Med.*, 10, 8, 1981.

167. Andriano, K.P., Change, M.K.O., Daniels, A.U., and Heller, J., Preliminary effects of *in vitro* lipid exposure on absorbable poly(ortho ester) films, *J. Appl. Biomater.*, 6, 129, 1995.

168. Barber, F.A. and Gurwitz, G.S., The effect of synovial fluid on suture strength, *Am. J. Knee Surg.*, 1, 189, 1988.

169. Barber, F.A. and Gurwitz, G.S., Inflammatory synovial fluid and absorbable suture strength, *Arthroscopy*, 4, 272, 1988.

170. Arnoczky, S.P. and Warren, R.F., The microvasculature of the meniscus and its response to injury: an experimental study in the dog, *Am. J. Sports Med.*, 11, 131, 1983.

171. Howell, D.S., Carreno, M.R., Pelletier, J.P., and Muniz, O.E., Articular cartilage breakdown in a lapine model of osteoarthritis, *Clin. Orthop. Relat. Res.*, 213, 69, 1986.

172. Mainardi, C.L., Biochemical mechanisms of articular destruction, *Rheum. Dis. Clin. North Am.*, 13, 215, 1987.

173. Loh, I.H., Lin, H.L., and Chu, C.C., Plasma surface modification of synthetic absorbable sutures, *J. Appl. Biomater.*, 3, 131, 1992.

174. Ratner, B.D., in *Comprehensive Polymer Science*, Vol. 7, Aggarwal, S.L., Ed., 1989, 201.

175. Yasuda, H., *Plasma Polymerization*, Academic Press, New York, 1985, 356.

176. Greisler, H., Kim, D.U., Price, J.B., and Voorhees, A.B., Anerial regenerative activity after prosthetic implantation, *Arch. Surg.*, 120, 315, 1985.

177. Greisler, H.P., Arterial regeneration over absorbable prostheses, *Arch. Surg.*, 117, 1425, 1982.

178. Greisler, H.P., Kim, D.U., Dennis, J.W. et al., Compound polyglactin 910/polypropylene small vessel prostheses, *J. Vasc. Surg.*, 5, 572, 1987.

179. Greisler, H.P., Ellinger, J., Schwarcz, T.H. et al., Arterial regeneration over polydioxanone prostheses in the rabbit, *Arch. Surg.*, 122, 715, 1987.

180. Greisler, H.P., Endean, E.D., Klosak, J.J., Ellinger, J., Dennis, J.W., Buttle, K., and Kim., D.U., Polyglactin 910/polydioxanone bicomponent totally resorbable vascular prostheses, *J. Vasc. Surg.*, 7, 697, 1988.

181. Yu, T.J., Ho, D.M., and Chu, C.C., Bicomponent vascular grafts consisting of synthetic biodegradable fibers. II. *In vivo* healing response, *J. Invest. Surg.*, 7, 195, 1994.

182. Greisler, H.P., Tattersall, C.W., Klosak, J.J. et al., Partially bioresorbable vascular grafts in dogs, *Surgery*, 110, 645, 1991.

183. Greisler, H.P., Small diameter vascular prostheses: macrophage-biomaterial interactions with bioresorbable vascular prostheses, *Trans. ASAIO*, 34, 1051, 1988.

184. Greisler, H.P., Dennis, J.W., Endean, E.D. et al., Derivation of neointima of vascular grafts, *Circul. Suppl. I*, 78, I6, 1988.

185. Pratt, L.M. and Chu, C.C., Dimethyltitanocene induced surface chemical degradation of synthetic biodegradable polyesters, *J. Polym. Sci. Chem. Ed.*, 32, 949, 1994.

186. Petasis, N.A. and Bzowej, E.I., Titanium-mediated carbonyl olefinations. I. Methylenations of carbonyl compounds with dimethyltitanocene, *J. Am. Chem. Soc.*, 112, 6392, 1990.

187. Postlethwait, R.W., Long-term comparative study of nonabsorbable sutures, *Ann. Surg.*, 171, 892, 1970.

188. Greenwald, D., Shumway, S., Albear, P., and Gottlieb, L., Mechanical comparison of 10 suture materials before and after *in vivo* incubation, *J. Surg. Res.*, 56, 372, 1994.

189. Van Winkle, W. and Salthouse, T.N., Biological Response to Sutures and Principles of Suture Selection, Ethicon, Somerville, NJ, 1976.

190. Sato, O., Tada, Y., Miyata, T., and Shindo, S., False aneurysms after aortic operations, *J. Cardiovasc. Surg.*, 33, 604, 1992.

191. Postlethwait, R.W., Dillion, M.L., and Reeves, J.W., Experimental study of silk suture, *Arch. Surg.*, 84, 698, 1962.

192. Harrison, J.H., Synthetic materials as vascular prostheses. II. A comparative study of nylon, Dacron, Orlon, Ivalon sponge and Teflon in large blood vessels with tensile strength studies, *Am. J. Surg.*, 95, 16, 1958.

193. Kronenthal, R.L., Intraocular degradation of nonabsorbable sutures, *Am. Intra-Ocular Implant Soc. J.*, 3, 222, 1977.

194. Schwertassek, K. and Dvorak, J., Contribution to degradation studies of synthetic fibers in living organisms, *Faserforsch. Textiltech.*, 21, 78, 1970.

195. Mehta, H.K., Biodegradation of nylon loops of intraocular implants in children, *Trans. Ophthalmol. Soc. (U.K.)*, 99, 183, 1979.

196. Williams, D.F., Effects of cellular enzymes on polymers, *Plast. Rubber Mater. Appl.*, 5, 179, 1980.

197. Blanksma, L.J. and Siertsema, J.V., Changes in the structure of intraocular nylon, *Doc. Ophthalmol.*, 44, 223, 1977.

198. Jongebloed, W.L., Figueras, M.J., Humalda, D. et al. Mechanical and biochemical effects of man-made fibers and metals in the human eye, a SEM study, *Doc. Ophthalmol.*, 61, 303, 1986.

199. Cohan, B.E., Pearch, A.C., and Schwartz, S., Broken nylon iris fixation sutures, *Am. J. Ophthalmol.*, 88, 982, 1979.

200. Drew, R.C., Smith, M.E., and Okun, N., Scanning electron microscopy of intraocular lenses, *Ophthalmology*, 85, 415, 1978.

201. Kronenthal, R.L., Nylon in the anterior chamber, *Ophthalmology*, 88, 965, 1981.

202. Anderson, J.M., Kline, S.A., and Hiltner, P.A., *In vitro* studies on the degradation of nylon 6, *Biomaterials '84 Transactions*, Vol. 7, 2nd World Biomaterials Congress, Washington, D.C., April 27-May 1, 1984, 211.

203. Troutman, R.C., Microsurgery of the anterior segment of the eye, in *Introduction and Basic Techniques*, Vol. 1, C.V. Mosby, St. Louis, 1974, 123.

204. Taylor, D., Intraocular lenses: 100 consecutive cases of intracapsular cataract extraction with Copeland iris plane lens implantation, *Ophthalmic Surg.*, 6, 28, 1975.

205. Boruchoff, S.A. and Donshik, P.C., Degradation of nonabsorbable sutures, *Ophthalmic Surg.*, 8, 42, 1977.

206. Cook, S.D., Kester, M.A., Brunet, M.E. et al., A histologic and mechanical evaluation of carbon-coated polyester suture, *J. Biomed. Mater. Res.*, 20, 1347, 1986.

207. McClellan, K.A. and Billson, F.A., Long-term comparison of Novafil and Nylon in corneoscleral sections, *Ophthalmic Surg.*, 22, 74, 1991.

208. Uemichi, Y., Makino, Y., and Kanazuka, T., Degradation of polypropylene to aromatic hydrocarbons over Pt- and Fe-containing activated carbon catalysts, *J. Anal. Appl. Pyrol.*, 16, 229, 1989.

209. Audisio, G., Silvani, A., Beltrame, P.L., and Carniti, P., Catalytic thermal degradation of polymers. Degradation of polypropylene, *J. Anal. Appl. Pyrol.*, 7, 83, 1984.

210. Uemichi, Y., Ayame, A., Noguchi, N., and Kanoh, H., Degradation of polypropylene over activated carbon catalyst, *Nippon Kagaku Kaishi*, 1429, 1985.

211. Liebert, T.C., Chartoff, R.P., Cosgrove, S.L. et al., Subcutaneous implants of polypropylene filaments, *J. Biomed. Mater. Res.*, 10, 939, 1976.

212. Cacciari, I., Quatrini, P., Zirletta, G. et al., Isotactic polypropylene biodegradation by a microbial community: physicochemical characterization of metabolites produced, *Appl. Environ. Microb.*, 59, 3695, 1993.

213. Pometto, A.L., Lee, B., and Johnson, K.E., Production of an extracellular polyethylene-degrading enzyme(s) by *Streptomyces* species, *Appl. Environ. Microbiol.*, 58, 731, 1992.

214. Wasserbauer, R., Beranova, M., and Vancurova, D., Biodegradation of polyethylene foils by bacterial and liver homogenates, *Biomaterials*, 11, 36, 1990.

215. Altman, A.J., Gorn, R.A., Craft, J., and Albert, D.M., The breakdown of polypropylene in the human eye: is it clinically significant?, *Ann. Ophthalmol.*, 18, 182, 1986.

216. Drews, R.C., Polypropylene in the human eye, *Am. Intra-Ocular Implant Soc. J.*, 9, 137, 1983.

217. Lerman, S., Effect of ultraviolet radiation (300-400nm) on polypropylene, *Am. Intra-Ocular Implant Soc. J.*, 9, 25, 1983.

218. Fechner, P.U., Hartmann, E., and Wehmeyer, K., Ultraviolet light and suture material, *Am. Intra-Ocular Implant Soc. J.*, 6(4), 349–351, 1980.

219. Apple, D.J., Mamalis, N., and Brady, S.E., Biocompatibility of implant materials: a review and scanning electron microscopic study, *Am. Intra-Ocular Implant Soc. J.*, 10, 53, 1984.

220. Jongebloed, W.L. and Worst, J.F.G., Degradation of polypropylene in the human eye: a SEM study, *Doc. Ophthalomol.*, 64, 143, 1986.

221. Garton, A., Carlsson, J.D., and Sturgeon, P.Z., The photo-oxidation of polypropylene monofilaments. III. Effects of filament morphology, *Text. Res. J.*, 47, 1977.

222. Oz, M.C., Johnson, J.P., Parangi, S., Chuck, R.S., Marboe, C.C., Bass, L.S., Nowygrod, R., and Treat, M.R., Tissue soldering by use of indocyanine green dye-enhanced fibrinogen with the near infrared diode laser, *J. Vasc. Surg.*, 11, 718, 1990.

223. Moazami, N., Oz, M.C., Bass, L.S., and Treat, M.R., Reinforcement of colonic anastomoses with a laser and dye-enhanced fibrinogen, *Arch. Surg.*, 125, 1452, 1990.

224. Poppas, D.P., Schlossberg, S.M., Richmond, I.L., Gilbert, D.A., and Devine, C.J., Laser welding in urethral surgery: improved results with a protein solder, *J. Urol.*, 139, 415, 1988.

225. Wider, T.M., Libutti, S.K., Greenwald, D.P., Oz, M.C., Font, D., Treat, M.R., and Hugo, N.E., Skin closure with dye-enhanced laser welding and fibrinogen, *Plast. Reconstr. Surg.*, 88(6), 1018, 1991.

226. Oz, M.C., Bass, L.S., Williams, M.R., Libutti, S.K., Benvenisty, A.I., Hardy, M., Treat, M.R., and Nowygrod, R., Initial clinical experience with laser assisted solder bonding of human vascular tissue, *Lasers Surg. Med.*, 3, 73, 1991.

227. Grubbs, P.E., Wang, S., Marini, C., Basu, S., Rose, D.M., Cunningham, J.N., Enhancement of CO_2 laser microvascular anastomoses by fibrin glue, *J. Surg. Res.*, 45, 112, 1988.

228. Muto, Y., Dupree, J.J., Duemler, S., Yang, Y., Koyanagi, N., Cuffari, W.J., and Matsumoto, T., Effects of argon laser on vascular materials, *J. Vasc. Surg.*, 7, 562, 1988.

229. Ashton, R.C., Libutti, S.K., Oz, M.C., Lontz, J.F., Lemole, G.M., and Lemole, G.M., The effects of laser-assisted fibrinogen bonding on suture materials, *J. Surg. Res.*, 53, 39, 1992.

Chapter 8

Biological Properties of Suture Materials

M. K. Hirko, P. H. Lin, H. P. Greisler, and C. C. Chu,

CONTENTS

I. GENERAL TISSUE REACTIONS AND CELLULAR RESPONSE

The presence of foreign materials like wound closure biomaterials or devices and surgical trauma from operation can induce inflammatory tissue reactions. Although the inflammation due to surgical trauma subsides within 7 to 14 d postoperation, inflammatory tissue reactions due to the presence of wound closure biomaterials persist as long as they remain present within the tissue. Excessive inflammatory reaction is undesirable because it lowers body defense mechanisms against infection, delays the subsequent proliferative phase of wound healing, and leads to inferior wound strength due to excessive scar tissue formation.

When implanted in living tissues, suture materials inevitably elicit a wide range of tissue reactions and cellular responses. The degree of tissue reaction depends largely on the chemical nature and physical configuration of the various suture materials. Suture materials of a protein or cellulose nature produce more marked tissue reactions than those of a synthetic nature, while a greater response is caused by multifilament sutures than by monofilament sutures.

There are two basic approaches to evaluating these tissue reactions: histology and enzyme histochemistry. The former evaluates cellular responses which can be assessed according to the reaction degree and area by microscopic observation of the type and population size of the responding cells, as well as edema and necrosis. The latter is particularly useful in the evaluation of the *in vivo* absorption mechanisms of absorbable suture materials. All histologic evaluation has some subjective component and, therefore, some type of numerical scoring system should be used in order to achieve a more independent and objective evaluation. Salthouse[1] suggested using the method of Sewell et al.,[2,3] for assessing the tissue

Table 8.1 Sewell Score System for Semiquantitative Histological Evaluation of Suture Materials

Histologic Grading of Tissue Reaction	
Characteristic	Weighting Factor
Width of zone	5
Overall cell density	3
Neutrophils	6
Giant cells	2
Lymphocytes-plasma cells	1
Macrophages	1
Eosinophils	1
Fibroblasts-fibrocytes	2
Edema	2
Necrosis	3

A Sample Score			
Parameter	Grade	Weighting Factor	Score
Zone	2	5	10
Cell density	2	3	6
Macrophages	2	1	2
Giant cells	1	2	2
Fibroblasts	2	1	2
Total score			22

From Sewell, W.R., Wiland, J., and Craver, B.N., *Surg. Gynecol. Obstet.*, 100, 483, 1955. With permission.

response to implanted sutures, and this approach was well accepted. In the Sewell method, reported in 1955, scores for the width of the reaction zone, cellular density, cell type, subsequent edema, and necrosis are combined, as illustrated in Table 8.1.[2,3] The degree of reaction depends on the total score: 0, no reaction; 1 to 8, minimal; 9 to 24, slight; 25 to 40, moderate; 41 and above, marked reaction. The general picture of cellular response to both absorbable and nonabsorbable suture materials involves various types of cells. For the first few d, neutrophils predominate and are eventually replaced by a macrophage population with a varying content of eosinophils, lymphocytes, and plasma cells. Blood vessels gradually infiltrate the wound area and fibroblasts proliferate. After a few weeks, the reaction subsides and a band of fibrous connective tissues forms, encapsulating the suture material. The width of the band and the number of surrounding macrophages and giant cells are related to the severity of the tissue reaction. It is generally true that the more inert the suture material, the narrower the fibrous connective tissue band and the less cellular reaction appears. However, individual variation among animals and patients does exist. If the suture material is of a multifilament nature, the filaments are widely separated and surrounded by invading cells. In the case of absorbable sutures, only residual monocytic cells and occasional fat cells are found at the suture site subsequent to complete absorption.

Almost all of the reported tissue reactions to suture materials are described either qualitatively and/or semiquantitatively by a score system originally developed by Sewell and coworkers in 1955, as noted previously.[3] Recently, Smit et al.[4] raised the issue of applying this scoring system to modern suture materials. Their major criticism was that the weighing factors of several inflammatory parameters are subjective and should be revised based on more than 30 years of published suture research information. They concluded that the development of an adapted, reliable, and reproducible scoring system is needed to assess tissue reactions to modern suture materials. In their recent study of tissue reaction to 10 suture materials (silk, Tevdek®, Ti-Cron®, Ethibond®, Prolene®, plain catgut, chromic catgut, Dexon®, Vicryl®, and Maxon®) in male Wistar rats (in the abdominal facial layer) using conventional histologic criteria, Smit found that the data obtained failed to demonstrate any systematic differences in tissue reaction to these 10 suture materials at 7 d postimplantation. They speculated that the major reason for their unexpected observations was the large tissue reaction caused by surgical trauma during the first 7 d postsurgery, thus masking any differences in tissue reaction caused by different suture materials. Their data suggest that a longer period (>7 to 14 d) should be used to assess any difference in tissue reaction of different suture materials. However, they argued that longer periods of assessment were not clinically relevant because the basis of physiological wound healing is established within the first 7 to 14 d

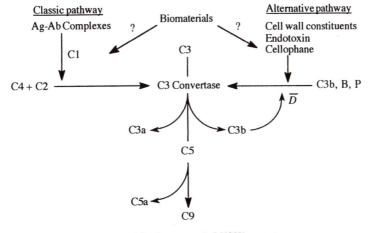

Figure 8.1 Complement activation pathway. (From Shepard, A.D. et al., *J. Vasc. Surg.*, 6, 829, 1984. With permission.)

postoperation, the same period in which surgical complications, including wound infection and adhesions, develop. Overall, they came to the conclusion that the best means of achieving normal wound healing without complication is to minimize surgical trauma through careful tissue handling and surgical manipulation, rather than the selection of biocompatible suture materials for wound closure.

In addition to the above general tissue reactions, it is interesting to note that suture materials and their base polymers have been reported to induce complement[5] and leukocyte activation.[6] Complement activation is known to be partially responsible for the host defense and acute inflammatory response to foreign materials via a production of plasma proteins serving as defense and inflammatory mediators. This complement activation leads to the adherence and activation of polymorphonuclear leukocytes (PMNs) which may trigger platelet aggregation by the release of platelet aggregating factor[7] or a direct neutrophil-platelet interaction,[8] and contributes to vascular graft thrombosis by promoting coagulation.[9] Shepard et al.[10] suggested that there are two pathways of complement activation, as illustrated in Figure 8.1: (1) classical, stimulated by antibody-antigen complexes; and (2) alternative, initiated by highly repetitive biochemical structures like complex lipopolysaccharides found in microorganism cell walls. Highly repetitive synthetic structures like certain polymeric surfaces could also activate both classical and alternative complement pathways leading to the deposition of leukocyte and platelets, with the release of cytokines like interleukin-1 (IL-1).[11–13] Coleman et al.[5] found that monofilament Prolene and Gore-Tex® sutures induced significant (*P* <.01) activation of C5a compared to controls, while Novafil® monofilament suture did not, as shown in Figure 8.2. The combination of the suture materials (Prolene, Gore-Tex, and Novafil) with Gore-Tex graft materials, however, did not result in a significant increase in the C5a levels above Gore-Tex graft controls alone. On the contrary, the combination of Prolene or Novafil sutures with Dacron graft materials resulted in a significant (*P* <.01) increase in C5a levels above Dacron graft controls, while the addition of Gore-Tex suture to Dacron grafts did not. It is unclear why Novafil suture alone did not induce complement activation (in terms of C5a production level), while a combination of Novafil® suture and Dacron® graft material led to a significant complement activation. Since C5a induces the adhesion of PMNs with subsequent generation of thromboplastin and oxygen radicals,[15,16] increased C5a production by the presence of some types of sutures and their combination with graft materials may lead to neointimal hyperplasia at the anastomotic site, and undesirable thrombotic vascular graft occlusions. Hayashi et al.[14] added to this theory with their report that platelet and leukocyte adhesion is related to *in vivo* thrombus formation resulting from polymer-induced complement activation.

In terms of leukocyte activation, Devereux et al.[6] recently reported PGA mesh and a composite mesh consisting of a PGA constituent, implanted into rats, induce functional activation of leukocytes. The level of hydrogen peroxide present was used to indicate the extent of functional leukocyte activation at 1, 2, 8, and 14 d postimplantation of PGA and other biomaterials onto the posterior rectus sheath of rats. Figure 8.3 summarizes the relative amounts of hydrogen peroxide production by leukocytes adherent

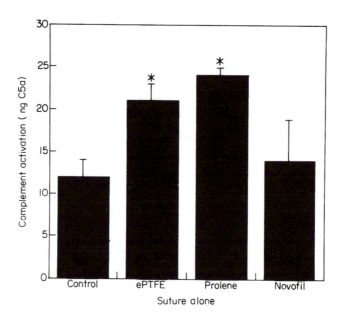

Figure 8.2 *In vitro* C5a generation by suture materials. * $p < .01$. (From Coleman, J.E. et al., *Eur. J. Vasc. Surg.*, 5, 287, 1991. With permission.)

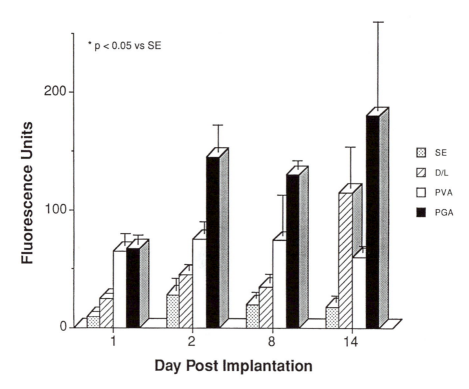

Figure 8.3 Hydrogen peroxide production by cells adherent to the four mesh materials from 1 to 14 d postoperation. (From Devereux, D.F. et al., *Am. J. Surg.*, 162(9), 243, 1991. With permission.)

onto PGA and other biomaterials. PGA mesh showed a continuous increase in functional activation of leukocytes in relation to the duration of implantation. At the end of 14 d, the level of leukocyte activation by PGA mesh was close to 200× that of the nonabsorbable silicone elastomer. The authors believed that this high level of induction of leukocyte activation may be responsible for the clinical observation

(80 patients) of the lack of infections or abscesses following "intestinal sling" surgical procedures. These surgical procedures incorporate either an absorbable material like polyglycolide (PGA) or Vicryl mesh, or nonabsorbable materials like silicone or metal to elevate the small bowel out of the true pelvis for safer postoperative radiation therapy without the complications associated with radiation-induced small bowel injury: (1) bowel cramps, (2) diarrhea, (3) malabsorption, (4) gastrointestinal (GI) tract hemorrhage, (5) stricture, and (6) perforation.[17] The total dosage of irradiation experienced by the pelvic organs, particularly small bowel, would affect the severity of the complications. Besides absorbable Dexon® and Vicryl mesh[18–21] used to lift small bowel loops from the pelvis, the use of other nonabsorbable materials like silicone, metal, omentum, and peritoneum[22–24] have been reported. However, the success rate associated with these nonabsorbable materials was quite low (i.e., <30%).[25]

A. ABSORBABLE SUTURES

Absorbable sutures are generally defined as suture materials that lose most of their tensile strength within 60 d after implantation beneath the skin surface. However, this loss of strength does not indicate complete absorption, as catgut may persist for years in various tissues.[26] Some of the more commonly used absorbable sutures are derived from synthetic substances — Dexon (polyglycolide), Vicryl (polyglactin 910), PDS®, or PDSII (polydioxanone), Maxon® (polytrimethylene carbonate), Monocryl (poliglecaprone 25), and Biosyn® (glycomer 63D). Absorbable sutures are mainly used as buried sutures, reducing the tension on superficial wound edges. The ideal absorbable suture has low reactivity, high tensile strength, slow absorption rates, and reliable knot security.

1. Catgut and Reconstituted Collagen Sutures

Catgut sutures, derived from sheep or cattle intima, have been in use for centuries. Catgut sutures retain significant tensile strength during the first 4 to 5 d of implantation. After 2 weeks, the tensile strength is essentially gone.[26] However, catgut that is soaked in chromic acid salts will usually have a delayed absorption time and a reduction in tissue reactivity compared with untreated catgut. Chromic gut retains its strength for 2 to 3 weeks and can be used in the dermal layer of a skin closure. Fast absorbing gut (Ethicon) is a newer form of catgut not treated with chromic salts. This can also be used as a percutaneous suture in split-thickness skin grafts or in suturing wounds on children, where it is difficult to remove sutures.

Because of their foreign protein nature, catgut sutures have a less predictable absorption rate and elicit a far more intense tissue reaction than synthetic absorbable and most nonabsorbable sutures. Microscopically, catgut sutures appear the same as any monofilament suture with a thin connective tissue capsule, lymphocytes, and a few histiocytes. The cellular reaction, however, changes when absorption begins. Areas of catgut suture degradation contain dense accumulations of macrophages, lymphocytes, and foreign body giant cells. The suture itself is packed with masses of chronic inflammatory cells, most notably, large foreign body giant cells. After complete absorption these cells are replaced by a dense mass of macrophages, as shown in Figure 8.4.[27] This marked inflammatory reaction may be the cause of collagen breakdown (and hence, lower wound strength) and may bring about a predisposition to infection.

Plain catgut produces the most extensive reaction and is associated with an early, prolonged, and marked exudate with some tissue necrosis. Lawrie et al.[28] found that the most striking histologic feature of plain catgut was the brisk, sterile, pyogenic reaction, which at 3 d after implantation produced an abscess six times the original suture diameter, as shown in Figure 8.5. This reaction led to a rapid loss of tissue strength due to the proteolytic enzymes in the purulent exudate. The pyogenic reaction to chromic catgut sutures was much less. This unique feature, however, has not been reported by other investigators.[27,29,30]

Variations in tissue reaction are also species dependent. Postlethwait et al.[30] studied the tissue reaction to several sutures, including catgut in humans. It was found that the reaction to catgut was dependent on the stage of absorption; the absorbing cells were almost exclusively monocytic, with a few lymphocytes and few or no polymorphonuclear neutrophils. After the absorption was complete, the site was marked by a collection of monocytes with characteristic brown, foamy cytoplasm. The authors demonstrated that a wide range of apparent biologic variation existed. For example, two catgut sutures removed at 8 and 11 years showed no evidence of absorption or reaction and were surrounded by a connective tissue capsule, whereas most animal studies indicated that catgut sutures had been completely absorbed between 35 and 60 d.[27,28] Katz and Turner[27] found that intense local cellular infiltrations persisted for periods beyond the absorption of the suture. This severe infiltration of macrophages and neutrophils was recently also reported by Okada et al.[31] in the subdermal tissue of rabbits at 4 weeks postimplantation.

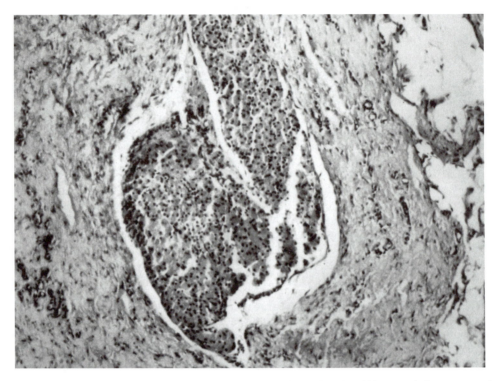

Figure 8.4 Histological section of 1/0 size chromic catgut suture in female rabbit at 75 d shows a complete resorption of the suture material. Implant was replaced by a large mass of macrophages located within a fibroconnective tissue collagen plaque. (From Katz, A.R. and Turner, R.J., *Surg. Gynecol. Obstet.*, 131, 701, 1970. Now known as *J. Am. Coll. Surg.* With permission.)

By using a modified Sewell tissue reaction grading system, Postlethwait[32] reported that the value of chromic catgut ranged from as low as 16.6 to as high as 48.4 (after 8 and 2 months in the muscles of rabbits), respectively, as indicated in Table 8.2.

Bergman et al.[33] examined the tissue and cellular responses to chromic catgut in three settings: intestinal anastomoses, urinary bladder closure, and abdominal wall closure. The histologic changes were essentially the same among the three tissues. The early inflammatory tissue reaction (i.e., after 7 to 10 d) was principally the same between catgut and PGA sutures. Fibrous-limited granulomas frequently formed around the catgut sutures. The granulomas contained PMNs, lymphocytes, and histiocytes with occasional single, multinuclear foreign body giant cells. Fragmented catgut sutures still persisted at the end of 4 months.

Salthouse et al.[34,35] examined the ophthalmic tissue response to catgut sutures by morphologic and enzyme histochemical observation. Table 8.3 summarizes these histologic responses to catgut as well as polyglactin 910 in the cornea, sclera, and ocular muscles of rabbits.[35] The pattern of cellular response varied somewhat in the three sites. Both suture types in the cornea were more rapidly absorbed vs. the scleral or ocular muscle sites. A much greater variation in suture reaction and absorption was found in the sclera than in either the cornea or ocular muscles. It was suggested that the distance of vascular elements to scleral suture sites was a factor involved in this variability. At corneal suture sites, the cellular population for both sutures consisted mostly of monocytic-type cells which did not appear to be macrophages of bone marrow origin. Neither lymphocytes nor fibroblasts were identified in the corneal suture site. Both lymphocytes and fibroblasts, however, appeared in sclera and ocular muscle catgut suture sites after 21 d. No lymphocytes were seen in any of the three collagen suture sites.

Bartone et al.[37] suggested that studies by Lawrie et al.[28] of the absorption rate of collagen-based sutures might be inaccurate, and they examined the tissue response of plain and chromic catgut and reconstituted collagen sutures in a variety of wounded and unwounded organs (kidney, bladder, liver, and muscle). The most important finding of this study was the increased duration for the absorption of collagen-based sutures. For example, 86.7% of the suture cross-sectional area still remained at the end of the study, 130 d. All sutures were encapsulated with a bilaminar fibrotic connective tissue capsule.

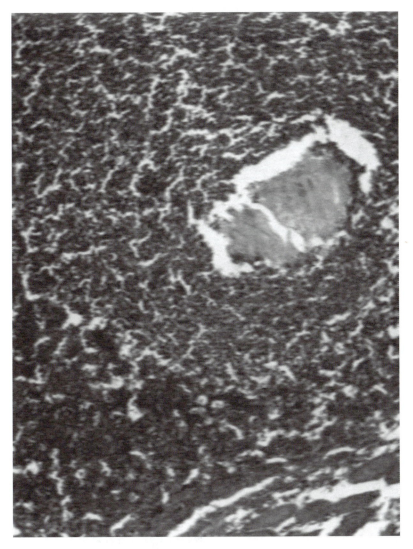

Figure 8.5 Histological picture of plain catgut 3 d after implantation in Wistar albino rats. The suture is reduced by half. The large abscess is divided into an inner zone of polymorphs and an outer zone of cell debris and blue "stringy" material. (From Lawrie, P. et al., *Br. J. Surg.*, 46, 638, 1959. With permission.)

The inner zone of the capsule contained numerous fibroblasts, histiocytes, neutrophils, lymphocytes, and eosinophils scattered throughout both the inner cellular and outer fibrous zones which was the thickest portion of the capsule. As shown in Figure 8.6, lymphoid nodules were occasionally found in the pericapsular zones of liver and bladder tissues and appeared to be independent of the suture type and duration of implantation. Multinucleated giant cells were most common in bladder and muscle tissues, and most numerous around catgut sutures, as shown in Figure 8.7. The outer fibrous zone consisted of concentric layers of fibroblasts and collagenous elements. The space originally occupied by the suture, after its absorption, was replaced by mononuclear cells, as shown in Figure 8.8. Urinary calculi were found to attach to the suture loop exposed to the bladder lumen of the unwounded series, as shown in Figure 8.9, while the tightly closed collagen-based sutures in the wounded tissues did not have bladder calculi because the tightly drawn (into bladder wall) sutures were subsequently covered by epithelium that protected the sutures from contact with urine.

Catgut sutures have been reported to be associated with clinically identifiable calcification in women who underwent lumpectomy and radiation therapy for breast cancer.[38–42] This type of suture calcification is considered to be benign and has a distinctive morphological appearance as a suture or suture loop. This unique mammographic morphological appearance should not be mistakenly identified as malignant

Table 8.2 Sewell Grading of Tissue Reactions of a Variety of Sutures in New Zealand White Rabbits

Grade of Tissue Reaction

Interval	No. of Animals	PGA 0[a]			PGA 3-0			Chromic 0		
		No. of Sutures	Range	Ave.	No. of Sutures	Range	Ave.	No. of Sutures	Range	Ave.
3 d	12	54	22.53	35.6	47	23.59	35.7	36	23.54	36.9
7 d	16	77	28.60	43.2	71	26.59	42.0	48	28.53	37.9
14 d	10	46	15.50	31.9	31	19.45	29.1	36	19.69	43.0
28 d	13	59	20.40	29.4	55	14.44	26.5	54	20.67	41.8
42 d	13	33	10.30	24.2	48	15.31	24.7	36	26.65	42.2
2 months	11	34	6.34	25.1	26	6.34	21.3	39	23.82	48.4
4 months	10	11	9.15	10.2	4	9.11	10.5	35	9.48	26.4
6 months	16	6	9.9	9.0	2	9.11	10.0	38	9.53	21.1
8 months	7	0	—	—	2	9.11	10.0	24	9.37	16.6

Interval	No. of Animals	Chromic 3-0			Silk			Dacron		
		No. of Sutures	Range	Ave.	No. of Sutures	Range	Ave.	No. of Sutures	Range	Ave.
3 d	12	38	14.50	34.1	38	29.54	41.1	28	12.53	36.5
7 d	16	63	23.53	38.9	60	28.63	43.4	60	23.58	40.9
14 d	10	46	24.58	42.2	40	20.47	31.9	37	19.47	31.8
28 d	13	47	26.63	42.0	52	20.44	26.2	38	11.43	25.9
42 d	13	56	21.75	44.6	52	15.39	28.2	62	15.45	25.2
2 months	11	39	28.71	46.6	51	15.40	24.0	39	15.34	22.4
4 months	10	21	9.46	21.3	52	15.27	18.5	52	11.25	17.5
6 months	16	31	9.33	12.1	69	5.23	13.1	65	5.25	15.2
8 months	7	15	9.48	18.8	32	15.32	19.2	32	5.28	16.7

[a] PGA, polyglycolide.

From Postlethwait, R.W., *Arch. Surg.*, 101, 489, 1970. With permission.

Table 8.3 Histologic Response of Absorbable Sutures in Ophthalmologic Tissues

Suture and Site	Histologic Response: Absorbable Sutures[a]						
	7 d	14 d	21 d	28 d	35 d	42 d	60 d
Chromic surgical gut, size 7-0; cornea	Slight P++ M++	Moderate P+ M++	Moderate absorbing M+++	Slight M++	Nearly absorbed M+	Absorbed M+	Only slight evidence of site
Chromic surgical gut; sclera	Slight P++ M+	Moderate M++	Moderate absorbing M+++	Slight M++ F+	Slight M+ F+, L+	Absorbed	A few residual cells
Chromic surgical gut; ocular muscle	Slight P+ M++	Moderate M++	Moderate M++ F+	Moderate M++ L+, F+	Slight M+ M+, F+	Nearly absorbed	Absorbed
Chromic collagen, size 7-0; cornea	Minimal P+ M+	Slight M+	Slight M+	Slight M+	Absorbed M+		
Chromic collagen; sclera	Minimal P+ M+	Slight M++	Slight M++ F	Slight M++ F+	Absorbed		
Chromic collagen; ocular muscle	Slight P+ M++	Moderate M++	Slight M++ F+	Slight M++ F+	Nearly absorbed M++ F+	Absorbed	
Polyglactin 910, size 7-0; cornea	Minimal P+ M++	Minimal M+	Minimal M++	Slight M++	Absorbed; a few residual cells		
Polyglactin 910, sclera	Minimal P+ M++	Slight M+	Slight M++ G+	Slight M++ F+, G+	Slight M++ F+	Slight M+ F+	Absorbed
Polyglactin 910; ocular muscle	Slight P+ M+	Moderate M++	Slight M++ G+, F+	Slight M++ F+, G+	Slight M++ F+, G+	Absorbed	

[a] M, monocytic type cells; P, polymorphonuclear cells (heterophils in rabbit); L, lymphocytes; F, fibroblasts; G, giant cells; and C, collagen fibers forming around suture sites. Cell population is composed of occasional cells (+); moderate population (++); and numerous cells (+++). Arbitrary designations compare tissue response at the suture sites; minimal, slight, moderate, and marked.

From Salthouse, T.N., Matlaga, B.F., and Wykoff, M.H., *Am. J. Ophthalmol.*, 84(2), 224, 1977. With permission.

calcifications. Stacey-Clear et al.[38] reported that 50% (21/42) of female patients who developed clinically evident calcifications were associated with calcified catgut sutures. This represented about 6% of the 335 women who had previously undergone irradiation therapy to the breast. The earliest case of calcified catgut suture in irradiated breast tissue was 2 years postoperation, but calcified catgut sutures had existed in one patient for as long as 13 years postimplantation. Calcium precipitation on sutures rarely happens in the nonirradiated breast. The actual relationship between calcified catgut sutures and radiation therapy of the breast is not clear. Stacey-Clear suggested that delayed healing in breast tissue secondary to irradiation therapy was responsible for this observation. They found that delayed healing might lead to delayed biodegradation and absorption of catgut suture. This delayed suture absorption, coupled with the conducive nature of the breast chemical microenvironment toward calcium precipitation, promoted the calcification of catgut sutures subsequent to irradiation therapy. This report of suture line irradiation-induced soft tissue calcification has not been reported in other similarly treated tissues.

Stone et al.[43] reported that glycerin treatment of chromic catgut suture (Softgut®) elicited the same degree of inflammatory reaction as untreated chromic catgut during the first 7 d postimplantation. Figure 8.10 shows the histologic pictures of both glycerin-treated and untreated chromic catgut sutures at 7 d postimplantation. The inflammatory response was graded as moderate to severe. Studies (one was

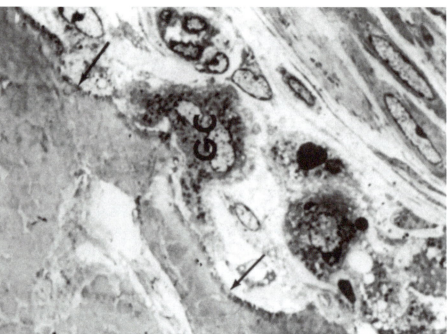

Figure 8.7 Histological picture of plain catgut suture in the bladder at 20 d postimplantation. There is erosion of the suture surface (arrow). Multinucleated giant cells (GC) may be observed. ×1030 with toluidine blue stain. (From Bartone, F.F. et al., *Invest. Urol.*, 13(6), 390, 1976. With permission.)

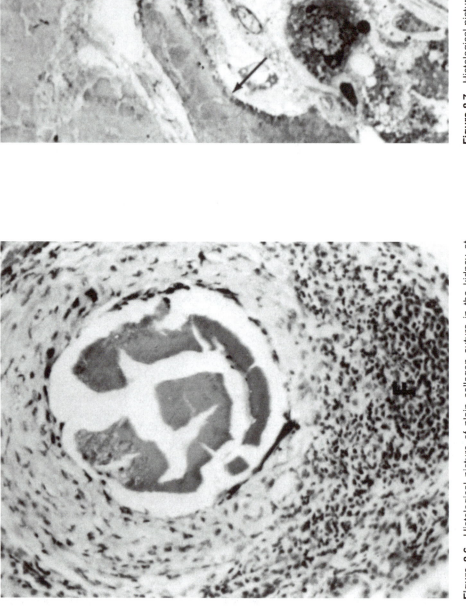

Figure 8.6 Histological picture of plain collagen suture in the kidney at 100 d postimplantation. A lymphoid follicle (F) is observed in the outer portion of the capsule near the bottom of this photo. ×125 with hematoxylin and eosin stain. (From Bartone, F.F. et al., *Invest. Urol.*, 13(6), 390, 1976. With permission.)

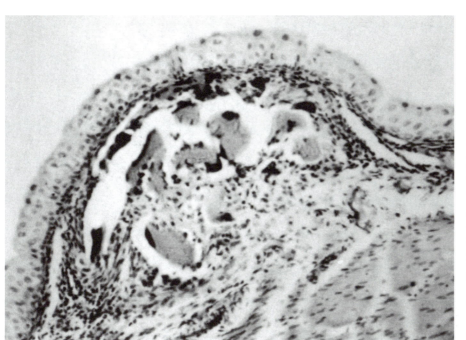

Figure 8.9 Histological picture of plain catgut suture in the bladder at 70 d postimplantation. Epithelium has overgrown the suture. ×125 with H&E stain. (From Bartone, F.F. et al., *Invest. Urol.*, 13(6), 390, 1976. With permission.)

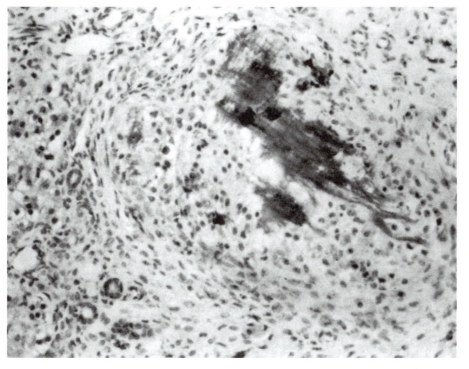

Figure 8.8 Histological picture of chromic catgut suture in the liver at 130 d postimplantation. There is a marked absorption of the suture fragment and proliferation of mononuclear cells of the inner portion of the capsule. ×125 with H&E stain. (From Bartone, F.F. et al., *Invest. Urol.*, 13(6), 390, 1976. With permission.)

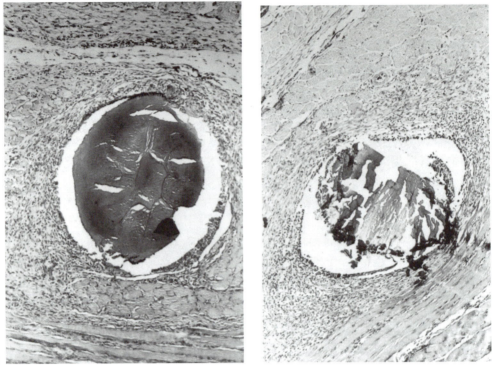

A   B

Figure 8.10 Histological pictures of glycerin-treated (A) and regular chromic gut (B) 7 d postimplantation in rats. (From Stone, I.K. et al., *Am. J. Obstet. Gynecol.*, 151, (8), 1087, 1985. With permission.)

epidemiological) of the glycerin-treated chromic catgut by Grant[44] and Spencer,[44,45] however, indicated some adverse effects due to the glycerin treatment. Table 8.4 summarizes the results of a 3-year follow-up. Female patients with perineal wounds repaired with glycerin-impregnated chromic catgut experienced dyspareunia 1.7× (*P* <.02) that of those without glycerin-treated chromic catgut sutures. The perineal pain occurred at 10 d postoperation, while dyspareunia occurred at 3 months and persisted at 3 years. As many as 8% of surveyed patients experienced dyspareunia 3 years after the initial perineal repair. Grant suggested that the most likely cause of this reported adverse reaction was the increased fibrosis with glycerin-treated chromic catgut sutures. Therefore, Grant suggested that glycerin-treated chromic catgut should not be used in the repair of perineal wounds.

2. Polyglycolide (Dexon) and Polyglactin 910 (Vicryl) Sutures

Dexon suture, first introduced in 1970, is made of polymers of glycolic acid (PGA). This suture material is renowned for its superb tensile and knot strengths as well as having delayed absorption and diminished tissue reactivity when compared to catgut. In animal studies, Dexon sutures were found to have a tensile strength loss of about 40% after 7 d.[46] By 15 d it had lost more than 80% of its original strength.[32,47] Finally, by 28 d, this material had only 5% of its original tensile strength, and is completely dissolved by 90 to 120 d.[48] There is less of an inflammatory response secondary to the absorption of PGA by hydrolysis when compared with the proteolytic absorption of catgut. In the monofilament form, Dexon is stiff and hard to work with; therefore, it is supplied in braided form for ease of handling. Dexon is also available with a synthetic coating (Dexon Plus®) in order to smooth knot tying and passage through tissue. Dexon II, with a new synthetic coating of polycaprolate, is a recent product designed to have more desirable handling qualities than Dexon Plus in terms of smoothness and knot security.

Vicryl suture, first introduced in 1974, is made of a copolymer of lactide and glycolide with a coating consisting of polyglactic acid and calcium stearate. This lubricant coating provides Vicryl with its superb handling and smooth tie-down properties. Technical studies have shown Dexon to have slightly greater tensile and knot strength than Vicryl,[49] but these differences are insignificant by clinical standards. Vicryl, like Dexon, retains only 8% of its original tensile strength by 28 d. However, a complete absorption of Vicryl is more expedient, occurring between 60 and 90 d.[50] Vicryl is degraded by hydrolysis like all

Table 8.4 Results of 3-Year Follow-Up of Women Repaired
with Glycerol-Coated Catgut Suture

Variable	Allocated Group	
	Softgut	Catgut
No. in original trial	377	360
No. who replied to questionnaire	263	253
Babies born since study *n* (% respondents)		
0*	147(56)	156(62)
1	109(41)	94(37)
2	7(3)	3(1)
Management of first subsequent delivery *n* (%)		
Mode of delivery		
Spontaneous vaginal	111(96)	94(97)
Instrumental	3(3)	1(1)
Cesarean section	2(2)	2(2)
Episiotomy performed *n* (% vaginal deliveries)	28(25)	13(14)*
Perineum sutured *n* (% vaginal deliveries)	82(72)	69(73)
Sexual intercourse painful *n* (% respondents)	51(19)	29(11)**
Soreness	43	28
Tightness	2	0
Other	6	1
Subanalysis based on women with no subsequent deliveries		
Sexual intercourse painful *n* (%)	28/146(19)	15/155(11)***
Soreness	23	14
Tightness	1	0
Other	4	1

* χ^2 (1 d.f.) = 3.89; P = .05.

** χ^2 (1 d.f.) = 6.18; P <.02.

*** χ^2 (1 d.f.) = 5.54; P <.02.

From Grant, A., *Am. J. Obstet. Gynecol.*, 96(6), 741, 1989. With permission.

synthetic polyesters and thus causes minimal tissue reaction. Vicryl is braided and comes in either a clear undyed or violet-dyed form. In cutaneous surgery, the dyed form is often visible beneath the skin surface. Buried Vicryl or Dexon sutures can rarely be extruded through the suture line.

Both Dexon and Vicryl sutures elicit minimal tissue reactions. Cellular reactions are mainly mononuclear in character and appear to be limited to the immediate surroundings of the suture strands. Katz and Turner[27] found that at 7 d in rabbits, Dexon sutures were surrounded by a narrow band of fibrous connective tissue with a few infiltrating mononuclear cells. By day 50, the histologic pattern was unremarkable: membranes of flattened macrophages, with occasional foreign body giant cells, surrounded and adhered closely to each fibril. This is believed to be responsible for the suture absorption. Pavan et al.[29] showed that this surrounding cellular reaction was attenuated by day 50 and that bundles of collagen fibrils appeared around the passage of the suture, replacing the physiologic tissue.

Postlethwait[32] evaluated Dexon tissue reaction by a modification of Sewell's criteria. As indicated in Table 8.2, the reaction reached a peak around the end of the first week and then subsided to as low as a 10.0 grade by 6 months. Polymorphonuclear leukocytes and lymphocytes were rare; giant cells were more common. Craig et al.[49] used an unmodified Sewell grading system with rats. Their mean score pattern was different from Postlethwait's data. Craig's data indicated that the highest tissue response scores occur around 2 months after implantation, while Postlethwait's results showed this to occur at 7 d. Craig also compared tissue response to PGA with that to polyglactin 910 sutures and found that they were both quantitatively and qualitatively similar.[49] Figure 8.11 details such a comparison. Bergman et al.[33] examined tissue reactions to PGA sutures in three tissues: the intestine, urinary bladder, and abdominal muscle of rabbits. In the intestine, the suture was found to be embedded in fibroblast-rich granulation tissue with multinuclear giant cells of a foreign body type, but without a fibrous capsule, at the end of 1 month. No fibrous granulomas, as observed with catgut suture, were found around the PGA sutures. The histologic changes in the muscle and bladder were essentially the same as those in the intestine.

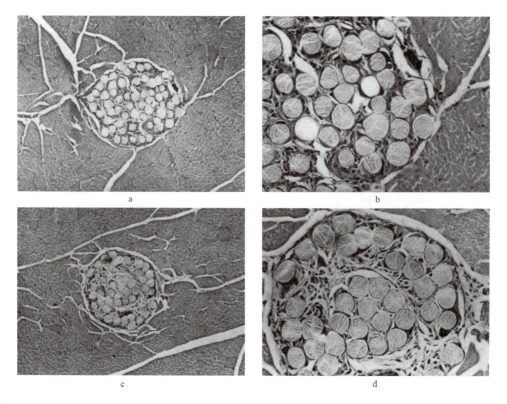

Figure 8.11 Tissue reaction and absorption profiles of 4/0 polyglactin 910 and polyglycolide sutures at 42 d postimplantation in rat. (a) Polyglactin 910 is extensively infiltrated by cells at ×85; (b) polyglactin 910: the cell population consists of an admixture of fibroblasts and macrophages at ×212; (c) polyglycolide: the cell population occupies the spaces between the filaments at ×85; (d) same as (c) except at ×212. In both (b) and (d), the cross sections of the filaments are eosinophilic and extensively fissured. (From Craig, P.H. et al., *Surg. Gynecol. Obstet.*, 141(1), 1, 1975. With permission.)

In the three ophthalmic tissues, Salthouse et al.[35] showed polyglactin 910 sutures induced similar cellular populations as chromic collagen sutures before 21 d, as shown in Table 8.3. Except in the cornea, giant cells along with fibroblasts were found with polyglactin 910 after 21 d. Giant cells, however, were not observed with either catgut or collagen sutures in the cornea, sclera, and ocular muscle of rabbits. However, the recent study by Yamanaka[36] may raise the concern of using PGA sutures in ophthalmology. Yamanaka in Japan reported two clinical cases of Dexon suture-induced chorioretinitis in squint surgery and he suggested that PGA sutures may act as strong antigens that could lead to inflammation of delayed hypersensitivity. The lesions included macula edema, granulomatous uveitis (caused by macrophages), and capillary occlusions. Based on a mouse animal model, Yamanaka found that macrophage blocking with carrageenin and an incomplete adjuvant were necessary to evoke the delayed hypersensitivity of ophthalmologic tissue to PGA sutures. There were a large number of lymphocytes and monocytes surrounding the PGA while much fewer lymphocytes were noted in the control group animals. Thus, Yamanaka concluded that PGA suture is not completely safe in ophthalmologic use.

The data reported on the reaction of nerve tissue to sutures are not as frequent as that for other tissues. It has been shown that the presence of sutures in a nerve repair site elicit two distinct tissue responses: cellular and fibroplastic.[50,51] The former reaches maximum activity in the early stage, is directed to removing the implanted material, and is composed of PMNs, lymphocytes, giant cells, and histiocytes. The latter seeks to wall off foreign suture materials, and reaches maximum stimulation during the later stages of healing. This fibroplastic reaction, however, impedes the regeneration of nervous tissues more severely than the cellular infiltration reaction.[51] DeLee et al.[55] examined the reaction of nerve tissue to sutures. They found that PGA, along with Prolene sutures, grossly appeared to evoke the least amount of scarring in rabbits during three types of nerve reconstruction: repaired nerve, nerve substance pass-through only, and epineurium only. In contrast, catgut sutures elicited only a minimal fibrous reaction, which was consistent with Guttman's finding.[50] Hudson et al.[56] reported that PGA sutures placed in peripheral nerves in rats resulted in minimal reaction; the degradation and absorption of PGA sutures were extremely local events and did not interfere with the histology of the nerve. No damage to neighboring nerve fibers secondary to tissue response to PGA sutures was found. Bratton et al.[57] used monofilament PGA in fascicular repair of peripheral nerves in dogs and monkeys. The cellular reaction was identical to Hudson's data for rats. At the suture line, the overall appearance was that of a traumatic neuroma. It was unusual to see a coherent fascicle with an intact perineurium. Both the electrophysiologic and histologic data indicate that repair of nerves with PGA sutures is similar to the use of nylon suture of identical caliber. This suggests that the absorption of PGA sutures and the subsequent cellular response do not interfere with the regeneration of axon units. One theory is that the main regenerative wave of axon sprouts passes the suture line before any significant changes in the histologic picture occurred at the suture lines.[57]

When sutures are used to close dura mater, it is important that cicatrix and adhesions be minimal. The absence of subdural adhesions is an advantage if reoperation proves necessary. Vallfors et al.[58] used dogs to study the quality of healing with both PGA and polyglactin 910 sutures for the closure of dura mater with respect to the smoothness of the subdural surface, the presence of adhesion between the sutures and the brain surface, the degree of absorption, and brain tissue reaction to the sutures. They found that both sutures elicited minimal cellular reaction as observed in other tissues. Polyglactin 910 sutures were, however, absorbed to a higher degree than PGA at 60 d; the remaining polyglactin 910 material at 60 d was only one fifth that found with PGA sutures. Polyglactin 910 sutures were considered to be better than PGA, because the proliferative changes it elicited in the surrounding tissue protruded from the subdural surface, resulting in strong adhesion to the underlying brain surface, eventually creating holes in the brain surface upon dural separation. When dura mater was separated, the effect was to tear off the leptomeninges with their vascular supply to the cortex. No significant subdural protrusions or adhesions were found under polyglactin 910 sutures.

In rat muscle, Matlaga and Salthouse[59] observed that macrophages closely adhered to the polyglactin 910 suture and appeared to surround the filaments by extension of thin lamellapodia as early as 1 d postimplantation. This type of cell-implant interaction was not generally observed with nonhydrolyzable suture materials. Fibroblasts and collagen were evident at 5 d and reached their highest concentration at 28 d. Absorption was evident from 35 to 53 d and was accompanied by the appearance of large numbers of mitochondria in the close vicinity of the plasma membranes of macrophages and foreign body giant cells adjacent to the filaments. Such increased metabolic activity was believed to be related to the metabolism of the hydrolytic degradation products of polyglactin 910, glycolate, and lactate.

There are relatively fewer reported studies on the *in vivo* tissue reactions of absorbable sutures in orthopedics. The most interesting one is probably from Barber and Deck, in their study of a new absorbable suture anchor, Expanding Suture Plug (ESP) made of 100% poly-L-lactide (PLLA) (Arthrex, Inc., Naples, Florida) for securing tendons and ligaments to bone.[60] There are some very important advantages of using biodegradable suture anchors rather than nonbiodegradable metallic staples, screw-washer combinations, and plates. The biodegradability of absorbable suture anchors would eliminate the need for any additional surgery to remove the implant in the event that the anchor migrates to an unexpected position and results in late infection or patient discomfort. Other advantages include their radiographic translucency which would not interfere with clinical diagnosis utilizing X-rays or MRI (magnetic resonance imaging). Absorbable suture anchors for the fastening of ligament or tendon on bones would also reduce the possibility of invasion of potential fragments of the implant into joints. Barber and Deck[60] reported that, during the 12 weeks of implantation of EPS in Barbados rams, there was a lack of foreign body reaction or inflammatory infiltrate. Contrary to the general belief that the rate of biodegradation of any absorbable implant must bear some relationship to the level of inflammatory and foreign body reactions it elicits, they argued that the well-known, much slower biodegradation rate of PLLA was not the cause for the lack of the observed classic pattern of inflammatory and foreign body reactions associated with the much faster absorbable polymers like PGA, glycolide-lactide copolymers, and polydioxanone during the 6 to 12 weeks postimplantation.

The cellular response to the absorption of these synthetic absorbable sutures in terms of cellular enzymes was also studied by Salthouse and Matlaga[61] in the skeletal muscle of rats. As shown in Table 7.15 in the last chapter, hydrolytic enzymes played no apparent role in the initial hydrolysis of polyglactin 910 sutures, but cellular oxidative enzyme systems associated with macrophages and giant cells were active from 28 to 42 d after implantation. This period coincided with the large increase in the numbers of mitochondria found inside macrophages, as mentioned above. It was thus hypothesized that the increase in enzymes associated with the citric acid cycle in cells which come in close contact with synthetic absorbable suture is involved in the active metabolism and degradation of lactic and glycolic acids to carbon dioxide and water.

3. Polydioxanone (PDS®) Sutures

PDS® suture is made of a paradioxanone polymer and was marketed as having prolonged tensile strength *in vivo* compared with Vicryl or Dexon. PDS suture retains 74% of its original tensile strength at 2 weeks, and 41% after 6 weeks.[62] Therefore, PDS can prove useful in situations where extended wound tensile strength is required. PDS is hydrolyzed more slowly than Vicryl or Dexon. Complete absorption of PDS occurs about 180 d postimplantation. PDS is available in either undyed or a violet-dyed thread. Unlike Vicryl or Dexon, PDS is manufactured as a monofilamentous suture and should have decreased affinity in harboring bacterial organisms. A disadvantage of using PDS is that it is more difficult to use than the braided synthetics because of intrinsic stiffness. In addition, PDS costs about 14% more than either Vicryl or Dexon. Polydioxanone II is a newer product that has decreased stiffness and smoother handling characteristics than PDS, while keeping the original tensile strength qualities.

PDS suture has been found to elicit minimal to slight foreign body reaction, which is confined to the vicinity of the implant site. Ray et al.[62] reported that the cell population was mainly mononuclear in character, consisting of macrophages and proliferating fibroblasts throughout the entire period of implantation (182 d) in the dorsal subcutis of Long-Evans rats. At the end of 5 d, the tissue reaction consisted mainly of a few macrophages and proliferating fibroblasts; other inflammatory cells like neutrophils, foreign body giant cells, eosinophils, and lymphocytes were rarely seen at this period of implantation. No neutrophils were seen throughout the whole study period. Figure 8.12 illustrates the histological finding of 2-0 dyed PDS at various periods of implantation in rats.[62] At the late period of implantation (>90 d), only macrophages and fibroblasts are consistently present at the implantation sites. After absorption, only a few enlarged macrophages or fibroblasts were found localized between normal muscle cells. Foci of fat cells occasionally occupy the suture implant site. Such tissue responses were similar to those for PGA and polyglactin 910 sutures. Between 5 and 91 d postimplantation, the anisotropy of the suture fiber remains and the cross sections of the suture are unstained and refractile.

Although standard histologic evaluation of sutures and biomaterials is usually performed in the subcutis or gluteal muscles of rats, the study of sutures is not limited to these sites. As a result, deviations from the above standard histologic data can be found. Cameron et al.[63] compared the performance of no.1 PDS and no.1 Prolene in abdominal closure. One hundred forty-three patients had abdominal closures with PDS and 141 others with Prolene; 0.7% of the patients with PDS and 15.5% of the patients with Prolene had wound infection. Later, 190 of these 284 patients were interviewed within 12 months. Eleven percent of these 190 patients had an incisional hernia; these were generally asymptomatic and evenly distributed among the two groups. The PDS group had a lower incidence of wound pain and palpable knots. Overall, these results indicated that PDS was easier to handle, caused less wound pain, and retained its strength for a considerable length of time. Cameron et al. also reported that wounds closed with PDS were more convenient in terms of fewer knots required and fewer patients suffering wound pains. Therefore, they concluded that PDS, in the long term, may have advantages over Prolene, although the true incidence of incisional herniation will require longer follow-up. Cameron et al. suggested that PDS may be an alternative to a nonabsorbable suture for laparotomy closure.

Taylor[64] compared PDS with nylon in a two-layer continuous closure of midline wounds and found that PDS was superior to nylon. Leaper et al.[65] did the same trial and found that a greater number of wound infections occurred with PDS, which is contrary to the Cameron series.[63] Schoetz et al.[66] used PDS to close abdominal wounds in 200 consecutive operative procedures. All the patients were followed for up to 1 year. He found that, despite a high incidence of risk factors for impaired wound healing, the incidence of dehiscence and evisceration was zero, while incisional hernia occurred in 2.9% of vertical midline wounds and in 3.6% of transverse incisions. They concluded that PDS is safe and effective for abdominal wound closures.[66]

In cardiovascular surgery, Torsello et al.[67] did experiments to evaluate absorbable and nonabsorbable sutures with continuous or interrupted suture technique on venous anastomoses in dogs. Eight venous anastomoses were performed with either an interrupted or continuous suture technique, using polypropylene or polydioxanone sutures, according to a randomized experimental model. Anastomosis morphology was monitored by venography directly after closure of the wound and at weekly intervals for 2 months and monthly intervals thereafter until 24 months. In 10 cases, venography was followed by transluminal angioscopy in the early postoperative period and after 1, 2, 4, 8, and 12 weeks. In the first 2 months, moderate and high degree stenosis was found in all groups by venography. After 2 months, there was a significant decrease in the incidence of stenosis; no significant decrease in the incidence of stenosis and no significant narrowing could be identified in any group except that using continuous nonabsorbable suture. Using angioscopy, a marked swelling of the intima at the site of the anastomoses could be detected in the early postoperative period in all experimental groups.

Aarnio et al.[68] conducted an experiment using six beagle dogs to evaluate PDS suture on free internal mammary artery grafts. Free internal mammary artery grafts, 3 cm long, were harvested via a median sternotomy and were implanted as arterial bypasses in femoral arteries (12 end-to-end anastomoses) and as arteriovenous shunts in the carotid artery-contralateral jugular vein position (12 end-to-side anastomoses). Twenty-four anastomoses were made with monofilament nonabsorbable suture material to serve as control grafts. After 6 months the grafts and anastomoses were explanted and studied with light and scanning electron microscopy (SEM). Macroscopically, the polydioxanone sutures had disappeared. No aneurysms or dilations were observed with either PDS or polypropylene closure. According to this study, polydioxanone is a suitable suture material for small luminal arterial anastomoses and is superior to polypropylene suture because PDS causes no tissue or other late changes on flow surfaces.

Zannini et al.[69] found, in the case of nonabsorbable vs. polydioxanone sutures tested in human anastomoses, some disadvantages, such as severe inflammatory changes, necrosis, calcifications, and intimal roughening. They predicated that polydioxanone can be absorbed completely after wound healing. This characteristic allows the perfect healing of the anastomosis without residual stenosis. Zannini et al. suggested that the use of PDS suture in repair of hypoplasia of the aortic arch would be helpful in reducing the incidence of repeat coarctation. However, Peleg et al.[70] felt that, in the case of tracheal and bronchial anastomoses, PDS suture should be used with caution, for its "bristly" knots can perforate adjacent blood vessels. Friberg et al.[71] also evaluated the fate of the subclavian flap repairs of aortic coarctation using PDS suture. All the young animals which underwent aortoplasties survived and grew normally. During the 6 to 26 weeks postoperative observation, there was no sign of flap destruction, and tissue reaction to PDS suture was minimal. All parts of the flap grew normally. This study indicated that PDS seems to be a good alternative for repair of aortic coarctation in early infancy.[71]

Recently, Myers[72] and Gersak[73] separately reported that tissue reactions between suture materials and arterial walls of young patients or animals led to greater fibrosis and calcification in arterial walls closed with absorbable sutures than those with nonabsorbable sutures. The physical form of sutures, i.e., multifilament vs. monofilament, also affected the level of fibrosis in the vessel walls. Gersak reported that monofilament sutures resulted in less fibrosis in vessel walls vs. multifilament suture. Along with the fibrosis of arterial walls, Gersak also found a higher level of persistent calcification in the vessel walls closed with absorbable PDS sutures than nonabsorbable Prolene sutures. On the contrary, Myers found that resolution of calcification occurred by 6 months postoperation, although microscopic calcification started to appear at 1 and 4 weeks postoperation. However, the issue of suture-induced calcification in vessel walls reported in the literature is frequently conflicting. In a more recent reported study by Gersak,[74] he found that there was no statistical difference in calcium density of arterial vessel walls of growing German shepherd dogs using either 6/0 PDS or Prolene sutures via end-to-end interrupted anastomoses. Irrespective of the type of suture materials, the sutured arterial vessel walls, however, showed statistically significant higher calcium density than the corresponding sutureless vessel parts. Therefore, Gersak's latest data suggested that the prevalence of calcification in the sutured arteries of young patients appears to be independent of the biodegradability of suture materials. It is the authors' opinion that the lack of statistically significant differences in calcium density of growing arterial walls between absorbable PDS and nonabsorbable Prolene sutures might be related to the very long biodegradation rate of PDS sutures described in the previous chapter. This very long biodegradation rate of PDS sutures would make them behave like nonabsorbable sutures from the tissue reaction point of view during the first few months postoperation. This suggests that rapidly absorbed sutures like Monocryl®, Dexon, or Vicryl may show different calcium densities within growing arterial vessel walls, compared to nonabsorbable sutures. There are no data in the literature to verify such a speculation at this time.

In a study by Mavroudis et al.,[76] eight infants were subjected to orthotopic cardiac transplantation with PDS suture. One died 6 h after diagnosis, one was allowed to die after 60 d because of acquired neurologic complications, and another had congenital cytomegalovirus infection. The remaining five patients had orthotopic cardiac transplantation performed with PDS and were followed-up for 17 months. The results showed appropriate graft growth, no aortic or pulmonary anastomotic strictures, normal right and left ventricular function, and no coronary artery disease. They concluded that infant orthotopic cardiac transplantation with PDS is an acceptable procedure for severe forms of untreatable congenital heart disease.

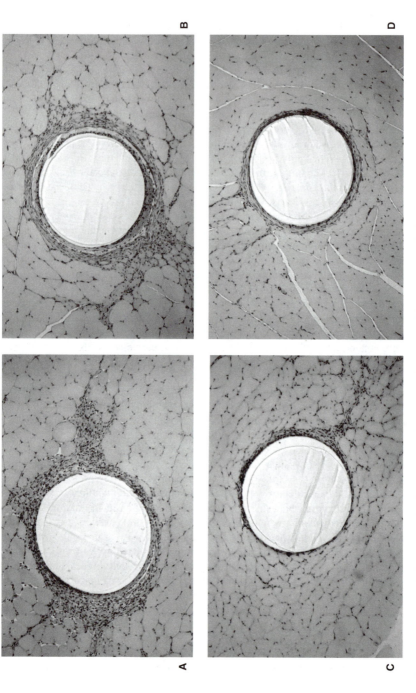

Figure 8.12.1 Tissue reactions and absorption of 2/0 dyed monofilament polydioxanone (PDS) suture at 5, 7, 14, and 28 d postimplantation in the gluteal muscles of rats. Hematoxylin and eosin stain. (A) PDS at 5 d surrounded by slightly irregular zone of inflammatory cells, consisting primarily of macrophages, with a scattering of neutrophils. Eosin-stained surrounding tissue is gluteal muscle. ×68. (B) PDS sutures at 7 d surrounded by a band of fibroblastic cells which has begun to orient around the periphery of the suture. A narrow band of macrophages and a few degenerated cells are seen at the interface between the reaction zone and the suture. The reaction is judged as slight. ×69. (C) PDS suture at 14 d. The reaction has become a thin band of proliferating fibroblasts and reaction is minimal. ×68. (D) PDS suture at 28 d. The reaction has become fibrocytic and a collagenous capsule encircles the monofilament strand. ×68. (From Ray, J.A. et al., *Surg. Gynecol. Obstet.*, 153, 497, 1981. With permission.)

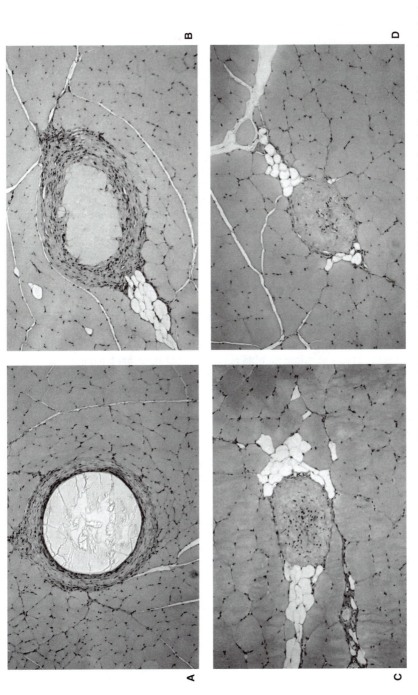

Figure 8.12.2 Tissue reactions and absorption of 2/0 dyed monofilament PDS sutures at 90, 168, 180, and 210 d postimplantation in the gluteal muscles of rats. Hematoxylin and eosin stain. (A) PDS at 90 d which has fragmented, indicating degradation. The suture strand is encased in a well-organized collagenous capsule, with a few macrophages at the suture-capsule interface. ×68. (B) At 168 d. Extensive fissuring of the suture has occurred and a substantial amount of the strand has absorbed. A zone of macrophages immediately surrounds the suture, which in turn, is encircled by collagenous fibers. ×68. (C) At 180 d. PDS suture is no longer visible. Large macrophages are present at the implant site. Fat cells occupy the space adjacent to the implant site. ×68. (D) At 210 d. PDS suture has completely absorbed. Only a few fibrocytes and macrophages are present. The site is essentially devoid of reaction at this time. ×68. (From Ray, J.A. et al., *Surg. Gynecol. Obstet.,* 153, 497, 1981. With permission.)

In ophthalmologic surgery, PDS was successfully used. In a study by Biardzka and Kaluzny,[77] PDS was used for cerclage of the eyeball on rabbits and it was proved that it was well tolerated by surrounding eye tissues. It did not cause side effects, and had a sufficiently long period of absorption to ensure chorioretinal cicatrization. In fact, 81.25% of reattachments were achieved in humans after primary repair, and 87.5% after the second operation. Biardzka and Kaluzny thus suggested that PDS is a good ocular cerclage material.

Autogenous lamellar corneal grafts were performed by Brightman et al.[78] on nine clinically normal dogs (one eye in each of two dogs and both eyes in each of seven dogs) and seven dogs with corneal disease (one eye in each dog). Nylon, PGA, polyglactin 910, and PDS suture materials were used in 8/0 to 10/0 sizes. The eyes of the normal dogs were examined weekly for up to 16 weeks; corneal endothelium was reestablished in all eyes by 6 weeks after surgery. The eyes of the dogs with corneal disease were reexamined periodically for up to 9 months. Twenty-two of 23 (95.7%) grafts were considered successful in that they were translucent, and the dogs were able to see after surgery. They found that nylon and polyglactin 910 caused the least tissue reactions.

Willatt et al.[79] conducted a study in aural wound closure to compare synthetic monofilament suture materials with chromic catgut and silk in aural wound closure. Forty patients undergoing mastoidectomy or tympanoplasty were randomized for either 3/0 PDS closure of fascia plus 3/0 Prolene closure of skin, or 2/0 chromic catgut closure of fascia plus 3/0 silk closure of skin. Known or suspected factors affecting wound healing were recorded. Nine patients had postoperative wound infections. The infection rate was significantly lower in wounds closed with PDS and Prolene, and in the tympanoplasty operation. Four patients closed with catgut and silk suffered wound dehiscence. No other complication of wound healing was noted in the trial. In conclusion, PDS and Prolene are superior suture materials compared to catgut and silk in the closure of aural wounds.

In subcutaneous tissue closure, Kirby et al.[80] reported two cases of calcinosis circumscripta associated with polydioxanone suture material diagnosed in two young dogs. In each case, the dog's owner noticed a firm mass at the site of a previous surgical incision. Mineralization of soft tissue was visible radiographically. At excision, multiple chalky white nodular masses within the subcutis extended in a linear pattern along the length of the suture incision, but not beyond it. Polydioxanone suture was identified within the center of the nodules, which were identified histologically as calcinosis circumscripta. The characteristic of calcinosis circumscripta is single or multiple, hard, painless subcutaneous nodules that consist of noncrystalline deposits of calcium salts surrounded by a granulomatous reaction. There are two types of calcification of tissues other than bone and teeth: metastatic and dystrophic. Abnormal calcium or phosphorus metabolism is associated with metastatic calcification. Dystrophic calcification, however, occurs in injured or necrotic tissues under the normal metabolism of calcium or phosphorus. The calcinosis circumscripta associated with PDS sutures reported by Kirby et al. was of the dystrophic type. The exact pathogenesis for this dystrophic calcification was unknown, but several possibilities were suggested. They include the presence of PDS suture as a site for catalytic nucleation of minerals, the acidic microenvironment resulting from the degradation products of PDS suture, and/or just coincidence.

In addition to the suture form, polydioxanone was also used as a "clip" in performing appendectomy during pelvic reconstructive surgery. Bellina and Lee[75] applied polydioxanone clips on 32 patients undergoing surgical management of endometriosis. Twelve patients had surgical reconstructions for pelvic adhesive disease and endometriosis with pelvic adhesive disease. After the procedure, among the 32 patients with endometriosis, 12 appendices were confirmed by histology to contain endometriosis; 1 contained a benign carcinoid tumor. Of the 12 patients with pelvic adhesive disease, 2 had associate endometriosis. Twenty-four appendices were histologically normal.

Polydioxanone has also been applied as a "staple" form in severely emphysematous lungs. Juettner et al.[81] reported a mechanical suture line reinforced by a polydioxanone ribbon is a simple, safe, and effective method for closure of air leaks, reactions, or biopsies. They have reported their experience with 14 patients (two cases of substantial panlobular emphysema, one of lymphangioleiomyomatosis, two of destroyed lungs as a result of generalized bullous disease, seven of bullous deformities of the upper lobe, and two of silicosis) and have been satisfied with the results. In particular, there were no bronchopleural fistulas or infectious complications during the median follow-up of 8.3 months (range 2 to 14 months). Because the polydioxanone ribbon is absorbed within a few weeks, there is little risk of implant infection compared with nonabsorbable material.

4. Polytrimethylene Carbonate Sutures (Maxon)

Maxon suture was developed to combine the excellent tensile strength retention qualities of PDS with improved handling properties. The first reported biocompatibility studies of Maxon sutures involved subcutaneous testing in rabbits.[82] Maxon provides wound support over an extended period of time, like PDS, with an average strength retention of 81% at 2 weeks and 30% at 6 weeks. Complete absorption by hydrolysis occurs between 6 and 7 months. There was no acute inflammatory infiltration, abscess formation, or tissue necrosis over the 9-month period of study. Neither cellular mobilization nor tissue reactivity was present distant from the implantation site. Due to the long period of suture mass absorption (7 months), chronic inflammation persisted before complete suture absorption, and the degree of such inflammation was dependent on the duration following implantation. At 3 months, the implant site was surrounded with a well-characterized and nourished mature fibrous connective tissue capsule. As the duration of implantation proceeded to $4 \frac{1}{2}$ months, no appreciable difference in tissue reaction vs. the 3-month period was found, except for the presence of multinuclear foreign body giant cells due to suture fragmentation. At 6 months, most of the Maxon suture mass was degraded and absorbed with a transition process of the Maxon-host reaction found. This involved an increasing deposition of collagen due to the absorption of the suture mass and partial resorption of macrophages. Those macrophages at the site of the implant exhibited vacuoles and granules indicative of phagocytized suture fragments. Eventually, at 9 months, all macrophages were replaced by a narrow, dense cord of collagen at the former site of suture repair.

Sanz et al.[83] evaluated 4/0 Maxon, Vicryl, chromic catgut, and PDS in fascial closure in rats with respect to tissue inflammatory reaction, knot security, suture tensile strength, and absorption. Two hundred ten rats were randomized into five groups, and 120 of these were used to evaluate tissue reactions and knot security, and 90 others were used to test suture tensile strength. They found that Maxon and Vicryl were statistically significantly stronger than PDS and chromic catgut during the critical 2-week period of wound healing. However, PDS and Maxon continued to retain significant tensile strength during the late postoperative periods. Maxon was evaluated as being the best suture material for abdominal fascial closures and pelvic surgery since it is relatively inert, has higher tensile strength retention, and can support healing wounds for longer time periods.

The failure load and maximum tensile strength of chromic catgut and two monofilament synthetic absorbable suture materials (PDS and Maxon) were measured up to 6 weeks after implantation in sheep using the following models: (1) a suture securing a synovial incision; and (2) coils located either within the synovial cavity of the knee or intramuscularly.[84] Although all synovial wounds healed satisfactorily, the performance of the different materials varied. The strength of chromic catgut was largely lost within a week and fragmentation occurred at the fourth week. The synthetic absorbable sutures lost their strength relatively more slowly. Maxon degraded in a linear manner, remaining intact but with little strength by week 6. PDS, though losing its strength at a slower rate, tended to fragment early, which may be of clinical importance in situations of delayed wound healing.

Metz et al.[85] examined *in vivo* tissue reactivity and degradation of both Maxon and PDS sutures in rabbit peritoneum and rectus fascia for intervals of 2 to 70 d for the purpose of identifying whether the complications of abdominal surgery (i.e., intraperitoneal inflammation and adhesion formation) relate to suture-induced tissue reaction. As shown in Figure 8.13, the inflammatory response of tissue (defined as the number of inflammatory cells/mm^2) to both Maxon and PDS sutures was similar. Inflammation reached a maximum at 4 d postimplantation and then subsided to preoperative levels by day 21. The inflammatory response was more intense in peritoneum than in fascia. The report by Metz et al. was also one of the few reports that examined the surface morphology of retrieved Maxon and PDS sutures. Figure 8.14 illustrates SEM of both Maxon and PDS sutures retrieved from rabbit peritoneum or fascia at 21 and 35 d postimplantation. Maxon sutures in both fascia and peritoneum tissues for 35 d (Figure 8.14 C and D) exhibited the familiar surface morphology, as in the *in vitro* study: generation of surface cracks and subsequent peeling of the outermost layer. In conjunction with these surface morphologic observations, Maxon suture became very fragile and disintegrated easily after 14 d, but PDS sutures retained structural integrity for at least 35 d implantation.

5. Poliglecaprone 25 Sutures (Monocryl®)

There is only one reported study of this latest synthetic absorbable monofilament suture from Ethicon. Bezwada et al.[86] implanted Monocryl® sutures in gluteal muscles of female Long-Evans rats for up to 119 d. Table 8.5 summarizes the median tissue reaction scores of a Monocryl suture based on a modified

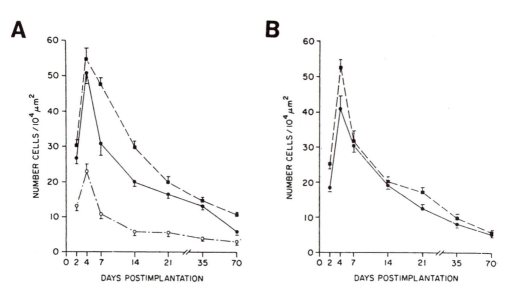

Figure 8.13 Inflammatory response of tissue to implanted sutures. (A) Response to Prolene and PDS; (B) response to Maxon. (○) Prolene implanted in fascia; (●) PDS implanted in fascia; (■) PDS implanted in peritoneum. (From Metz, S.A. et al., *J. Gynecol. Surg.*, 5(1), 37, 1989. With permission.)

Sewell score system. It appears that tissue reactions exhibited two stages: a high level of tissue reaction at 3 d postimplantation, followed by a low level of tissue reaction between 7 and 28 d postimplantation. However, there was a surge in tissue reactions between 28 and 91 d postimplantation which reached the lowest level at the time of complete absorption. Morphologically, the tissue reactions elicited by Monocryl are mainly characterized by the presence of fibroblasts and macrophages and fewer numbers of lymphocytes, plasma cells, and leukocytes, as shown in Figure 8.15. Occasionally, giant cells were present. The concentrations of these cells decreased with time of implantation.

A pharmacokinetic study of the absorption of ^{14}C-labeled caproyl moiety of Monocryl sutures in rats indicated that the bulk of the implanted dose (about 96%) was eliminated from rats within 98 d postimplantation.[86] The major routes of elimination of the radiolabeled Monocryl sutures were through urinary excretion (49%) and pulmonary expiration (41%). The remaining amounts were eliminated through feces (5%).

B. NONABSORBABLE SUTURES

Nonabsorbable sutures are generally defined as filamentous material that is appropriately resistant to the degradation mechanisms of living tissues. However, the term nonabsorbable is relative because some of these sutures are eventually degraded. The most common nonabsorbable sutures used today include silk, nylon, polypropylene, polyesters, polybutester, and Gore-Tex.

1. Silk and Cotton Sutures

Silk suture is made from natural protein filaments spun by the silkworm larva as it builds a cocoon. Among the nonabsorbable suture materials, silk and cotton are considered to be the worst in terms of tissue and cellular response. In a 2-year long-term comparative study in rabbit muscles, Postlethwait found that the predominant cell type present after 1 week were histiocytes and fibroblasts.[87] A firm fibrous tissue capsule was found after 1 year and some histiocytes were still present. The mononuclear response was variable and, in some sections, clearly marked. Giant cells were seen at all time intervals. The suture generally remained a compact bundle with occasional penetration by cells. As shown in Table 8.6, Sewell tissue reaction grades remained moderate even after 1 year.

Postlethwait et al.[88] also examined five different types of silk sutures in rabbits: regular (wax-coated), uncoated black, uncoated white, Teflon-coated black, and Teflon-coated white. The histologic changes in the healing wounds were essentially the same over a period of 42 d. Coating materials seemed not to affect the healing of the wound significantly. Giant cells were observed only occasionally. Granuloma formation could not be found with the regular, uncoated black or uncoated white silk.

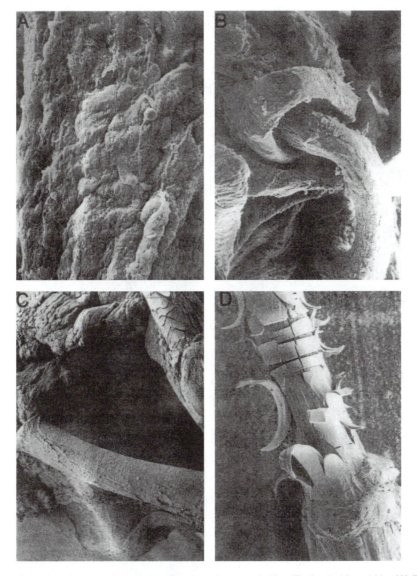

Figure 8.14 Scanning electron micrographs of implanted sutures in New Zealand white rabbits. (A) PDS suture in peritoneum at 21 d, ×175; (B) PDS suture in peritoneum at 21 d, ×43; (C) Maxon suture in fascia at 35 d, ×11; (D) Maxon suture in peritoneum at 35 d, ×21. (From Metz, S.A. et al., *J. Gynecol. Surg.*, 5(1), 37, 1989. With permission.)

Table 8.5 Median Tissue Reaction Scores for Monocryl Sutures after Intramuscular Implantation in Rats

Size	Days Postimplantation						Time to Complete Absorption (d)
	3	7	28	63	91	119	
2-0	17	9	7.5	15	20	2.5	119
6-0	10	12.5	6	11.5	0	0	91

Note: Scores are as follows: 0, no reaction; 1–8, minimal reaction; 9–24, slight reaction; 25–40, moderate reaction; 41–56, marked reaction; 56+, extensive reaction.

From Bezwada, R.S et al., *Biomaterials*, 16, 1141, 1995. With permission.

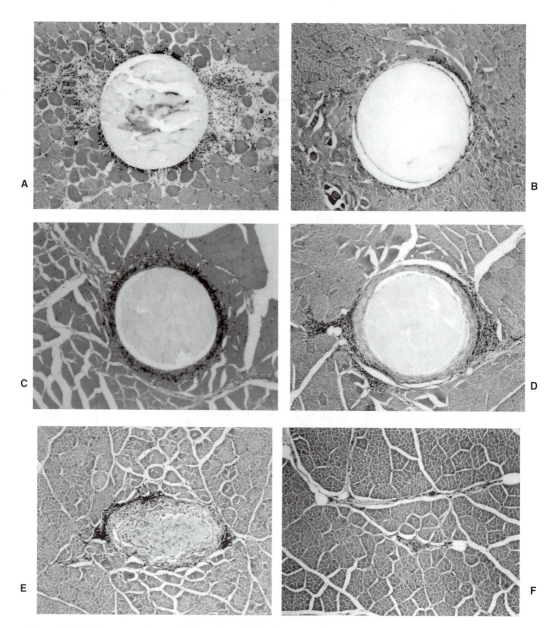

Figure 8.15 Tissue reaction and absorption of 2/0 dyed monofilament Monocryl suture at 3, 7, 28, 63, 91, and 119 d postimplantation. H&E stained, paraffin-embedded rat gluteal muscle at ×150. (A) Monocryl suture at 3 d surrounded by an irregular zone of edema and inflammatory cells, primary macrophages, and neutrophils, separating skeletal muscle cells. (B) Monocryl suture at 7 d with a minimal inflammatory reaction zone composed of macrophages and fibroblasts. (C) Monocryl suture at 28 d with a slight inflammatory reaction zone composed primarily of macrophages and fibroblasts with a scattering of eosinophils. (D) Monocryl suture at 63 d with a slight inflammatory reaction zone composed primarily of macrophages, fibroblasts, lymphocytes, and plasma cells. (E) At 91 d, the Monocryl suture has been completely absorbed. There is a slight inflammatory reaction zone composed of large, foamy macrophages centrally with fibroblasts, lymphocytes, and plasma cells at the periphery. (F) At 119 d, the Monocryl suture has undergone complete absorption. There is a minimal inflammatory reaction composed of macrophages, fibroblasts, lymphocytes, and plasma cells. (From Bezwada, R.S. et al., *Biomaterials*, 16, 1141, 1995. With permission.)

Table 8.6 Average Sewell Histological Grading of a Variety of Nonabsorbable Sutures

	Silk	Cotton	Nylon	Polypropylene	Dacron	Polydek	Tevdek
Weeks							
1	43.9	47.9	37.5	38.2	39.9	40.6	39.9
2	44.1	48.6	32.8	33.3	31.6	32.2	39.4
4	44.9	45.7	28.8	32.2	29.9	37.8	40.6
Months							
3	38.1	38.6	24.4	19.3	25.4	29.0	40.2
6	35.0	38.9	17.6	20.3	24.6	36.5	35.4
12	32.7	32.6	12.6	22.3	22.2	27.7	22.7
18	31.7	34.5	13.5	15.8	18.8	30.6	30.5
24	33.1	35.4	13.4	21.3	20.2	33.1	25.5

Note: The lowest grade attainable is 9.

From Postlethwait, R.W., *Ann. Surg.*, 171(6), 892, 1970. With permission.

The reaction to cotton in the early periods was similar to that of silk, but cotton evoked a little greater cellular reaction than silk as Postlethwait reported.[87] Granulation tissue was still present at the end of 4 weeks. Foreign body giant cells were also more prominent than with silk. After 1 year, cellular reaction continued and was marked around those sutures whose cotton fibers had begun to separate. This separation and resulting response accounted for the relatively high Sewell tissue reaction grade. There was no evidence of disappearance in the cotton suture.

A more acute reaction to cotton suture was also reported by Castelli et al.[89] in the gingival tissue of rhesus monkeys. Neither silk nor cotton provoked an inflammatory response, but the macrophage and giant cell response was more precocious and pronounced with cotton, especially in the first week of implantation. Castelli et al. suggested that the ability of cotton to induce a more rapid and broad cellular response probably derived from its ability to affect the gingival microenvironment to a more significant degree than did silk and other nonabsorbable sutures.[89] With both cotton and silk, however, there was neither a significant increase in local vascular permeability nor a leukocytic margination and migration into the gingival tissue around the suture tracts.

Postlethwait et al.[30] observed that the tissue reaction to silk and cotton in humans generally was similar to, but less intense, than that seen in experimental animals. The first and most frequent reaction included the development of a fibrous tissue capsule of variable thickness, consisting of layers of histiocytes and giant cells varying in both occurrence and numbers. The second reaction occurred when the suture interstices were invaded by fibroblasts and histiocytes. Evidence of absorption was found in silk as well as cotton.

Salthouse et al.[35] evaluated a series of sutures implanted into rabbit eyes. Silk provoked the greatest cellular reaction and infiltration among all the sutures tested. Table 8.7 summarizes their data. When compared with other nonabsorbable sutures, numerous populations of monocytic and giant cells were seen over most of the periods of implantation (42 d), particularly in sclera and ocular muscle. Tissue reaction associated with monofilament nylon and polypropylene sutures was minimal at all times in cornea, sclera, and ocular muscle. By 90 d, sutures encapsulated with a thin band of fibrous tissue were seen in both sclera and ocular muscle, but not in the cornea. Similar reactivity to polypropylene and nylon sutures was also found in a study by Kelly et al.[91]

Silk suture has been reported to be intensely thrombogenic.[92–94] Because of this characteristic, along with its ready availability, ease in delivery via microcatheters, and soft pliability, silk sutures have been used experimentally as embolic agents for the preoperative treatment of cerebral arteriovenous malformations. Such an endovascular therapy could facilitate the surgical removal of the lesions by reducing blood loss at surgery. However, the intensive inflammatory response of silk sutures has raised concerns in several clinical cases. In a recent study by Deveikis et al., patients using silk suture as an embolic agent revealed prominent intravascular acute inflammatory cell accumulations, extravascular inflammation, and, occasionally, vessel wall necrosis.[94] These intense local inflammatory reactions extended to systemic signs of inflammation like fever and diaphoresis in one clinical case. The symptoms disappeared after the removal of the silk suture. The details of the thrombogenic nature of silk will be given in Section IV.

Table 8.7 Histologic Response of Nonabsorbable Sutures in Ophthalmologic Tissues

Suture and Site	7 d	14 d	21 d	42 d	90 d
Nylon, 10-0 monofilament; cornea	Minimal to slight M+	Minimal M+	Minimal	Minimal	Minimal
Nylon; sclera	Minimal P+ M+	Minimal M+ F+	F+ C	C	C
Nylon; ocular muscle	Minimal to slight P+ M++	Minimal M+ F+	C M+ F+	M++ F+	
Polypropylene, 9-0 monofilament; cornea	Minimal to slight M+	Minimal to moderate M+	Minimal	Minimal	Minimal
Polypropylene; sclera	Minimal P+ M+	Minimal M+ F+	C F+	C	C
Polypropylene; ocular muscle	Minimal M+	Minimal M+ F+	M+ F+	C	C
Silk, black braided 8-0; cornea	Moderate P+ M++	Moderate to marked M++	Moderate to marked M++	Suture degrading M+	Suture absorbed or extruded
Silk; sclera	Moderate P+ M++	Moderate P+ M++	Moderate to marked M+++	Moderate M+ G+	Suture degrading
Silk; ocular muscle	Moderate P+ M++	Moderate to marked M+++ G+'	Moderate to marked M+++ G++ F+	Moderate M++ G+	Suture degrading or degraded

Note: M, monocytic type cells; P, polymorphonuclear cells (heterophils in rabbit); lymphocytes; F, fibroblasts; G, giant cells; and C, collagen fibers forming around suture sites. Cell population is composed of occasional cells (+); moderate population (++); and numerous cells (+++). Arbitrary designations compare tissue response at the suture sites: minimal, slight, moderate, and marked.

From Salthouse, T.N., Matlaga, B.F., and Wykoff, M.H., *Am. J. Ophthalmol.*, 84(2), 225, 1977. With permission.

2. Nylon Sutures

Nylon suture, first introduced in 1940, is a synthetic polyamide polymer fiber. The monofilament form of this suture (Ethilon®, Dermalon®) is the most frequently used nonabsorbable suture in cutaneous wound closure. Nylon suture is renowned for its high tensile strength, excellent elastic properties, minimal tissue reactivity, and low cost. The main disadvantage of using nylon is its prominent memory, which subsequently leads to an increased number of knots needed to hold a given stitch in place. Ethilon can be ordered soaked in alcohol to decrease its memory and increase its pliability. Multifilamentous braided nylon sutures (Nurolon®, Surgilon®) are seldom used in cutaneous wound closure because of a slightly higher infection rate and an increased cost. Nonetheless, the braided design makes them more pliable and easier to handle.

Although nylon is considered a nonabsorbable suture, it still undergoes partial degradation through hydrolysis at a very slow rate. Studies in rabbits have shown that implanted nylon retains 89% of its original tensile strength at 1 year and 72% by 2 years.[86] At this time, the degradation process is apparently stabilized. Moloney[53] found nylon sutures to retain approximately 66% of their original strength after 11 years. Hartman[52] compared monofilament nylon and Vicryl suture as buried sutures and found less

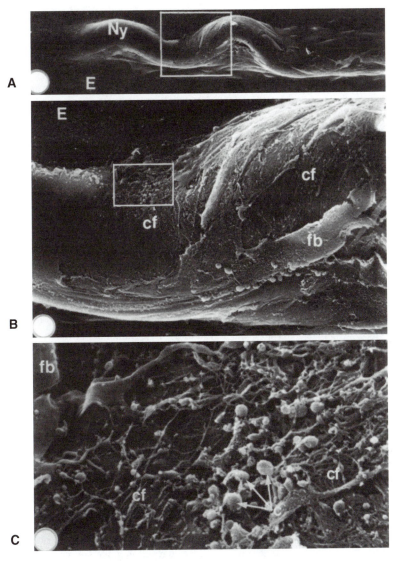

Figure 8.16 Nylon suture partly below and partly above endothelium of rabbit corneas after a 6 week residence. A – 190x. The □ region was magnified and shown in B, 1050x. The suture was covered with a kind of network of collagen fibrils (cf) and inflammatory cells (c) with some fibroblasts (fb) on top, growing in from the bordering endothelium. (E) Normal endothelium. C – is the region marked by □ in B at 5200x. (From Jongebloed, W.S. et al., *Doc. Ophthalmol.*, 75, 351, 1990. With permission.)

clinical inflammatory response with nylon than with similarly placed Vicryl sutures. Clear buried nylon sutures are used by some surgeons to prevent "scar spread" since it retains its tensile strength for such a long time.

Recent reported studies of the tissue reactions of nylon sutures in rabbit cornea, however, indicated that monofilament nylon sutures exhibited far more extensive tissue reaction than stainless steel sutures within a few days postimplantation and the reaction persisted for 4 to 6 weeks.[95–97] This persistent tissue reaction to nylon sutures in cornea showed a unique phenomenon that the nylon sutures must be slowly covered by inflammatory cells, proteinacious organic materials, and collagen fibers before the deposition of fibroblast cells (Figure 8.16).[95] Contrary to nylon sutures, the stainless steel suture was covered with fibroblast cells immediately without the preliminary deposition of collagen materials and showed no inflammatory reaction of epithelium. Jongebloed et al. attributed the observed different level of tissue reactions in rabbit cornea to the different surface free energy of sutures.[97] nylon has low surface free energy, which should discourage cell adhesion and spreading. Thus, nylon requires preadsorbed protein and collagen materials to make its surface more favorable for attracting fibroblasts. High surface free energy materials like stainless steel could promote fibroblast adhesion with or without the presence of preadsorbed organic materials.

3. Polypropylene Sutures

Polypropylene (Prolene, Surgilene®) is an extremely inert suture with a low tissue reactivity and an excellent tensile strength. It has a slippery surface with low adherence to tissue which is ideal for a running intradermal stitch because it tends to slide out smoothly at the time of suture removal. When wound swelling occurs, Prolene suture will stretch to accommodate the wound, thus there will be no cutting through the tissue. When wound swelling recedes, the suture will remain loose. The long-term tissue and cellular responses to the synthetic nonabsorbable sutures were studied by Postlethwait.[87] As shown in Table 8.6, the reaction to monofilament Prolene was similar to that for monofilament nylon with a little more cellular reaction through all time intervals. During the first week, histiocytes and fibroblasts predominated with a few lymphocytes and neutrophils surrounding these two sutures. Clear zones containing mainly unattached histiocytes were seen around both sutures at 2 weeks. Cellular reaction was minimal after 6 months.

Kronenthal,[98] however, reported that monofilament polypropylene sutures caused the least reaction among all available sutures. This difference was attributed to the fact that the polypropylene sutures used by Postlethwait fragmented. Each fragment stimulated its own cellular reaction and increased the overall grade of tissue reaction. Miller[99] reported that polypropylene sutures were biologically inert. Soon after implantation, an early, acute inflammatory reaction, dominated by PMNs, was observed. It was very mild and more transient than for most synthetic nonabsorbable sutures. Connective tissue encapsulation of the suture was early, rapid, and stayed thin for the remainder of the implantation period. Monofilament polypropylene sutures aroused less tissue reaction than stainless steel, which evoked a moderate-to-marked cellular response. Clayman,[100] on the other hand, reported polypropylene sutures to be slightly more reactive than wire. He also found that polypropylene is more rigid than nylon 6 (Supramid®) and may be associated with a higher incidence of sphincter erosion and papillary laceration in eyes receiving iridocapsular, iris clip, or medallion-style lenses.

4. Polyester Sutures

Polyester fibers are polymers that are formed by condensation polymerization. Braided polyesters were manufactured to provide the same high tensile strength and low tissue reactivity as the monofilaments, but with improved qualities in handling and knot security. Polyester sutures are either coated or uncoated. Mersilene® and Dacron are uncoated, braided polyesters that have a rough surface that produces drag when pulled through tissues and when knots are set. In order to ameliorate this problem, coated polyesters such as Ethibond were developed. They are not commonly used, due to relatively higher costs and the susceptibility of the coatings to "cracking" after knots are tied.[90]

Uncoated multifilament Dacron sutures produced a tissue reaction grade similar to those of polypropylene and nylon during the first month of implantation.[87] By 3 months, the sutures were surrounded by a rim of connective tissues with one or two layers of histiocytes next to the suture. Giant cells were rarely seen. Most sutures were tightly encased in fibrous tissue with little cellular reaction after 6 months. The sutures remained compact at 2 years. The Teflon-coated Dacron sutures, Polydek® and Tevdek®, however, elicited more tissue reaction than the uncoated Dacron, due to the occasional dislodged fragments of Teflon. Each fragment of Teflon stimulated an intense cellular reaction. The differences in reaction between Teflon-coated and uncoated Dacron sutures may not be of clinical significance. The reaction consisted mainly of a fibrous tissue capsule as long as no shedding of Teflon occurred.

Postlethwait[87] also examined the tissue reaction of the synthetic nonabsorbable sutures in human beings. All of these sutures were encapsulated by narrow, compact fibrous tissues with occasional histiocytes or giant cells present. Monofilament nylon still produced the least reaction of all sutures examined. No fragmentation was detected after 10 years. Cellular invasion between the filaments of uncoated Dacron did not occur even after 10 years. Teflon-coated Dacron sutures were more reactive due to the Teflon particles mentioned previously.

In other special incidences, such as peripheral nerve repair, nonabsorbable sutures like silk, stainless steel, nylon, and Mersilene were also used in preference to absorbable sutures, based on the lesser degree of cellular infiltration that is often associated with a higher degree of tissue response.[50,57,101,102] Bratton et al.[57] found that both monofilament nylon and PGA sutures were adequate in the performance of perineural intrafascicular suturing. This is because both sutures were in monofilament form and hence did not arouse extracellular reaction due to cellular infiltration into the suture strands.

5. Polybutester Novafil® Suture

Novafil nonabsorbable suture, introduced in 1983, is a thermoplastic copolymer composed of polyglycol terephthalate and polybutylene terephthalate (polybutester).[103] It is a monofilamentous suture that was designed to be stronger, less stiff, and possess a lower friction coefficient then either polypropylene or nylon. Being monofilamentous, it induces little inflammatory reaction when surgically implanted. A unique feature of this copolymer is its elasticity. This suture has the capacity to stretch 50% of its length at loads of only 25% of its knot breaking level.[103] This elasticity at low loads has the clinical advantage of elongation of the suture when wound edema occurs and maintenance of this tension when the edema recedes, which reduces the potential for suture marks and cut-throughs.

In a randomized clinical trial comparing the cosmetic outcome of midline abdominal laparotomy scars using either nylon or Novafil suture for skin closure, Trimbos et al.[104] reported that Novafil sutures caused significantly less scar hypertrophy within 18 months following surgery when compared with nylon sutures. This difference may be explained by the unique elastic properties of Novafil sutures, which allow the sutures to adapt to a far greater extent to increased tension on wound edges. This elastic suture profile was also demonstrated in experiments studying the role of suture materials in abdominal wound dehiscence. Using Novafil, nylon, and PGA sutures to close abdominal wounds in rats, Rodeheaver et al.[103] measured the abdominal wound bursting pressure using a water-filled balloon implanted in the peritoneal cavity. He found a significantly higher intra-abdominal rupture volume with the use of Novafil than with nylon and PGA. Because of its elastic nature, Novafil suture provided an extra margin of safety in closure of abdominal wounds.

6. Polytetrafluoroethylene (Gore-Tex®) Suture

Because Gore-Tex sutures are used mainly in the cardiovascular system, most of the published biocompatibility studies have used such a system to evaluate their tissue reactions. Cavallaro et al. recently reported that Gore-Tex sutures used in the end-to-end anastomoses of the infrarenal aorta of beagle dogs showed tissue reactions as satisfactory as, or even better than polypropylene sutures during the period of 15 to 150 d postoperation.[105] They found that Gore-Tex sutures appeared to be rapidly and fairly accepted by the host tissues and surprisingly no connective tissue ingrowth within Gore-Tex suture fiber was found. An example is illustrated in Figure 8.17.

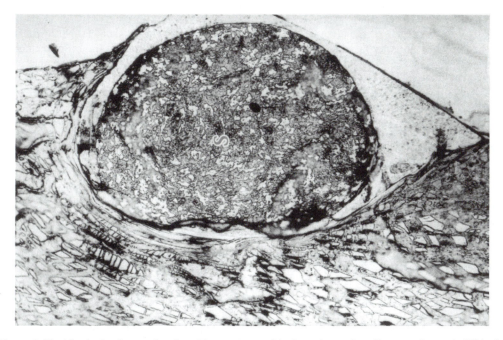

Figure 8.17 Histologic picture of a Gore-Tex suture used in fastening a Gore-Tex vascular graft. "S" is the location of the suture. (Courtesy of W.L. Gore & Associates.)

Recently, Revuelta et al.[106] and David et al.[107] used Gore-Tex sutures for the surgical repair of ruptured or elongated chordae tendineae of the anterior leaflet of the mitral valves by replacing the chordae tendineae with the Gore-Tex sutures. After 3 months of implantation in sheep, the chordae made of Gore-Tex suture was completely surrounded by a sheath with either no adverse tissue reaction or a mild inflammatory cell reaction of the mononuclear type at the sheath-suture interface.[106] There was no sign of microscopic calcification at the Gore-Tex chordae. The sheath had three layers: an inner dense concentric core of collagenous tissue with bundles arranged parallel to the longitudinal direction of the Gore-Tex suture, a loose spongiosa as the middle layer, and endothelium on the surface of the regenerated chorda without platelet accumulation or thrombus formation. Revuelta et al. thus suggested that owing to the good biocompatibility and tissue regeneration capability, Gore-Tex suture could be a viable alternative as a stent for the formation of chordae tendineae with a structure similar to the native one. When experimenting in human beings, David et al. reported that the replacement of diseased chordae tendineae of 43 patients with Gore-Tex sutures is a simple means to reconstructing mitral valves in patients who would otherwise require a more tedious, complicated, and costly surgical replacement of mitral valves by prosthetic valves.[107] Histologic evaluation of a 9-month-old Gore-Tex chordae retrieved from a patient showed that the interstices of Gore-Tex suture had plasma proteins. Contrary to the histologic findings in animals, the portion of the Gore-Tex chordae in human beings that was not in contact with the leaflets and papillary muscles was not covered by any cellular components. No thrombi were found on the surface of Gore-Tex suture chordae.

7. Carbon Fiber Sutures

Information on the tissue response to carbon fiber sutures, particularly at the cellular level, is sparse due to the infrequent use of carbon fiber sutures for wound closure. Most of the biocompatibility data on carbon fibers have been obtained from carbon implants for orthopedic and dental purposes. Although carbon implants are generally recognized to elicit minimal foreign body reaction,[108] it is premature to extrapolate these data to carbon fiber sutures, even given the well-established fact that the physical form of a material largely determines the type and extent of tissue response to that material. Carbon fibers for suture use experience mechanical forces different from most carbon implants. This difference in mechanical forces could induce a different type of tissue response.

One of the most representative works on the biocompatibility of carbon fiber sutures was the study by Brown and Pool[109] of the use of braided carbon fiber sutures to repair surgically transected or lacerated digital flexor tendons in 20 mature horses. After 1 month, foreign body reaction was found to be limited to a 1 mm wide zone of granulation tissue surrounding the carbon sutures. Histiocytes and lymphocytes were the predominant cell types. Foreign body giant cells were not frequently observed. Carbon filaments were occasionally separated and infiltrated by fibroblasts, histiocytes, and lymphocytes. No eosinophils, however, were found. They noted a few fragments of carbon fiber in the cortical sinuses of the cubital lymph nodes by 1 month. The number of fragments increased with time, and as time went on, they came to be found in the axillary lymph nodes, where they were not initially observed. Free carbon fragments, up to 300 mm in size, were also found in the sinuses and cortical parenchyma of the nodes. There was, however, no inflammatory response immediately around the fragments. This lack of an inflammatory reaction in the lymph nodes, identified by Brown and Pool,[109] indicates that the stimulation was peripheral. Because carbon fibers were washed with acetone to remove polymers prior to autoclaving, their study did not find reactions such as tissue eosinophilia normally associated with carbon implants.

II. GRANULOMA FORMATION

A suture granuloma is a granulomatous reaction around buried suture material, of clinical relevance particularly in the superficial layers of the skin. Most granulomas are minor and consist of a layer of macrophages adherent to the suture material, surrounded by a few fibroblast cells and a thin fibrous capsule. The formation of granulomas is related to the chronic inflammatory reaction caused by suture materials. The amount of cellular invasion between suture materials varies and seems to increase with time. This response is not usually clinically apparent and does not interfere with successful wound healing. When an amplified response occurs, it generally presents as a draining tract or superficial area of inflammation along the suture line during the postoperative period. In a microscopic study of healed human wounds, Postlethwait[87] noted that there was significantly more inflammatory reaction to silk and cotton, less so with Dacron, and least with nylon and wire, as evidenced by the presence of histiocytes, giant cells, and suture invasion by monocytes. LoCicero et al.[110] noted that following abdominal fascial closure, there was a significant increase in suture granuloma formation with braided nonabsorbable sutures compared with monofilament materials. Absorbable sutures do not usually give rise to suture granulomas except for catgut sutures, particularly chromic catgut.[111]

With a more intense inflammatory reaction, or in a chronic suture granuloma, a discharging sinus or a mass can form, which only resolves when the suture is removed or extruded. This could be undesirable following herniorrhaphy. Several investigators have reported that chronic inflammatory reactions secondary to suture granulomas following herniorrhaphy may lead to the erosion of nonabsorbable sutures into surrounding urinary tract structures. Flood and Beard[112] noted two patients who complained of dysuria, hematuria, and suprapubic pain following either inguinal or femoral hernia repair with silk sutures eventually developed large paravesical masses. Histological examination of the paravesical masses revealed chronic granulomatous changes with silk sutures noted within the center of these granulomas, and erosion of suture materials into the urinary bladder walls. Symptoms improved with the removal of silk sutures and the drainage of associated abscesses. Lynch et al.[113] reported a patient with inguinal pain and a pelvic mass following herniorrhaphy which mimicked a carcinoma. Biopsy revealed a suture granuloma involving bladder wall, further emphasizing the importance of considering a suture granuloma in the differential diagnosis complicating previous inguinal surgery.[114]

Since suture granulomas are a common entity secondary to nonabsorbable suture materials,[87] they can occur anywhere in the body. Several investigators have reported that suture granulomas in the gastrointestinal tract may be asymptomatic and found incidentally in routine X-ray studies. Sander and Woesner[115] observed a case of suture granuloma of the stomach following splenectomy. Belleza and Lowman[116] reported a similar case of a silk suture granuloma occurring in the stomach following total colectomy. Both of these cases emphasized the possibility of suture granuloma formation away from an organ that underwent primary surgery. Al-tawil et al.[117] reported an incidentally discovered esophageal suture granuloma following a fundoplication for chronic gastroesophageal reflux. Gueler et al.[118] reported four patients with suture granulomas of the stomach following repairs of perforated duodenal ulcers using silk sutures. Suture granulomas were discovered using either endoscopic examinations or contrast X-ray studies.

Occasionally, physicians are faced with a diagnostic challenge in patients with suture granulomas in the biliary tract who develop symptoms of biliary tract obstruction mimicking signs of a neoplasm. Murphy et al.[119] reported a patient who developed jaundice, weight loss, and abdominal pain 17 years following the resection of a duodenal leiomyosarcoma. With preoperative endoscopy and contrast X-rays suggesting a cholangiocarcinoma, the patient underwent surgical exploration and was found to have a suture granuloma with surrounding fibrosis within the common bile duct, without any evidence of malignancy. Gleeson and McMullin[120] reported a similar case in which a patient developed symptoms of obstructive jaundice suggestive of a cholangiocarcinoma 18 years following cholecystectomy. Histological analysis of the mass revealed a silk suture granuloma with surrounding fibrosis and foreign body giant cells without any evidence of malignancy. Therefore, with the clinical presentation and a cholangiogram showing signs consistent with a cholangiocarcinoma, one should consider suture granuloma of the biliary tract in the differential diagnosis in patients with prior history of biliary or upper abdominal surgery.

The presence of suture granuloma due to nonabsorbable sutures in head and neck surgery has also been found to cause considerable tissue reaction and morbidity. In a retrospective study over an 8-year period, Eldridge and Wheeler[121] noted no granulomas among 193 patients who underwent thyroid surgery using absorbable sutures. However, among 526 patients who underwent thyroid surgery using silk sutures, 40 patients developed suture granulomas; an incidence of 8%. Over 65% of these patients required one or more operations due to complications arising from suture granulomas. Eldridge and Wheeler also noted a high incidence of suture granuloma following surgery for Grave's disease — 13% compared with 8% overall. This high incidence of suture granuloma formation following subtotal thyroid procedure may be related to the use of silk ligatures as a technique of achieving hemostasis.

Suture granulomas have also been reported as a result of dental procedures. Manor and Kaffe[122] reported a case of suture granuloma from a fragment of silk suture left in place 6 weeks following a free gingival autograft. Brunsvold et al.[123] also reported a similar case of suture granuloma from a silk suture left accidentally in the alveolar mucosa following a dental procedure. The granuloma later became infected and developed into a drainage tract. The wounds were healed uneventfully following the removal of the offending suture.

Suture granulomas were also found in pulmonary operations. Baumgartner and Mark[124] reported an incidence of 4.4% of this type of complication in 181 pulmonary resections using Tevdek suture materials to close the bronchial stumps. Granulation tissue around the loosened sutures was observed. The authors attributed the inflammatory reaction to the suture material, which led to the emergence of new symptoms, such as hemoptysis, wheezing, nonproductive cough, and the expectoration of suture materials. The suture-induced tissue reaction, which impairs bronchial stump healing, has been recognized since the beginning of pulmonary operations. Absorbable sutures have been considered to be more suitable than nonabsorbable ones in bronchial closure. Sherman and Conant[125] reported that fewer bronchopleural fistulas occurred with the use of chromic catgut suture for bronchial closure than with silk. Jack[126] reported a similar trend of reduction in the number of bronchopleural fistulas when chromic catgut was used in pulmonary resections. Albertini[127] was also observed that exposed endobronchial sutures were responsible for the persistent cough of five patients with histories of resectional lung surgery. He pointed out that suture materials, like any other foreign body in the bronchus, could likely migrate to the bronchial lumen during the healing process and lead to infection, granuloma formation, and cough.

Other uncommon presentations of suture granulomas include fine needle aspirates of breast tissue mimicking malignancy.[128] Maygarden et al.[128] reported three cases of suture granulomas of the breast area following surgical resection of carcinoma. Fine needle aspiration cytology hinted at disease recurrence. The predominance of spindled cells and dissimilarity to the original tumors helped in cytologically distinguishing these granulomas from recurrent carcinoma. Frumkin et al.[129] also reported a delayed tissue inflammatory reaction to absorbable suture material simulating melanoma following severe scalp and facial trauma. Nodular melanoma was suspected, but further microscopic examination proved the lesion to be a granuloma with transepidermal elimination of exogenous filamentous suture material.

III. WOUND INFECTION

A. FREQUENCY OF WOUND INFECTION

The development of postoperative wound infection often retards normal wound healing. It has been well established that the presence of foreign materials of either synthetic or natural origin in a wound significantly enhances the susceptibility of surrounding tissues to infection. Among all foreign materials, suture materials are the most important, because they are used in almost all wound closures, and many distressing complications such as infection, wound disruption, and chronic sinus formation occur in sutured wounds. The majority of surgical infection begins in the vicinity of the suture lines, and then extend to other portions of the body via the vascular and/or lymphatic systems. In other words, suture materials may contribute greatly to the genesis of surgical infections. It has been shown by Elek and Conen[130] that the number of *Staphylococcus aureus* that are needed to establish infection can be reduced 10,000-fold by the presence of silk suture. The concentration of *S. aureus* necessary to induce pus formation dropped to 1×10^2 from 1×10^6 due to the presence of silk sutures. It is also important to recognize that even the most biocompatible suture materials tend to elicit some degree of surgical infection in tissues contaminated with microorganisms. Edlich et al.[131] reported that the percentage of gross infection in mice with nylon-sutured surgical wounds was considerably higher than in needle tracks of control mice (53.7% and 0%, respectively, for *S. aureus* and 70.8% and 0%, respectively, for *Escherichia coli*).

B. ROLE OF SUTURES IN WOUND INFECTION

Suture materials vary in their propensity to produce bacterial infection in surgical wounds. The physical configuration of the suture thread has been suggested to be an important factor in determining its susceptibility to surgical infection.[132–134] Alexander et al.[132] found no significant difference in the severity of infection by *S. aureus* among multifilament nonabsorbable sutures, silk (braided, uncoated, and siliconized), braided nylon, twisted cotton, and stainless steel. Sutures in multifilament form resulted in higher wound infection than the same sutures in monofilament form, as shown in Figure 8.18. Twisted silk sutures produced more infection than braided silk because of the rather loose arrangement of the fibers in the twisted form.

Blomstedt and Osterberg[133] also observed that surgical infection rates were higher for multifilament sutures with high capillary capacity than for noncapillary sutures. The viable bacterial count recovered from the implanted monofilament noncapillary polypropylene sutures, after 41 d in rat muscle, showed a significant decrease from the initial injected amount (i.e., from 2.5×10^7 to 2.1×10^3), while with multifilament twisted nylon sutures that support capillary action, the bacteria roughly maintained their

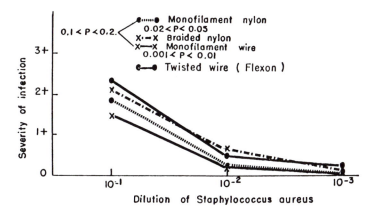

Figure 8.18 Comparison of severity of wound infection of monofilament nylon, braided nylon, monofilament wire, and multifilament twisted wire. (From Alexander, J.W. et al., *Ann. Surg.*, 165, 192, 1967. With permission.)

initial numbers (1.2×10^7 to 0.3×10^7).[133] The corresponding number of viable bacteria recovered from controls (no sutures) was significantly lower (<25) than with either suture. The results of these viable bacterial counts were consistent with the study by Osterberg and Blomstedt[134] of the level of inflammatory cell reaction near implanted and infected suture sites. Both a greater intensity and a longer duration of reaction were found around capillary threads than around noncapillary materials. Bucknall and Ellis[135] also examined the role of the physical structure of sutures on the number of bacteria (*S. aureus*) taken up by four types of sutures (silk, PGA, multifilament and monofilament nylon) and found that braided sutures like silk and nylon took up three times more *S. aureus* than monofilament nylon suture. They concluded that it is the physical structure of a suture that controls the amount of bacteria that a suture attracts.

The data reported above demonstrate that the physical structure of the nonabsorbable sutures is more important in inducing wound infection than the chemical constituents (including coating materials). It has been postulated that due to the topology of the multifilament suture, it is difficult for inflammatory cells to reach the bacteria hiding deep in the interstices of the multifilament suture. Hence, phagocytic activity is retarded. It has also been suggested that multifilament sutures induce stronger tissue reactions, and hence weaken the tissue's defense toward bacteria. Thus, the degree of enhancement of infection by a suture is parallel to the degree of inflammatory reaction caused by the suture. The superior resistance to infection of chromic and iodized catgut sutures, compared to plain catgut sutures, further demonstrates this point of view. The capillarity of the multifilament sutures, of course, is also related to their propensity to wound infection.

Edlich et al.[131] achieved contrary results and concluded that the chemical structure of suture materials appeared to be the most important factor in the development of surgical infection, while physical configuration played a relatively unimportant role. Nylon and polypropylene sutures had the lowest incidence of infection among all the nonabsorbable sutures. Dacron sutures elicited the next lowest degree of infection in contaminated subdermal wounds, followed by stainless steel. Silk and cotton sutures were the worst performers, with a distinct propensity toward wound infection. Among the absorbable sutures, the infection rate for contaminated tissues containing PGA was significantly lower than for catgut sutures. Suture coatings did not alter the incidence of early infection in the contaminated tissue. Edlich's conclusion was further supported by the work of Varma et al.,[136,137] in which seven suture materials were implanted in surgical wounds inoculated with three dilutions of *S. aureus*. Mono- and multifilament steel, irrespective of physical configuration, elicited the least acute infection of all sutures. Varma et al.[138] also conducted a comparative histopathologic study of different sutures in infected wounds of dogs at various stages. In general, neutrophils were the predominant cell until 6 d after the onset of acute infection, but macrophages and fibroblasts predominated later, as shown in Table 8.8. However, there were large numbers of neutrophils present even in chronic implantation (at 40 d) of plain and chromic catgut, silk, and Mersilene sutures. This suggests a persistence of local infection. These sutures also elicited the greatest tissue response, as evidenced grossly by suture-induced granulomas. At the same time interval (40 d), neutrophils were minimal in the infected surgical wounds with steel, Dexon, and monofilament nylon.

Table 8.8 Mean Relative Cell Counts in Infected Surgical Wounds Implanted with Various Suture Materials

Dilution of Inoculum	Cell Type	Suture Materials							
		Control	Steel	Nylon	Silk	Mersilene	Dexon	Plain Catgut	Chromic Catgut
1:1	Neutrophils	78, 55, 40, a	44, 42, 5, 1	48, 15, 5, 0	59, 55, 59, 31	73, 66, 68, 40	83, 52, 36, 1	63, 51, 42, 33	63, 47, 40, 34
	Macrophages	11, 34, 40, a	45, 40, 52, 45	34, 53, 58, 50	20, 30 26, 38	20, 20, 22, 39	3, 32, 46, 33	11, 20, 24, 37	20, 25, 27, 34
	Fibroblasts	9, 6, 16, a	10, 17, 38, 45	15, 28, 32, 49	15, 13, 12, 23	4, 10, 10, 20	3, 11, 10, 57	17, 25, 30, 26	15, 22, 30, 26
1:10	Neutrophils	78, 50, 28, a	33, 13, 8, 1	60, 8, 3, 3	65, 60, 56, 40	53, 30, 46, 35	69, 35, 28, 1	56, 54, 40, 20	67, 58, 35, 13
	Macrophages	17, 35, 43, a	48, 60, 58, 40	30, 38, 35, 32	14, 13, 23, 36	21, 50, 42, 38	17, 48, 57, 57	28, 26, 30, 42	27, 28, 30, 33
	Fibroblasts	2, 15, 24, a	16, 23, 26, 58	8, 48, 60, 57	15, 18, 16, 20	20, 15, 10, 21	6, 12, 11, 30	16, 18, 21, 34	6, 10, 23, 44
1:100	Neutrophils	a, a, a, a	20, 10, 41, 1	60, 20, 3, 1	58, 25, 20, 37	55, 20, 5, 3	58, 41, 14, 1	56, 61, 38, 3	62, 52, 33, 4
	Macrophages	a, a, a, a	47, 54, 50, 31	15, 30, 39, 28	30, 56, 60, 37	30, 40, 52, 54	12, 29, 60, 44	24, 15, 37, 42	20, 24, 35, 45
	Fibroblasts	a, a, a, a	31, 32, 43, 67	25, 40, 57, 67	5, 15, 16, 20	12, 25, 34, 33	12, 18, 21, 49	10, 20, 20, 47	16, 21, 25, 45

Note: Data are expressed as mean for each of four different times after implantation (6, 10, 20, and 40 d). Each mean is expressed as a percentage of five microscopic fields (0.135 mm) in each of four dogs.

a, no detectable lesions in the histopathologic sections.

From Varma, S., Johnson, L.W., Ferguson, H.L., and Lumb, W.V., *Am. J. Vet. Res.*, 42(4), 563, 1981. With permission.

Table 8.9 Suture Resistance to Infection

Suture	Points
Plain catgut	58
Chromic catgut	46
Dexon	12
Dexon-S	18
Vicryl	20
Silk (Multil.)	38
Cotton	47
Surgilon (Multil.)	24
Nurolon (Multil.)	22
Ethibond (Multil.)	22
Ti-Cron (Multil.)	23
Stainless steel (Multil.)	21
Stainless steel (Mono.)	17
Surgilene (Mono.)	21
Prolene (Mono.)	20
Ethilon (Mono.)	20

Data from Sharp, W.V., Belden, T.A., King, P.H., and Teague, P.C., *Surgery*, 91(1), 61, 1982.

Using Edlich's mouse model, Sharp et al.[139] studied the resistance of 16 types of 3/0 natural and synthetic suture materials to both *S. aureus* and *E. coli*. They used a point system for both macroscopic and microscopic observations; the final grade for a suture was a summation of both observations. The lower the point total, the more resistant the suture was to infection. Table 8.9 summarizes their results and demonstrates the superiority of the synthetic sutures in resistance to infection. The synthetic monofilament nonabsorbable and braided absorbable sutures performed better than synthetic braided nonabsorbable sutures. Among all the suture materials tested, plain catgut was the worst offender, followed by chromic catgut. Dexon sutures were the most resistant (the lowest in score). The presence or absence of suture coatings did not appear to have any effect on their propensity toward infection. Sharp et al.[139] consequently advised against the use of natural sutures in the presence of infection.

C. BACTERIAL ADHERENCE

Recently, it has been suggested by several investigators that the preferential adherence of bacteria to suture materials might be linked to their propensity toward wound infection.[140–143] Chu and Williams[140] used radiolabeled *E. coli* and *S. aureus* and scanning electron microscopy to examine the preferential adherence of bacteria to ten sutures quantitatively and qualitatively. A wide range of bacterial adherence to suture materials was observed according to the variety of suture material, the type of bacteria, and the duration of contact. Among the absorbable suture materials, as shown in Figure 8.19, polydioxanone (PDS) suture had the least affinity toward *S. aureus* and *E. coli* due to its monofilament configuration and hydrophobicity. Dexon sutures, however, had the highest affinity toward these two bacteria because of their braided structure and relative hydrophilicity. The data also indicated that the chemical nature of the suture was the major factor contributing to bacterial attachment. *S. aureus* was found to adhere to sutures more readily than *E. coli*, which may be due to the difference in cell wall structure and cell motility. The attachment of bacteria on a suture surface was not time-independent, but, in fact, a dynamic phenomenon. This suggests that the process of bacterial attachment is reversible. The mechanism of this reversible adherence was thought to be the balance between the electrical double-layer repulsion energies at different electrolyte concentrations and van der Waals attractive energies. The motility of the bacteria, of course, could also contribute to this reversible mechanism.

Sugarman and Musher[141] reported a similar time-dependent bacterial adherence, but a nonlinear continuous increase in adherent bacteria with the duration of contact was observed. The magnitude of this increase was largest during the early period of exposure. They also found that more than 100× as many bacteria adhered to plain catgut as to monofilament nylon sutures of the same diameter. Adherence to PGA or silk was intermediate. This indicates again that surface area, or physical configuration, is not the major factor of bacterial adherence.

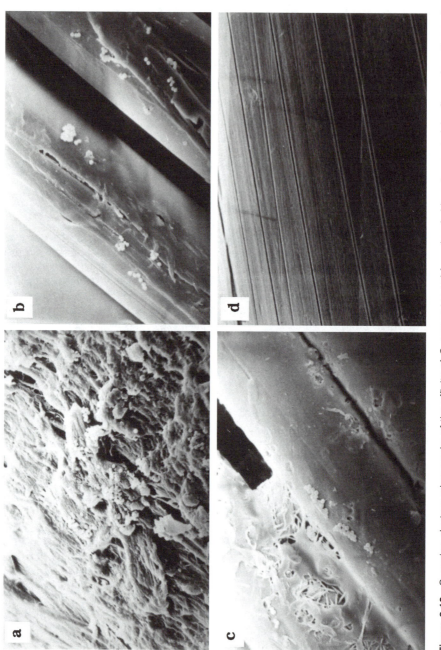

Figure 8.19 Scanning electron micrographs of the affinity of *S. aureus* toward four absorbable suture materials after various times of contact. (a) Catgut, (b) Dexon, (c) Vicryl, (d) PDS. (From Chu, C.C. and Williams, D.F., *Am. J. Surg.*, 147, 19, 1984. With permission.)

Katz et al.[142] used *in vitro* adherence assays and revealed that monofilament nylon sutures supported the fewest of adherent bacteria, whereas the affinity of bacteria to other suture materials was found to increase in the following order: Nurolon, Surgilon, chromic catgut, Ti-Cron, linen, silk, plain catgut, and Dexon, as indicated in Table 8.10. The adherence data correlated well with the degree of infection obtained in mice in the presence of different sutures. Recently, Howell et al.[143] compared the effects of nonabsorbable suture (nylon, Prolene) and cyanoacrylate tissue adhesive on bacterial counts in contaminated wounds and found wounds closed with adhesive alone had significantly lower bacterial counts than wounds containing suture material. The results of this time-kill study were consistent with a bacteriostatic adhesive effect of the cyanoacrylate against *S. aureus*.

Does the recently developed expanded polytetrafluoroethylene (Gore-Tex) suture have a different propensity toward suture-related wound infection compared to other sutures? Paterson-Brown et al.[144] recently examined the role of five suture materials (Gore-Tex, Prolene, PDS, Dexon, and Vicryl) in *E. coli-* and *Bacteroides fragilis*-contaminated (5×10^5 microorganisms) wounds of female guinea pigs. They demonstrated that Gore-Tex suture was no different from other suture materials in terms of its ability to increase the incidence of infection. All sutures, except Dexon, showed about 50% wound infection rate, while controls had only 26%. This difference between the sutures and controls was statistically significant at $P < .01$. Dexon suture had the lowest incidence of wound infection (41%) among all five sutures tested, but the difference was not statistically significant.

D. INFECTION-RELATED SINUS FORMATION

Infected wounds can develop sinuses. Although suture sinuses delay the full recovery of patients from operations, they have received little attention in recent surgical literature. Cutler and Dunphy[145] showed that the frequency of this complication was directly related to the degree of contamination: 2.3% in clean wounds, 11% in contaminated wounds, and 80% in infected wounds closed with silk. Bucknall and Ellis[146] showed a highly significant relationship between sinus formation and postoperative wound infection. Up to 86.4% of the patients who developed sinuses had a proven postoperative wound infection prior to the development of the sinus. With clean wounds, Shouldice et al.[147] showed that even monofilament stainless steel suture rarely produced suture sinuses; but sinuses formed when the suture broke.[148]

As the name implies, suture sinuses are associated with the presence of suture materials in the wound, with nonabsorbable sutures a particular problem. Corman et al.[149] reported that 9% of 102 patients whose wounds were closed with multifilament or monofilament nonabsorbable sutures developed suture sinuses, whereas no sinuses were found in 59 wounds closed with Vicryl suture. Bucknall et al.,[146] however, found that the incidence of sinus formation with absorbable sutures (i.e., 11.5% with PGA) was statistically similar to that with nonabsorbable sutures (i.e., 9.4% with monofilament nylon) in abdominal wound closure, presumably due to infection delaying the absorption of PGA sutures, and hence making them act as foreign bodies. Their results appear to be contradictory to those of Leaper et al.[148] and Bentley et al.[150] Leaper et al.[148] reported that there were no occurrences of suture sinuses in 121 cases of abdominal wound closure with PGA suture, while there was one occurrence with nylon suture and three occurrences with stainless steel suture. Bentley et al.[150] found only one occurrence among 814 abdominal wounds closed with PGA sutures where a suture sinus developed.

Among the nonabsorbable sutures, multifilament forms have long been considered to induce suture sinuses more frequently than monofilament ones.[151–155] For example, Haxton[155] closed 300 abdominal wounds without a single sinus developing, even though some of the wounds were infected. This classical observation has recently been challenged by several studies which indicate that monofilament nonabsorbable sutures also induce a high percentage of suture sinuses.[149,156] Greaney[156] reported that 26 of 31 suture sinuses (84%) in abdominal wounds were associated with monofilament nylon and polypropylene suture. Corman et al.[149] reported that 5.7% of wounds closed with monofilament Prolene sutures developed suture sinuses.

An important question is why bacteria enter wounds and remain beyond the reach of the host defense system in the presence of monofilament suture materials. Several hypotheses have been proposed. Greaney[156] suggested that the interstice of the knots, particularly large ones, often associated with monofilament sutures, may be responsible for the isolation of bacteria from host defense mechanisms, but no experimental data available in the literature prove the hypothesis that a knot could serve as a nidus of infection from which a wound sinus may develop. Bucknall[157] believed that movement of a monofilament suture produces a space between the suture and the surrounding fibrous capsule in which bacteria can survive. The problem with this hypothesis is that it is difficult to understand how bacteria

Table 8.10 Adherence of Bacteria to Surgical Sutures

Suture Type	Nature of Material	S. aureus[a] Cells per 3 cm	E. coli[b] Cells per 3 cm	S. marcescens[c] Cells per 3 cm	S. dysentariae[c] Cells per 3 cm	B. fragilis[a] Cells per 3 cm
Chromic (monofilament)	Natural catgut (absorbable)	$(1.5 \pm 0.2) \times 10^7$	$(3.6 \pm 0.4) \times 10^6$	$(6.8 \pm 1.0) \times 10^6$	$(1.7 \pm 0.2) \times 10^5$	$(1.3 \pm 0.2) \times 10^7$
Dexon (braided)	Polyglycolide (absorbable)	$(5.1 \pm 0.5) \times 10^7$	$(1.2 \pm 0.2) \times 10^7$	$(2.7 \pm 0.4) \times 10^7$	$(3.9 \pm 0.5) \times 10^6$	$(2.6 \pm 0.5) \times 10^7$
Nurolon (braided)	Polyamide (6,6) (nonabsorbable)	$(7.5 \pm 1.0) \times 10^4$	$(1.6 \pm 0.3) \times 10^6$	$(6.1 \pm 1.0) \times 10^6$	$(1.9 \pm 0.2) \times 10^6$	$(1.1 \pm 0.2) \times 10^7$
Nylon (monofilament)	Polyamide (6,6) (nonabsorbable)	$(7.1 \pm 0.8) \times 10^6$	$(1.2 \pm 0.3) \times 10^6$	$(3.4 \pm 0.5) \times 10^6$	$(5.4 \pm 0.7) \times 10^6$	$(4.3 \pm 0.4) \times 10^6$
Silk (braided)	Natural fiber (nonabsorbable)	$(2.5 \pm 0.4) \times 10^7$	$(5.2 \pm 0.6) \times 10^6$	$(1.6 \pm 0.2) \times 10^7$	$(2.0 \pm 0.2) \times 10^6$	$(1.5 \pm 0.2) \times 10^7$
Ti-Cron (braided)	Silicone treated	$(2.4 \pm 0.5) \times 10^7$	$(5.0 \pm 0.6) \times 10^6$	$(1.4 \pm 0.2) \times 10^7$	$(1.8 \pm 0.2) \times 10^6$	$(1.4 \pm 0.2) \times 10^7$

[a] $n = 20$.
[b] $n = 6$.
[c] $n = 4$.

From Katz, S., Izbar, M., and Mirelman, D., *Ann. Surg.*, 194(1), 35, 1981. With permission.

could survive in the presence of the host defense before the formation of the fibrous capsule. This could happen only if a fibrous capsule encloses the suture very early in the healing process so that bacteria are protected from body defenses. Everett[152] suggested that a mechanical property of the suture (rigidity) appears to determine the development of a wound sinus in some cases. This concept of mechanical irritation due to the stiffness of the suture was also reported by Haxton,[155] who revealed that chronic sinuses were almost never found in wounds closed with fine monofilament nylon sutures (number 3/0 and 5/0), but were common with a thicker gauge. Everett[151] also suggested that the ends of a knot, if they protrude, may also cause irritation and hence sinus formation. This is most likely to occur if the ends project into the mobile subcutaneous tissues. He concluded that the danger of sinus formation exists with all nonabsorbable suture materials, and to a greater extent with multifilament sutures. The incidence of sinuses when monofilament sutures are used, however, is small, provided fine and flexible sutures are used and the ends are buried or cut flush with the knot. It is important, however, that the ends should not be cut too short, otherwise the knot may unravel.

The stiffness of nonabsorbable suture cut ends has also been found to cause considerable tissue reaction, particularly in ophthalmic surgery. In a retrospective study of 18 patients, Nirankari et al.[158] found that the exposed, stiff 10-0 monofilament nylon and Prolene suture ends produced conjunctival granuloma, tarsal ulceration, giant papillary conjunctivitis, corneal infiltrate, corneal vascularization, contact lens intolerance, foreign body sensation, and pain. Trimming the suture ends or removing the offending sutures resulted in the immediate relief of all symptoms. Sugar and Meyer[159] also reported similar symptoms of giant papillary conjunctivitis after keratoplasty and attributed this to mechanical irritation produced by the stiff protruding ends of monofilament sutures. This suture-end irritation has also been found in other branches of surgery. Reynolds[160] found that no. 1 nylon suture tail was responsible for femoral nerve injury after inguinal herniorrhaphy. The suture tail stuck through the substance of the femoral nerve and a neurological defect was observed. Removal of the offending suture cleared the defects.

IV. THROMBOGENICITY

The success of cardiovascular surgery, including anastomoses of arteries and veins, and the anchorage of prosthetic heart valves, partially depends on the thrombogenicity of suture materials. Due to the broad range of chemical, physical, and biological characteristics of currently available suture materials, a wide range of thrombogenicity of these suture materials would be expected. A study of five 10/0 suture materials (Prolene, Mersilene, Vicryl, silk, and Ethilon) by Dahlke et al.[161] using scanning electron microscopy, has shown that polypropylene was the most blood-compatible material and silk the most thrombogenic. Ethilon showed deposits of platelets and fibrin on its surface during the first 3 weeks after implantation. Uncoated polyester sutures exhibited a fairly satisfactory nonthrombogenicity and displayed minimal traces of fibrin on their surface at 14 d after implantation. Vicryl sutures showed a thrombogenicity similar to Mersilene at 3 d, as evident in Figure 8.20, and were covered extensively by platelets with slender extrusions and irregularly shrunken erythrocytes at 7 d and thereafter. At 56 d, Vicryl sutures were entirely covered by neointima. It is believed that the degradation properties, particularly the chemical nature of the degradation products of Vicryl sutures, may modify their thrombogenicity according to the length of implantation. Table 8.11 summarizes the thrombogenicity of the five sutures. The difference in thrombogenicity among the five sutures, however, became small with an increase in the duration of implantation. It appears that the chemical characteristics of the sutures and their surfaces contribute to the large differences in thromboresistance, particularly in the early period of implantation. Pham et al.[162] illustrate this point by describing a case of thrombus formation at the left atrial Prolene suture line of a patient after undergoing a bilateral sequential single lung transplantation.

Although the blood biocompatibility of carbon sutures has not been reported in the literature, blood-carbon interaction has been investigated extensively. Because the thromboresistance of a material is largely a function of chemical factors, the results of blood biocompatibility with carbon implants could provide an indication of the biocompatibility of carbon sutures and blood. Bokros et al.[163] have reported that smooth polished LTI (low temperature isotropic) pyrolytic carbons have excellent thromboresistance when implanted in the canine superior vena cava. Salzman et al.[164] used the amount of adherence of platelets to carbon as an indicator of blood biocompatibility. They found that adherence to carbon was high, but release of platelet constituents was minimal. Surface treatment of carbon beads with albumin led to both low retention of platelets and low release of platelet constituents. Thus, the carbon surface

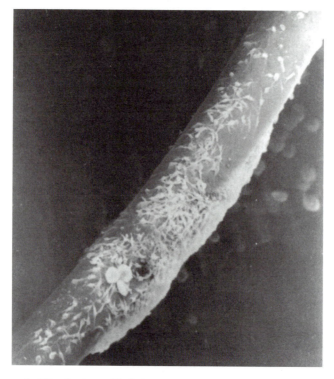

Figure 8.20 A fragment of Vicryl suture with distinct deposition of platelets with dendritic processes 3 d after implantation. ×700. (From Dahlke, H. et al., *J. Biomed. Mater. Res.*, 14, 251, 1980. With permission.)

Table 8.11 Comparison of Thrombogenicity of Five Suture Materials

Suture Material	Days Postimplantation				
	3	**7**	**14**	**28**	**56**
Prolene	±	±	±	+	+
Silk	++++	++++	++	+	±
Ethilon	+++	+++	++	++	±
Vicryl	+++	++	++	++	±
Mersilene	+++	+	+	±	±

Note: Thrombogenicity grading: ++++, strong; +++, moderate; ++, slight; +, poor; ±, trace; -, none.

From Dahlke, H., Dociu, N., and Thurau, J.J., *J. Biomed. Mater. Res.*, 14, 251, 1980. With permission.

is modified, after contact with blood, toward a more thromboresistant condition, through a mechanism that is not fully understood. If the oxidation of the carbon in the finishing stage is too severe, hence making the surface of the carbon fiber rough, this could impair thromboresistance by producing a rough surface.[165] It is believed, however, that surface energy alone does not dictate the thromboresistance of a material.

Biomaterials, when exposed to flowing blood either *in vivo* or *in vitro*, are rapidly covered with a dense coating of platelets. Johnson et al.[166] found that lower-molecular-weight proteins such as hemoglobin and albumin, when administered to a polypropylene (7/0 Prolene) suture during vessel passage, play a role in the prevention of fibrinogen adsorption to sutures, hence reducing the ability of platelet suture attachment. These results suggest that vessel-passed sutures are relatively protected from platelet deposition, at least in the short term, and that this effect is more powerful than prostaglandin E_1, one of the most potent soluble platelet antagonists.[167]

Table 8.12 Incidence of Urinary Concretions in Rabbit Bladders Repaired with
Various Suture Materials

Suture Material	Days						
	3	7	14	30	60	90	120
Polyglycolide	4/4	4/4	0/2	0/2	0/2	0/2	0/2
Medium chromic catgut	3/4	4/4	0/2	0/2	0/2	0/2	0/2
Black braided silk	0/4	3/4	2/2	5/5	2/2	2/2	2/2
Braided polyester, silicone treated	—	—	—	1/2	2/2	2/2	2/2
Braided polyester, Teflon coated	—	—	—	2/2	0/2[a]	2/2	2/2
Monofilament polyethylene	—	—	—	1/2[b]	1/2	1/2[b]	1/2
Monofilament polypropylene	—	—	—	1/2	0/2[a]	2/2	2/2

[a] Suture not present in either bladder.
[b] Suture not present in one bladder.

From Kaminski, J.M., Katz, A.R., and Woodward, S.C., *Surg. Gynecol. Obstet.*, 146, 353, 1978. With permission.

V. FORMATION OF URINARY CALCULI

The peculiar environment of the urinary and biliary tracts present unique requirements for suture materials. Due to the high concentration of salts and inorganic compounds in both tracts, the presence of any foreign body may act as a nidus for calculus formation. Because of this concern, absorbable suture materials have been used almost exclusively in these physiologic tracts of the body.

Kaminski et al.[168] conducted a study of urinary bladder calculus formation on both absorbable and nonabsorbable sutures in rabbits, cats, and dogs. As shown in Table 8.12, irrespective of suture materials, calculi were found with regularity in rabbits, but not in cats or dogs. No calculi were found after 7 d when the bladder was closed with the absorbable sutures (PGA and chromic catgut), whereas the incidence of calculus formation associated with the nonabsorbable sutures (braided silk, polyester, and monofilament polyethylene and polypropylene) were very high and approached 100% at a later period. Kaminski and co-workers concluded that surface characteristics and cross-sectional geometry appeared to be less important than the absorbability of a suture material in the formation of persistent urinary calculi. Similar findings were reported by Gorham et al.[169] in their *in vitro* incubation study of both absorbable (Vicryl, plain and chromic catgut) and nonabsorbable sutures (Mersilk, Mersilene, and Ethilon) in both healthy and stone-forming human patients and rabbits. Case et al.[170] studied three absorbable sutures (Vicryl, PGA, and chromic catgut) on experimental cystotomy wounds in dogs for 30 d. Tables 8.13 and 8.14 summarize the incidence of urinary stone formation for various types of sutures after 2 to 4 weeks of incubation in human urine.[171] Considerably less urinary stone deposits were associated with absorbable than with nonabsorbable sutures. Of the nine patients, only three had urinary stone deposits in Vicryl sutures as determined by X-ray elemental analysis. Among this group, only one had an abnormally high calcium content. Chromic catgut sutures had only one case of severe calculi deposits among eight patients. No inorganic stone deposits were found in patients with known history of urinary stone formation, except one who showed slight calcium deposits at 1 week. The lack of stone formation with chromic catgut sutures was also confirmed by Bartone and Shires.[171,172] Subsequently, however, they reported that if chromic catgut or collagen sutures projected into the bladder lumen (i.e., exposed to urine), calculi formation occurred.[37] None of these absorbable sutures in the study by Gorham[169] showed any stone deposit in rabbit urine at pH 8.2 for 7 to 17 d at 37°C. Nonabsorbable sutures, however, had a much higher incidence of stone deposits (Table 8.14). In monofilament nylon suture (Ethilon), more than half of the population (4/7) had slight to severe stone crystal deposits. This same ratio was also maintained among the five patients with history of clinical stone formation. Mersilene suture (braided polyester) exhibited no urinary depositions after 2 weeks, but 100% of the Mersilene sutures showed urinary stone deposits at 3 weeks incubation.

Other investigators, however, have reported that the interstices of a braided suture can serve as foci for the precipitation and growth of salt crystals. Yudofsky and Scott[173] found that a nonabsorbable multifilament suture with crevices and irregularities in its surface, such as silk and coated and uncoated polyester, enhanced stone growth on sutures by three distinct mechanisms: (1) nonuniform surfaces provide ideal foci for ion concentration, which results in restricted ion kinetics and more frequent local ion collisions, and thereby increases the possibility of salt formation; (2) irregular surfaces provide sites

Table 8.13 Deposition of Urinary Salts of Three Absorbable Sutures After Incubation in Human Urine

Patient No.	Vicryl	Chromic Catgut	Plain Catgut
1[a]	—	Clean	—
4[a]	—	Clean	—
5[a]	—	Clean	—
7[a]	—	Clean	—
9 (2 samples)	+(Ca, P)‡	—	—
(2 samples)	+++(Ca, P)‡		
10	Clean	—	—
11	Clean	—	—
12	Clean	+++(Ca, Cr)‡	+++(Ca, P)
13	—	Clean	Clean†
14[a]	—	+(Ca, P, S)†	Clean†
		Clean‡	+(Ca, Fe)‡
15	Clean	—	Clean
16	Clean	Clean†	—
18[a]	++(Ca, P)	—	—
19[a]	+(Ca)	—	—
22[a]	Clean	—	—

Note: Incubations were carried out at 37°C for 2 weeks unless otherwise indicated († = 1 week, ‡ = 3 weeks). +, light deposition of urinary salts; ++, medium deposition; +++, heavy deposition. The elemental composition of these crystals is shown in brackets.

[a] Known clinical stone former.

From Gorham, S.D., Anderson, J.D., Monsour, M.J., and Scott, R., *Urol. Res.*, 16, 111, 1988. With permission.

Table 8.14 Deposition of Urinary Salts of Three Nonabsorbable Sutures After Incubation in Human Urine

Patient No.	Ethilon	Silk	Mersilene
1[a]	+(Ca, P, Na)	—	—
4[a]	Clean	—	—
5[a]	Clean	—	—
7[a]	+++(Ca, P)	—	—
12	+(Ca)‡	++(Ca, S, P, K, Cr)	Clean
		+(Ca, K, Cr)	
		(2 samples)	
13	+(No elements found, presumably organic)†	—	Clean
14[a]	+++(Ca, P)	Clean†	Clean (2 samples)
15	—	+++(Ca, Cr)‡	Clean
16	Clean	—	—

Note: Incubations were carried out at 37°C for 2 weeks unless otherwise indicated († = 1 week, ‡ = 3 weeks). With the Mersilene sutures, calcium-containing deposits were found with urine from patients no. 12, 13, and 15 when incubations were extended to 3 weeks. +, light deposition of urinary salts; ++, medium deposition of urinary salts; +++, heavy deposition of urinary salts. The elemental composition of these crystals is shown in brackets.

[a] Known clinical stone former.

From Gorham, S.D., Anderson, J.D., Monsour, M.J., and Scott, R., *Urol. Res.*, 16, 111, 1988. With permission.

into which crystals already present in the urine stream can lodge and wedge; and (3) the crevices shelter the crystals from the natural scrubbing action of urine flow. For the same reasons, nonabsorbable monofilament suture would elicit the least amount of crystallization in supersaturated urine. Monofilament nylon and polypropylene sutures induced crystallization of salts only after 7 d in supersaturated urine, while it took only 2 hours for silk and polyester to show evidence of stone formation. The lower incidence of urinary stone formation associated with monofilament sutures was also observed by Bartone and Stinson[174] in a study in which there were only three cases of calculi formation among 99 cystotomies of guinea pigs closed with 5/0 polypropylene sutures. These cases occurred in the early time periods, within 28 d after the operation.

It appears that the geometric structure of a suture is important in inducing stone formation only if the suture is a nonabsorbable one. In other words, absorbable sutures, irrespective of their construction, behave similarly in terms of stone formation. This hypothesis is supported by the work of Bergman and Holmlund.[175] They compared the incidence of salt crystal precipitation in rabbits with the use of catgut and PGA sutures. No differences were found between the two sutures and it appeared that precipitation was independent of the type of absorbable suture material. This was attributed to the fact that the suture material was covered by an organic matrix, probably mucous substances, before a layer of salt crystals was deposited upon it. As soon as the underlying suture was covered by such a matrix, further precipitation was independent of the properties and structure of the core, i.e., of suture. Milroy[176] also demonstrated that there was no difference in the rate or amount of calcification between catgut and PGA looped sutures in sterile and infected rat bladders.

Bartone and Gardner[177] observed, however, that the number of calculi produced on 5/0 PGA sutures (4/100) was higher than with catgut and collagen sutures (1/230) in guinea pigs. They also concluded that the rate of growth of the transitional epithelium determined whether the suture would act as a nidus for calculi formation. If the rate of such growth was inhibited by the chemical or physical properties of the suture or by infection, the naked suture would provide the site for calculi formation. Marrow et al.[178] demonstrated that PGA seemed to have less propensity toward calculogenesis than chromic catgut and silk sutures in the bladders of mongrel dogs. The earlier appearance of slough with PGA sutures may explain the absence of stone formation. Stewart et al.[179] compared polydioxanone, polyglactin, and chromic catgut suture in 120 rat bladders, studying propensity for calculogenic potential, changes in urine pH, and suture absorption. They found that none of the sutures predisposed to infection, and there was wide variability but no correlation in urine pH. Although initially the polydioxanone incited a greater inflammatory response, by 6 months all three suture types were similar. There was no significant difference in calculogenic potential between these materials over the 6 month course of study. Based on this study in rats, it would appear that polydioxanone suture is equal to catgut and polyglactin suture in bladder surgery.

VI. CARCINOGENICITY

The role of suture materials in the local recurrence of cancer following primary resection and anastomosis was documented as early as 1907 when Ryall[180] presented 11 cases of suture hole cancer and stated his belief that contaminated needles or sutures were the cause. He and other investigators attributed a majority of local recurrences to the mechanical transplantation of cancer in suture materials from the involved to the uninvolved area.[180–182] More cases of cancer implantation in suture wounds and surgical scars after operation were found in the bladder, ovaries, and colon.[183–185] In Knox's study,[186] the recurrence of colon cancer, especially at the suture line, has been found to reach as high as 77.5%, the result of suture implantation. Certain suture materials are known to enhance anastomotic tumor cell growth in various experimental animal models.[187,188] Reinbach et al.[189] determined that tumor cell adherence at sites of colonic injury is dependent on the suture material used and not on the injury itself. More specifically, colonic injury repaired with silk sutures resulted in significantly more intraperitoneal tumor cells than colonic injury alone, or injury repaired with Prolene.[189]

Haverback and Smith[181] found that when a suture was pulled through a solid mast cell tumor, enough viable malignant cells adhered to the suture to cause tumor growth in 50% of the total animals tested, whereas the frequency of developing tumors approached 100% when the suture was passed through a suspension of cancer cells. It is not understood why tumor cells that have adhered to suture materials grow, even though the substrates do not have the vascular system to provide nutrients to the cells. Yu and Cohn[190] suggested that tumor cells tend to grow better on injured serosal surfaces (anastomotic sites) than on normal ones. This suggests that injured segments of the serosa at suture hole locations provide

Table 8.15 Results of Using Four Different Organic Acids with a 1:20 Dilution of Cytosieved Mast Cell Tumor Suspension and Chromic Catgut Sutures

	Suture Position			
Treatment of Suture[a]	Left In	Pulled Through	Total no. of Mice	No. of Mice that Developed Tumor
None	+	−	15	12
	−	+	15	15
17.0% picric acid[b]	+	−	15	0
	−	+	15	0
20.8% *ortho*-phthalic acid	+	−	15	0
	−	+	15	0
24.4% *ortho*-chlorobenzoic acid	+	−	15	0
	+	−	15	0
24.4% *ortho*-nitrobenzoic acid	+	−	15	0
	−	+	15	0

[a] The sutures were dipped in the respective acid solution for 5 min and then dried in air for 24 h prior to use. Methyl alcohol was the solvent for the picric and *ortho*-phthalic acids. Absolute alcohol was the solvent for the *ortho*-chlorobenzoic and *ortho*-nitrobenzoic acids.

[b] Strictly speaking, picric acid is not a true organic acid.

From Haverback, C.Z. and Smith R.R., *Cancer*, 12, 1029, 1959. With permission.

an ideal environment for the newly implanted tumor cells to grow. Those cells that adhere to the part of the suture material away from the suture holes are believed to be less or not important in the subsequent recurrence of cancer. Other studies have implied that actual tissue injury may have an effect on tumor localization onto suture materials.[191,192] In fact, one theory proposes that secretion of adhesive glycoproteins (laminin and fibronectin) by regenerating vascular endothelial cells coupled with exposure of basement membrane collagen following surgical injury may provide a suitable environment that will attract and support the growth of tumor cells.[189]

However, these models have failed to adequately compare the influence of structural and chemical properties of sutures on tumor cell adherence. Uff et al.[193] studied the relationship of malignant cell adherence between chemically similar but topographically dissimilar materials. They found that significantly more cells adhered to both protein-based and multifilament sutures compared with monofilament, synthetic, or metal sutures. Of particular interest is the author's observation that stainless steel, currently used in colorectal anastomotic stapling devices, and PDSII, adhere to the least number of cells.

In order to minimize the mechanical transplantation of malignant cells via a suture vector, a variety of organic compounds have been used to coat the surface of the suture. Haverback and Smith[181] used four different organic acids. Their results are summarized in Table 8.15. Acid-treated catgut sutures were effective in inhibiting tumor growth. There was no evidence of local or systemic toxic effects of the acids used at the concentrations utilized during the experiment. Among the four organic acids, orthophthalate, orthochlorobenzoate, and orthonitrobenzoate were found to be much less soluble in water than picric acid, and hence, dissolved less readily in a wet, aqueous, operative field.

Suture materials serve not only as the vehicles for the mechanical transplantation of tumor cells, but also can interact biologically with the surrounding tissue and create a predisposition to the growth of cancer cells. The degree of potentiation of tumor growth by a suture material appears to parallel its effect in wound infection. In a recent study of the use of B16 melanoma tumor model in mice, Pendergrast et al.[194] found that all tested suture types (chromic catgut, PGA, silk, nylon, and steel) predispose to early tumor occurrence and growth when the inoculating dose of B16 melanoma tumor cells is 1×10^5 or higher, as shown in Figure 8.21. With the normal subclinical cell inoculum dose, namely, 1×10^3, only silk and steel sutures consistently increase the rapidity of onset and the total number of tumors. In comparison, chromic catgut and PGA do not increase tumor occurrence at this cell dose inoculum level. Monofilament nylon suture is the only subtype which does not cause earlier occurrence or a greater number of tumors. This discussion indicated that silk sutures elicit the greatest incidence of wound infections among the nonabsorbable suture materials; monofilament nylon and polypropylene elicited the least. It is believed that the excessive inflammatory response elicited by silk may impair the ability of the injured tissue to resist both bacterial infection and tumor cell growth.

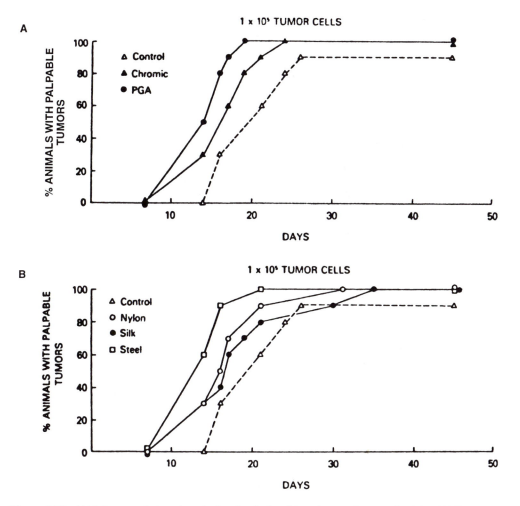

Figure 8.21 (A) Influence of chromic catgut and polyglycolide suture on the growth of 1×10^6 B16 melanoma cells; (B) influence of nylon silk and steel suture on the growth of 1×10^5 B16 melanoma cells. (From Pendergrast, W.J., Jr. et al., *J. Surg. Oncol.*, 8, 223, 1976. With permission.)

Another avenue of interest in regard to suture carcinogenicity is surgical technique. O'Donnell et al.[195] tried to determine whether suture technique affected the incidence of perianastomotic tumors in experimentally induced colonic cancers in rats. They compared transmural vs. seromuscular closures in experimentally created colotomies. Findings included an increased incidence of tumor formation in the transmural group compared to the seromuscular group. Buhr et al.[196] noted that gastrointestinal tumor formation was elevated in rats whose intestines were stapled compared to hand-sewn Vicryl suture technique. The only difference was noted to be nickel found within the staple structure. Nickel is a potent carcinogen and is felt to demonstrate a potential hazard of stapling techniques.

Stainless steel is the exception to the above theories: stainless steel sutures elicit minimal tissue reaction but cause a relatively significant incidence of wound infections and tumor occurrence. It has been proposed that the physical properties of this suture material may explain this paradoxical effect.[131] Because stainless steel sutures are "stiff," they may incite additional tissue damage due to their inability to conform to the topology of the wound tissue. Such tissue damage renders this tissue less resistant to both bacterial infection and tumor growth.

Surgeons, thus, should be aware that even the most inert suture material enhances tumor occurrence and growth at tumor cell burdens of 1×10^4 cells or higher. At clinical levels, surgeons should practice the best possible suturing techniques to minimize or even eliminate tumor seeding in the operative wound. When only a relatively low tumor cell count is present (1×10^3 and less), the type of suture material utilized in surgical wound reapproximation determines the degree of tumor growth facilitation.

REFERENCES

1. Salthouse, T.N., Biocompatibility of sutures, in *Biocompatibility in Clinical Practice,* Vol. 1, Williams, D.F., Ed., CRC Press, Boca Raton, FL, 1981, chap. 12.
2. Chu, C.C., The degradation and biocompatibility of suture materials, *Crit. Rev. Biocompatibility,* 1(3), 261, 1985.
3. Sewell, W.R., Wiland, J., and Craver, B.N., New method of comparing sutures of bovine catgut in three species, *Surg. Gynecol. Obstet.,* 100, 483, 1955.
4. Smit, I.B., Witte, E., Brand, R., and Trimbos, J.B., Tissue reaction to suture materials revisited: is there argument to change our views? *Eur. Surg. Res.,* 23, 347, 1991.
5. Coleman, J.E., McEnroe, C.S., Gelfand, J.A., Connolly, R.J., and Callow, A.D., Complement activation by vascular sutures both alone and in combination with synthetic vascular prostheses, *Eur. J. Vasc. Surg.,* 5, 287, 1991.
6. Devereux, D.F., O'Connell, S.M., Liesch, J.B., Weinstein, M., and Robertson, F.M., Induction of leukocyte activation by meshes surgically implanted in the peritoneal cavity, *Am. J. Surg.,* 162, 243, 1991.
7. Ostermann, G., Till, U., and Thielmann, K., Studies on the stimulation of human blood platelets by semi-synthetic platelet-activating factor, *Thromb. Res.,* 30, 127, 1983.
8. Redl, H., Hammerschmidt, D.E., and Schlag, G., Augmentation by platelets of granulocyte aggregation in response to chemotaxins: studies utilizing an improved cell preparation technique, *Blood,* 61, 125, 1983.
9. Niemetz, J., Mulfelder, T., Chiereg, M.E., and Troy, B., Procoagulant activity of leukocytes, *Ann. N.Y. Acad. Sci.,* 283, 208, 1977.
10. Shepard, A.D., Gelfand, J.A., Callow, A.D., and O'Donnell, T.F., Complement activation by synthetic vascular prostheses, *J. Vasc. Surg.,* 1, 829, 1984.
11. Hertzlinger, G.A. and Cumming, R.D., Role of complement activation in cell adhesion to polymer blood contact surfaces, *Trans. Am. Soc. Artif. Intern. Organs,* 26, 165, 1980.
12. Okusawa, S., Dinarello, C.A., Yancey, K.B., Endeers, S., Lawley, T.J., Frank, M.M., Burke, J.F., and Gelfand, J.A., C5a induction of human interleukin 1: synergistic effect with endotoxin or interferon, *J. Immunol.,* 139, 2635, 1987.
13. Okusawa, S., Yancey, K.B., van der Meer, J.W., Endeers, S., Lonnemann, G., Hefter, K., Frank, M.M., Burke, J.F., Dinarello, C.A., and Gelfand, J.A., C5a stimulates secretion of tumor necrosis factor from human mononuclear cells in vitro: comparison with secretion of interleukin 1b and interleukin 1a, *J. Exp. Med.,* 168, 443, 1988.
14. Hayashi, K., Fukumura, H., and Yamamoto, N., In vivo thrombus formation induced by complement activation on polymer surface, *J. Biomed. Mater. Res.,* 24, 1385, 1990.
15. Muhlfelder, T.W., Niemetz, J., and Kreutzer, D., C5 chemotactic fragment induces leukocyte production of tissue factor activity. A link between complement and coagulation, *J. Clin. Invest.,* 63, 147, 1979.
16. Sacks, T., Moldow, C.F., and Craddock, P.R., Oxygen radicals mediate endothelial cell damage by complement stimulated granulocytes, *J. Clin. Invest.,* 61, 1161, 1978.
17. Trimbos, J.B., Snijders-Keiholz, T., and Peters, A.A.W., Feasibility of the application of a resorbable polyglycolic acid mesh (Dexon mesh) to prevent complications of radiotherapy following gynaecological surgery, *Eur. J. Surg.,* 157, 281, 1991.
18. Deutsch, A.A. and Stern, H.S., Technique of insertion of pelvic Vicryl mesh sling to avoid postradiation enteritis, *Dis. Colon Rectum,* 32, 628, 1989.
19. Rodier, J.F., Janser, J.C., Roy, C., and Rodier, D., Exclusion pelvienne par treillis de polygalactine 910 (Vicryl) pour la prevention des radiolesions du grele. A propos d'une serie du 24 cas, *Bull. Cancer,* 76, 1121, 1989.
20. Sener, S.F., Imperato, J.P., Blum, M.D., Ignatoff, J.M., Soper, T.G., Winchester, D.P., and Meiselman, M., Technique and complications of reconstruction of the pelvic floor with polyglactin mesh, *Surg. Gynecol. Obstet.,* 168, 475, 1989.
21. Soper, J.T., Clarke-Pearson, D.L., and Creasman, W.T., Absorbable synthetic mesh (910-polyglactin) intestinal sling to reduce radiation-induced small bowel injury in patients with pelvic malignancies, *Gynecol. Oncol.,* 29, 283, 1988.
22. Caspers, R.J.L. and Hop, W.C.J., Irradiation of true pelvis for bladder and prostatic carcinoma in supine, prone or trendelenburg position, *Int. J. Radiat. Oncol. Biol. Phys.,* 9, 589, 1983.
23. Bakare, S.C., Shafir, M., and McElhinney, A.J., Exclusion of small bowel from pelvis for postoperative radiotherapy for rectal cancer, *J. Surg. Oncol.,* 35, 55, 1987.
24. Green, N., The avoidance of small intestine injury in gynecologic cancer, *Int. J. Radiat. Oncol. Biol. Phys.,* 9, 1385, 1983.
25. Kavanah, M.T., Feldman, M.I., Devereux, D.F., and Kondi, E.S., New approach to minimizing radiation associated small bowel injury in high dose irradiation: a preliminary report, *Cancer,* 56, 1300, 1985.
26. Bennett, R., Selection of wound closure materials, *J. Am. Acad. Dermatol.,* 18, 619, 1988.
27. Katz, A.R. and Turner, R.J., Evaluation of tensile and absorption properties of polyglycolic acid sutures, *Surg. Gynecol. Obstet.,* 131, 701, 1970.
28. Lawrie, P., Angus, G., and Reese, A.J.M., The absorption of surgical catgut, *Br. J. Surg.,* 46, 638, 1959.
29. Pavan, A., Bosio, M., and Longo, T., A comparative study of polyglycolic acid and catgut as suture materials. Histomorphology and mechanical properties, *J. Biomed. Mater. Res.,* 13, 477, 1979.
30. Postlethwait, R.W., Willigan, D.A., and Ulin, A.W., Human tissue reaction to sutures, *Ann. Surg.,* 181, 144, 1975.
31. Okada, T., Hayashi, T., and Ikada, Y., Degradation of collagen suture *in vitro* and *in vivo, Biomaterials,* 13, 448, 1992.
32. Postlethwait, R.W., Polyglycolic acid surgical suture, *Arch. Surg.,* 101, 489, 1970.

33. Bergman, F.O., Borgstrom, S.J.H., and Holmlund, D.E.W., Synthetic absorbable surgical suture material (PGA). An experimental study, *Acta Chir. Scand.,* 137, 193, 1971.
34. Salthouse, T.N., Kaminska, G.Z., and Murphy, M.L., Suture absorption in rabbit cornea and sclera: enzyme histochemical and morphologic observations, *Invest. Ophthalmol.,* 9, 844, 1970.
35. Salthouse, T.N., Matlaga, B.F., and Wykoff, M.H., Comparative tissue response to six suture materials in rabbit cornea, sclera, and ocular muscle, *Am. J. Ophthalmol.,* 84, 224, 1977.
36. Yamanaka, T., Chorioretinitis caused by synthetic absorbable sutures, *Lens Eye Toxicity Res.,* 9 (3,4), 559, 1992.
37. Bartone, F.F., Shervey, P.D., and Gardner, P.J., Long term tissue responses to catgut and collagen sutures, *Invest. Urol.,* 13, 390, 1976.
38. Stacey-Clear, A., McCarthy, K.A., Hall, D.A., Pile-Spellman, E.R., Morose, H.E., White, G., Cardenosa, G., Sawicka, J., Mahoney, E., and Kopans, D.B., Calcified suture material in the breast after radiation therapy, *Radiology,* 183, 207, 1992.
39. Rebner, M., Pennes, D.R., Adler, D.D., Helvie, M.A., and Lichter, A.S., Breast microcalcifications after lumpectomy and radiation therapy, *Radiology,* 170, 691, 1989.
40. Davis, S.P., Stomper, P.C., Weidner, N., and Meyer, J.E., Suture calcification mimicking recurrence in the irradiated breast: a potential pitfall in mammographic evaluation, *Radiology,* 172, 247, 1989.
41. Solin, L.J., Fowble, B.L., Troupin, R.H., and Goodman, R.L., Biopsy results of new calcifications in the post irradiated breast, *Cancer,* 63, 1956, 1989.
42. Dershaw, D.D., Shank, B., and Reisinger, S., Mammographic findings after breast cancer treatment with local excision and definite irradiation, *Radiology,* 164, 455, 1987.
43. Stone, I.K., von Fraunhofer, J.A., and Masterson, B.J., A comparative study of suture materials: chromic gut and chromic gut treated with glycerin, *Am J. Obstet. Gynecol.,* 151, 1087, 1985.
44. Grant, A., Dyspareunia associated with the use of glycerol-impregnated catgut to repair perineal trauma. Report of a 3 year follow-up study. Short Communication, *Am. J. Obstet. Gynecol.,* 96, 741, 1989.
45. Spencer, J.A.D., Grant, A., Elbourne, D., Garcia, J., and Sleep, J., A randomized comparison of glycerol-impregnated chromic catgut with untreated chromic catgut for the repair of perineal trauma, *Br. J. Obstet. Gynecol.,* 93, 426, 1986.
46. Morgan, M.N., New synthetic absorbable suture material, *Br. Med. J.,* 2, 308, 1969.
47. Herman, J.B., Kelly, R.J., and Higgin, G.A., Polyglycolic acid sutures, *Arch. Surg.,* 100, 486, 1970.
48. Blomstedt, B. and Jacobson, S., Experiences with polyglactin 910 in general surgery, *Acta Chir. Scand.,* 143, 259, 1977.
49. Craig, P.H., Williams, J.A., and Davis, K.W., A biologic comparison of polyglactin 910 and polyglycolic acid synthetic absorbable sutures, *Surg. Gynecol. Obstet.,* 141, 1, 1975.
50. Guttman, L., Experimental study on nerve suture with various suture materials, *Br. J. Surg.,* 30, 370, 1983.
51. Sunderland, S. and Smith, G.K., Relative merits of various suture materials, *Br. J. Surg.,* 30, 370, 1983.
52. Hartman, L.A., Intradermal sutures in facial lacerations. Comparative study of clear monofilament nylon and polyglycolic acid, *Arch. Otolaryngol. Head Neck Surg.,* 103, 542, 1977.
53. Moloney, G.E., The effect of human tissues on the tensile strength of implanted nylon sutures, *Br. J. Surg.,* 48, 528, 1961.
54. Nordstrom R.A. and Nordstrom, R.M., Absorbable vs. nonabsorbable sutures to prevent postoperative stretching of wound area, *Plast. Reconstr. Surg.,* 78, 186, 1986.
55. DeLee, J.C., Smith, M.T., and Green, D.P., The reaction of nerve tissue to various suture materials: a study in rabbits, *J. Hand Surg.,* 2, 38, 1977.
56. Hudson, A.R., Bilbar, J.M., and Hunter, D., Polyglycolic acid suture in peripheral nerve: an electron microscopic study, *Can. J. Neurol. Sci.,* 2, 17, 1975.
57. Bratton, B.R., Kline, D.G., and Hudson, A.R., Use of monofilament polyglycolic acid suture for experimental peripheral nerve repair, *J. Surg. Res.,* 31, 482, 1981.
58. Vallfors, B., Hansson, H.-A., and Svensson, J., Absorbable or nonabsorbable suture materials for closure of the dura mater, *Neurosurgery,* 9, 407, 1981.
59. Matlaga, V.F. and Salthouse, T.N., Electron microscopic observations of polyglactin 910 suture sites, in *First World Biomaterials Congress,* Abstr., Baden, Austria, April 8 to 12, 1980.
60. Barber, F.A. and Deck, M.A., The in vivo histology of an absorbable suture anchor: a preliminary report, *Arthroscopy: J. Arthroscopic Relat. Surg.,* 11(1), 77, 1995.
61. Salthouse, T.N. and Matlaga, B.F., Polyglactin 910 suture absorption and the role of cellular enzymes, *Surg. Gynecol. Obstet.,* 142, 544, 1976.
62. Ray, J.A., Doddi, N., Regula, D., Williams, J.A., and Melveger, A., Polydioxanone (PDS), a novel monofilament synthetic absorbable suture, *Surg. Gynecol. Obstet.,* 153, 497, 1981.
63. Cameron, A.E., Parker, C.J., and Field, E.S., A randomised comparison of polydioxanone (PDS) and polypropylene (Prolene) for abdominal wound closure, *Ann. R. Coll. Surg.,* 69, 113, 1987.
64. Taylor, T.V., The use of polydioxanone suture in midline incisions, *J. R. Coll. Surg. (Edinburgh),* 30, 191, 1985.
65. Leaper, D.J., Allan, A., May, R.E., Corfield, A.P., and Kennedy, R.H., Abdominal wound closure: a controlled trial of polyamide (nylon) and polydioxanone sutures (PDS), *Annu. J. R. Coll. Surg.,* 67, 273, 1985.
66. Schoetz, D.J., Jr., Coller, J.A., and Veldenheimer, M.C., Closure of abdominal wounds with polydioxanone. A prospective study, *Arch. Surg.,* 123, 72, 1988.

67. Torsello, G., Schwartz, A., Aulich, A., and Sandmann, W., Absorbable polydioxanone suture for venous anastomoses: experimental studies using venography and transluminal angioscopy, *Eur. J. Vasc. Surg.*, 1, 319, 1987.

68. Aarnio, P.H., Lehtola, A., Sariola, H., and Mattila, S., Polydioxanone and polypropylene suture material in free internal mammary artery graft anastomoses, *J. Thorac. Cardiovasc. Surg.*, 96, 741, 1988.

69. Zannini, L., Galli, R., Alampi, G., Santorelli, M.C., Nuzzo, F., Galassi, A., and Pierangeli, A., The use of absorbable suture: morphological findings in a newborn three months after coarctation repair, *Italian J. Surg. Sci.*, 16, 297, 1986.

70. Peleg, H., Pai, U.N.M., and Emrich, L.J., An experimental comparison of suture materials for tracheal and bronchial anastomoses, *Thorac. Cardiovasc. Surg.*, 34, 384, 1986.

71. Friberg, L.G., Mellgren, G.W., Eriksson, B.O., and Soren, B., Subclavian flap angioplasty with absorbable suture polydioxanone (PDS), *Scand. J. Thorac. Cardiovasc. Surg.*, 21, 9, 1987.

72. Myers, J.L., Invited letter concerning: calcification after end-to-end arterial anastomosis, *J. Thorac. Cardiovasc. Surg.*, 99, 380, 1990.

73. Gersak, B., Fibrous changes and presence of calcium in the vessel walls six months after end-to-end arterial anastomoses in growing dogs, *J. Thorac. Cardiovasc. Surg.*, 99, 379, 1990.

74. Gersak, B., Presence of calcium in the vessel walls after end-to-end arterial anastomoses with polydioxanone and polypropylene sutures in growing dogs, *J. Thorac. Cardiovasc. Surg.*, 106(4), 587, 1993.

75. Bellina, J.H. and Lee, F.L., Clip appendectomy, *J. Reprod. Med.*, 34, 475, 1989.

76. Mavroudis, C., Harrison, H., Klein, J.B., Gray, L.A., Ganzel, B.L., Wellhausen, S.R., Elbl, F., and Cook, L.N., Infant orthotopic cardiac transplantation, *J. Thorac. Cardiovasc. Surg.*, 96, 912, 1988.

77. Biardzka, B. and Kaluzny, J., Experimental and clinical investigation on the suitability of PDS threads for cerclage of the eyeball, *Ophthalmology*, 197, 47, 1988.

78. Brightman, A.H., McLaughlin, S.A., and Brogdon, J.D., Autogenous lamellar corneal grafting in dogs, *J. Am. Vet. Med. Assoc.*, 195, 469, 1989.

79. Willatt, D.J., Durham, L., Ramadan, M.F., and Bark-Jones, N., A prospective randomized trial of suture material in aural wound closure, *J. Laryngol. Otol.*, 102, 788, 1988.

80. Kirby, B.M., Knol, J.S., Manley, P.A., and Miller, L.M., Calcinosis circumscripta associated with polydioxanone suture in two young dogs, *Vet. Surg.*, 18, 216, 1989.

81. Juettner, F.M., Kohek, P., Pinter, H., Klepp, G., and Friehs, G., Reinforced staple line in severely emphysematous lungs, *J. Thorac. Cardiovasc. Surg.*, 97, 362, 1989.

82. Katz, A., Mukherjee, D.P., Kaganov, A.L., and Gordon, S., A new synthetic monofilament absorbable suture made from polytrimethylene carbonate, *Surg. Gynecol. Obstet.*, 161, 213, 1985.

83. Sanz, L.E., Patterson, J.A., Kamath, R., Willett, G., Ahmed, S.W., and Butterfield, A.B., Comparison of Maxon suture with Vicryl, chromic catgut and PDS sutures in fascial closure in rats, *Obstet. Gynecol.*, 71, 418, 1988.

84. Walton, M., Strength retention of chromic gut and monofilament synthetic absorbable suture materials in joint tissues, *Clin. Orthop. Relat. Res.*, 242, 303, 1989.

85. Metz, S.A., Chegini, N., and Masterson, B.J., *In vivo* tissue reactivity and degradation of suture materials: a comparison of Maxon and PDS, *J. Gynecol. Surg.*, 5, 37, 1989.

86. Bezwada, R.S., Jamiolkowski, D.D., and Erneta, M., Monocryl suture, a new ultra-pliable absorbable monofilament suture, *Biomaterials*, 16, 1141, 1995.

87. Postlethwait, R.W., Long-term comparative study of nonabsorbable sutures, *Ann. Surg.*, 171, 892, 1970.

88. Postlethwait, R.W., Dillion, M.L., and Reeves, J.W., Experimental study of silk sutures, *Arch. Surg.*, 84, 698, 1962.

89. Castelli, W.A., Nasjleti, C.E., and Caffesse, R.E., Gingival response to silk, cotton, and nylon suture materials, *Oral Surg. Oral Med. Oral Pathol.*, 45, 179, 1978.

90. Macht, S.D. and Krized, T.J., Sutures and suturing: current concepts, *J. Oral Maxillofac. Surg.*, 36, 710, 1978.

91. Kelly, S.E., Ehlers, J., and Llovera, J., Comparison of tissue reaction to nylon and Prolene sutures in rabbit iris and cornea, *Ophthalmic Surg.*, 6, 105, 1955.

92. Eskridge, J.M. and Scott, J.A., Preoperative embolization of brain AVMs using surgical silk and polyvinyl alcohol, *Am. J. Euroradiat.*, 10, 882, 1989.

93. Barth, K.H., Strandberg, J.D., Kaufman, S.L., and White, R.L., Chronic vascular reactions to steel coil occlusion devices, *Am. J. Roentgenol.*, 131, 455, 1978.

94. Deveikis, J.P., Manz, H.J., Luessenhap, A.J., and Patronas, N., A clinical and neuropathologic study of silk suture as an embolic agent for brain arteriovenous malformations, *Am. J. Neuroradiat.*, 15, 263, 1994.

95. Jongebloed, W.L. and Van Der Veen, G., Reaction of the rabbit corneal endothelium to nylon sutures: a SEM study, *Doc. Ophthalmol.*, 75, 351, 1990.

96. Wijneveld, W.J., Jongebloed, W.L., Worst, J.G.F., and Houtman, W.A., Comparison of the reaction of the cornea to nylon and stainless steel sutures: an animal study, *Doc. Ophthalmol.*, 74, 297, 1989.

97. Jongebloed, W.L., Kalicharan, D., and Worst, J.G.F., Behavior of nylon sutures in corneal endothelium, a TEM and SEM study, *Elektronenmikroskop Direktabb. Oberfl.* 28, 143, 1995.

98. Kronenthal, R.L., Intraocular degradation of nonabsorbable sutures, *Am. Intra-Ocular Implant Soc. J.*, 3, 222, 1977.

99. Miller, J.M., Evaluation of a new surgical suture (Prolene), *Am. Surg.*, 39, 31, 1973.

100. Clayman, H.J.M., Polypropylene, *Ophthalmology*, 88, 959, 1981.

101. Seddon, H., *Surgical Disorders of the Peripheral Nerves*, Williams & Wilkins, Baltimore, 1972, 271.

102. Cilento, R., Schwartz, S.J., and Hinshaw, J.R., Evaluation of suture material and bio-electric environment in nerve anastomosis, *Surg. Forum*, 14, 412, 1963.

103. Rodeheaver, G.T., Nesbit, W.S., and Edlider, R.F., Novafil: a dynamic suture for wound closure, *Am. Surg.*, 204, 193, 1986.

104. Trimbos, J.B., Smeets, M., Verdel, M., and Hermans, J., Cosmetic result of lower midline laparotomy wounds: polybutester and nylon skin suture in a randomized clinical trial, *J. Obstet. Gynecol.*, 82, 390, 1993.

105. Cavallaro, A., Sciacca, V., Cisternino, S., and Gallo, P., Experimental evaluation of tissue reactivity to vascular sutures: Dacron, polypropylene and PTFE, *J. Vasc. Surg.*, 21(2), 82, 1987.

106. Revuelta, J.M., Garcia-Rinaldi, R., Gaite, L., Val, F., and Garijo, F., Generation of chordae tendineae with polytetrafluoroethylene stents, *J. Thorac. Cardiovasc. Surg.*, 97(1), 98, 1989.

107. David, T.E., Bos, J., and Rakowski, H., Mitral valve repair by replacement of chordae tendineae with polytetrafluoroethylene sutures, *J. Thorac. Cardiovasc. Surg.,* 101, 495, 1991.

108. Forster, L.W., Rali, Z.A., and McKibbin, B., Biological reaction to carbon fiber implants: the formation and structure of a carbon-induced neotendon, *Clin. Orthop.,* 131, 299, 1978.

109. Brown, M.P. and Pool, R.R., Experimental and clinical investigations of the use of carbon fiber sutures in equine tendon repair, *J. Am. Vet. Med. Assoc.,* 182, 956, 1983.

110. LoCicero, J., Robbin, J.A., and Webb, W.R., Complications following abdominal fascial closures using various nonabsorbable sutures, *Surg. Gynecol. Obstet.*, 157, 25, 1983.

111. Holmlund, D., Tera, H., and Wiberg, Y., *Suture and Techniques for Wound Closure*, Naimark and Barba, New York, 1976, 13.

112. Flood, H.D. and Beard, R.C., Post-herniorrhaphy paravesical granuloma, *Br. J. Urol.*, 61, 266, 1988.

113. Lynch, T.H., Waymont, B., Beacock, C.J., and Wallace, D.M., Paravesical suture granuloma: a problem following herniorrhaphy, *J. Urol.*, 147(2), 460, 1992.

114. Nagar, H., Stitch granulomas following inguinal herniotomy; a 10-year review, *J. Pediatr. Surg.*, 28, 1505, 1993.

115. Sander, I. and Woesner, M.E., "Stitch" granuloma: a consideration in the differential diagnosis of the intramural gastric tumor, *Am. J. Gastroenterol.,* 57, 558, 1972.

116. Belleza, N.A. and Lowman, R.M., Suture granuloma of the stomach following total colectomy, *Radiology*, 127, 84, 1978.

117. Al-tawil, Y.S., Gilger, M.A., Hawkins, E.P., and Pokorny, W.J., Esophageal suture granuloma as a complication of a fundoplication, *J. Pediatr. Gastroenterol. Nutrit.*, 18, 104, 1994.

118. Gueler, R., Shapiro, H.A., Nelson, J.A., and Bush, R., Suture granuloma simulating tumors, *Digest. Dis.*, 21, 223, 1976.

119. Murphy, J.R., Shay, S.S., Moses, F.M., Braxton, J., Jaques, D.P., and Wong, R.K., Suture granuloma masquerading as malignancy of the biliary tract, *Digest. Dis. Sci.*, 35, 1176, 1990.

120. Gleeson, M.J. and McMullin, J.P., Suture granuloma simulating a cholangiocarcinoma, *Br. J. Surg.*, 74, 35, 1987.

121. Eldridge, P.R. and Wheeler, M.H., Stitch granuloma after thyroid surgery, *Br. J. Surg.*, 74, 345, 1987.

122. Manor, A. and Kaffe, I., Unusual foreign body reaction to a braided silk suture: a case report, *J. Periodontol.*, 53, 86, 1982.

123. Brunsvold, M.A., Reding, M.E., and Kornman, K.S., Infected suture granuloma: a case report, *Int. J. Oral Maxillofac. Implants*, 6, 215, 1991.

124. Baumgartner, W.A. and Mark, J.B.D., Bronchoscopic diagnosis and treatment of bronchial stump suture granuloma, *J. Thorac. Cardiovasc. Surg.*, 81, 553, 1991.

125. Sherman, P.H. and Conant, J.S., Bronchial closure with catgut sutures, *J. Thorac. Surg.*, 35, 363, 1958.

126. Jack, G.D., Bronchial closure, *Thorax*, 20, 8, 1965.

127. Albertini, R.E., Cough caused by exposed endobronchial suture, *Ann. Int. Med.*, 94, 205, 1981.

128. Maygarden, S.J., Novotny, D.B., and Johnson, D.E., Fine needle aspiration cytology of suture granulomas of the breast: a potential pitfall in the cytologic diagnosis of recurrent breast cancer, *Diag. Cytopathol.*, 10(2), 175, 1994.

129. Frumkin, A., Gorbacz, S., and Lifschitz-Mercer, B., Delayed reaction to suture material simulating melanoma, *Cutis*, 49(1), 59, 1992.

130. Elek, S.D. and Conen, P.E., The virulence of Staphylococcus pyogenes for man. Study of the problems of wound infection, *Br. J. Exp. Pathol.*, 38, 573, 1957.

131. Edlich, R.F., Paneka, P.H., and Rodeheaver, G.T., Physical and chemical configuration of sutures in the development of surgical infection, *Ann. Surg.,* 177, 679, 1973.

132. Alexander, J.W., Kaplan, J.Z., and Altemeier, W.A., Role of suture materials in the development of wound infection, *Ann. Surg.,* 165, 192, 1967.

133. Blomstedt, B. and Osterberg, B., Suture materials and wound infection, *Acta Chir. Scand.,* 144, 269, 1978.

134. Osterberg, B. and Blomstedt, B., Effect of suture materials on bacterial survival in infected wounds, *Acta Chir. Scand.,* 145, 431, 1979.

135. Bucknall, T.E. and Ellis, T.H., Infectivity of suture materials used in abdominal wound closure, *Eur. Surg. Res.*, 13, 64, 1981.

136. Varma, S., Lumb, W.V., and Johnson, L.W., Further studies with polyglycolic (Dexon) and other sutures in infected experimental wounds, *Am. J. Vet. Res.,* 42, 571, 1981.

137. Varma, S., Ferguson, H.L., and Breen, J., Tissue reaction to suture materials in infected surgical wounds: an experimental study, *J. Surg. Res.*, 17, 165, 1974.

138. Varma, S., Johnson, L.W., Ferguson, H.L., and Lumb, W.V., Tissue reaction to suture materials in infected surgical wounds — a histopathologic evaluation, *Am. J. Vet. Res.*, 42, 563, 1981.

139. Sharp, W.V., Belden, T.A., King, P.H., and Teague, P.C., Suture resistance to infection, *Surgery*, 91, 61, 1981.

140. Chu, C.C. and Williams, D.F., The effects of physical configuration and chemical structure of suture materials on bacterial adhesion — a possible link to wound infection, *Am. J. Surg.*, 147, 197, 1984.

141. Sugarman, B. and Musher, D., Adherence of bacteria to suture materials, *Proc. Soc. Exp. Biol. Med.*, 167, 156, 1981.

142. Katz, S., Izbar, M., and Mirelman, D., Bacterial adherence to surgical sutures, *Ann. Surg.*, 194, 35, 1981.

143. Howell, J.M., Bresnahan, K.A., and Stair, T.O., Comparison of the effects of suture and cyanoacrylate tissue adhesive on bacterial counts in contaminated lacerations, *Antimicrob. Agents Chemother.*, 39(2), 559, 1995.

144. Paterson-Brown, S., Cheslyn-Curtis, S., Biglin, J., Eye, J., Easmon, C.S.F., and Dudley, H.A.F., Suture materials in contaminated wounds: a detailed comparison of a new suture with those currently in use, *Br. J. Surg.*, 74, 734, 1987.

145. Cutler, E.C. and Dunphy, J.E., The use of silk in infected wounds, *N. Engl. J. Med.*, 224, 101, 1941.

146. Bucknall, T.E. and Ellis, H., Abdominal wound closure — a comparison of monofilament nylon and polyglycolic acid, *Surgery*, 89, 672, 1981.

147. Shouldice, L.E., Glassow, F., and Black, N., A study of sinuses occurring after the use of silk only, wire only or a combination of the two, *Can. Med. Assoc. J.*, 84, 576, 1961.

148. Leaper, D.J., Pollock, A.V., and Evans, M., Abdominal wound closure: a trial of nylon, polyglycolic acid and steel sutures, *Br. J. Surg.*, 64, 603, 1977.

149. Corman, M.L., Veidenheimer, M.C., and Coller, J.A., Controlled trial of three suture materials for abdominal wound closure after bowel operations, *Am. J. Surg.*, 141, 510, 1981.

150. Bentley, P.G., Owen, W.J., Girolami, P.L., and Dawson, J.L., Wound closure with Dexon (PGA) mass suture, *Ann. R. Coll. Surg. Engl.*, 60, 125, 1978.

151. Everett, W.G., Suture materials in general surgery, *Prog. Surg.*, 8, 14, 1970.

152. Hewett, A.L., Jones, B.W., and Headstream, J.W., Experience with wire closure of lumbodorsal incision, *J. Urol.* (Baltimore), 85, 320, 1961.

153. Crawford, D.T. and Ketcham, A.S., Late complications of wire sutures and some causative factors, *Am. J. Surg.*, 100, 898, 1963.

154. McCullum, G.T. and Link, R.F., The effect of closure techniques on abdominal disruption, *Surg. Gynecol. Obstet.*, 119, 75, 1964.

155. Haxton, H., Nylon darn repairs of hernia, *Lancet*, 1, 428, 1958.

156. Greaney, M.G., A clinical and experimental study of suture sinuses in abdominal wounds, *Surg. Gynecol. Obstet.*, 155, 712, 1982.

157. Bucknall, T.E., Abdominal wound closure: choice of sutures, *J. R. Soc. Med.*, 74, 580, 1981.

158. Nirankari, V.S., Karesh, J.W., and Richards, R.D., Complications of exposed monofilament sutures, *Am. J. Ophthalmol.*, 95, 515, 1983.

159. Sugar, A. and Meyer, R.F., Giant papillary conjunctivitis after keratoplasty, *Am. J. Ophthalmol.*, 91, 239, 1981.

160. Reynolds, A., Femoral nerve injury, *J. Neurosurg.*, 58, 459, 1983.

161. Dahlke, H., Dociu, N., and Thurau, K., Thrombogenicity of different suture materials as revealed by scanning electron microscopy, *J. Biomed. Mater. Res.*, 14, 251, 1980.

162. Pham, S.M., Armitage, J.M., and Katz, W.E., Left atrial thrombus after lung transplantation, *Ann. Thorac. Surg.*, 59(2), 513, 1995.

163. Bokros, J.C., LaGrange, L.D., Fadali, A.M., Vos, K.D., and Ramos, M.D., Correlations between blood compatibility and heparin adsorptivity for an important impermeable isotropic pyrolytic carbon, *J. Biomed. Mater. Res.*, 3, 497, 1969.

164. Salzman, E.W., Lindon, J., Baier, D., and Merril, E.W., Surface-induced platelet adhesion, aggregation, and release, *Ann. N.Y. Acad. Sci.*, 283, 114, 1977.

165. Schoen, F.J., Carbons in heart valve prostheses. Foundations and clinical performance, in *Biocompatible Polymers, Metals, and Composites,* Szycher, M., Ed., Schuster & Schuster, Technomic, PA, 1983, chap. 11.

166. Johnson, P.C., Garrett, K.O., Brash, J.L., and Cornelius, R.M., Delivery of proteins to sutures during passage through the vessel wall reduces subsequent platelet deposition by blocking fibrinogen absorption, *Arteriosclerosis Thromb.*, 12, 727, 1992.

167. Johnson, P.C., Platelet-mediated thrombus in microvascular surgery: new knowledge and strategies, *Plast. Reconst. Surg.*, 86, 359, 1990.

168. Kaminski, J.M., Katz, A.R., and Woodward, S.C., Urinary bladder calculus formation on sutures in rabbits, cats, and dogs, *Surg. Gynecol. Obstet.*, 146, 353, 1978.

169. Gorham, S.D., Anderson, J.D., Monsour, M.J., and Scott, R., The in vitro assessment of a collagen/Vicryl (polyglactin) composite film together with candidate suture materials for use in urinary tract surgery, *Urol. Res.*, 16, 111, 1988.

170. Case, G.D., Glenn, J.F., and Postlethwait, R.W., Comparison of absorbable sutures in urinary bladder, *Urology*, 7, 165, 1976.

171. Bartone, F.F. and Shires, T.K., The reaction of the urinary tract to catgut and reconstituted collagen sutures, *J. Urol.*, 101, 411, 1969.

172. Bartone, F.F. and Shires, T.K., The reaction of kidney and bladder tissue to catgut and reconstituted collagen sutures, *Surg. Gynecol. Obstet.*, 128, 1221, 1969.

173. Yudofsky, S.C. and Scott, F.B., Urolithiasis in suture materials — its importance, pathogenesis and prophylaxis: an introduction to the monofilament Teflon suture, *J. Urol.*, 102, 745, 1969.

174. Bartone, F.F. and Stinson, W., Reaction of the urinary tract to polypropylene sutures, *Invest. Urol.*, 14, 44, 1976.

175. Bergman, F. and Holmlund, D.E.W., Intravesical urinary salt precipitations on catgut and Dexon sutures, *Acta Chir. Scand.*, 139, 487, 1973.

176. Milroy, E., An experimental study of the calcification and absorption of polyglycolic acid and catgut sutures within the urinary tract, *Invest. Urol.*, 14, 141, 1976.

177. Bartone, F.F. and Gardner, P.J., Polyglycolic acid suture in the urinary tract, a light and electron microscopic study, *Urology*, 2CD, 43, 1973.

178. Marrow, F.A., Kogan, S.J., and Freed, S.Z., In vivo comparison of polyglycolic acid, chromic catgut and silk in tissue of the genitourinary tract: an experimental study of tissue retrieved and calculogenesis, *J. Urol.*, 112, 655, 1974.

179. Stewart, D.W., Buffington, P.J., and Wacksman, J., Suture material in bladder surgery: a comparison of polydioxanone, polyglactin, and chromic catgut, *J. Urol.*, 143(6), 1261, 1990.

180. Ryall, C., Cancer infection and cancer recurrence: danger to avoid in cancer operations, *Lancet*, 2, 1311, 1907.

181. Haverback, C.Z. and Smith, R.R., Transplantation of tumor by suture thread and its prevention, *Cancer*, 12, 1029, 1959.

182. Leinhardt, D.J., Smart, P.J., and Howat, J.M., Jejunal carcinoma associated with nonabsorbable suture material, *Postgrad. Med. J.*, 64(755), 717, 1988.

183. Chester, J.F., Gaissert, H.A., Ross, J.S., Malt, R.A., and Weitzman, S.A., N-[4-(5-nitro-2-furyl)-2-thiazolyl] forma-mide-induced bladder cancer in mice: augmentation by suture through the bladder wall, *J. Urol.*, 137, 769, 1987.

184. Calderisi, R.N. and Freeman, H.J., Differential effects of surgical suture materials in 1,2-dimethylhydrazine-induced rat intestinal neoplasia, *Cancer Res.*, 44(7), 2827, 1984.

185. Akyol, A.M., McGregor, J.R., Galloway, D.J., Murray, G., and George, W.D., Recurrence of colorectal cancer after sutured and stapled large bowel anastomoses, *Br. J. Surg.*, 78, 1297, 1991.

186. Knox, L.C., Relationship of massage to metastasis in malignant tumors, *Ann. Surg.*, 75, 129, 1972.

187. McGregor, J.R., Galloway, D.J., Jarrett, F., Brown, I.L., and George, W.D., Anastomotic suture materials and experimental colorectal carcinogenesis, *Dis. Colon Rectum*, 34, 987, 1991.

188. Appleton, G.V., Davies, P.W., and Williamson, R.C., Effect of defunction on cytokinetics and cancer at colonic suture lines, *Br. J. Surg.*, 77, 768, 1990.

189. Reinbach, D., McGregor, J.R., and O'Dwyer, P.J., Effect of suture material on tumor cell adherence at sites of colonic injury, *Br. J. Surg.*, 80, 774, 1993.

190. Yu, S.K. and Cohn, I., Tumor implantation on colon mucosa, *Arch. Surg.*, 96, 956, 1968.

191. McCue, J.L., Sheffield, J.P., Uff, C., and Phillip, R.K., Experimental carcinogenesis at sutured and sutureless colonic anastomoses, *Dis. Colon Rectum*, 35, 902, 1992.

192. Hubens, G., Totte, E., Verhulst, A., Van Marck, E., and Hubens, A., The influence of the interaction of sutures with the mucosa on tumor formation at colonic anastomoses in rats, *Eur. Surg. Res.*, 25, 213, 1993.

193. Uff, C.R., Yiu, C., Boulos, P.B., and Philips, R.K., Influence of suture physicochemical and surface topographic structure on tumor cell adherence, *Dis. Colon Rectum*, 36, 850, 1993.

194. Pendergrast, W.J., Jr., Futrell, J.W., and Mardiney, M.R., Differences in potentiation of melanoma growth by absorbable and nonabsorbable suture, *J. Surg. Oncol.*, 8, 223, 1976.

195. O'Donnell, A.F., O'Connell, P.R., and Royston, D., Suture technique affects perianastomotic colonic crypt cell production and tumour formation, *Br. J. Surg.*, 78(6), 671, 1991.

196. Buhr, H.J., Hupp, T., and Beck, N., Gastrointestinal tumours after stapler vs. vicryl anastomoses in carcinogen-treated rats, *Eur. J. Surg. Oncol.*, 16(6), 493, 1990.

Chapter 9

Suture Techniques and Selection

S.S. Kang, W. Irvin, J.R. Perez-Sanz, and H. P. Greisler

CONTENTS

This chapter briefly reviews the merits of different types of sutures and suturing techniques in a variety of clinical environments. The use of absorbable and nonabsorbable monofilament or multifilament sutures and continuous or interrupted suturing techniques for repairs of various tissues in the human body as these relate to clinical outcomes are addressed. Because the focus of this chapter is of a clinical nature, the majority of the papers discussed are clinical studies, but some experimental data are also included as necessary.

I. SURGICAL PRINCIPLES

As described in Chapter 2, several factors that favorably influence wound healing can be controlled to some extent by the surgical team at the time of the procedure. Without a doubt, the single most important component of successful wound healing is maintenance of sterile and aseptic technique to prevent infection. Whatever its source, infection in the wound is a serious deterrent to wound healing. To promote optimum wound healing and to achieve the best possible results for the patient, the surgeon must keep the following principles in mind.

1. A properly planned incision is just long enough to afford sufficient operating space.
2. A clean incision is made through the skin with one stroke of evenly applied pressure on the scalpel.
3. All tissues should be handled gently and as little as possible throughout the operative procedure. Care must be taken in placing and handling retractors to prevent undue pressure on tissues.
4. Meticulous hemostasis is essential, for blood not only obscures the operative field and makes accurate dissection more difficult, blood can also act as a culture medium for microbial growth leading to wound infection, abscess, etc.
5. Preservation of blood supply is important in all tissues. Adequate debridement of all devitalized and necrotic tissue, and removal of inflicted foreign bodies, is essential to healing.
6. Periodic irrigation with warm physiologic saline, or covering exposed surfaces with saline-moistened sponges helps avoid drying of tissues during long procedures.
7. Tissue should be approximated without tension or strangulation to prevent ischemic necrosis. The surgeon must evaluate each patient and choose the wound closure material most likely to promote healing under each particular surgical circumstance.

No wound will remain approximated with an inadequate closure technique or improper choice of wound closure material.

II. CARDIOVASCULAR SYSTEM

Artery-to-artery anastomoses, including primary closure of arteriotomies, are said to heal by 28 d[1] and vein-to-artery anastomoses to heal by 6 to 8 weeks.[2] Therefore, in patients with normal vascular healing, the suture used for these situations may not need to be permanent. What is more important is tensile strength during the healing phase and lack of significant inflammation. A suture used for vascular anastomoses should also have a low coefficient of friction to minimize injury to the intima and the disruption of plaques.[3]

Polyglycolide (Dexon®) and polyglactin 910 (Vicryl®) have been shown in experimental animal models to be suitable for vascular anastomoses.[4,5] However, these sutures have not been used clinically because of concerns about their premature loss of tensile strength and their tendency to drag through the vessel wall. In addition, many vascular reconstructions are performed on elderly, infirm patients likely to exhibit a broad spectrum of healing characteristics. As a consequence, although a nonabsorbable suture may not be required, polypropylene (Prolene®) is the most widely used suture for arterial anastomoses. Coated polyester, another nonabsorbable suture, is also commonly used. Both of these sutures have minimal drag in tissues and maintain their tensile strength permanently.

The use of nonabsorbable sutures in pediatric cardiovascular operations may be a major factor in the development of anastomotic strictures.[6] The development of polydioxanone (PDS®) and polyglyconate (Maxon®) sutures has generated interest in these absorbable materials for arterial anastomoses, particularly in growing children. These sutures are monofilament and exhibit minimal tissue drag and maintain tensile strength for a prolonged period of time. The traditional approach to arterial repairs in growing children has been to employ interrupted nonabsorbable suture to allow circumferential growth of the artery. This is time consuming. A suitable absorbable suture may allow a faster continuous suture technique.

Stillman and Sophie[7] compared continuous Maxon with partially interrupted Prolene to repair aortic transections in 1-month-old pigs. Histologic analysis revealed no stenoses in the Maxon group, but an average of 5.8% and 3.5% stenoses at 6 and 9 months, respectively, in the Prolene group.

End-to-end repairs of iliac arteries in growing pigs were performed with interrupted PDS or Prolene by Steen et al.[8] In their study, the use of an all interrupted suture technique resulted in no stenoses in either group. However, Prolene was said to elicit a more pronounced inflammatory tissue response in that model and for that reason, PDS was recommended.

Load-bearing healing of a prosthetic graft-to-artery anastomosis does not occur following implantation of currently clinically available vascular grafts and the anastomosis remains dependent on its sutures to maintain integrity.[9] Resorption or breakage of these sutures may therefore result in disruption of the anastomosis and subsequent pseudoaneurysm formation. Therefore, prosthetic grafting should always be performed with nonabsorbable sutures. In the early era of vascular surgery, silk suture was widely used and has been implicated in the subsequent high prevalence of pseudoaneurysm formation. The tensile strength of silk decreases by as much as 20% to 40% after 1 month, and is nearly gone by 2 years.[10] Because of the inadequacy of silk, polyethylene suture was widely used in the 1960s. Although polyethylene had been considered to be nonabsorbable, it fractured, hydrolyzed, and underwent enzymatic digestion, and it too led to the development of many pseudoaneurysms.[11] As stated above, Prolene is the most widely used, but coated polyester and Gore-Tex®[12] sutures also perform adequately.

Prolene seems to have some advantages over multifilament polyester. Roy et al.[13] evaluated different sutures used to anastomose prosthetic aortic grafts in dogs. Prolene exhibited less inflammatory reaction and less thrombogenicity than polyester. On the other hand, Prolene, being a monofilament, is liable to fracture if the outer shell is injured. It can be easily damaged by any instrument or sharp-edged surface, such as a calcified plaque. Care must be taken to prevent such damage, which may not be noticed intraoperatively and may later cause suture failure.

For aortic grafting, 3/0 Prolene is commonly used. At the other range of arterial size, such as tibial, peroneal, and pedal arteries, 7/0 suture is appropriate. There are experimental data that indicate that for carotid arteriotomies, 6/0 Prolene is suitable but that 7/0 Prolene may not exhibit sufficient tensile strength at this location because of the additional stress on the suture line caused by cervical motion.[14,15]

III. ABDOMINAL SYSTEM

A. ABDOMINAL WALL CLOSURE

There are numerous clinical studies, prospective and retrospective, on the optimal suture methods for closure of the abdominal fascia after laparotomy. Although the merits of different kinds of incisions can be argued, the vast majority of studies concerns the closure of the midline vertical incisions. The time required for continuous closure is always less than for interrupted closure. The debate most frequently concerns the use of absorbable vs. permanent suture and the use of continuous vs. interrupted suturing technique. Most studies have addressed the rate of wound infection, early wound dehiscence, late herniation, sinus formation, and other late wound complications. Some studies have tried to determine the degree of wound pain in the late postoperative period.

A common problem with many of the studies is the comparison of different suture techniques using different suture materials. Nonetheless, the large number of published reports makes available some conclusions: continuous suture technique is as reliable as interrupted technique; late hernias might be more common with quickly absorbed Vicryl or Dexon compared to slowly absorbed Maxon or PDS or nonabsorbable sutures; and late wound pain and sinus formation is more common with nonabsorbable sutures. Chromic (and therefore, plain) catgut has been found to be unacceptable because of its early loss of tensile strength.[16] Taking deep bites of tissue is important and for continuous closure, a suture length to wound length ratio of at least 4:1 is recommended.[17] This is easily done when closing the abdominal wall by placing sutures 2 cm from the fascial wound edge and 2 cm apart, which will result in a ratio of 4.2:1 (Figure 9.1).[18] Results of some of the more recent randomized studies follow.

Wissing et al.[19] compared four techniques to close the fascia after midline laparotomy incisions in a randomized prospective study of 1491 patients. All four techniques used mass closure and differed by the use of either interrupted no. 2 Vicryl, continuous no. 1 Vicryl, continuous 0 PDS, or continuous no. 1 nylon. There was no significant difference in the rate of early wound infection or wound dehiscence among the four groups. At 1 year, continuous nylon had a significantly higher incidence of wound pain and suture sinus formation. The rate of incisional hernia was also lowest in the nylon group (10.4%), which was significantly lower than continuous Vicryl (20.6%), which was the highest. Continuous PDS was the second lowest (13.2%).

Interrupted no. 1 Vicryl was compared to continuous 0 Maxon by Trimbos et al.[20] in a randomized study of 340 women undergoing midline laparotomy. No significant differences could be found in the incidence of early wound infection and dehiscence or in late suture sinuses, incisional hernias, or wound pain, comparing the interrupted and continuous closure groups.

Richards et al.[21] randomized 571 patients with various abdominal incisions, most commonly midline vertical incisions, to either closure with continuous 0 Prolene or with interrupted 0 Dexon in a single layer for vertical incisions and in two layers for oblique incisions. In midline incisions, the dehiscence rate was 2% (5 of 244) for the continuous closure group, vs. 0.9% (2 of 229) for the interrupted closure group. Hernias developed in 2% of the continuous and 0.5% of the interrupted closure group. For oblique incisions, dehiscence occurred in 0% (0 of 39) of the continuous and 2% (1 of 50) of the interrupted

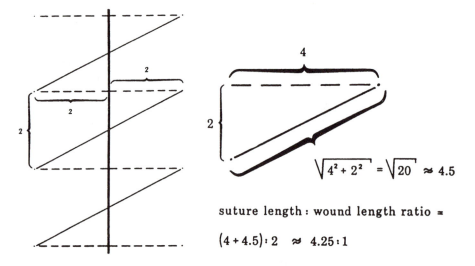

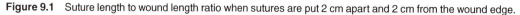

$$\sqrt{4^2 + 2^2} = \sqrt{20} \approx 4.5$$

suture length : wound length ratio =

$$(4 + 4.5) : 2 \approx 4.25 : 1$$

Figure 9.1 Suture length to wound length ratio when sutures are put 2 cm apart and 2 cm from the wound edge.

closure group. There were no late hernias. None of the differences were statistically significant. Continuous closure required an average of 20 min vs. 40 min for the interrupted closure.

A comparison of different suture materials using the same technique was performed by Krukowski et al.[22] They randomized 757 consecutive patients undergoing midline laparotomy to either continuous mass closure with no. 1 PDS or with no. 1 Prolene. There was only one dehiscence in each group. The incidence of late hernias was similar (7.7% for PDS, 9.7% for Prolene), but Prolene suture required removal from five patients for late wound pain or sinus formation.

Israelsson and Jonsson[23] compared continuous nylon vs. continuous PDS in a randomized trial of 813 patients with midline laparotomies. There were no differences in wound dehiscence, wound infection, or incisional hernia rates between the two groups.

A comparison of the same suture using different techniques was performed by Fagniez et al.[24] Dexon was used to close midline laparotomies in 3135 patients who were randomized between continuous and interrupted suture techniques. The dehiscence rate was not different: 1.6% with continuous sutures and 2% with interrupted sutures. Continuous closure was preferable because it was more economical and less time consuming.

Randomized trials have shown no differences in dehiscence or hernia rates when the peritoneum is closed as a separate layer, included in the mass closure, or ignored.[25] Subcutaneous sutures have been shown to increase the risk of wound infection and are generally not recommended.[26]

B. GASTROINTESTINAL SUTURE

Traditional teaching on gastrointestinal anastomoses has maintained that serosal apposition is preferred. This has been commonly performed by using a two-layer technique. The inner layer is usually through the entire bowel wall using an absorbable suture, such as chromic catgut, Vicryl, or Dexon, and is either continuous or interrupted. The outer layer is placed through the seromuscular layer in an inverting fashion using nonabsorbable material, most commonly silk, and also using either continuous or interrupted technique.

Recently, single-layer techniques have been championed by some to be as effective, less time consuming, and associated with the development of fewer anastomotic strictures. Both absorbable and nonabsorbable sutures have been shown to be satisfactory. Although some experimental studies have shown interrupted sutures to be preferable to continuous sutures,[27] a clinical advantage is not evident.

Irvin et al.[28] performed the earliest randomized prospective clinical trial of single-layer vs. two-layer intestinal anastomoses. Both ileal and colonic anastomoses were included, but none were to the rectum. The radiologic leak rate (not necessarily an indication of an untoward clinical response) was 17% in the single-layer group and 16% in the two-layer group. They were able to conclude that the single-layer technique was as good as the two-layer method.

A randomized trial of single-layer vs. two-layer colorectal anastomoses was reported by Everett.[29] The single-layer anastomosis was performed with interrupted braided nylon and the two-layer with full thickness continuous chromic catgut and seromuscular interrupted braided nylon. The clinical leak rate was 1% in both groups. Radiologic leak rates were similar in the two groups when the anastomosis was to the intraperitoneal rectum (15.4% vs. 15.8%), but for those anastomoses below the pelvic reflection, the radiologic leak rate was significantly greater for the group using the two-layer technique (9% vs. 46%). On the other hand, Goligher et al.[30] did not find any advantage in a single-layer technique over a two-layer technique for either high or low rectal anastomoses.

McDonald and Baird[31] demonstrated good results in 327 small intestinal and colonic anastomoses using a single layer of interrupted Vicryl sutures. There were only two clinically apparent leaks, for a rate of 0.6%.

Bardini et al.[32] performed a randomized prospective study comparing the efficacy of a single layer of continuous Maxon vs. a single layer of interrupted Vicryl for cervical esophagogastric anastomoses. There were 21 patients in each group. One asymptomatic anastomotic leak and two anastomotic strictures developed in the interrupted suture group. Operative time and suture cost were significantly less with the continuous suture technique.

A continuous single layer anastomosis constructed of either PDS or Maxon was compared to endoluminal circular stapling in various esophageal anastomoses in 580 patients by Fok et al.[33] The rates of clinical anastomotic leaks was 5% in the sutured group and 3.8% in the stapled group, which were not statistically different. However, anastomotic strictures developed in 10.5% of the patients with sutured anastomoses and 29.2% of the patients with stapled anastomoses, which was statistically significant. Thus, the single-layer continuous suture technique was preferred.

A similar comparison was made by Seufert et al.[34] Eighty patients undergoing total gastrectomy were randomized to have the esophagojejunostomy performed with an endoluminal stapler or with a single layer of continuous Maxon. Both methods gave good results. Of the 40 patients with stapled anastomoses, anastomotic leakage was apparent intraoperatively in 3 patients, leading to surgical correction. Technical failure occurred in one patient who then required a sutured anastomosis. One patient developed a leak. None of the sutured anastomoses developed a leak. There was one transient late stenosis in the sutured group which resolved spontaneously.

The single-layer continuous suture technique has been shown to be safe for gastric anastomoses. Demartines et al.[35] performed 96 gastroduodenostomies and gastrojejunostomies with a continuous single layer of 4/0 Maxon. A 2.1% clinical leakage rate was noted, all in patients who had perforated ulcers with peritonitis.

Saran and Lightwood[36] used a single layer of continuous Dexon for anastomoses in 66 upper gastrointestinal and 65 colonic resections. Clinical anastomotic failure was seen in 4.5% and 6.2% of the patients in each group, respectively.

Continuous single-layer Prolene anastomosis for colon resections has been compared to double-layer anastomosis and stapling.[37] There was a 6.8% (3/44) anastomotic leak rate for continuous single layer Prolene, 9.5% (2/21) for double layer, and 0 percent (0/19) for stapling. These differences were not statistically significant. Two of three leaks in the single-layer group and one of two in the double-layer group were in patients taking steroids. The average cost was $4 for single layer, $8 for double layer, and $35 for stapling.

A much larger series of continuous single-layer Prolene colocolic, colorectal, ileocolic, and iliorectal anastomoses was reported by Max et al.[38] Out of 1000 anastomoses, the clinically evident leak rate was 1% and the anastomotic stricture rate was 1%, with no deaths due to anastomotic complications.

IV. BRONCHIAL, TRACHEAL, AND CHEST SYSTEM

A. BRONCHIAL SUTURE

Bronchial closure after pneumonectomy has been performed with a variety of sutures such as stainless steel wire, Dexon, Vicryl, or Prolene, and with stapling devices. Some authors believe that absorbable sutures are preferred because they will not persist as foreign bodies which may cause excessive granulation.[39] Interrupted suture technique with knots tied on the outside has been recommended.[40]

Sarsam and Moussali[41] constructed a posterior flap from the pliable membranous bronchus using 2/0 chromic catgut. They believe that bronchial healing is not affected by the type of suture material as long as there is no tension at the suture line.

Excellent results have been obtained by Al-Kattan et al.[42] using 2/0 Prolene. They approximated the membranous portion to the cartilaginous wall and placed a double row of continuous horizontal sutures followed by a third row of over and over continuous suture. There were 7 fistulas (1.3%) out of 530 consecutive patients. They did not condemn staplers but noted that the use of staplers is limited when dealing with thickened airways or in close proximity to a tumor and that a stapler is much more expensive.

Another method of bronchial stump closure was reported by Sato et al.[43] They apposed the cartilaginous walls and placed horizontal mattress sutures with Teflon pledgets near the corners and interrupted sutures in between using 2-0 coated braided polyester. One patient out of 288 developed a bronchopleural fistula.

B. TRACHEAL SUTURE

Repair of a circumferential defect of the trachea resulting either from trauma or from surgical resection of tumor or stricture is best performed by end-to-end anastomosis.[44] This is usually performed by suturing the tracheal cartilages on either side of the anastomosis to each other. With this technique, long segments of the trachea can be resected and the ends approximated by extensive mobilization, although some tension may exist.

The best suture material for tracheal reconstruction is debated. Interrupted suture technique is usually used. Some authors prefer absorbable sutures for this anastomosis. Alstrup and Sorenson[45] used interrupted Dexon or chromic catgut with good results in a small series of pediatric patients. Maasen et al.[46] also favor absorbable sutures. The use of nonabsorbable suture is thought to lead to suture granulomas with subsequent stenosis at the anastomotic site. However, Nordin and Ohlsen[47] contend that nonabsorbable sutures are *less* likely to induce the formation of granulation tissue. In their experimental studies, the use of nonabsorbable suture was associated with more suture granulomas but the use of 3/0 Dexon led to separation of the anastomotic lines because of early loss of tensile strength. These diastases were filled in with granulating scar tissue that later caused significant stenoses. Perhaps PDS or Maxon would cause fewer suture granulomas as well as fewer anastomotic strictures.

In an experimental study by McKeown et al.[48] on growing rabbits, tracheal transection and anastomosis was performed using continuous or interrupted PDS or continuous or interrupted Prolene sutures. Although all methods of anastomosis produced some degree of tracheal stenosis, the use of interrupted PDS resulted in significantly less tight stenosis. Friedman et al.[49] conducted similar experiments in lambs, comparing PDS and Vicryl sutures. They found little difference between continuous or interrupted suture techniques but found more intense inflammatory reaction, more rapid resorption, and greater subsequent fibrosis with Vicryl sutures.

Grillo et al.[50] have accumulated one of the largest clinical series of patients with tracheal resection and reconstruction with 521 tracheal reconstructions from 1965 through 1992. Before 1978, they used braided polyester or Prolene and had suture line granulation develop in 23.6% of the patients (44 of 186). Since then, they switched to Vicryl and found anastomotic granulation formation in only 1.6% (5 of 317). PDS was used briefly by these surgeons but was abandoned because they felt that it showed no advantages and was more cumbersome to use.

C. CHEST WALL CLOSURE

Major wound complications after median sternotomy are infrequent, occurring in less than 2% of patients,[51] and the most common complication is sternal dehiscence.[52] Closure of a median sternotomy is commonly accomplished using monofilament stainless steel wire, either placed through the sternum away from the divided edge or passed completely around the sternum.

Stoney et al.[52] placed an average of six wires through the sternum in simple loops and found a dehiscence rate of 1.7% (17 out of 1000) with wires that were twisted tight manually, and a rate of 0.3% (3 out of 1000) when wires were affixed with a crimped locking plate. In their experience, with complete dehiscence the wires were found to have cut completely through the sternum, and with partial separation the wires had partially cut into the sternum. Dehiscence caused by breakage of the wires was unusual.

Because of this, other authors have advocated figure-eight suture techniques. Goodman et al.[53] placed wires through the sternum three fourths the distance laterally from the cut edge, in interrupted figure-eight fashion. One suture was placed in the manubrium and two or three sutures in the body of the sternum. They felt that the figure-eight suture placement was more stable because the tension on the wires was oriented obliquely on the sternum instead of horizontally as would occur with simple sutures. Their dehiscence rate was 0.4% (5 out of 1200 consecutive closures).

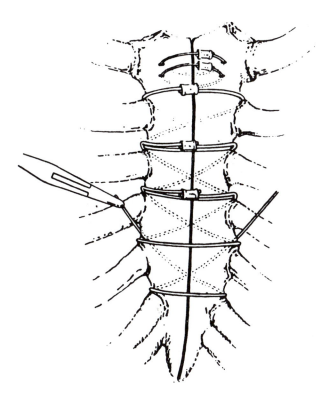

Figure 9.2 Closure of the sternum using interlocking figure-eight sutures. (From March, R.F., Jr. et al., *Ann. Thorac. Surg.*, 47, 928, 1989. With permission.)

A further modification was reported by Di Marco et al.[54] They placed two simple transmanubrial sutures. Remaining sutures were in a parasternal figure-eight fashion, each suture going through two adjacent intercostal spaces. These figure-eight sutures were interlocked by placing the upper loop of a subsequent suture around the same intercostal space that was encircled by the bottom loop of the previous suture and by placing the upper loop of the subsequent suture superior to the lower loop of the previous suture (Figure 9.2). This method prevented sternal fracture and dehiscence by imparting a lateral reinforcement on the sternum and by distributing the tension over a larger area of each interspace. In 978 consecutive patients, they did not have any sternal dehiscence.

The use of alternative suture materials, such as Teflon-coated Dacron®,[55] nylon bands,[56] and Silastic® bands,[57] have been abandoned. However, a report by Pastorino et al.[58] demonstrated the safety of Maxon for sternal closure. No. 1 Maxon was used as a double strand around the sternum through the intercostal spaces either as simple or figure-of-eight suture placement. Out of 216 consecutive sternotomies closed with this suture material, there were no cases of sternal dehiscence or infection.

V. OBSTETRIC AND GYNECOLOGIC SYSTEM

A. CRITERIA FOR CLOSURE OF A VARIETY OF TISSUES
1. Subcutaneous Layer
Unless the cautery unit is used to seal subcutaneous blood vessels, free ties will be needed almost immediately following the skin incision. Typically, a rapidly absorbed suture material with adequate short-term tensile strength is desired (such as chromic).

2. Gastrointestinal Tract
The principal concern in closing wounds of the gastrointestinal tract is leakage, for leakage can result in localized or generalized peritonitis. A leak-proof anastomosis or closure is essential. A practicing gynecologist most frequently encounters the need for knowledge and skill in basic intestinal surgery when there is unexpected trauma at the time of surgery. Most commonly, such trauma occurs secondary

to the laceration to an adhesed loop of bowel upon entering the peritoneal cavity; less frequently, the trauma may occur during intraabdominal dissection of adhesions or possibly excessive pressure of a retractor upon a loop of bowel. Whatever the etiology, the critical part of the problem is immediate recognition of the trauma and correction of the damage to the intestine.

3. Small Intestine

The small intestine heals very rapidly and maximal strength is reached in about 14 d. For injuries involving the seromuscular layer only, interrupted 4/0 silk or synthetic nonabsorbable suture may be utilized, with the primary suture line made perpendicular to the long axis of the intestine to minimize narrowing of the bowel lumen. For small antimesenteric perforations or tears less than 1 cm in diameter, an inner purse string of 4/0 absorbable synthetic suture is imbricated inside of an outer purse string of 4/0 silk or other nonabsorbable suture such as Prolene. Neither suture layer should penetrate the mucosa, but rather only the submucosa, muscularis, and serosa of the bowel.

Linear lacerations greater than 1 cm are corrected with a two-layer closure. The primary suture lines should run perpendicular to the long axis of the intestine, again to minimize narrowing of the bowel lumen. It should be a full-thickness closure employing 4/0 absorbable synthetic suture placed in either a continuous closure or in a closure with interrupted sutures. The continuous closure will result in a tighter seal. It is important not to lock continuous sutures in the intestine because this may produce ischemia along the suture line. A second seromuscular outer layer of interrupted silk is then placed to invert the primary suture line. For longer linear lacerations, typically loop closures are utilized to repair these defects unless tissue necrosis or interruption of blood supply has occurred. In the latter case, resection of the impaired segment with reanastomosis is performed with either loop closure or resection. The same general principals of suture closure apply as for any other small bowel repair. Namely, the inner full-thickness primary suture line should consist of 4/0 absorbable synthetic suture, and the outer seromuscular imbricating suture line consist of permanent 4/0 silk or synthetic nonabsorbable interrupted sutures.

4. Large Bowel

The principles that apply to repair of damage to the small bowel are similarly applied in the setting of damage to the large bowel. For seromuscular linear lacerations that are not full thickness, the defect should be picked up in the transverse direction and closed with a primary seromuscular suture line of interrupted 4/0 silk or similar synthetic nonabsorbable suture sewn perpendicular to the long axis of the colon. Again, such an orientation is designed to avoid narrowing of the lumen. When a full-thickness laceration has occurred, it is wise to use a two-layer closure. Given the high microbial content of the colon, any time that it is violated some degree of contamination of the surrounding tissue is unavoidable. Braided or multifilament sutures are contraindicated in the setting of potential infection; therefore, the inner primary suture line for a full-thickness colon defect should consist of an interrupted layer of monofilament synthetic absorbable suture such as coated Vicryl (ideally suited because of its reliable rate of absorption after 28 d). An outer seromuscular layer of interrupted 4/0 silk or Prolene is perfectly acceptable, followed by thorough irrigation of the closure area to dilute the bacterial content remaining.

In the setting in which the bowel has been unprepared preoperatively and gross fecal contamination has occurred, the wisest approach is to exteriorize the damaged segment of colon.

5. Bladder

The reported incidence of urinary tract injury in gynecologic surgery (excluding radical hysterectomy) is 0.2% to 2.5%.[59] The most common injury is cystotomy during abdominal hysterectomy. If a bladder injury is recognized interoperatively, primary repair is almost always successful. If the damage is not appreciated, a vesicovaginal fistula may result.

Permanent sutures should not be used in cystotomy repairs, as they may serve as a nidus for the development of bladder stones. Many surgeons employ 3/0 chromic catgut for bladder repairs. However, given the fact that studies indicate 3 weeks are required for complete bladder healing following damage, a more logical suture of choice would be the synthetic absorbable sutures Dexon or Vicryl. They maintain 60% of their tensile strength after 10 to 14 d, and have a reliable rate of absorption after 28 d. The repair itself consists of a primary running continuous suture line through the mucosa and muscularis of the bladder, designed to invert and reapproximate the mucosa. A second layer of interrupted 3/0 synthetic absorbable sutures is then placed through all muscle layers, with the interrupted suture placed 1 cm apart and in such a fashion that they imbricate the bladder muscle over the primary suture line. The bladder should be closed without tension over the suture line. In a healthy patient with an uncomplicated closure in the dome of the bladder, 5 d of catheter drainage is adequate. In a patient with dependent cystotomy or risk factors for poor healing (radiation, steroid use, poor nutrition, etc.) 10 to 14 d of catheter drainage is required. Whenever a catheter remains in the bladder for 72 h or longer, cystitis will result after removal. Therefore, an antibiotic is given upon removal of the catheter in this setting. If the repair is close to the trigon, inspection of the trigon area should be performed prior to attempting the repair and once the repair is complete as well. This can be accomplished via cystoscopy in the dorsal lithotomy position, or through a small cystotomy incision in the dome of the bladder if employing the abdominal supine approach.

6. Rectum
The rectum is notoriously slow to heal. Because the lower portion is retroperitoneal, it does not have a serosal covering. When suturing the rectum, monofilament sutures are indicated because of the potential microbial contamination in the rectum. Synthetic absorbable monofilament sutures with prolonged tensile strength and minimal reactivity are the sutures of choice.

7. Fascia
The fascia is the strongest tissue in the abdominal wall, as well as many other sites of the body, yet it heals very slowly, regaining only 40% of its original strength in 2 months following incision. Seventy-five percent of the strength is regained within 9 months, and generally restoration of maximal strength usually requires more than 1 year. Even then, the fascia will never again be as strong as it was prior to surgical incision.

8. Muscle
Sutures, when placed in abdominal muscle tissue, are usually of the same material as that used for fascial closure.

9. Subcutaneous Fat
Placing sutures in the subcutaneous fat layer for any reason is of questionable benefit and must be examined critically. Fat is mostly water and as such has no tensile strength. The placement of subcutaneous sutures to obliterate dead space and to prevent hematoma formation carries with it a significant infectious risk to the wound closure, because the presence of a single suture of any type will drastically reduce the size of the inoculum required to produce infection. If one is concerned about hematoma formation impairing wound healing by preventing tissue approximation, a more prudent course of action than suture placement would be to assure meticulous hemostasis prior to skin closure.

10. Subcuticular Layer
The subcuticular layer of tough connective tissue in the dermis, when sutured, will hold the skin edges in close approximation when good cosmetic results are required. Studies have shown that single subcuticular layer closures produce less evidence of scar gaping or expansion at 6 and 9 months after surgery than do simple skin closures.

Either absorbable or nonabsorbable sutures may be used. If nonabsorbable suture is chosen, the suture strand must come out through the skin at each end of the incision. Prolene is a good choice for the latter, in that it displays minimal tissue adhesiveness and may be easily "pulled through" once the critical period of collagen synthesis is complete.

The size of suture employed will depend upon the degree of tension upon the skin. When skin tension is great, such as in abdominal closures, larger size should be used. Where skin tension is not great, such as in the face and neck, very fine sizes of subcuticular sutures can be used. In general, the closer the approximation of the skin edge being sutured, the more hairline the scar that will result.

11. Skin
Most wound stress is taken up by the fascia. Therefore, in closing most wounds, particularly abdominal wounds, reliance is placed upon fascial closure to hold the wound together, not the skin closure. Thus, the skin or subcuticular stitches need only be strong enough to overcome the natural skin tension and keep the wound edges in apposition. Suture technique for skin closure may be either continuous or interrupted, with either absorbable or nonabsorbable material. Since we are not able to sterilize the skin preoperatively, rather only cleanse it with an antiseptic agent, in theory the same suture strand should

not be repeatedly passed through the skin and thereby introduce the risk of cross-contamination along the entire suture line in so doing. For this, as well as other reasons, interrupted technique in the skin is usually preferred.

Monofilament sutures are superior to multifilament sutures in skin closure, for two reasons. First, monofilament sutures induce significantly less tissue reaction than multifilament sutures, and hence yield a cosmetically superior result. Second, it must be remembered that skin sutures are exposed to the external environment. Contamination with exogenous microorganisms in the wound and suture track is a potential hazard leading to wound infection or stitch abscess. Unlike monofilament sutures, multifilament sutures may provide a haven for microorganisms that can penetrate the interstices of suture, into areas too tightly braided or twisted for granulocytes and macrophages to work their way into. Thus, it can be appreciated that monofilament sutures are usually preferred for skin closure.

Nonabsorbable skin sutures are always removed postoperatively. A general rule regarding timed removal is as follows:

1. Skin about face and neck, 2 to 5 d
2. Other skin sutures, 5 to 8 d
3. Retention sutures, 10 to 14 d

The difference in time is related to the rate of healing in individual areas and the purpose for which the sutures were initially placed. The key to successful cosmetic closure is suture removal prior to epithelialization of the suture track with subsequent "railroad track" scar formation, and before contamination is converted into infection.

B. INCISION AND CLOSURE IN THE ABDOMINAL SYSTEM
1. Incision
Preoperative clinical trials have shown that in respect to the types of abdominal incisions employed and the incidence of wound dehiscence or hernia formation, there is little or no difference between paramedian, oblique, or transverse incisions.[60] The only approach having an undoubted advantage is the wide or lateral paramedian incision, shown to reduce the incidence of postoperative incisional hernia formation from 10% to 1% of major laparotomies.[61]

2. Closures
A variety of wound closure techniques have been popularized, including the layered closure, Smead-Jones mass closure, the interrupted mass closure, and the continuous mass closure. It has been demonstrated repeatedly that the mass closures, incorporating anterior fascia, rectus muscle, posterior sheath if present, and peritoneum in each bite, are stronger and more secure wound closures than layered closures.[62] This is a result of the sutures being placed farther from the fascial edges and incorporating more tissue, thereby reducing the pressure per unit area around the suture.

3. Suture
The abdominal wound may break down either completely or partially, for one or more of the following reasons:

1. The knot may break or come undone. This results from a problem in suture technique.
2. The suture may rupture, either because it is too weak for the tension placed on it or because it is rapidly destroyed in the tissues before adequate wound healing has taken place. This factor should be avoidable if suture of the correct size and type is selected.
3. The sutures may cut through the tissues. This may occur either because they are placed too close to the wound edge, because they are tied too tightly, resulting in ischemic necrosis, or because of excessive weakening of the tissues from such factors as jaundice, uremia, protein depletion, or most importantly, infection.

The most common finding in wound dehiscence is that the suture and surgical knot remain intact but that one or more of the sutures cuts or pulls through the tissue.[63] Several factors can contribute to this complication. Sutures that are placed too far apart cause increased tension on each suture. Sutures should be placed 1 to 2 cm from each fascial edge and 1 cm apart. The sutures should be tied with enough tension to loosely reapproximate the fascial edges. The wound becomes swollen and edematous shortly after it is inflicted; sutures tied with too much tension initially may cause pressure necrosis of the intervening tissues and thereby increase the risk of suture "cut through."

It has been shown repeatedly that chromic catgut should not be used for abdominal closures because it loses most of its tensile strength in less than 1 week.[64] Because of the slow healing time of fascia and because a fascial suture must bear the maximum stress of the wound, a moderate size nonabsorbable suture (i.e., Prolene) or delayed absorbable synthetic suture (i.e., PDS, Maxon) should be used.[65] In the absence of infection or gross contamination, either multifilament or monofilament sutures may be used. In the presence of infection, however, a monofilament delayed absorbable or an inert monofilament nonabsorbable suture is indicated.

Interrupted technique is employed most frequently to close fascia. Recent data show that running continuous sutures are faster and are as effective and safe as interrupted sutures.[62–64,66] Continuous sutures have the theoretical advantage of distributing wound tension evenly across the suture line, more so than is the case with interrupted sutures. With running continuous closures, the ratio of suture length to wound length should be at lease 4:1.[67] The surgeon must understand the suture material being used and its characteristics, because knot integrity with continuous running closures is essential.

In general, the best way to reduce the incidence of wound dehiscence and herniation is to (1) do all that is possible to prevent wound infection, (2) use good surgical technique, and (3) use appropriate sutures placed the correct distance apart and tied down with appropriate tension with secure knots.

C. STAPLE AND CLIP DEVICES FOR WOUND CLOSURE

Beginning with the earliest d of surgery, surgeons have been concerned about the time required for, and the extent of, trauma associated with certain surgical procedures. In an effort to address both of these issues, in 1908 a Hungarian surgeon, Professor Hamer Hültl of Budapest, introduced the first mechanical wound closure device for internal use. This instrument was used to place straight double rows of staples in an alternating fashion across the stomach. Hültl recognized the importance of two principles: the need for a B-shaped formation of the staples, and fine wire as the basic staple material.[68] The Soviet Union actively researched and further developed these instruments during the 1950s. The first American-made stapling devices were manufactured by the US Surgical Corporation and introduced in the late 1960s. Since that time, there have been many improvements and new staplers developed, with current stapling devices available as single- or multi-fire instruments, or as reusable instruments with disposable cartridges. Surgical staplers generally operate upon a two-step process. In the first step, no significant tissue damage occurs. This step involves compression and immobilization of the tissue, and is reversible. The second step places the staples and may also cut the tissue. Each instrument is designed for stapling specific tissues. The surgeon selects the correct instrument for the desired application. Relative to conventional suturing technique, stapling offers two significant advantages. (1) Stapling is faster than conventional suturing, and hence can reduce operating time and blood loss. (2) Stapling can result in less tissue trauma because tissue handling is minimized. Surgical staplers have also been shown to decrease peritoneal contamination during bowel surgery, for studies have demonstrated improved blood flow to the gastrointestinal anastomosis when stapling instruments are used compared to hand-sewn anastomosis.[69] This has been attributed to less tissue trauma and less localized necrosis, which favors angiogenesis at the anastomotic site.[69] The "B" shape of the closed staples is noncrushing, yet it provides for adequate hemostasis and approximation. Given the noncrushing staple configuration, how-ever, it is therefore necessary to visually inspect each staple line for hemostasis after staples are placed. Any small areas of bleeding can be controlled with cautery or fine absorbable suture.

There are two types of staples currently available: permanent staples of stainless steel or titanium and absorbable staples made of a lactide-glycolic polymer absorbed by hydrolysis. Permanent staples are inert and have much less tissue reaction than currently available sutures.[70] Absorbable staples can be used at sites where permanent staples may be undesirable, such as in the vaginal cuff closure, cystotomy repair, and bowel segments for urinary conduits. Absorbable clips retain over 50% of their tensile strength at 60 d.[71] The details of clips and staples will be given in Chapter 10.

1. Skin

Skin staples have been used extensively to close surgical incisions[72] and have recently been advocated for the closure of lacerations.[73] They have been utilized extensively to hold skin grafts in place.[72] To understand the advantages of skin staples, it is necessary to keep in mind specific aspects of skin closure. The two basic requirements for apposing skin are that:

1. The edges of the cuticular and subcuticular layers are everted (i.e., aligned with the edges slightly raised in an outward direction). As the skin incision heals, the tissue will slowly flatten out and form an even surface.
2. The skin edges must be aligned as close to their original configuration as possible. If one edge is placed in a location higher or lower than its original location relative to the apposing edge, the best cosmetic result will not be obtained and unnecessary scars can form.[74]

The rectangular design of skin staples minimizes tissue trauma; approximation of the skin edges by stapling minimizes tissue compression. The space between the crown of the staple (top) and the skin surface immediately beneath reduces the incidence of cross-hatching marks so commonly seen with incisions closed with too much tension on an incision line or because of postoperative edema.

Skin staplers can be used virtually anywhere, regardless of body contour. Applications include routine operative skin closure, graft fixation, or for laceration repairs that present to the emergency room. Most studies have documented that staples are cosmetically superior or equal to suture closure. At the same time, patients' acceptance of stapled incisions is good and they have been reported to be less painful to remove than sutures in most studies.[75]

Recently, a subcuticular skin stapler utilizing absorbable staples has been introduced, with excellent cosmetic results. This is a significant step forward in skin closure, and will likely replace current conventional mechanical skin closure devices.

2. Viscera
A variety of mechanical closure devices have been introduced recently for application in abdominal surgery.

1. TA (transverse anastomosis) stapling instruments place a double row of staggered staples, and can be used with either metal or absorbable staples. The TA instruments have multiple applications, including repair of enterotomies, appendectomies, repair of cystotomies, and vaginal cuff closure. Some surgeons have also used the TA-55 (with small staples and narrow staple spacing) to secure the infundibulopelvic ligament.
2. GIA (gastrointestinal anastomosis) instrument — the GIA is a surgical staple instrument that places two double staggered rows of staples and cuts the tissue between the two double rows. This device is most often used for dividing bowel and in the formation of functional end-to-end anastomosis. As with all visceral staplers, hemostasis should be verified along the staple line after staple placement. This instrument is not designed and should not be used for stapling bowel mesentery. This stapling device can be used safely on irradiated intestine.[76]
3. EEA (end-to-end anastomosis) stapling instrument — the EEA instrument is used for end-to-end and end-to-side anastomosis of the alimentary tract. It minimally inverts the mucosal edges and has been used extensively for low rectal anastomoses. The use of this instrument has been reported to allow even lower anastomosis and can be performed manually.[77]

It is important to avoid tension on all bowel anastomoses, regardless of technique used (sutures or staples). If the omentum is present, it can be taken down from the right side of the colon and stomach and sutured in the pelvis over the site of the anastomosis. This is most often performed when the patient has previously received high-dose pelvic radiation therapy.

D. SURGICAL MESH PRODUCTS
Primary closure of large abdominal wall defects generally places such repair under sufficient tension that the incidence of wound infection and necrosis is significantly increased. Surgical meshes are viable alternatives to primary wound closure of large abdominal wall defects when the addition of a reinforcing or bridging material is needed to obtain the desired surgical result. Suture placement of a sheet of mesh to bridge the defect will serve to maintain the viscera within the abdominal cavity until the mesh has become infiltrated, and ultimately overgrown with reparative granulation tissue.

Surgical mesh for these purposes is made of four different materials: (1) stainless steel, (2) polyester fiber, (3) polypropylene, and (4) polyglactin 9/0. The first of these, steel mesh, is biologically inert, yet exhibits inflexible handling characteristics that make it difficult and stiffer to work with than the synthetic fabric meshes. Polyester and polypropylene synthetic fiber mesh are bidirectionally elastic, permitting these meshes, once in place, to adapt to various stresses encountered in the body. The fiber junctions are not subject to the same work fatigue exhibited by more rigid metallic mesh (surgical steel). Both polyester and polypropylene elicit a minimum to slight inflammatory reaction, transient, followed by deposition of a thin fibrous layer of tissue. The mesh remains soft and pliable, and is not absorbed, degraded, nor weakened by the activity of tissue enzymes.

Synthetic absorbable mesh (polyglactin 9/0) is intended for use as a buttress to provide support during the healing process. Significant support is provided for at least 14 d postoperatively, but being absorbable, it should not be used when extended wound support is required.

For secure placement of surgical mesh, sutures should be placed approximately $1/4$ in. from the edge of the mesh, and should be spaced $1/4$ to $1/2$ in. apart. Nonabsorbable suture, preferably of the same material as the mesh, should be used to secure the nonabsorbable mesh. When the meshes are used in infants and children likely to experience further growth, the surgeon should be aware that these materials are limiting and will not expand to accommodate future growth potential.

E. SUMMARY

Over the years, as new synthetic suture materials have come into use, it is of interest to see how hard old habits die. Catgut sutures, with clearly limited tensile strength, moderately rapid absorption, and marked tissue reactivity, are still the most largely used sutures in this country. The surprising thing about this fact is that the newer synthetic sutures are clearly superior. They retain tensile strength longer, are minimally reactive and, therefore, minimize infectious risk while providing excellent wound strength. In addition, the multifilament synthetic sutures, given their limited "memory," exhibit excellent handling characteristics as well as greater knot security.

In general, when it comes to suture selection, the surgeon today has a vast array from which to choose for use in different body tissues. Adequate strength of suture material will prevent suture breakage, while ensuring adequate knot security (sufficient number of flat, square throws) will prevent knot slippage. Of paramount importance, however, is the fact that the surgeon must understand the nature of various suture materials, the biologic forces in the healing wound, and the interaction of the sutures with the tissues. The following general principles should guide the surgeon in suture selection.

1. When a wound has reached maximal strength following healing, sutures are then no longer necessary. Thus:
   a. Tissues that heal slowly, such as the skin and fascia, should usually be closed with nonabsorbable or delayed absorbable synthetic suture.
   b. Tissues that heal rapidly, such as the stomach, colon, and bladder may be closed with absorbable sutures.
2. Foreign bodies in potentially contaminated tissue may convert contamination to infection. Therefore:
   a. Avoid multifilament sutures that may convert a contaminated wound into an infected one.
   b. Use monofilament sutures in potentially contaminated tissues.
3. Where cosmetic results are important, close and prolonged apposition of wounds and avoidance of irritants will produce the best results. Therefore:
   a. Use the smallest inert monofilament suture materials such as nylon or polypropylene.
   b. Avoid skin sutures and close subcuticularly whenever possible.
   c. Under certain circumstances to maximize skin edge apposition, skin closure tape may be used.
4. Foreign bodies in the presence of fluids containing high concentration of crystalloids may act as nidus for precipitation and stone formation. Therefore:
   a. In the biliary and urinary tract, use rapidly absorbed sutures.
5. Regarding suture size:
   a. Use the finest size possible commensurate with the natural strength of the tissue.
   b. If the postoperative course of the patient may produce sudden strains on the suture line, reinforce it with retention sutures. Remove these as soon as the patient's condition has stabilized.

VI. ORTHOPEDIC SYSTEM

The principal objective of wound closure after a surgical procedure is to enhance and speed healing, as well as to restore and preserve function of the surgically treated part. Essentially, the surgeon attempts to repair or minimize tissue injury caused by accidental trauma or by the surgical procedure itself. Closure of a surgical wound is not absolutely necessary, as spontaneous healing by secondary intention (wound contraction, granulation, and epithelialization) will typically proceed to yield a well-healed wound.[78] However, successful surgical wound closure with healing by primary intention will provide

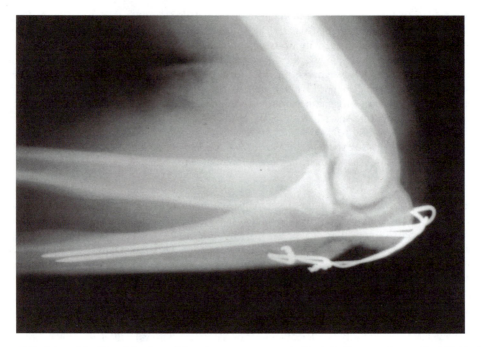

Figure 9.3 Internal fixation of fracture of the olecranon process to illustrate the use of smooth straight wires with figure-eight wire to convert distraction forces to compressive forces after an osteotomy of the olecranon.

much speedier healing and sealing of the wound from bacterial contamination.[79] Healing by primary intention is also more aesthetically pleasing and less painful. Moreover, prosthetic components are particularly susceptible to infection, making an effective closure essential.[80]

A wide variety of suture techniques are commonly used by orthopedic surgeons without a significant clinical discrepancy in results. The goal of a safe, effective, and cosmetic closure can be achieved by adherence to surgical principles; the specific choice of suture technique is not as important. Wound closure should be done in a clean environment and the tissues should be gently but securely approximated. Attention to hemostasis is important. Dead space should be avoided since it is a potential repository of blood or serous fluid and thus could provide a favorable environment for the development of infection.[78]

Specific wound closure problems in orthopedic surgery include repairs of osteotomies as well as repair of muscle or tendons to bone after their detachment for a surgical exposure. The most frequently seen examples of osteotomies in surgical exposure to joints include the olecranon process at the elbow and the greater trochanter at the hip. Secure fixation is necessary to maintain joint stability and function as well as to promote rapid healing. Because of the hardness of the tissue, metallic devices such as pins, staples, wires, and cables are the materials of choice. The olecranon process is most commonly repaired by pins or a screw with application of a tension band. In this manner, tensile forces are converted to dynamic compressive forces (Figure 9.3).[81] The principle behind repair of an osteotomy of the greater trochanter is similar, but the forces involved are greater; consequently, the materials are heavier (Figure 9.4).

Muscle or tendon is detached from bone in several instances. Usually the repair for muscle is not critical, since the tendency to retraction is not great as long as the origin and insertion are not disturbed; here the muscle or its aponeurosis would be loosely approximated with braided absorbable suture in interrupted or continuous technique. In some cases, however, the muscle detached is too likely to retract or would be too precious for its function to be compromised; this is the case with the anterior portion of the deltoid — loss of the function of this muscle would cause loss of arm elevation. Consequently, after careful dissection and protection throughout the operation, this muscle is reattached with interrupted nonabsorbable braided sutures (for longer lasting, stronger fixation) tied in figure-eight fashion.[82] Tendons detached from their insertions on bone are usually repaired in similar manner, frequently to drill holes in a roughened area of bone. Again because of greater forces, hip rotator insertions are repaired with braided tape. Protected motion can then be started immediately.

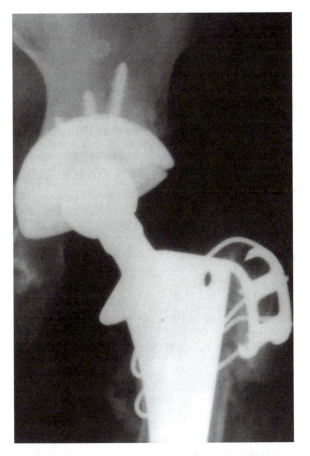

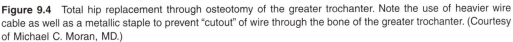

Figure 9.4 Total hip replacement through osteotomy of the greater trochanter. Note the use of heavier wire cable as well as a metallic staple to prevent "cutout" of wire through the bone of the greater trochanter. (Courtesy of Michael C. Moran, MD.)

Suture of other deep tissues involves repair of joint capsule, tendons, and muscle to preserve joint stability and function. A well-reasoned surgical approach aims to incise these structures along the course of their fibers or along lines of minimal tension. In this way, the repair bears less tension and nonabsorbable or slowly absorbable sutures are applied in continuous manner.

Closure of fascia and subcutaneous tissues is done to eliminate dead space to minimize the risk of hematoma formation and the development of infection. While studies report that the strength of a fascial repair increases slowly over several months, the empiric convention is to suture this tissue with either running or interrupted braided absorbable material. Subcutaneous closure, either continuous or interrupted, helps provide eversion of the tissue and prolonged wound support.[83] Despite the lack of scientific basis to justify closure of subcutaneous fatty tissue because of poor suture holding qualities, many surgeons place sutures at this site without significant difference in the incidence of subcutaneous hematomas in hip replacement surgery, with authors of one study recommending careful hemostasis.[84]

Skin repair is accorded special importance because of the desirability of accurate skin edge apposition for a cosmetically pleasing result. It is generally felt that a patient is more likely to be satisfied with a fine smooth line than with a wide scar with multiple "railroad track" hatch marks which are caused by prolonged pressure of a suture across the line of the incision. Again, the first step of a cosmetic closure lies in the making of the incision, which should ideally be within skin tension lines. This is not always practicable, however, and somehow the finest of incisions can heal into broad scars in the extremities of young people.[82]

Skin repair can be effected with the use of tape strips, various forms of suture techniques, or with staples. Tape strips have the advantage of not interfering with host defenses and therefore can minimize the risk of infection, but they require more meticulous subcutaneous apposition and hemostasis to be effective.[85–87]

Suture techniques are considered by many to be superior from a cosmetic viewpoint, as more precise skin edge coaptation can frequently be achieved. Subcuticular sutures are especially effective as they provide uniform tension on the skin edges while avoiding "railroad track" marks or other marks from suture entry points alongside the wound. In that respect they are preferable to other suture and stapling techniques.[79,88] Skin staples have the great advantage of ease and speed of application combined with acceptable cosmetic results. This makes them ideal for long linear incision.[89] "Railroad track" marks may occur, and staple insertion sites are more prominent after delayed staple removal.[79] Some studies consider skin stapling equivalent to suture techniques in this respect,[90] but this is controversial.[79] Their effect on host defenses is minimal.[86,87] Staples are more expensive than sutures[91] and current cost considerations in the U.S. may inhibit their future use.

In summary, the rationale supporting the choice of suture technique in orthopedic surgery is based on the tissues and their function. A wide variety of techniques are in use and these seem to be dependent on careful consideration as well as on anecdotal experience.

REFERENCES

1. Lowenberg, R.I. and Shumacker, H.B., Jr., Experimental studies in vascular repair. II. Strength of arteries repaired by end-to-end suture, with some notes on growth of anastomoses in young animals, *Arch. Surg.,* 59, 74, 1979.
2. Moore, W.S. and Malone, J.M., Vascular repair, in *Fundamentals of Wound Management*, Hunt, T.K. and Dunphy, J.E., Eds., Appleton-Century Crofts, New York, 1979, 476.
3. Reul, G.J., Jr., The role of sutures in complications in vascular surgery and their relationship to pseudoaneurysm formation, in *Complication in Vascular Surgery,* Bernhard, V.M. and Towne, J.B., Eds., Grune & Stratton, New York, 1980, 615.
4. Pae, W.E., Waldhausen, J.A., Prophet, G.A., and Pierce, W.S., Primary vascular anastomosis in growing pigs, *J. Thorac. Cardiovasc. Surg.,* 81, 921, 1981.
5. Myers, J.L., Waldhausen, J.A., Pae, W.E., Abt, A.B., Prophet, G.A., and Pierce, W.S., Vascular anastomoses in growing vessels: the use of absorbable sutures, *Ann. Thorac. Surg.,* 34, 529, 1982.
6. Haluck, R.S., Richenbacher, W.E., Myers, J.L., Miller, C.A., Abt, A.B., and Waldhausen, J.A., Results of aortic anastomoses made under tension using polydioxanone suture, *Ann. Thorac. Surg.,* 50, 392, 1990.
7. Stillman, R.M. and Sophie, Z., Repair of growing vessels, *Arch. Surg.,* 120, 1281, 1985.
8. Steen, S., Andersson, L., Lowenhiem, P., Stridbeck, H., Walther, B., and Holmin, T., Comparison between absorbable and nonabsorbable, monofilament sutures for end-to-end arterial anastomoses in growing pigs, *Surgery,* 95, 202, 1984.
9. Moore, W.S., Hall, A.D., and Allen, R.E., Tensile strength of arterial prosthetic anastomoses, *J. Surg. Res.,* 13, 209, 1972.
10. Courbier, R. and Larranaga, J., Natural history and management of anastomotic aneurysms, in *Aneurysms: Diagnosis and Treatment,* Bergen, J.J. and Yao, J., Eds., Grune & Stratton, New York, 1982, 567.
11. Starr, D.S., Weatherford, S.C., Lawrie, G.M., and Morris, G.C., Jr., Suture material as a factor in the occurrence of anastomotic false aneurysms, *Arch. Surg.,* 114, 412, 1979.
12. Dang, M., Thacker, J.G., Hwang, J.C., Rodeheaver, G.T., Melton, S.M., and Edlich, R.F., Some biomechanical considerations of polytetrafluoroethylene sutures, *Arch. Surg.,* 125, 647, 1990.
13. Roy, J., Guidon, R., Cardou, A., Blais, P., Theriault, Y., Marois, M., Noel, H.P., Gosselin, C., and Gerardin, H., Cardiovascular sutures as assessed by scanning electron microscopy, *Scan. Electron Microscopy,* 3, 203, 1980.
14. Landymore, R.W., Marble, A.E., and Cameron, C.A., Effect of force on anastomotic suture line disruption after carotid arteriotomy, *Am. J. Surg.,* 154, 309, 1987.
15. Dobrin, P.B., Polypropylene suture stresses after closure of longitudinal arteriotomy, *J. Vasc. Surg.,* 7, 423, 1988.
16. Goligher, J.C., Irvin, T.T., Johnston, D., De Dombal, F.T., Hill, G.L., and Horrocks, J.C., A controlled clinical trial of three methods of closure of laparotomy wounds, *Br. J. Surg.,* 62, 823, 1975.
17. Israelsson, L.A. and Jonsson, T., Suture length to wound length ratio and healing of midline laparotomy incisions, *Br. J. Surg.,* 80, 1284, 1993.
18. Wadstrom, J. and Gerdin, B., Closure of the abdominal wall: how and why, *Acta Chir. Scand.,* 156, 75, 1990.
19. Wissing, J., van Vroonhoven, T.J.M.V., Schattenkerk, M.E., Veen, H.F., Ponsen, R.J.G., and Jeekel, J., Fascia closure after midline laparotomy: results of a randomized trial, *Br. J. Surg.,* 74, 738, 1987.
20. Trimbos, J.B., Smit, I.B., Holm, J.P., and Hermans, J., A randomized clinical trial comparing two methods of fascia closure following midline laparotomy, *Arch. Surg.,* 127, 1232, 1992.
21. Richards, P.C., Balch, C.M., and Aldrete, J.S., Abdominal wound closure: a randomized prospective study of 571 patients comparing continuous vs. interrupted suture technique, *Ann. Surg.,* 197, 238, 1983.
22. Krukowski, Z.H., Cusick, E.L., Engeset, J., and Matheson, N.A., Polydioxanone or polypropylene for closure of midline abdominal incisions: a prospective comparative clinical trial, *Br. J. Surg.,* 74, 828, 1987.
23. Israelsson, L.A. and Jonsson, T., Closure of midline laparotomy incisions with polydioxanone and nylon: the importance of suture technique, *Br. J. Surg.,* 81, 1606, 1994.

24. Fagniez, P.L., Hay, J.M., Lacaine, F., and Thomsen, C., Abdominal midline incision closure: a multicentric randomized prospective trial of 3,135 patients, comparing continuous vs. interrupted polyglycolic acid sutures, *Arch. Surg.,* 120, 1351, 1985.

25. Hugh, T.B., Nankivell, C., Meagher, A.P., and Li, B., Is closure of the peritoneal layer necessary in the repair of midline surgical abdominal wounds? *World J. Surg.,* 14, 231, 1990.

26. De Holl, D., Rodeheaver, G., Edgarton, M.T. et al., Potential of infection by suture closure of dead space, *Am. J. Surg.,* 127, 716, 1974.

27. Jibron, H., Ahonen, J., and Zederfeldt, B., Healing of experimental colonic anastomoses: effects of suture technique on collagen metabolism in the colonic wall, *Am. J. Surg.,* 139, 406, 1980.

28. Irvin, T.T., Goligher, J.C., and Johnston, D., A randomized prospective trial of single-layer and two-layer inverting intestinal anastomoses, *Br. J. Surg.,* 60, 457, 1973.

29. Everett, W.G., A comparison of one layer and two layer techniques for colorectal anastomosis, *Br. J. Surg.,* 62, 135, 1975.

30. Goligher, J.C., Lee, P.W.G., Simpkins, K.C., and Lintott, D.J., A controlled comparison of one- and two-layer technique of suture for high and low colorectal anastomoses, *Br. J. Surg.,* 64, 609, 1077.

31. McDonald, C.C. and Baird, R.L., Vicryl intestinal anastomosis, *Dis. Colon Rectum,* 28, 775, 1985.

32. Bardini, R., Bonavina, L., Asolati, M., Ruol, A., Castoro, C., and Tiso, E., Single-layered cervical esophageal anastomoses: a prospective study of two suturing techniques, *Ann. Thorac. Surg.,* 58, 1087, 1994.

33. Fok, M., Ah-Chong, A.K., Cheng, S.W.K., and Wong, J., Comparison of a single layer continuous hand-sewn method and circular stapling in 580 oesophageal anastomoses, *Br. J. Surg.,* 78, 342, 1991.

34. Seufert, R.M., Schmidt-Matthiesen, A., and Beyer, A., Total gastrectomy and oesophagojejunostomy — a prospective randomized trial of hand-sutured versus mechanically stapled anastomoses, *Br. J. Surg.,* 77, 50, 1990.

35. Demartines, N., Rothenbuhler, J.M., Chevalley, J.P., and Harder, F., The single-layer continuous suture for gastric anastomosis, *World J. Surg.,* 15, 522, 1991.

36. Saran, S. and Lightwood, R.G., Continuous single-layer gastrointestinal anastomosis: a prospective audit, *Br. J. Surg.,* 76, 493, 1989.

37. Ceraldi, C.M., Rypins, E.B., Monahan, M., Chang, B., and Sarfeh, I.J., Comparison of continuous single layer polypropylene anastomosis with double layer and stapled anastomoses in elective colon resections, *Am. Surg.,* 59, 168, 1993.

38. Max, E., Sweeney, W.B., Bailey, H.R., Oommen, S.C., Butts, D.R., Smith, K.W., Zamora, L.F., and Skakun, G. B., Results of 1,000 single-layer continuous polypropylene intestinal anastomoses, *Am. J. Surg.,* 162, 461, 1991.

39. Baumgartner, W.A. and Mark, J.B.D., Bronchoscopic diagnosis and treatment of bronchial stump suture granulomas, *J. Thorac. Cardiovasc. Surg.,* 81, 553, 1981.

40. Hood, R.M., *Techniques in General Thoracic Surgery,* 2nd ed., Lea & Febiger, Philadelphia, 1993.

41. Sarsam, M.A. and Moussali, H., Technique of bronchial closure after pneumonectomy, *J. Thorac. Cardiovasc. Surg.,* 98, 220, 1989.

42. Al-Kattan, K., Cattalain, L., and Goldstraw, P., Bronchopleural fistula after pneumonectomy with a hand suture technique, *Ann. Thorac. Surg.,* 58, 1433, 1994.

43. Sato, M., Saito, Y., Naganoto, N., Endo, C., Usuda, K., Takahashi, S., Kan'ma, K., Sagawa, M., Ota, S., Nakada, T., and Fujimura, S., An improved method of bronchial stump closure for prevention of bronchopleural fistula in pulmonary resection, *Tohoku J. Exp. Med.,* 168, 507, 1992.

44. Grillo, H.C., Surgical treatment of postintubation tracheal injuries, *J. Thorac. Cardiovasc. Surg.,* 78, 860, 1979.

45. Alstrup, P. and Sorenson, H.R., Resection of acquired tracheal stenosis in childhood, *J. Thorac. Cardiovasc. Surg.,* 87, 547, 1984.

46. Maassen, W., Greschuchna, D., Vogt-Moykopf, I., Toomes, H., and Lullig, H., Tracheal resection — state of the art, *Thorac. Cardiovasc. Surg.,* 33, 2, 1985.

47. Nordin, U. and Ohlsen, L., Prevention of tracheal stricture in end-to-end anastomosis, *Arch. Otolaryngol.,* 108, 308, 1982.

48. McKeown, P.P., Tsuboi, H., Togo, T., Thomas, R., Tuck, R., and Gordon, D., Growth of tracheal anastomoses: advantage of absorbable interrupted sutures, *Ann. Thorac. Surg.,* 51, 636, 1991.

49. Friedman, E., Perez-Atayde, A.R., Silvera, M., and Jonas, R.A., Growth of tracheal anastomoses in lambs: comparison of PDS and Vicryl suture material and interrupted and continuous techniques, *J. Thorac. Cardiovasc. Surg.,* 100, 188, 1990.

50. Grillo, H.C., Donahue, D.M., Mathisen, D.J., Wain, J.C., and Wright, C.D., Postintubation tracheal stenosis: treatment and results, *J. Thorac. Cardiovasc. Surg.,* 109, 486, 1995.

51. Goldman, G., Nestel, R., Snir, E., and Vidne, B., Effective technique of sternum closure in high-risk patients, *Arch. Surg.,* 123, 386, 1988.

52. Stoney, W.S., Alford, W.C., Jr., Burrus, G.R., Frist, R.A., and Thomas, C.S., Jr., Median sternotomy dehiscence, *Ann. Thorac. Surg.,* 26, 421, 1978.

53. Goodman, G., Palatianos, G.M., and Bolloki, H., Technique of closure of median sternotomy with trans-sternal figure-of-eight wires, *J. Cardiovasc. Surg.,* 27, 512, 1986.

54. Di Marco, R.F., Jr., Lee, M.W., Bekoe, S., Grant, K.J., Woelfel, G.F., and Pellegrini, R.V., Interlocking figure-of-8 closure of the sternum, *Ann. Thorac. Surg.,* 47, 927, 1989.

55. Macmanus, Q., Okies, J.E., Phillips, S.J., and Starr, A., Surgical considerations in patients undergoing repeat median sternotomy, *J. Thorac. Cardiovasc. Surg.*, 69, 138, 1975.

56. Sanfelippo, P.M. and Danielson, G.K., Nylon bands for closure of median sternotomy incisions: an unacceptable method, *Ann. Thorac. Surg.*, 13, 404, 1972.

57. Okies, J.E. and Phillips, S.J., Sternal approximation, *Ann. Thorac. Surg.*, 17, 423, 1974.

58. Pastorino, U., Muscolino, G., Valente, M., Andreani, S., Travecchio, L., Infante, M., Terno, G., and Ravasi, G., Safety of absorbable suture for sternal closure after pulmonary or mediastinal resection, *J. Thorac. Cardiovasc. Surg.*, 107, 596, 1994.

59. Buchsbaum, H.J. and Schmidt, J.G., *Gynecologic and Obstetric Urology*, W.B. Saunders, Philadelphia, 1978.

60. Guillou, P.J., Hall, T.J. et al., Vertical abdominal incisions: a choice? *Br. J. Surg.*, 67, 395, 1980.

61. Ellis, H., Bucknall, T., and Cox, P., Abdominal incisions and their closure. *Curr. Prob. Surg.*, 22, 1985.

62. Humphries, A.L., Corley, W.S., and Moretz, W.H., Massive closure versus layer closure for abdominal incisions, *Am. Surg.*, 30, 700, 1964.

63. Wadstrom, J. and Gerdiw, B., Closure of the abdominal wall; how and why? *AOTA Chir. Scand.*, 156, 75, 1990.

64. Sanz, L. and Smith, S., Mechanisms of wound healing, suture material and wound closure, in *Strategies in Gynecologic Surgery*, Buchsbaum, H.J. and Walten, L., Eds., Springer-Verlag, New York, 1986, 53.

65. Van Winkle, W. and Salthouse, T.N., *Biological Response to Sutures and Principles of Suture Selection*, Ethicon, Somerville, NJ, 1976.

66. Ellis, H., Bucknall, T., and Cox, P.J., Abdominal incisions and their closure, *Curr. Prob. Surg.*, 22, 1985, 3–51.

67. Jenkins, T.P.W., The burst abdominal wound: a mechanical approach, *Br. J. Surg.*, 63, 873, 1976.

68. Steichen, F.M., Staplers in intestinal surgery, *Contemp. Surg.*, 14, 51, 1979.

69. Wheeless, C.R. and Smith, J.J., A comparison of the flow of iodine 125 through three different intestinal anastomoses: standard, Gambee and stapler, *Obstet. Gynecol.*, 62, 513, 1983.

70. U.S. Surgical Corporation, Stapling Techniques — General Surgery with Auto Suture Instruments, 3rd ed. U.S. Surgical Corporation, Norwalk, CT, 1988.

71. Steckel, R.R. and Jann, H.W., Experimental evaluation of absorbable copolymer staples for hysterectomy, *Obstet. Gynecol.*, 68, 404, 1986.

72. Edlich, R.F., Beclar, D.G., Thacker, J.G., and Rodeheaver, G.T., Scientific basis for selecting staple and tape closures, *Clin. Plast. Surg.*, 17, 571, 1990.

73. Johnson, A., Rodeheaver, G.Y., and Durand, L.S., Automatic dispensable stapling devices for wound closure, *Ann. Emerg. Med.*, 10, 631, 1981.

74. Ethicon, Inc., Wound Closure Manual, Ethicon, Somerville, NJ, 1994, p. 57.

75. Gildert, H.W. and Everett, W.G., Clips or sutures for herniorrhophy wounds? *Br. J. Clin. Pract.*, 44, 306, 1990.

76. Berek, J.S., Hacker, N.F., and Lagasse, L., Rectosigmoid coloetomy and reanastamosis to facilitate resection of primary and recurrent gynecologic cancer, *Obstet. Gynecol.*, 64, 715, 1984.

77. Nelson, J.H. and Morgan, L., Stapling techniques, in *Manual of Basic Pelvic Surgery*, Nelson, J.H. and Morgan, L., Eds., McGraw-Hill, New York, 1994, 108.

78. Cohen, J.K., et al., Wound care and wound healing, in *Principles of Surgery*, 6th ed., Schwartz, S., Shires, G.T., Spencer, F.C., and Husser, W.C., McGraw-Hill, New York, chap. 8, 1994.

79. Clayer, M. and Southwood, R.T., Comparative study of skin closure in hip surgery, *Aust. NZ J. Surg.*, 61,363, 1991.

80. Gristina, A.G. and Costerton, J.W., Bacterial adherence to biomaterials and tissue: the significance of its role in clinical sepsis, *J. Bone Joint Surg.*, 67A, 264, 1985.

81. Muller, M.E., Allgower, M., Schneider, R., and Willenegger, H., *Manual of Internal Fixation*, 2nd ed., Springer-Verlag, Berlin, 1979.

82. Neer, C.S., *Shoulder Reconstruction*, W.B. Saunders, Philadelphia, 1990.

83. Ratner, D., Nelson, B.R., and Johnson, T.M., Basic suture materials and suturing techniques, *Semin. Dermatol.*, 13, 20, 1994.

84. Strange-Vognsen, H.H., Torhom, C., Lebech, A., and Hancke, S., Hematomas and subcutaneous suture techniques in total hip replacement, *Arch. Orthop. Trauma Surg.*, 111, 51, 1991.

85. Bunker, T.D., Problems with the use of op site sutureless skin closures in orthopedic procedures, *Ann. R. Coll. Surg. Engl.*, 1983, 65, 260, 1983.

86. Johnson, A., Rodeheaver, G.T., Durand, L.S., Edgerton, M.T., and Edlich, R.F., Automatic disposable suture devices for wound closure, *Ann. Emerg. Med.*, 10, 631, 1981.

87. Stillman, R.M., Marino, P.A, and Seligman, S.J., Skin staples in potentially contaminated wounds, *Arch. Surg.*, 119, 821, 1984.

88. Angelini, G.D., Butchart, E.G., Armistead, S.H., and Breckenridge, I.M., Comparative study of leg wound skin closure in coronary artery bypass graft operations, *Thorax*, 39, 942, 1984.

89. Chamas, P.J. and Crager, M.D., The use of skin stapling in podiatric surgery: a review and update, *J. Foot Ankle Surg.*, 32, 536, 1993.

90. Harvey, C.F. and Hume Logan, C.J., A prospective trial of skin staples and sutures in skin closure, *Irish J. Med. Sci.*, 155, 194, 1986.

91. Gatt, D., Quick, G.R.G., and Owen-Smith, M.S., Staples for wound closure: a controlled trial, *Ann. R. Coll. Surg. Engl.*, 67, 318, 1982.

Chapter 10

Ligating Clips and Staples

J. A. von Fraunhofer

CONTENTS

I. INTRODUCTION

The primary function of any ligating device is to occlude the lumen of a vessel or tubular organ and maintain occlusion until there is permanent closure from natural healing.[1] Ligation of blood vessels to ensure hemostasis has been performed for centuries and, with advances in surgery and available armamentarium, the surgical applications of ligating clips and staples has increased markedly. These applications include the extensive ligation of vessels in gynecological and urological (GU) procedures, such as tubule ligation for female sterilization, prevention of pulmonary emboli by ligation of the inferior vena cava, ligation of the cystic duct and artery during cholecystectomy and, increasingly, closure of surface wounds.[1] Despite the widespread and growing surgical use of ligating clips, there is a paucity of literature on the subject.

Traditionally, filamentous materials such as sutures have been used for ligation and wound closure but there are certain inherent problems with sutures, as discussed extensively elsewhere within this monograph. Examples of such problems are given in Table 10.1, but probably the most important limitations to the use of sutures for vessel ligation are the difficulty the surgeon has in gaining good access and tying a secure knot within a deep cavity or confined surgical area and the time required to tie a secure knot, especially in sutures that require complex knotting techniques (see Chapter 6). Other potential problems such as the risk of the suture carrying microorganisms into the wound, suture breakage during surgery, postsurgical knot slippage, and reduced control during suturing due to slippage, rotation, and even loss of the needle from the needle holder are very real, but can be minimized by good surgical technique. Uncontrolled or accelerated dissolution of absorbable sutures can also occur but, again, untoward effects are controllable by good technique and appropriate selection of the suture material. Nevertheless, current surgical preference in many situations is to use mechanical clips for ligation and staples for many types of wound closure.

The primary requirements for ligating clips, as for all materials and devices used within the human body, are absence of toxicity and immunogenicity, biocompatibility, and the ability to be tolerated by many different types of tissue without eliciting adverse reactions and/or responses, Table 10.2. Likewise,

Table 10.1 Problems Associated with Surgical Sutures

Time-consuming nature of secure knot tying
Need for secure knots under all conditions with all sutures
Difficulty of access in deep wounds and confined areas
Risk of suture breakage during surgery
Loss of control due to needle slippage or rotation within needle holder
Postsurgical slippage of the knotted suture or ligature
Early or pathologically induced dissolution of absorbable sutures

Table 10.2 Requirements for Ligating Devices

Nontoxic and biocompatible
Absence of allergic and immunogenic effects
Tolerated by wide variety of tissues
High strength and low solubility
Finite longevity in the body
Secure fastening system

the need for a simple, secure, and easily operated fastening or locking mechanism is obvious. However, an important question is how long should the ligating device remain *in situ* before it can safely be removed, dislodged, or dissolved by physiological processes? Surprisingly, there is little data in the literature on the time required for secure occlusion of vessels and tubular organs, but a recent study[2] showed that permanent hemostasis in canine femoral arteries requires ligation for 96 h. Other work[3] performed with absorbable ligating clips suggests that secure blood vessel occlusion is attained within 24 h. Since most absorbable suture materials retain adequate strength and integrity for at least 2 to 3 weeks, foreshortened tissue longevity is not a problem in secure ligation. However, excessive durability and extended device lifetimes within the body could present problems, particularly in GU applications. Such considerations affect the selection of materials and devices for surgical applications.

This chapter describes the three classes of ligating clips and staples based on the materials from which these devices are made: metallic, polymeric, and others. This chapter also describes the numerous and far-reaching applications for ligating clips and staples in surgical practice. These devices are convenient, reasonably easy to use, and can be placed rapidly while not requiring the same surgical skill necessary for accurate and secure placement of sutures. Their radiolucency is an added advantage. Nevertheless, the indications are that these devices, even those manufactured from absorbable polymeric materials, may remain in the body for extended periods of time. As yet, there do not appear to be any report of adverse reactions resulting from such effects and, at this stage, the advantages may outweigh the disadvantages.

II. METALLIC LIGATING CLIPS

Initially, only metallic ligating clips were available, primarily because they were introduced into surgery considerably before synthetic polymeric materials were discovered. In fact, the first ligating clips were hand-formed, U-shaped, round silver wire clips used for neurosurgery.[4] The basic Cushing neurosurgery clip design remained largely unchanged for many years, although there were such advances as the use of flattened silver wire and forceps that simultaneously formed clips while cutting the wire.[5] Given the desirable properties of metallic materials used to fabricate ligating clips, shown in Table 10.3, the use of silver would appear to be a good choice at first glance. Silver is reasonably corrosion resistant, has acceptable strength, is malleable and ductile so that it can be shaped easily, and, after closing into a loop, the metal will not spring open. However, it was found that silver could provoke intense inflammatory reactions in both nerve tissue and the meninges, with the clips eventually becoming surrounded by dense encapsulation. As a result, other, less reactive metallic materials, i.e., metals with greater corrosion resistance, were sought for this application.

The tantalum neurosurgical clip was developed in the 1940s and was a significant advance over silver in terms of corrosion resistance and, particularly, biocompatibility, since the biological response to tantalum consists of minimal investment by connective tissue and/or neurolagia fibrils.[6,7] Being a refractory metal, tantalum components are fabricated by powder metallurgical techniques, namely sintering

Table 10.3 Desirable Properties of Metals for Ligating Clips

High strength
Malleability and ductility
Capacity for work-hardening
Corrosion resistance

Table 10.4 Properties of Implantable Metal Alloys

Metal	Tensile Strength (MPa)	Elongation (%)	Modulus of Elasticity (GPa)
Cobalt-chromium (cast)	650–700	4–12	210
Cobalt-chromium (wrought)	860–1700	5–30	230
Cobalt-nickel	650–800	2–10	200
Type 316L stainless steel (wrought)	500–750	12–40	193
Type 316L stainless steel (cold worked)	960–1500	10–50	200
Tantalum	34–125	1–40	186
Titanium	300–550	25–30	110
Ti-6Al-4V	830–970	12–15	112

Data from von Fraunhofer, J.A., *Clin. Obstet. Gynecol.*, 31, 718, 1988.

the metal powder into the desired shape. Pure tantalum is extremely corrosion resistant, has a high tensile strength, and is very ductile and malleable, these characteristics ensuring that the clips will close reasonably easily around a vessel and, following closure, they will stay closed with little risk of springing open. Tantalum clips have a variety of surgical uses and were used extensively, particularly in tubule ligation,[1,8,9] but, since the 1960s, a variety of other metals have also been used to fabricate ligating clips. The physical properties of these metals are summarized in Table 10.4 and it can be seen that these alloys are basically identical to those used for the fabrication of orthopedic and oromaxillofacial implants. Until recently, the vast majority of ligating clips and staples were fabricated from tantalum and stainless steel. Now, stainless steel staples and clips are being phased out and replaced by titanium because of the greater tendency of stainless steel to distort computed tomography (CT) scans by a "starburst effect".[10] The great advantage of metal ligating clips is that once they are closed around a vessel, their inherent malleability precludes the clip springing open when the seating/closing pressure is released.

Various designs of composite metal-plastic spring clips have been developed recently, primarily for laparoscopic sterilization.[11–13] Typically, these devices are plastic- or silicone-coated titanium strips, coated stainless steel springs, or plastic systems using spring closure. Metal and metal-plastic ligating clips are easy to use, stable, insoluble, and provide secure ligation, but they possess certain inherent disadvantages. Certain metals, e.g., nickel, cobalt, and alloys containing these elements, can induce inflammatory and/or allergic reactions; all metals are radio-opaque, which can present problems in radiological, CT, and magnetic resonance imaging (MRI) examinations and, when used in the female GU tract, have the potential for causing penile lacerations. As a result, there has been a trend in recent years to use nonmetallic and, indeed, biodegradable ligating devices for internal or buried use, although there is a widespread application of metal clips in primary skin closure. These devices are manufactured from the same materials used for surgical implants (primarily titanium) and suffer from the same limitations, although the fact that they are not maintained in place for extended periods avoids many of the problems associated with buried metallic devices.

III. POLYMERIC LIGATING DEVICES

The advantages of filamentary ligatures are obvious, namely minimal bulk, material softness, radiolucency, and, depending upon the suture material, minimal tissue response and biodegradability although the problems of tying sutures in deep cavities or confined spaces remain. The latter consideration led to the development of smooth Teflon® (polytetrafluoroethylene, PTFE) clips to narrow the inferior vena cava to trap emboli without interruption of blood flow.[14–16] These clips do not appear to have been used for tubal ligation or hemostasis while the chemical inertness of PTFE prevents the absorption of these clips under physiological action. However, absorbable ligating clips have been developed from the biodegradable polymers used to fabricate suture materials, see Chapter 4. Two absorbable clips and one absorbable staple are currently available and in clinical use.

The Absolok® clip is fabricated from poly-*p*-dioxanone (the polymer utilized for PDS suture) while the Lactomer® clip and staple are fabricated from a 70:30 copolymer of glycolic and lactic acids.[17–20] Since Absolok clips are fabricated from poly-*p*-dioxanone, the clips should exhibit very similar chemical

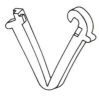

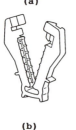

(a)

(b)

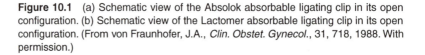

Figure 10.1 (a) Schematic view of the Absolok absorbable ligating clip in its open configuration. (b) Schematic view of the Lactomer absorbable ligating clip in its open configuration. (From von Fraunhofer, J.A., *Clin. Obstet. Gynecol.*, 31, 718, 1988. With permission.)

and physical properties to PDS sutures. The Lactomer products are fabricated from a modification of the polymer used in the manufacture of Vicryl but the polymer differs from polyglactin 910 in its proportion of lactide copolymer units. As a result of these chemical differences, the mechanical and hydrolytic behavior of Lactomer is not the same as that observed with Vicryl and, in fact, the hydrolytic behavior is closer to that of Dexon (polyglycolide) within the pH range of 5.0 to 9.0.[17] Both resins are thermoplastic and, therefore, are moldable into complex shapes and will exhibit stress relaxation. The fabrication of ligating devices from polyester-based polymers should ensure a regular and predictable hydrolytic breakdown *in vivo* and although they will induce a typical foreign body tissue reaction, it should be of limited duration and of relatively minor intensity. Clinical studies on Absolok clips[18–20] and Lactomer staples[21] clearly indicate a number of superior attributes to those of metallic clips while providing comparable efficiency in hemostasis.

Since both the absorbable clips and the absorbable staple are manufactured from viscoelastic materials, they will exhibit elastic recovery under rapidly imposed loading but permanent deformation under static loading. Additionally, they will continue to deform (creep) under continuous loading and, as discussed in Chapter 6, will reorganize their internal structure to neutralize externally applied forces, i.e., exhibit stress relaxation. As a result of these viscoelastic effects, if these devices are closed by compression in the clinical setting, there will be a tendency for them to reopen. Consequently, these devices incorporate an integral locking mechanism to ensure that the clip, once closed, will be securely locked around the ligated structure upon release of the placement force. The locking mechanisms of the two clips differ (Figure 10.1), in that the Absolok clip has a latch-type system while interlocking teeth are used for the Lactomer clip. These differences in locking mechanism are reflected in the lock strengths of the two clips. The lock mechanism for the large Lactomer clip was stronger than that for the large Absolok clip but there were no differences between the medium and small sizes of the two clips.[22] The two types of clips showed differences in their *in vivo* behavior.

In vivo studies (subcutaneous implantation in rabbits) showed little change in the lock mechanism strength for Absolok clips over a period of 21 d but, depending upon the clip size, there was a decrease of 25% to 27%, compared to controls, at 28 d, see Figure 10.2.[22] In contrast, the Lactomer clip showed a decrease in lock strength within 7 d of implantation, with a much lower decrease with continuing exposure, Figure 10.3.[22] The small and medium Lactomer clips showed their greatest change (about. 60% and 40%, respectively) in lock strength over 7 d, with little change thereafter, while the large clip showed a 65% decrease in lock strength over 14 d. The Lactomer staple, Figure 10.4,[22] showed a behavior similar to that of the Lactomer clip, namely a large and progressive decrease in lock strength over 21 d with little change in strength over the implantation period of 21 to 27 d. However, it should be noted that, although the lock strength of Lactomer clips and staples exhibited marked change in strength over 21 d implantation, the actual strengths were comparable to those of the somewhat weaker Absolok staples at the same time period. Given the fact that hemostasis appears to be established within 96 h or less,[2,3] the observed *in vivo* loss in strength of these absorbable clips due to hydrolytic breakdown over a period of 7 to 21 d should not be a clinical problem. In fact, there are indications that these devices may have an unexpectedly long *in vivo* life.

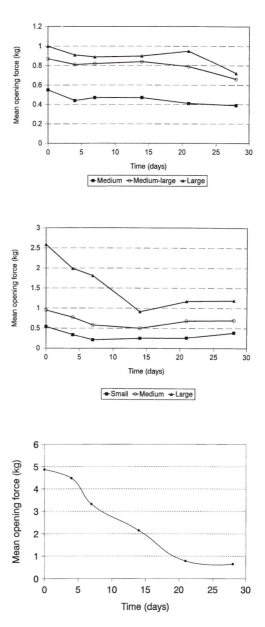

Figure 10.2 Change in *in vivo* lock mechanism strength of Absolok clips. (Data from Hay, D.L. et al., *J. Biomed. Mater. Res.*, 22, 179, 1988.)

Figure 10.3 Change in *in vivo* lock mechanism strength of Lactomer clips. (Data from Hay, D.L. et al., *J. Biomed. Mater. Res.*, 22, 179, 1988.)

Figure 10.4 Change in *in vivo* lock mechanism strength of Lactomer staples. (Data from Hay, D.L. et al., *J. Biomed. Mater. Res.*, 22, 179, 1988.)

Studies of the decomposition of Absolok and Lactomer clips[23] indicated quite early onset of degradation *in vivo*, as early as 7 d in the case of the Absolok clip and 2 weeks for Lactomer clips. The *in vitro* breakdown, however, was considerably slower for clips (and staples) manufactured from both materials, although the Absolok clips showed a faster rate of breakdown. The Lactomer devices showed little sign of degradation after 10 weeks incubation in a phosphate-buffered saline solution (pH 7.3) at 37°C. Breakdown appeared to occur via surface cracking and fissuring, which deepened and widened with time. The latter process and associated surface roughening appeared to encourage cellular attachment and possibly permitted the ingress of microorganisms in the presence of bacterial infection.[24,25] Bacterial infection of Absolok and Lactomer clips *in vivo* resulted in attachment and rapid growth of bacteria over the clips, with no apparent initiation of surface breakdown. With time, the bacterial layers on the clip surfaces formed a progressively thickening plaque-like material, possibly representing accumulation of inhibited bacteria since polyglycolide is known to inhibit bacterial growth.[26] The plaque-like layer on the clips appeared to significantly reduce the rate of *in vivo* clip degradation, an occurrence that might compromise wound healing.[25] In clean wounds, the initial reaction to the absorbable clips was attachment of numerous inflammatory cells and some fibroblasts to the clip surface but, over time, there was a reduction in inflammatory cells and an increase in fibroblasts.[24] Proliferation of the latter resulted in the formation of a fibrous tissue capsule around the clips which gradually increased with time. As a result of tissue capsule formation, residues of the clips were found to be present within the encapsulating tissue after 25 weeks implantation, while clips that were implanted in porous protective nylon pouches were totally degraded and residue-free at the same period. These findings indicate that the polymers used to fabricate Absolok and Lactomer devices permit tissue adhesion to their surfaces and this appears to restrict, and possibly prevent, enzyme access to the clips so that biodegradation is inhibited. At this stage, the clinical significance of these findings is uncertain but it does suggest that biodegradability is a relative term and absorbable materials and devices may have a longer than anticipated longevity in the body.

IV. OTHER LIGATING DEVICES

In recent years a new device, known as the pelviscopic loop ligature or PLL, has been introduced for gynecological and general surgical procedures such as the ligation of arterial bleeders, vascular pedicles, the uteroovarian ligament, and the infundibulopelvic ligament.[27,28] The PLL consists of US/P O gauge chromic gut suture encased in a polymeric sheath, one end of the suture being tied in a slip knot while the other is imbedded in a plastic tail. The loop is placed over the structure to be ligated and, as the sheath covering the length of the suture is held in one hand, the loop is tightened by pulling on the plastic tail. The PLL has been used extensively for the past 25 years in Germany and its use in the U.S. is steadily increasing. There have been no reports of hemorrhagic complications in the use of the device.[25,29] In clinical use, after abdominal insufflation with carbon dioxide, the device is introduced into the abdominal cavity through a 5 mm laparoscopic trocar sheath. Tensile testing of the PLL[26] clearly showed that there was no difference in the strength of the chromic gut suture itself and that of the bond between the suture and the plastic tail (Table 10.5). The strength of the ligating slip knot was dependent upon surgical technique. In particular, one or two pulls on the plastic after seating the loop around the structure to be ligated had no effect on loop security. However, additional pulls on the plastic tail resulted in a marked drop in failure load (over 50%) while the mode of failure appear to be primarily by slippage. The PLL when used optimally would appear to be a useful addition to the surgical armamentarium in that it is of low cost and provides secure hemostasis, while the fact that it is used through a trocar reduces the surgical invasion, particularly in such procedures as tubule ligation.

V. SURGICAL STAPLES

Surgical stapling was introduced in the late 1970s and has grown in popularity and scope of application over the years,[30,31] being used widely in human and veterinary gynecological, cardiovascular, gastrointestinal, esophageal, and pulmonary surgery. Surgical stapling is a mechanical method of apposing tissue and despite certain technical advantages such as convenience, speed, and accessibility (see Section VI), similar surgical principles to those for suturing must be adhered to in use. Surgical staples formerly were fabricated from stainless steel but, as discussed earlier for clips, titanium is predominating as the material of choice for this application. The staple is very similar to the familiar office staple and in use,

Table 10.5 Tensile Strength of the Pelviscopic Loop Ligature (PLL)

Test Subject	Failure Load (kg)
PLL, 1 pull	1.36 ± 0.25*
PLL, 2 pulls	1.21 ± 0.21
PLL, 3 pulls	0.60 ± 0.40
Suture-tail junction	1.46 ± 0.11
Chromic gut suture	1.43 ± 0.12

* Mean value ± standard deviation.

Data from Hay, D.L. et al., *J. Reprod. Med.*, 35, 260, 1990.

Table 10.6 Metallic Staple Dimensions

Crown Width (mm)	Leg Length (mm)	Closed Height (mm)	Wire Diameter (mm)
3.0	2.5	1.0	0.20
3.0	3.85	1.5	0.20/0.21
3.0	4.85	2.0	0.24
4.0	3.0	1.25	0.20
4.0	3.5	1.5	0.23
4.0	4.0	1.75	0.20
4.0	4.5	1.0–2.5[a]	0.23
4.0	4.8	2.0	0.28
4.0	5.5	1.0–2.5[a]	0.28

[a] Closure range.

it is placed or seated in a similar manner, namely the staple is forced through the tissue and is folded or bent into a B-shape by means of an anvil. Clearly, for any given application, the leg length of the staple must be sufficient to penetrate completely the tissue to be stapled and, accordingly, there is a range, though limited, of staple dimensions (Table 10.6). Larger staples are generally required for the thicker gastric walls while smaller staples can be applied to other alimentary tract organs.[10]

A wide variety of stapling instruments are now available and the range of surgical procedures in which they can be applied is still expanding, reflecting both advances in armamentarium and surgical technique. At present both single-use (disposable) and reusable devices are available. Originally, the staples were propelled through tissue by an integral CO_2 cylinder,[32] but now the majority of staplers are manually operated by squeezing a pair of handles together. All staplers carry a cartridge of staples to permit numerous staplings in a single procedure and disposable staplers with reloadable cartridges are also available.[33] Further, staplers that place single and multiple rows of staples, typically in a staggered configuration, are in use together with end-to-end and end-to-side anastomosis devices, the latter categories having a circular configuration that place concentric staggered rows of staples and incorporate a blade to remove redundant tissue and create a new lumen.[10] A diversity of stapling instruments is available, as indicated by the number of manufacturers (Table 10.7), and reflects the many applications of surgical stapling as well as differences in design and construction of staplers.

Lactomer absorbable staples were introduced into gynecologic surgery for hysterectomies and cesarean sections to avoid the postoperative complication of dyspareunia that can accompany the use of metallic staples, as well as any radiological complications. Unlike metal staples, polymeric staples cannot be bent around an anvil into a B-shape. Accordingly, the staple is composed of two parts, a U-shape fastener and a figure 8-shape retainer, and in use the fastener is forced through the tissue to lock into the retainer on the other side. There are, however, certain inherent disadvantages with polymeric clips and staples, namely their size. Since polymers are mechanically weaker than the metals used for staple and clip fabrication (stainless steel, tantalum, and titanium), clips and staples manufactured from polymers must have greater bulk. Consequently, precautions must be taken during surgery to prevent their dislodgment while the greater thickness of the polymeric staple prohibits crossing of staple lines which is possible with metallic staples.[10]

Table 10.7 Manufacturers of Staples and Staplers

Manufacturer	Address
Davis & Geck, Cyanamid Canada, Inc.	88 McNabb Street, Markham, ON L3R6E6
Ethicon Inc.	US Route 22, P. O. Box 151, Somerville, NJ 08876
General Medical Corp.	8741 Landmark Road, Richmond, VA 23228
Howmedica, Pfizer Hospital Products	359 Veterans Blvd., Rutherford, NJ 07070
3M Co., 3M Health Care	3M Center Bldg 275-4E-01, St. Paul, MN 55144
National Wire and Stamping, Inc.	2801 S Vallejo Street, Englewood, CO 80110
Pilling-Weck, Teleflex, Inc.	1 Weck Drive, Research Triangle Pk., NC 27709
United States Surgical Corp., Auto Suture Co.	150 Glover Avenue, Norwalk, CT 06856

The latest advance in skin stapler technology has been the development of a disposable device that delivers an absorbable Lactomer pin into the subcutaneous layer of tissue just below the dermis, that is, it effects subcuticular closure of skin.[34] The device incorporates a pair of gripper blades that approximate and evert the wound edges, after which a pin is pushed into the dermis, the pin penetrating the dermis twice on each side of the wound to hold the tissue together. A comparison of staple pin and suture closure showed that dermal closure by sutures approximated the divided dermis without noticeable eversion of the skin edges, while the stapler everted and interdigitated the tissue edges.[34] However, the stapler inserted three separate dermal staples in 1.4 ± 0.8 min, while it required 6.2 ± 0.6 min for placement of six interrupted dermal sutures, that is, subcuticular stapling was some five times faster and was claimed to require considerably less psychomotor skills. Further, it was found that the inflammatory response and amount of purulent discharge for staple pin dermis closure was significantly less than for suture closure when exposed to the same bacterial inocula. Likewise, the numbers of viable bacteria recovered from dermal pin closed wounds was significantly less. However, suture dermis closure provided more immediate security, eight times greater, as determined by wound breaking strength, but no statistical significant difference in wound strength was claimed at 14 d.

VI. STAPLES AND CLIPS VS. SUTURES

As stated previously, surgical stapling is a mechanical method of apposing tissue and is considered to be the fastest method of closure of long skin incisions,[34,35] while providing faster attainment of secure occlusion and greater resistance to infection than suturing.[3,31] The subcutical pin likewise achieved closure of the dermis faster than suturing, with reduced localized infection although initial wound security was better for suture closure.[34] It is further thought that when properly performed, the cosmetic appearance of stapled wounds is equal to that of sutured wounds.[31,36]

A recent study of laparoscopic oophorectomies indicated that similar operating times and uniformly good results were obtained with pretied ligatures, bipolar coagulation, and automatic stapling devices.[37] Stapling techniques are claimed to be safe, easy, and quick to perform for hepatic, pulmonary, and cardiovascular surgery.[38–40] An evaluation of laparoscopic hemostasis using titanium clips, absorbable clips, and chromic gut sutures showed that all three methodologies were easily applied and effective in achieving hemostasis;[41] although no statistically significant difference was established, the authors indicated that the adhesion scores were lower for absorbable clips. Other workers, however, have indicated that there was greater adhesion formation associated with the use of absorbable staples than with absorbable sutures, and while Hyskon (Dextran-70) reduced peritoneal adhesions at sites of suturing, excision, and thermal injury there was no effect in the stapling area.[42]

The use of staples has also been found to save costs when compared with suturing.[36,43] Orlinsky et al.[43] recently reported that stapling is a less expensive means of skin closure than suturing with respect to emergency department repair of linear nonfacial lacerations. The average total cost per case was $21.58 for the suture group and $17.69 (with suture kit) and $7.84 (without suture kit) for the staple group. This cost advantage would increase with increasing laceration length.

Notwithstanding the advantages of speed, convenience, and reduced infection rates of stapling, there are some limitations and disadvantages, notably the need to slightly evert the wound edges.[34,35] Since the staple must penetrate all layers of the tissue being stapled, stapling of thick, inflamed, or edematous tissues may be contraindicated. Likewise, the contraindications to dermal pin wound closure are when strong skin tension effects are present and its use for thick or scarred dermal tissue.[34] While staples and dermal pins can be applied over bone and viscera, there needs to be a minimum clearance of 4 to 6.5 mm between the skin and the underlying structures.[30,35]

This section indicates that there are numerous, and far-reaching, applications for ligating clips and staples in surgical practice. These devices are convenient, reasonably easy to use, and can be placed rapidly while not requiring the same surgical skill necessary for accurate and secure placement of sutures, while their radiolucency is an added advantage. However, a learning curve does exist for successful clinical use of this technology. Further, the indications are that even staples and pins manufactured from absorbable polymeric materials may remain in the body for extended periods of time. As yet, there do not appear to be any reports of adverse reactions resulting, and, at this stage, the advantages may outweigh the disadvantages.

VII. SUMMARY

Ligation of blood vessels for hemostasis is a venerable procedure in surgery and the development of specialized ligating clips and staples has simplified and facilitated this procedure. Often, these devices may be used in preference to the traditional filamentary sutures. Further, the continued development and modification of clips, particularly the absorbable type, has stimulated their extensive use in gynecological and urological procedures, typically tubule ligation for female sterilization. The first ligating clips were manufactured from metals, for example the Cushing silver wire neurosurgery clip and the wide variety of tantalum, stainless steel, and composite metal-plastic spring clips used in general, GU, and OB/GYN surgery. The sometimes adverse tissue reactions induced by metals and their long-term residence in the body stimulated the search for alternative, specifically absorbable thermoplastic, clip materials. Two absorbable clips and an absorbable staple and dermal pin are currently in clinical use. The Absolok clip is fabricated from poly-p-dioxanone while the Lactomer clip, staple, and pin are fabricated from a 70:30 glycolic and lactic acid copolymer. These materials are radiolucent and exhibit predictable hydrolytic decomposition, but they are subject to stress relaxation, which necessitates the incorporation of locking mechanisms in the clip design to ensure security of closure. Although these clips will elicit a typical foreign body reaction, it should be of limited severity and duration. The degradation of these clips and staples is far more rapid under *in vivo* conditions than *in vitro*, while their exposure *in vivo* to bacterial infection indicated formation of a progressively thickening plaque-like layer on the surface which significantly reduced the rate of *in vivo* clip degradation. The residence time of these absorbable devices in the body would appear to be far longer than predicted. A promising new development has been the introduction of the pelviscopic loop ligature or PLL for a variety of gynecological and general procedures. This device appears to be a convenient and economical technique for a variety of ligation procedures.

Closure of skin, vessels, and other tissues by mechanical means (staples and pins) has made significant progress over the past 20 years and these devices are safe, effective, rapid in use, and reduce local infection levels. However, it appears that the initial wound tear strength for stapled or pinned wounds is lower than for sutures. Mechanical "suturing" can provide satisfactory esthetics and while it cannot be used in all situations, it is advantageous where rapid closure is required. It is uncertain whether there are any adverse effects resulting from the long residence time of absorbable clips and staples in the body.

REFERENCES

1. Von Fraunhofer, J.A., Mechanical properties of nonabsorbable and absorbable ligating clips, *Clin. Obstet. Gynecol.*, 31, 718, 1988.
2. Hay, D.L., von Fraunhofer, J.A., and Masterson, B.J., Hemostasis in blood vessels after ligation, *Am. J. Obstet. Gynecol.*, 160, 737, 1989.
3. Brohim, R.M., Foresman, P.A., and Rodeheaver, G.T., Development of independent vessel security after ligation with absorbable sutures or clips, *Am. J. Surg.*, 165, 345, 1993.
4. Cushing, H., The control of bleeding in operations of brain tumors with the description of silver "clips" for the occlusion of vessels inaccessible to the ligature, *Ann. Surg.*, 54, 1, 1911.
5. McKenzie, K.G., Some minor modifications of Harvey Cushing's silver clip outfit, *Surg. Gynecol. Obstet.*, 45, 549, 1927.
6. Prudenz, H., The use of tantalum clips for hemostasis in neurosurgery, *Surgery*, 12, 791, 1942.
7. Burke, G., The corrosion of metals in tissues: and an introduction to tantalum, *Can. Med. Assoc. J.*, 43, 125, 1940.
8. Kylberg, F., The use of tantalum clips in general surgery, *Acta Chir. Scand.*, 141, 242, 1975.
9. Haskins, A.L., Oviductal sterilization with tantalum clips, *Am. J. Obstet. Gynecol.*, 114, 370, 1972.
10. Pavletic, M.M. and Schwartz, A., Stapling instrumentation, *Vet. Clin. North Am.*, 24, 247, 1994.
11. Hulka, J.F. and Omran, K.F., Comparative tubal occlusion: rigid and spring-loaded clips, *Fertil. Steril.*, 23, 633, 1972.
12. Hulka, J.F., Omran, K.F., Lieberman, B.A., and Gordon, A.G., Laparoscopic sterilization with the spring clip: instrumentation development and current clinical experience, *Am. J. Obstet. Gynecol.*, 135, 1016, 1979.
13. Filshie, G.M., Casey, D., Pogmore, J.R., Dutton, A.G.B., Symonds, E.M., and Peake, A.B.L., The titanium/silicone rubber clip for female sterilization, *Br. J. Obstet. Gynaecol.*, 88, 655, 1981.
14. Moretz, W.H., Rhode, C.M., and Shepherd, M.H., Prevention of pulmonary embolism by partial occlusion of the inferior vena cava, *Am. Surg.*, 25, 617, 1964.
15. Hendricks, G.L. and Barnes, W.T., Experiences with the Moretz clip: 100 cases, *Am. Surg.*, 37, 558, 1971.
16. Moretz, W.H., Still, J.M., Griffin, L.H., Jennings, W.D., and Wray, C.H., Partial occlusion of the inferior vena cava with a smooth Teflon clip: analysis of long-term results, *Surgery*, 71, 710, 1972.

17. Reed, A.M. and Gilding, D.K., Biodegradable polymers for use in surgery poly(glycolic)/poly(lactic acid) homo and co-polymers: in vitro degradation, *Polymer*, 22, 494, 1981.
18. Schaefer, C.J., Colombani, P.M., and Geelhoed, G.W., Absorbable ligating clips, *Surg. Gynecol. Obstet.*, 154, 513, 1982.
19. Michel, F., Ponsot, Y., Roland, J., Thibault, P.H., Rouquette, A.M., and Gattegno, B., Biological tolerance to polydioxanone absorbable clips: a comparison with metallic ligating clips, *Eur. Surg. Res.*, 17, 383, 1985.
20. Clarke-Peterson, D.L. and Creasman, W.T., A clinical evaluation of absorbable polydioxanone ligating clips in abdominal and pelvic operations, *Surg. Gynecol. Obstet.*, 161, 250, 1985.
21. Steckel, R.R., Jann, H.W., Kaplan, D., Jakowski, R.M., and Schwartz, A., Experimental evaluation of absorbable copolymer staples for hysterectomy, *Obstet. Gynecol.*, 68, 404, 1986.
22. Hay, D.L., von Fraunhofer, J.A., Chegini, N., and Masterson, B.J., Locking mechanism strength of absorbable ligating devices, *J. Biomed. Mater. Res.*, 22, 179, 1988.
23. Chegini, N., Hay, D.L., von Fraunhofer, J.A., and Masterson, B.J., A comparative scanning electron microscopic study on degradation of absorbable ligating clips in vivo and in vitro, *J. Biomed. Mater. Res.*, 22, 71, 1988.
24. Chegini, N., von Fraunhofer, J.A., Hay, D.L., and Masterson, B.J., Tissue reactions to absorbable ligating clips, *J. Reprod. Med.*, 33, 187, 1988.
25. Chegini, N., Hay, D.L., von Fraunhofer, J.A., and Masterson, B.J., Effects of bacterial infection on absorbable vascular ligating clips, *J. Reprod. Med.*, 33, 25, 1988.
26. Thiede, A., Jostarndt, L., Lünstedt, B., and Sonntag, H.G., Controlled experimental, histological and microbiological studies on the inhibition of infection by polyglycolic acid, *Chirurg.*, 51, 35, 1980.
27. Semm, K., Pelvi-Trainer, Ein Übungsgerat für die operative Pelviskopie zum Erlemen endoskopischer Ligatur und Nahttechniken, *Geburtshilfe Frauenheilkd.*, 46, 60, 1986.
28. Hay, D.L., Levine, R.L., von Fraunhofer, J.A., and Masterson, B.J., Chromic gut pelviscopic loop ligature: effect of the number of pulls on the tensile strength, *J. Reprod. Med.*, 35, 260, 1990.
29. Levine, R.L., Economic impact of pelviscopic surgery, *J. Reprod. Med.*, 30, 655, 1985.
30. Steichen, F.M. and Ravitch, M.M., Mechanical sutures in surgery, *Br. J. Surg.*, 60, 191, 1973.
31. Schwartz, A., Historical and veterinary perspectives of surgical stapling, *Vet. Clin. North Am.*, 24, 225, 1994.
32. Phung, D., Abidin, M.R., Thacker, J.G., Rodeheaver, G.T., Westwater, J.J., Doctor, A., and Edlich, R.F., Evaluation of automatic disposable rotating cartridge skin staplers, *J. Burn Care Rehab.*, 9, 538, 1988.
33. Jones, K.C., Himmel, H.N., Towler, M.A., Thacker, J.G., and Edlich, R.F., New advances in automatic disposable rotating cartridge skin staplers, *Burns*, 19, 159, 1993.
34. Zachmann, G.C., Foresman, A., Bill, T.J., Bentrem, D.J., and Rodeheaver, G.T., Evaluation of a new absorbable Lactomer subcuticular staple, *J. Appl. Biomater.*, 5, 221, 1994.
35. Waldron, D.R., Skin and fascia staple closure, *Vet. Clin. North Am.*, 24, 413, 1994.
36. Brickman, K.R. and Lambert, R.W., Evaluation of skin stapling for wound closure in the emergency department, *Ann. Emerg. Med.*, 18, 122, 1989.
37. Daniell, J.F., Kurtz, B.R., and Lee, J.Y., Laparoscopic oophorectomy: comparative study of ligatures, bipolar coagulation and automatic stapling devices, *Obstet. Gynecol.*, 80, 325, 1992.
38. Jurim, O., Colonna, J.O. II, Colquhon, S.D., Shaked, A., and Busuttil, R.W., A stapling technique for hepatic resection, *J. Am. Coll. Surg.*, 178, 510, 1994.
39. Walshaw, R., Stapling techniques in pulmonary surgery, *Vet. Clin. North Am.*, 24, 335, 1994.
40. Monnet, E. and Orton, E.C., Surgical stapling devices in cardiovascular surgery, *Vet. Clin. North Am.*, 24, 367, 1994.
41. Grainger, D.A., Meyer, W.R., and DeCherney, A.H., Laparoscopic clips: evaluation of absorbable and titanium with regard to hemostasis and tissue reactivity, *J. Reprod. Med.*, 36, 493, 1991.
42. Ling, F.W., Stovall, T.G., Meyer, N.L., Elkins, T.E., and Muram, D., Adhesion formation associated with the use of absorbable staples in comparison to other types of peritoneal injury, *Int. J. Gynecol. Obstet.*, 30, 361, 1989.
43. Orlinsky, M., Goldberg, R.M., Chan, L., Puertos, A., and Slajer, H.L., Cost analysis of stapling versus suturing for skin closure, *Am. J. Emerg. Med.*, 13(1), 77, 1995.

Chapter 11

Tissue Adhesives

Y. Ikada

CONTENTS

Many approaches have been advocated to enhance the surgeon's ability to achieve a rapid and effective control of wound closures, which is one of the dominating variables in any surgical procedure. A rapid and satisfactory wound closure can minimize the time spent in the operation room, the time patients are under anesthesia, the need for transfusions, and complications that occasionally accompany wound closure. To date, the use of sutures has been the most widely used method for wound closure because of the high reliability of closure required for satisfactory wound healing. However, alternative wound closure techniques have long been sought since suturing procedures often require highly skilled and experienced surgeons, a relatively longer time for wound closure, and the need for postoperative removal of nonabsorbable suture materials on skin to reduce any risk that could lead to adverse reactions. Possible alternatives of sutures for wound closure include clips, staples, and tissue adhesives. Clips and staples are described in Chapter 10. This chapter focuses on the recent development of tissue adhesives used for wound closure. For readers who are interested in a more detailed discussion of tissue adhesives, there are two comprehensive monographs on tissue adhesives.[1, 1a]

Adhesives are ubiquitous for home and industrial use, but their use in surgery is still not widely accepted, even though their use requires less surgical skill than suturing, wound closure is effected more quickly, and tissue adhesives may simplify complex surgical procedures. What are the reasons for the lower use of adhesives for wound closure? A major reason is the specific environment where surgical

Table 11.1 Requirements for Tissue Adhesives

Before Curing	After Curing
1. Sterilizable	1. Strongly bondable to tissues
2. Easy in preparation	2. Biostable union until wound healing
3. Viscous liquid or liquid possible for spray	3. Tough and pliable
4. Nontoxic	4. Resorbable after wound healing
5. Rapidly curable under wet, physiological conditions (pH 7.3, 37°C, 1 atm)	5. Nontoxic
6. Reasonable cost	6. Not obstructive to wound healing or promoting wound healing

adhesives are applied, since tissues to be adhered with surgical adhesives are quite delicate and differ markedly from the nonbiological objects upon which conventional adhesives are used.

I. DESIGN PRINCIPLES OF TISSUE ADHESIVES

Adhesives to be applied to living tissues should meet specific requirements, which are summarized in Table 11.1. First, they must achieve a biostable union between tissue surfaces until proper wound healing is achieved. This first requirement is identical to those for sutures. However, contrary to most sutures, tissue adhesives must always be resorbed in the body so that the two edges of a wound can eventually meet and be physically reunited for a complete wound healing. Because of the biodegradation requirement, it is essential that the biodegradation products of cured tissue adhesives are not cytotoxic, as is the case for other resorbable biomaterials. It is also highly desirable that tissue adhesives should be readily applied to tissues in adequate amounts without the need for any elaborate techniques and devices.

Regardless of the application modality, tissue adhesives should always be in the flow state with adequate viscosity during application. This is the most remarkable characteristic of adhesives that differentiates them from other bonding means. Bonding of two identical or different objects can be achieved only when a viscous liquid adhesive is cured to become a solid. The flow characteristic of tissue adhesives permits them to wet and spread over the entire surface of the object to be adhered, resulting in effective and close contact between the adhesive molecules and the object surface. The curing or solidifying of liquid-state adhesives can be realized through either polymerization, chemical crosslinking, or solvent evaporation at ambient temperature. Tissue adhesives also should be solidified on tissues by one of these curing methods.

One of the greatest challenges to the use of tissue adhesives is the high water content of tissues. Even if the water on a tissue surface is removed just prior to the application of tissue adhesive, water beneath the tissue surface could migrate onto the bonding surface and adversely affect the curing process.

Another important requirement of tissue adhesives is the rapid formation of a strong bond on the tissue in the presence of moisture without retarding wound healing. If an impervious tissue adhesive layer covers the whole surface of an injured tissue to be closed, the tissue healing which requires cell migration, will be greatly delayed by the tissue adhesive barrier. Therefore, desirable application modes of adhesives to tissues may be those schematically illustrated in Figure 11.1. The spot application of tissue adhesives would not delay wound healing, but requires very strong adhesion capability in the adhesive. The sheet-aided application of tissue adhesives will cause insufficient wound closure because of only one-side adhesion. If the adhesive layer is composed of a resorbable hydrogel with a high water content or a resorbable porous material, cells will be able to infiltrate into the hydrogel or porous material, resulting in revascularization and tissue regeneration. The use of porous tissue adhesive would permit the whole surface of the approximated tissues to be covered with such tissue adhesives; however, the bonding strength of porous tissue adhesives like hydrogels is generally very low because of the high water content.

The availability of biodegradable biomaterials having adequate adhesion properties also imposes a challenge for the development of successful tissue adhesives. Although many synthetic biodegradable biomaterials were developed for surgical and pharmaceutical use in the last few decades, most do not have adhesion properties at body temperature. Most biodegradable biomaterials exhibiting adhesion properties are of biological origin, like collagen, denatured collagen (gelatin), and fibrin.

These challenging requirements for tissue adhesives may account for their far less frequent use than sutures for wound closure, which can be regarded as one type of spot closing coupled with very high

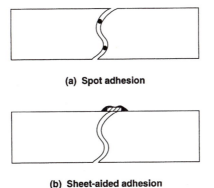

(a) **Spot adhesion**

(b) **Sheet-aided adhesion**

Figure 11.1 Two ideal modes of adhesive application to tissues.

bonding strength. This chapter describes the three types of tissue adhesives currently available: fibrin glue, poly-2-cyanoacrylates, and gelatin-resorcinol-formaldehyde. In addition, recent discoveries of some new experimental tissue adhesives are also briefly described.

II. NATURAL TISSUE ADHESIVE SYSTEM: FIBRIN GLUE

When human skin is slightly injured, e.g., to the extent that no suturing is necessary for its closure, bleeding will cease within minutes due to the formation of a blood clot which subsequently closes the small wound. This is the initial process of naturally occurring wound closure. Clot is formed as a product of the final common pathway of the blood coagulation cascade, illustrated in Figure 11.2. Fibrin glue mimics this final stage of the coagulation cascade for its adhesive capability. The major component of a blood clot is the fibrin network produced by polymerization of the fibrin monomer which is a product of partial hydrolysis of fibrinogen by thrombin. In the final stage of clot formation the fibrin network undergoes crosslinking by the catalytic action of factor XIII to reinforce the clot. Fibrinogen is a plasma protein with a molecular weight of 340,000 and is present in the plasma at concentrations of 2 to 6 mg/ml. Once the coagulation cascade is triggered by a lesion or some other reason, the activated factor X selectively hydrolyzes prothrombin to thrombin.

Naturally produced clot is an excellent adhesive for tissues, but the clot formation is insufficient in amount for urgent wound closure, unless the tissue incision is tiny. Therefore, an additional application of an "artificial" clot to a normal, surgically injured tissue is required for a proper wound closure. This is the principle behind the use of fibrin glue as a tissue adhesive. Besides this inherent adhesive property of fibrin glues, the clot formation during wound healing could also promote the healing process by causing an influx of fibroblasts, endothelial cells, inflammatory cells, and new blood vessels. Fibrin glues are now the most widely used tissue adhesives in surgery.

A. PREPARATION

The experimental trial of fibrin clots as tissue adhesives was first reported by Young and Medawar in 1940.[2] They prepared fibrin from an aqueous solution of fibrinogen and thrombin and applied it for the anastomosis of a peripheral nerve. Unfortunately, sufficiently high bonding strength was not achieved because of too low a fibrinogen concentration in the stock solution. Following the successful preparation of highly concentrated solutions of purified fibrinogen[3] by Blombäck and Blombäck, Matras et al. successfully approximated the rabbit sciatic nerve using a highly concentrated fibrinogen solution, in the 1970s.[4] Their work subsequently paved the way for using fibrins as a tissue adhesive.

The current commercially available fibrin glue is a two-component adhesive, generally consisting of four vials as shown in Figure 11.3. Vial 1 consists of fibrinogen powder and factor XIII, while vial 2 contains aqueous liquid for the preparation of fibrinogen and factor XIII solutions. Aprotinin, an inhibitor of fibrinolysis, is often included in vial 2. Vials 3 and 4 contain thrombin powder and an aqueous solution of $CaCl_2$, respectively, to prepare a thrombin solution. Ca^{2+} is required when thrombin selectively hydrolyzes fibrinogen through its catalytic action. Thrombin not only catalyzes the conversion of fibrinogen to fibrin but also initiates the activation of factor XIII.

320

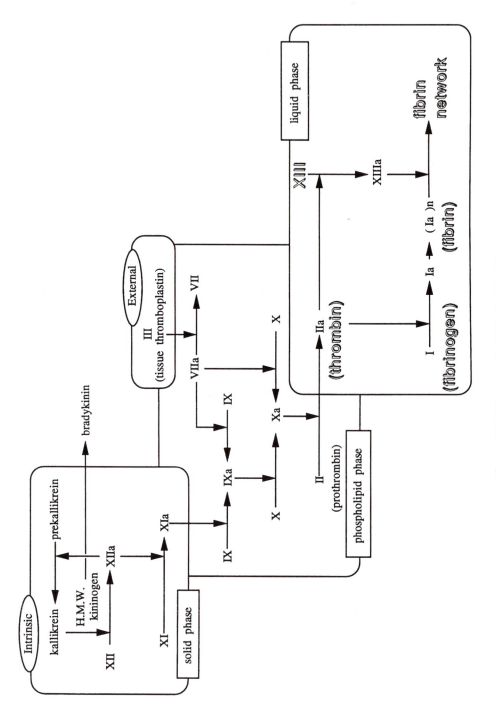

Figure 11.2 The cascade of blood coagulation.

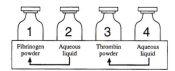

1. Prepare fibrinogen and thrombin solutions at room temperature

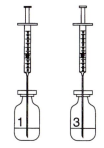

2. Fill the fibrinogen and thrombin solutions into syringes

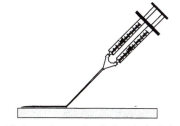

3. Connect the two syringes and apply the mixed solution to tissues

Figure 11.3 Application procedure of fibrin glue.

An example of how to prepare and apply a fibrin glue is the following procedure. A fibrin kit stored below 10°C is thawed to room temperature and then the whole aqueous liquid in vial 2 is transferred to vial 1 by a syringe to prepare the fibrinogen-factor XIII solution. At the same time, the aqueous liquid in vial 4 of the same volume as the aqueous liquid in vial 2 is introduced to vial 3 by use of a syringe to prepare the thrombin solution. After filling the fibrinogen solution and the thrombin solution into two different syringes in equal volumes, the solutions are mixed and applied to the wounded site to form a fibrin clot *in situ*. In the past, bubbles often formed during the preparation of the fibrinogen solution, but this problem has been overcome by keeping vial 1 under a negative pressure. Currently, devices with a gas-driven sprayer to apply the fibrinogen and thrombin solutions to tissues at the same time are available commercially (Figure 11.4). Owing to the development of this type of applicator, application of fibrin glue to tissues was greatly simplified and dripping of the precured solution was markedly minimized. Consequently, the surgical use of fibrin glue has become remarkably popular in Europe. Such pressurized spray systems are not practical for the application of small amounts, i.e., <1 ml of fibrin glue.

B. PHYSICAL PROPERTIES

The physical properties of cured fibrin glue are dependent primarily on the fibrinogen concentration in the precured fibrin glue. Tissue bonding is stronger with higher fibrinogen concentrations in the initial solution. The highly concentrated solutions, however, are too viscous and expensive. Generally, the fibrinogen concentration of the solution to be applied to tissues is 40 to 80 mg/ml and the thrombin concentration is 6 mg/ml. Mixing of these solutions in equal volumes yields a fibrin hydrogel with a water content around 90 wt% and tensile strength around 200 g/cm^2.

Bonding strength of the cured fibrin glue to tissues is markedly influenced by the nature of tissues and the extent of the wound. If the tissue is fatty, only poor bonding with fibrin glue is achieved, because fibrin glue is very hydrophilic. Figure 11.5 shows the bonding strength of a fibrin glue to different tissues of pig.[5]

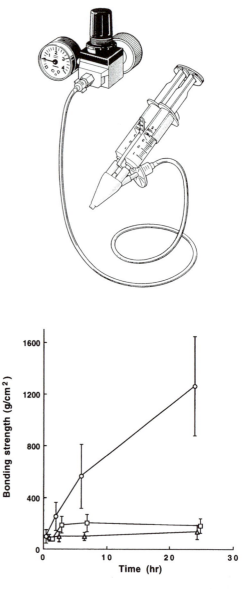

Figure 11.4 A spray set for application of fibrin glue.

Figure 11.5 Bonding strength of fibrin glue to porcine tissues as a function of time after application (○) rib; (△) tendon; (□) arterial aorta.

There have been few studies on the *in vivo* degradation of cured fibrin glues because of the difficulty in isolating and quantifying the fibrin glues remaining in the body. The resorption rate of cured fibrin glue in the body was found to depend on various factors, including the tissue water content, concentration of proteases and protease inhibitors present in the tissue, host cellular response to the fibrin clot, and the extent of crosslinking of fibrin molecules. Unless crosslinking is introduced, the fibrin clot would disappear from the body within a few weeks. Therefore, aprotinin is added to fibrin glue to retard the protease action, or fibrin is reinforced by crosslinking between the carboxyl and the amino groups in the fibrin molecules with factor XIII. Since sufficient factor XIII is present in the fibrinogen fraction to initiate adequate crosslinking of the fibrin clot, additional factor XIII does not appear to increase the binding strength of the preparation. Figure 11.6 shows the weight loss of cured fibrin glue subcutaneously and intraperitoneally implanted in rats.[6]

C. TOXICITY

Fibrin glue is nontoxic when pure human fibrinogen and thrombin are used. There has been no report that clearly shows tissue toxicity of fibrin glue. However, because the fibrinogen employed for commercial fibrin glue kits is obtained from the human blood of multiple donors utilizing precipitation techniques

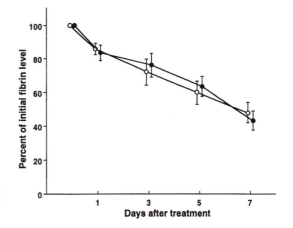

Figure 11.6 Resorption of fibrin glue in rat (○) subcutaneously implanted; (●) intraperitoneally implanted.

(e.g., cryoprecipitation, ethanol precipitation, cold ammonium sulfate precipitation, and poly(ethylene glycol) precipitation), cross-contamination remains a major concern. The most common method of concentrating fibrinogen is cryoprecipitation performed in closed sterile containers. There is, however, a risk of viral transmission, particularly hepatitis and acquired immunodeficiency syndrome (AIDS), although the latter has not been substantiated. In 1978, before the epidemic of AIDS, the U.S. Food and Drug Administration (FDA) banned the use of commercial homologous products of fibrinogen because of the extremely high risk of hepatitis contamination. This concern has led to the limited use of fibrin glues as tissue adhesives in the U.S.

To address this concern, bovine thrombin has been suggested because it is readily available without contamination. However, as this bovine material presents a xenogeneic component, the antibody against the bovine thrombin will be formed in the patient blood.[7] In fact, Banninger et al. showed that human application of fibrin glue containing bovine thrombin induced a marked prolongation of thrombin time because of the development of inhibitors of bovine thrombin.[8] Other methods like heat have also been used to reduce cross-contamination of blood-borne products by deactivating viruses.

D. APPLICATIONS

Fibrin glue prepared from donors' plasma has been used extensively in Europe and Japan for many years. The clinical application of fibrin glue covers all surgeries, as shown in Table 11.2. It should be pointed out, however, that the main purpose of the use of topical fibrin glue is not for tissue adhesion but for hemostasis. The reason for such a use may be the insufficient adhesive strength of fibrin glue. Although tissue closure by fibrin glue can be finished in minutes, the bonding strength is not high enough to ensure proper wound approximation until the wound heals completely. This is particularly important in those tissues subject to high pressure or loading. The lack of proper bonding strength with fibrin glues also makes their use for air- or liquid-tight closure questionable. Notwithstanding these drawbacks of fibrin glue, there are growing numbers of reports on the applications of fibrin glue as a tissue adhesive. One of the most common uses is to fasten grafts into positions when suture fixation is difficult. Some of the recent applications of fibrin glue are described below.

Table 11.2 Surgical Applications of Fibrin Glue

1. Gastroenterological surgery: hemostasis and reinforcement of intestinal anastomosis, prevention of bile leakage
2. Cardiovascular surgery: microvascular anastomosis, coating of artificial vessel, hemostasis of heparinized blood, reinforcement of vascular anastomosis, prevention of blood leakage
3. Thoracic surgery: prevention of air leakage after pneumonectomy, occlusion of tracheostoma, adhesion of pleura
4. Neurosurgery: prevention of cerebrospinal fluid leakage, neural anastomosis
5. Gynecology: end-to-end anastomosis of oviduct, adhesion of peritoneum and fascia
6. Plastic surgery: fixation of skin graft and wound cover, protection of oral mucosa, adhesion of bone and cartilage, hemostasis, filling, occlusion of traumatic tympanum defect
7. Orthopedics: fixation of bone fragments
8. Urology: adhesion of kidney, pelvis renalis, and ureter
9. Others: adhesion of substantial organs, hemostasis of hepatectomy

McKay et al. compared a laparoscopic resection and fibrin glue anastomosis with an open ureteral resection and suture anastomosis using female pigs.[9] The fibrin glue technique was performed by laparoscopically excising a ureteral segment, placing two transmural sutures over a stent and sealing the anastomosis with fibrin glues. At 4 weeks the stent was removed and at 8 weeks the animals were sacrificed for testing. The experimental group had one anastomotic breakdown, but all others had patent ureters. Radiographically, both groups demonstrated mild to moderate hydroureteronephrosis. It was concluded that laparoscopic ureteral reanastomosis with fibrin glue was feasible.

Seguin et al. reported aortic valve repair with fibrin glues for type A acute aortic dissection.[10] The repair is now generally done by resuspending the aortic valve using different types of suturing technique, usually passing through the aortic wall, which would cause bleeding at the suture sites. Seguin et al. suggested, instead, simply injecting fibrin glues between the two dissected layers of the aortic annulus, which achieves resuspension of the aortic valve and reinforces the proximal stump without the need for any sutures. To evaluate the efficacy of this simple technique, 15 cases of patients who underwent operative intervention for the treatment of type A aortic dissection associated with acute aortic insufficiency were reviewed. The mean follow-up time was 2.3 years. The computed tomography study in all patients showed closure of the dissecting process on the proximal ascending aorta.

The scleral pocket technique has dramatically changed wound closure after phacoemulsification with implantation of a posterior chamber lens. The use of single-stitch technique and wound closure by fibrin adhesive is now possible. Mester et al. conducted a comparative study of 385 consecutive patients; 167 received only fibrin glues for wound closure and 218 had the single-stitch procedure.[11] No complications were observed in either group. Surgically induced astigmatism was smaller in the fibrin group than in the single-stitch group. The results suggest that postoperative against-the-rule astigmatism can be prevented with fibrin glues.

As mentioned above, fibrin glues have been applied in surgery not only for wound closure but also for other purposes. One of the recent interesting applications of fibrin glues is to serve as a drug carrier for a sustained release. Fasol et al. used a modified fibrin glue to induce site-directed angiogenesis from aorta to heart.[12] They incorporated 1 μg of endothelial-cell growth factor into fibrin glues, implanted the modified fibrin glues in 10 experimental animals between the aorta and the myocardium of the left ventricle, and compared the results with those in 5 control animals that received normal fibrin glues without the growth factor. Nine weeks after implantation, angiography and histologic investigation showed newly grown vascular structures between the aorta and the myocardium in all experimental animals, but none in the control animals. This study shows the feasibility of initiating site-directed formation of new blood vessel structures to the heart by a modified fibrin glue implant containing angiogenic growth factor.

Postoperative adhesion formation in the abdominal and thoracic cavities is a serious problem in surgery. Sheppard et al. conducted a study, using 42 animals, to ascertain whether fibrin glues can inhibit adhesion formation in the peritoneal cavity of rats.[13] Bilateral circular peritoneal-muscular defects were created to induce adhesion formation. The right-sided defects were closed linearly with interrupted sutures, thus closing the peritoneum, and the left-sided defects were closed with a continuous suture placed circumferentially, leaving the peritoneal defect open. In 21 animals, the abdomen was closed with no further treatment, while in the other 21 animals, the defects were covered with fibrin glues. All rats were sacrificed at 30 d for evaluation. In the control group, 71% (15/21) rats had high graded adhesion to the closed defect, compared with 14% (3/21) in the fibrin glue group. For the left-sided lesions, 76% (16/21) animals in the control group had high grade adhesion compared with 9.5% (2/21) animals in the fibrin glue group.

E. IMPROVEMENTS

The most remarkable attempt to improve fibrin glues is the use of autologous blood components for preparing fibrin glues, to avoid the risk of viral contamination. Although multiple-donor blood used for the preparation of commercial fibrin glues is screened for infectious agents and is relatively safe, the risk for infectious transmission does exist. Park and Cha produced autologous fibrin glue from each of 30 human donors using the ammonium sulfate precipitation method.[14] The fibrinogen concentration ranged from 13 to 57 mg/ml with an average yield of 54.6%. There was a direct relationship between the level of fibrinogen in plasma and the autologous fibrin glue that was made from the same donor's plasma. The result suggests that the quality of this category of autologous fibrin glue depends partially on the fibrinogen level of the donor's plasma.

Tawes et al. obtained autologous fibrin glues through the same routine predonation procedures as with red blood cells before major elective surgery or, intraoperatively, from the platelet-rich plasma of patients.[15] They found that the autologous fibrin glues from predonation act more like an epoxy glue, while the autologous fibrin glue made during surgery is less viscous and acts more like a sealant because of the lower concentration of fibrinogen in platelet-rich plasma. An increase in viscosity of fibrin glues by adding sodium hyaluronate was reported by Wadstrom and Wik.[16] They approximated the femoral artery of rats with three conventional sutures and then sealed the artery with the modified fibrin glue. It was found that the increased viscosity of fibrin glues resulted in a significantly higher patency rate and a reduction in the amount of fibrin that entered the vessels.

In the future, fibrin glues composed of human recombinant components produced by biotechnology may appear, which should be much more effective and readily available, with no risk of infectious transmission.

III. SYNTHETIC TISSUE ADHESIVE SYSTEM: POLY-ALKYL-2-CYANOACRYLATES

A large number of synthetic adhesives have been manufactured for industrial and consumer uses, but most of them are not appropriate as tissue adhesives. The major reasons include the toxicity of adhesive ingredients, slow or no curing of adhesives in the presence of moisture at body temperature, and insignificant *in vivo* biodegradability of cured adhesives. As mentioned earlier, no adhesives can be applied in surgery if they have any of the above unfavorable characteristics. In restorative dentistry, some synthetic adhesives have been clinically applied, but they cannot be used for wound healing and are not resorbed into the body.

Among all existing synthetic adhesives, 2-cyanoacrylates (alkyl-2-cyanoacrylates or alkyl-α-cyanoacrylates) are the only ones which meet most of the requirements as tissue adhesives. Cyanoacrylates were discovered by H.W. Coover in 1951, through serendipity, at Tennessee Eastman Co.[17] He started research to develop tissue adhesives based on cyanoacrylates in 1960 through collaboration with Ethicon Co. (Somerville, NJ), and applied for FDA approval for the use of cyanoacrylates as tissue adhesives in 1964. Although his research group worked very hard for 6 years to achieve the improvements recommended by the FDA, they discontinued their work in tissue adhesive development because they failed to secure FDA approval for commercial use in the U.S. Alkyl-2-cyanoacrylates, with larger alkyl groups, have been tried clinically in humans in Canada, Europe, and Israel. The only cyanoacrylate tissue adhesive that has been used clinically in Europe is Histoacryl® from B. Braun. It may be available for human use in the U.S. under the name TraumaSeal® from Ethicon. 3M has Vetbond® tissue adhesive for veterinary use.

A. CHEMICAL STRUCTURE AND PHYSICAL PROPERTIES

2-Cyanoacrylates are acrylic monomers with the following chemical structure:

$$
\begin{array}{c}
\text{CN} \\
| \\
\text{CH}_2\!=\!\text{C} \qquad \text{(R:alkyl)} \\
| \\
\text{O}\!=\!\text{C-O-R}
\end{array}
$$

They are synthesized from formaldehyde and alkyl cyanoacetates, generally through the processes shown in Figure 11.7. The 2-cyanoacrylate monomers are highly polymerizable under neutral and basic conditions. They are purified by distillation in an acidic atmosphere, such as SO_2. Table 11.3 lists the boiling point, specific gravity, and viscosity of 2-cyanoacrylates. The detailed mechanism of polymerization of 2-cyanoacrylates is not fully understood, but it seems very probable that they polymerize via an ionic mechanism in which water molecules act as co-initiator. Cyanoacrylate polymers undergo hydrolytic degradation, which takes place through nonenzymatic reactions shown in Figure 11.8. The weight loss and formaldehyde formation from films of ethoxyethyl-2-cyanoacrylate polymer, when immersed in phosphate buffer solution of pH 7.4 at 37°C, are shown in Figures 11.9 and 11.10, respectively.[18] The linear formaldehyde production appears to support the degradation mechanism shown in Figure 11.8.

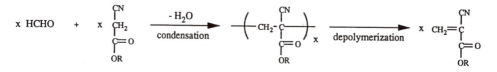

Figure 11.7 Synthetic route of 2-cyanoacrylate.

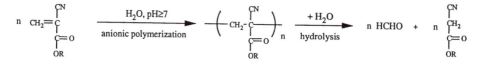

Figure 11.8 Polymerization of 2-cyanoacrylate and hydrolysis of the polymerization product.

Table 11.3 Physical Properties of Alkyl 2-Cyanoacrylates

Cyanoacrylate	Structure of Alkyl[a]	Boiling Point °C/mmHg	Specific Gravity (d_4^{20})	Viscosity (cp)
Methyl 2-cyanoacrylate	CH_3	55–57/5	1.0887	2.2
Ethyl 2-cyanoacrylate	CH_3CH_2	60–62/5	1.0452	2.9
n-Propyl 2-cyanoacrylate	$CH_3(CH_2)_2$	70–72/5		
n-Butyl 2-cyanoacrylate	$CH_3(CH_2)_3$	86–88/5		
Isobutyl 2-cyanoacrylate	$\overset{\displaystyle CH_3}{\underset{\displaystyle }{\vert}}$ $CH_3CH–CH_2$	77–80/5	0.9873	2.9
n-Hexyl 2-cyanoacrylate	$CH_3(CH_2)_5$	112–115/5		
n-Octyl 2-cyanoacrylate	$CH_3(CH_2)_7$	120–123/5		
Ethoxyethyl 2-cyanoacrylate	$CH_3CH_2OCH_2CH_2$	108/5	1.0652	4.5

[a] R of $\overset{\displaystyle CN}{\underset{\displaystyle }{\vert}}$ $CH_2=C–CO_2–R$

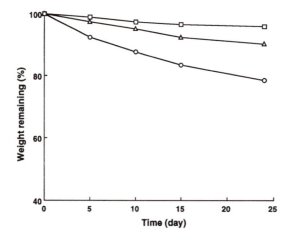

Figure 11.9 Weight loss of poly(ethoxyethyl 2-cyanoacrylate) films with different molecular weights (Mn) (○) 7,800; (△) 27,000; (□) 41,500.

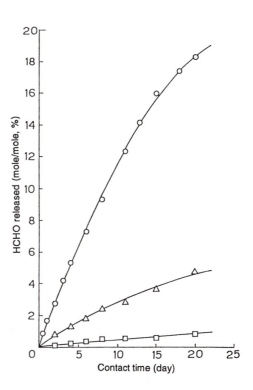

Figure 11.10 Release profiles of formaldehyde from poly(ethoxyethyl 2-cyanoacrylate) films with different molecular weights (Mn) (○) 7,800; (△) 27,000; (□) 41,500.

Table 11.4 Physical Properties of Cured 2-Cyanoacrylates

Cured Cyanoacrylate	Bonding to Stainless Steel		Softening Temperature °C	Glass Transition Temperature, °C
	Set Time, min	Strength, kg/cm²		
Poly (methyl 2-cyanoacrylate)	<1	136	123	136
Poly (ethyl 2-cyanoacrylate)	<1	137	116	140
Poly (isobutyl 2-cyanoacrylate)	5	121	108	130
Poly (ethoxyethyl 2-cyanoacrylate)	5–6	114	69	84

Table 11.4 gives the set time and bonding strength of cyanoacrylate adhesives applied to stainless steel plates.[18] Softening and glass transition temperatures of cyanoacrylate polymers are also shown in Table 11.4. As can be seen, cured cyanoacrylates are not pliable at body temperature, except for the ethoxyethyl-2-cyanoacrylate polymer.

B. BIODEGRADATION MECHANISM

The need for a biodegradable tissue adhesive is obvious. The presence of undegraded polymer fragments decreases the surface area available for collagenous union of the wound edges. Accordingly, the fibro-plasia phase is mechanically impaired and occurs only after enough adhesive has degraded to permit bridging of the fibroblasts. Poly(alkyl-α-cyanoacrylate)-based tissue adhesives biodegrade inside the body. In the presence of an aqueous environment, the polymer gives rise to its degradation products, notably formaldehyde and other breakdown products. The rate of degradation is the greatest for methyl α-cyanoacrylate, and diminishes as the size of the alkyl group increases at pH 7.0.[1,19] α-Cyanoacrylates with branched alkyl groups also degrade faster than their straight-chain homologs. The rate of degradation is higher in an alkaline solution (pH 8) for all homologous α-cyanoacrylates and differs only slightly from one to another. For example, the rate constants of both methyl and n-butyl α-cyanoacrylates at pH 7.0 are 3.0×10^{-3} and 1.0×10^{-5}, respectively. This alkaline-accelerated aqueous degradation suggests that the mechanism must involve the initial attack of hydroxyl ions on the chain methylene group and subsequent chain scission, as shown in Figure 11.11. The degradation *in vitro* would reach an equilibrium

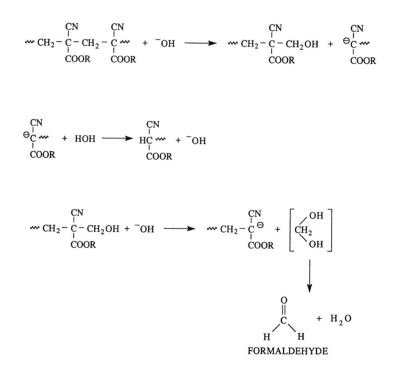

Figure 11.11 Degradation mechanism of poly (alkyl-α-cyanoacrylate) in aqueous medium. (Adapted from Refojo, M.F., Dohlman, C.H., and Koliopoulos, J., Adhesives in ophthalmology: a review, *Survey of Ophthalm.*, 15(4), 217, 1971.)

at which the concentration of formaldehyde produced remains constant. In addition to the dependence of the degradation rate on the pH of the medium and the size of the alkyl group, Vezin and Florence have reported that polymer particle specific surface, particle size, molecular weight, and molecular weight distribution also affect the *in vitro* heterogeneous phase degradation rate of the poly(alkyl α-cyanoacrylate).[20] The degradation occurs at the chain ends and travels along the polymer chain.

Other factors, such as the orientation and crystallinity of the polymer, could also affect its rate of degradation. A more oriented and crystallized polymer is expected to degrade more slowly and hence be less toxic. No data have been reported in this area.

C. TOXICITY

As shown in Figure 11.10, cyanoacrylate polymers yield formaldehyde as a by-product of hydrolytic degradation. Although the production rate of formaldehyde decreases with increase in the length of alkyl groups and the molecular weight of cyanoacrylate polymers, as shown in Table 11.5 and Figure 11.12, respectively,[21] the released formaldehyde is histotoxic and can cause acute and chronic inflammation unless the level accumulated in the treated area is below the threshold. The *in vitro* cytotoxicity of cyanoacrylate polymers can be studied using cultured cells. The percent growth inhibition of Swiss 3T3 cells induced by microspheres of various cyanoacrylate polymers is shown in Figure 11.13.[18] The cells were cultured in a modified Eagle's medium containing 10% fetal calf serum (FCS) in the presence of cyanoacrylate microspheres for 24 h at 37°C. It is apparent that methyl 2-cyanoacrylate polymer completely inhibits cell growth when added by 20 mg/well, whereas isobutyl 2-cyanoacrylate polymer has no effect on the cell growth, at least for the first 24 h. This suggests that the cytotoxicity of cyanoacrylate polymers greatly depends on the biodegradation rate of cyanoacrylate polymers and hence on the formaldehyde production rate. This assumption may be supported by the results shown in Figure 11.14, where the inhibition of cell growth is plotted against the concentration of formaldehyde released to the culture medium from the added cyanoacrylate polymers, together with the inhibitory effect of free formaldehyde.[21] It is apparent that the linear correlation between the inhibition of cell growth and the formaldehyde concentration of the medium must indicate that the formaldehyde released from the microspheres of cyanoacrylate polymer should be solely responsible for inhibiting the cell growth.

Table 11.5 Formaldehyde Release from Poly(2-Cyanoacrylate) Microspheres in Modified Eagle's Medium Containing 5% Fetal Calf Serum after Contact for 24 h

Poly(2-cyanoacrylate)	$\overline{M}w$	Formaldehyde ($\mu g/100 \, \mu g$)
Poly (methyl 2-cyanoacrylate)	3.8×10^4	3.621
Poly (ethyl 2-cyanoacrylate)	2.1×10^4	0.088
Poly (isobutyl 2-cyanoacrylate)	3.2×10^4	0.005
Poly (epoxyethyl 2-cyanoacrylate)	2.8×10^4	5.320

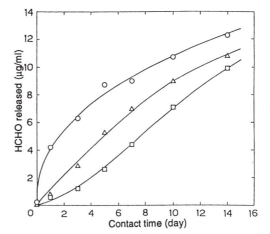

Figure 11.12 Release profiles of formaldehyde from poly(ethyl 2-cyanoacrylate) microspheres with different molecular weights (500 mg/ml) (○) 14,000; (Δ) 21,000; (□) 42,000.

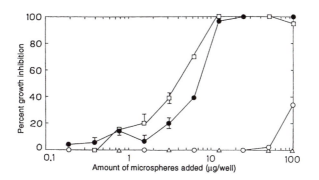

Figure 11.13 The inhibitory effect of different poly(2-cyanoacrylate) microspheres on cell growth (24 hr incubation) (□) poly(ethoxyethyl 2-cyanoacrylate) (Mw = 28,000); (●) poly(methyl 2-cyanoacrylate) (Mw = 38,000); (○) poly(ethyl 2-cyanoacrylate) (Mw = 21,000); (Δ) poly(isobutyl 2-cyanoacrylate) (Mw = 32,000).

Ciapetti et al. studied the *in vitro* cytotoxicity of cyanoacrylate monomers using drops of the monomers.[22] They employed two methods for the direct contact of cells with the cyanoacrylate liquids; one drop of each cyanoacrylate was placed onto a culture dish bottom and then L929 cells suspended in the culture medium were immediately added; conversely, after 1 or 2 d post-cell seeding, one drop of cyanoacrylate was added onto the semiconfluent monolayer. Crystal violet staining was used for determining the cell number. Figure 11.15 shows the result of crystal violet staining of viable cells after 6 h cell culture on the cyanoacrylate liquid monolayer. Apparently, cyanoacrylates do not allow the growth of L929 cells, as determined by crystal violet staining. Their cytotoxic effect is already evident at 6 h and confirmed at 24 h.

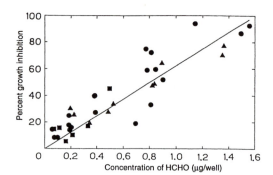

Figure 11.14 Relationship between the cell growth inhibition and the concentration of formaldehyde released from different poly(2-cyanoacrylate) microspheres (●) free formaldehyde; (▲) poly(ethyl 2-cyanoacrylate); (■) poly(isobutyl 2-cyanoacrylate) microspheres.

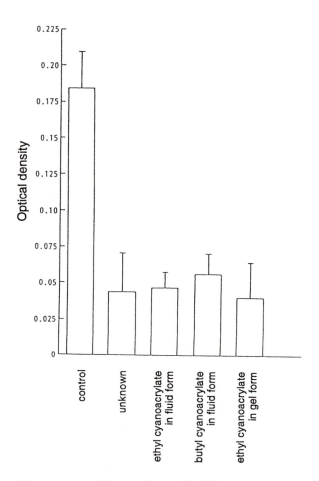

Figure 11.15 Cell growth on cyanoacrylate monolayers after 6 h exposure as measured by crystal violet stain uptake.

   In ophthalmology, the tissue response is also found to depend on the amount of adhesive material used.[23] The smaller the amount of adhesive used, the less the tissue reaction elicited. The fairly good tolerance reported in ocular surgery could be attributed to the small amount of adhesive used, ranging from half a microliter to several microliters per application. This tissue response is obviously related to the rate of build-up of degradation products and the ability of the tissue to metabolize them. The order of tolerance levels of the most commonly used synthetic tissue adhesives are as follows: *n*-decyl, *n*-octyl, *n*-heptyl, *n*-butyl, and isobutyl α-cyanoacrylates are well tolerated; methyl α-cyanoacrylate is least tolerated.[23]

A very recent advancement in α-cyanoacrylate tissue adhesives by Leung et al. may provide an innovative solution toward the concern of cytotoxicity of the formaldehyde released from α-cyanoacrylate tissue adhesives. Leung et al. used the concept of formaldehyde scavengers to neutralize the formaldehyde released. Readers are advised to read Chapter 12, "New Emerging and Experimental Materials for Wound Closure," Section IV, *New Tissue Adhesives*, for details.

D. APPLICATIONS

The possible applications of cyanoacrylate tissue adhesives were first reported by Coover. The following is a citation from the reminiscences of Coover.[17]

> Sutureless surgery, particularly rejoining veins, arteries, or intestines was indeed possible with the cyanoacrylates. They were equally useful in sealing and reinforcing suture lines in more conventional procedures. In ophthalmic surgery, these adhesives readily sealed small punctures or lesions in the eyeball, ordinarily very difficult to do, with sight-saving results. Corneal transplants were made safer and easier to perform. In cosmetic surgery, the use of cyanoacrylate to replace or supplement sutures greatly reduced scarring. Bleeding ulcers could be sealed with a coating of adhesive which protected the ulcer from stomach acids while healing proceeded, a procedure which could be accomplished through an endoscope without surgery. Repairs of soft organs, lung lesions, and other serious damage could be more easily done with these adhesives than by conventional methods. Cyanoacrylate adhesives were particularly useful in dental surgery in sealing tooth sockets after extractions and in periodontal surgery. An unexpected bonus in periodontal surgery was that cyanoacrylate greatly reduced the postoperative pain suffered by the patient. In all of these operations, the adhesive made the work easier and quicker for the surgeon, reduced the stress on the patient, promoted rapid recovery of function, or appearance, and sometimes, made possible otherwise impossible repairs, thus saving lives.

> Probably the most unusual and valuable use of the cyanoacrylates was as hemostatic agents, a use which departed somewhat from the original concept of a tissue-joining adhesive. Uncontrollable bleeding is a serious problem in surgery, particularly in the repair of soft organs such as the liver or spleen. It was found that a thin coating of cyanoacrylate sprayed on the bleeding surface almost instantly stopped the loss of blood. This was truly a life-saving procedure for it controlled bleeding when all other measures failed.

> The ultimate test for cyanoacrylate medical adhesive came in the Vietnam war. Medical evacuation helicopters brought the seriously wounded to battle-zone surgical units, sometimes within minutes after injury. Once there, all too often even the most skilled surgeon could not save many of those suffering grave wounds of the chest or abdomen. Uncontrollable bleeding killed them before the damage could be repaired. In 1966 a special surgical team trained and equipped with cyanoacrylate adhesive went to Vietnam and experienced almost miraculous results. A simple spray stopped the bleeding almost instantly, allowing time to treat the wounds by conventional means. Because of cyanoacrylate, many were saved who would otherwise have died. A revolutionary advance in surgery seemed to be at hand. But it was not to be in the United States, although Europe and Japan have reduced to successful practice the medical uses developed by our research teams. Technology had succeeded, but federal regulation was about to cancel that success.

> The first application for new drug approval went to FDA in 1964. Over the next six years, cyanoacrylates were tested and retested for safety. Every time approval seemed to be almost in hand, FDA changed their standards and requested new data. Each time retesting affirmed the safety and efficacy of the cyanoacrylate. Finally, the only concern was about possible carcinogenicity of the cyanoacrylates. The FDA proposed a third long-term, very costly study which might answer their objections. Ethicon and we faced a dilemma. The cost of this study would exceed the revenues for cyanoacrylates for years to come. On the other hand, the need for this unique life-saving adhesive was great. After much agonizing, it was finally concluded that the proposed multi-million dollar study was not an attractive gamble. This was based on the fact that there was no assurance that FDA would not propose a fourth carcinogenicity study and the general belief that there was little chance of obtaining approval even if the results were entirely favorable because of this cancer concern.

> What was the evidence for carcinogenicity? Only this — solid cyanoacrylate polymer disks implanted in rats, but not in other animals, caused tumors, some of which were malignant. Not only did this

test in no way approximate actual use of the adhesive, but rats were known to react in this way to implants of almost any insoluble material that blocks fluid flow — nearly all plastics, metals, ceramics — including many materials used routinely in prosthetic devices give the same effect. Neither humans nor animals treated with cyanoacrylate applied under normal surgical conditions developed tumors, but the questions raised by the rat implant tests were enough to prevent approval. Today, in the United States, an occasional Investigational Drug Permit is issued allowing the limited use of cyanoacrylate in special circumstances. A few surgeons risk using nonmedical cyanoacrylate without approval, purchasing industrial grade adhesive or even consumer adhesive. Could you choose for yourself, I am sure you'd accept a small risk of cancer in ten years or twenty years over bleeding to death on the operating table. After all, the benefit/risk equation looks pretty good. No choice, says FDA, the risk must be zero in our equation. By 1972, after twelve years of technical success and a record of saving lives, the cyanoacrylate medical adhesive was, for all practical purposes, dead.

Through animal experiments, Coover recognized that an adverse tissue reaction was induced by methyl 2-cyanoacrylate but not significantly by cyanoacrylates with longer side chains, such as the *n*-butyl and isobutyl esters. Since then, numerous papers have been published on animal studies and clinical trials of cyanoacrylates for various purposes, including tissue adhesion, tissue repair, embolization, sclerotherapy, hemostasis, and sealing. According to histochemical studies, methyl 2-cyanoacrylate invokes severe tissue damage in contrast to butyl 2-cyanoacrylate. A representative tissue reaction to cyanoacrylates applied to an incised site of rabbit skin is shown in Figure 11.16.[24] A significant inflammatory response is observed around the subcutaneous tissue glued with methyl and ethoxyethyl 2-cyanoacrylates. This response persisted for approximately 1 week. However, the inflammatory reaction in the skin tissue treated with ethyl and isobutyl 2-cyanoacrylates became mild at the second week postoperatively, and their polymers still remained at the wound site. The disappearance rate of cyanoacrylate polymers from the tissue was roughly in proportion to the degree of inflammatory tissue reaction.

The bonding strength of incised skins of rabbit glued with cyanoacrylates is higher than that of skins closed with silk suture for 1 week after closure, as shown in Figure 11.17.[24] After that, the bonding strength increases with time for both cyanoacrylate adhesives and silk suture, except for methyl 2-cyanoacrylate which degrades most rapidly. These findings suggest that wound closure using cyanoacrylate adhesives is better than that by suture at least for the first week postoperation, during which the bonding strength of wounds depends largely on wound closure biomaterials. Vanholder et al. undertook a comparative double blind randomized study using rats for closing skin wounds by a cyanoacrylate tissue adhesive (ethyl 2-cyanoacrylate) and a classical silk suture.[25] Skin incisions were made on both sides of the rat back; one side was closed by cyanoacrylate and the other side by silk suture. The external cosmetic and the morphologic aspects of skin wounds were photographically scored by independent observers. Evaluations were performed at 1, 2, 4, and 8 weeks. The morphological study demonstrated no adverse effects for the adhesive treatment with a minor inflammatory infiltrate. Sutured wounds had a higher tendency to develop abscesses and/or major inflammation. The evaluation results for an 8-cm incision are given in Tables 11.6 and 11.7. As can be seen, there was no difference in score between adhesive and suture closures: 8.3 ± 1.9 for adhesive vs. 8.3 ± 1.5 for silk suture. The adhesive-treated wounds scored better than nontreated wounds (8.9 ± 1.3 vs. 7.4 ± 3.3).

Caballero-Gómez and Ortega-Moreno performed experimental end-to-end uterine horn anastomosis in 20 rats with the conventional technique of microsurgery, *n*-butyl 2-cyanoacrylate, and cyanoacrylate in addition to one or two microsutures.[26] Only the cases of conventional approximation and of cyanoacrylate in combination with two microsutures showed a patency rate of 100%, whereas in the case of uterine horns approximated with cyanoacrylate adhesive alone the patency rate was 80%. Their findings indicate that tissue adhesive and two sutures used together may offer a viable alternative to sutures for genital duct anastomosis.

Quillen and Rosenwasser examined the efficacy of aerosolization as a means of applying cyanoacrylate to the cornea.[27] They created central corneal perforations in cadaver eyes and delivered a small amount of *N*-butyl-2-cyanoacrylate to the perforation site via aerosol. An adequate seal of 1 mm perforation was found following the aerosol application of cyanoacrylate adhesive. On the other hand, Leahey et al. evaluated the ocular clinical use of *N*-butyl cyanoacrylate for 44 patients for a 2-year period.[28] The complications of glue application included corneal perforation (19 eyes), descemetoceles (9 eyes), leaking filtering blebs (6 eyes), stromal thinning (5 eyes), wound leaks (4 eyes), and exposure keratopathy (1 eye). Outcome was penetrating keratoplasty (19 eyes), no further intervention (14 eyes), enucleation (4 eyes), surgical revision of a filter (2 eyes), scleral patch graft (1 eye), conjunctival transplant (1 eye), failed

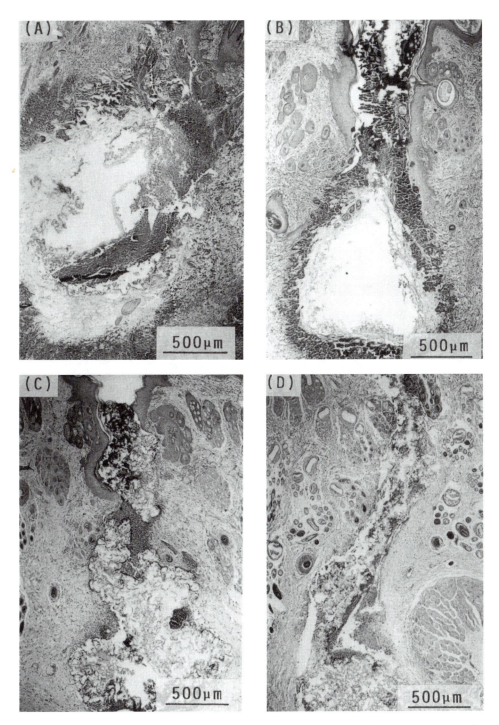

Figure 11.16 Photomicrographs 7 d after gluing the skin incision of rabbit with (A) methyl 2-cyanoacrylate, (B) ethoxyethyl 2-cyanoacrylate, (C) ethyl 2-cyanoacrylate, and (D) isobutyl 2-cyanoacrylate.

tarsorrhaphy (1 eye), suturing of wound (1 eye), and a lamellar graft (1 eye). Vision improved in 52% of eyes. These results demonstrate that this tissue adhesive provides an effective method of temporary or permanent closure of an impending or frank perforation.

In cardiothoracic surgery, 2-cyanoacrylates have often been used. For instance, Sabanathan et al. employed *N*-butyl 2-cyanoacrylate in pulmonary resections of 187 patients.[29] The glue reinforced the stapled bronchial stump (135 patients), the sutured bronchial anastomosis in sleeve resections

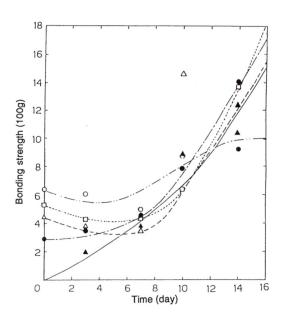

Figure 11.17 Bonding strength of incised rabbit skin closed with 2-cyanoacrylates and silk. (●) Methyl 2-cyanoacrylate; (○) ethyl 2-cyanoacrylate; (Δ) isobutyl 2-cyanoacrylate; (□) ethoxyethyl 2-cyanoacrylate; (▲) silk.

Table 11.6 Photographic Score of Large (8 cm) Wounds Closed with Ethyl 2-Cyanoacrylate (G) and Vicryl Suture (S)

Rat no.	Week 1		Week 2		Week 4		Week 8	
	G	S	G	S	G	S	G	S
1	2.8	6.7	9.6	10.0	8.7	9.8	9.4	8.9
2	8.8	6.4	9.4	7.7	9.6	9.9	8.9	10.0
3	2.4	6.5	9.3	6.0	6.0	8.0	9.4	8.9
4	8.9	5.9	7.8	9.7	9.6	10.0	9.7	10.0
5	6.6	7.8	9.8	9.2	6.7	8.0	9.2	8.6
6	4.9	6.4	9.5	8.6	8.7	9.4	8.8	8.8
7	7.0	6.7	9.0	7.3	9.2	9.3	9.4	9.1
8	9.9	7.6	9.1	9.1	9.8	9.5	9.4	9.2
9	6.1	3.9	9.2	7.7	7.2	8.5	9.3	9.1
Mean	6.4	6.4	9.2	8.4*+	8.4*+	9.1**	9.3*	9.2*
± S.D.	2.6	1.1	0.6	1.3	1.4	0.8	0.3	0.5

Note: $* P <.05$; $** P <.01$ vs. week 1, same treatment; $^+ P <.05$, glue vs. suture at the same week.

Table 11.7 Photographic Scores in Comparison of Ethyl 2-Cyanoacrylate (G) and No Treatment (Sh)

Rat no.	Week 1		Week 2		Week 4		Week 8	
	G	Sh	G	Sh	G	Sh	G	Sh
1	9.6	9.2	10.0	9.8	10.0	9.8	9.9	9.3
2	8.3	0.0	9.2	9.3	8.5	9.1	8.3	7.7
3	10.0	0.8	9.3	8.6	9.7	7.9	8.5	7.9
4	4.8	1.9	9.3	9.1	8.2	8.7	9.0	9.0
Mean	8.2	3.0	9.5	9.2	9.1	8.9	8.9	8.5
± S.D.	2.4	4.2	0.4	0.5	0.9	0.8	0.7	0.8

Note: Overall means ($n = 16$); G, 8.9 ± 1.3 vs. Sh, 7.4 ± 3.3. Overall means: $P <.01$.

(37 patients), or the staple lines of wedge resections (15 patients). Mortality was 1.6% overall and 5% among pneumonectomies (2 of 40). Bronchopleural fistulae occurred in 0.5% of all pulmonary resections and pneumonectomies (1/40). There were no cyanoacrylate adhesive-related complications. A follow-up of the patients up to 689 months has indicated not only its effectiveness but also its safety. They have concluded that N-butyl 2-cyanoacrylate glue is safe, offers protection to bronchial margins, and may be valuable in preventing bronchial stenosis after sleeve resections.

How do synthetic tissue adhesives like cyanoacrylates perform in the presence of contaminated wounds? An early study by Eiferman and Snyder indicated that cyanoacrylate tissue adhesives are bacteriostatic for Gram-positive microorganisms.[30] This unique antimicrobial property of cyanoacrylate tissue adhesives was confirmed recently by Noordzij et al.[31] and Howell et al.[32] In an animal study of the effect of tissue adhesives on wound infection, Noordzij et al. reported that wounds contaminated by *Staphylococcus aureus* at both 10^5 and 10^6 concentration and closed by N-butyl-2-cyanoacrylate tissue adhesive (Histoacryl® from B. Braun Melsungen AG, Germany) exhibited better resistance to wound infection (in terms of percent of gross infection and the number of viable bacteria count) than 5/0 polypropylene suture.[31] In the absence of bacterial contamination, however, the percutaneous suture closure resulted in a more secure wound than Histoacryl did right after the closure. There was no significant difference in wound strength between the Histoacryl and polypropylene suture closure at 7 d postsurgery. These findings by Noordzij et al. were also confirmed by a more recent study by Howell et al. of *S. aureus*-contaminated laceration in male albino guinea pigs.[32] The *S. aureus* contaminated wounds closed with N-butyl-2-cyanoacrylate (Nexaband® liquid from Veterinary Products Labs, Phoenix, AZ) had lower bacterial counts (about 1/2) than the same wound closed with Vicryl suture. In contrast, there is one reported study by Olson et al. which indicated that N-butyl-2-cyanoacrylate adhesive (Vetbond® from 3M) facilitated the colonization of *S. epidermidis*[33] and hence the adhesive had weak or no bacteriocidal property. Obviously, there is a need for additional study to resolve the conflicting reports.

E. IMPROVEMENTS

The medical use of cyanoacrylate adhesives for tissue bonding has been well established outside the U.S., although they are still under review by the FDA. For instance, their use in treating arterial aneurysms in neurosurgery and for tacking skin grafts into place are customary procedures because of their ease and speed of use. However, medical-grade cyanoacrylate adhesives are associated with several problems, such as toxicity of biodegradation by-products, difficult handling due to instantaneous polymerization and very low viscosity of cyanoacrylate monomers, and fairly high cost.

To improve these drawbacks, some modifications have been attempted on 2-cyanoacrylates. Matthews[34] proposed to use commercially available products for medical application to save on the cost, because commercial cyanoacrylate adhesives were found to be bacteriostatic.[30–32,34] Yoshitomi Pharmaceutical Co., Osaka, Japan is selling a modified cyanoacrylate adhesive, Biobond®. This is a mixture of ethyl cyanoacrylate monomer, nitrile rubber, toluene diisocyanate, and an organic solvent. Mixing of cyanoacrylate with nitrile rubber makes the cured adhesive much more pliable, but prolongs the set time and would increase toxicity. Addition of adequate polymers could increase the low viscosity of cyanoacrylate monomers and improve the pliability of the resulting cyanoacrylate polymers without any risk of additional toxicity.

Tseng et al. mixed cyanoacrylates with D,L-lactide/ε-caprolactone copolymers [P(LA-co-CL)], which are biodegradable and nontoxic to tissues.[35] The viscosity of cyanoacrylate monomers increased remarkably upon mixing with P(LA-co-CL), as shown in Figure 11.18, while the set time became longer with the increasing concentration of P(LA-co-CL) in the mixture, accompanied by decreased stiffness of the cured polymer and reduced cell growth inhibition. There was no substantial difference in the bonding strength *in vivo* between the pure cyanoacrylate monomers and the cyanoacrylates mixed with different concentrations of P(LA-co-CL) up to 15 wt%. The handling properties of the mixture during surgery were also greatly improved.

IV. HYBRIDIZED TISSUE ADHESIVE SYSTEM, GRFs

A. PREPARATION

Some aqueous polymer solutions are known to set through gel formation in minutes when a crosslinking agent is added to the solution. One such water-soluble polymer is gelatin which is absorbable in the body. The use of crosslinked gelatin for tissue adhesion was first described by Tatooles and Braunwald.[36] They further reported that a gelatin-resorcinol mixture crosslinked with a combination of formaldehyde (GRF)

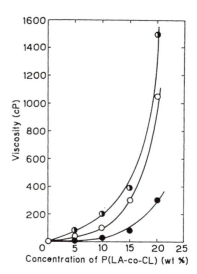

Figure 11.18 Viscosity of mixtures of 2-cyanoacrylate and D,L-lactide-ε-caprolactone copolymer [P(LA-co-CL)] with the ε-caprolactone content of 0.7. (◑) ethoxyethyl 2-cyanoacrylate – P(LA-co-CL) (Mw=102,000); (○) ethoxyethyl 2-cyanoacrylate – P(LA-co-CL) (Mw=62,000); (●) ethyl 2-cyanoacrylate – P(LA-co-CL) (Mw=62,000).

and sometimes glutaraldehyde (GRFG) gave a satisfactory bonding strength in hepatic and renal tissues of dogs.[37] It should be stressed that GRF is free from blood components, similar to cyanoacrylate adhesives.

In 1968, Cooper and Falb also studied gelatin crosslinked with formaldehyde as a tissue adhesive.[38] They added resorcinol to gelatin-formaldehyde mixtures to improve their very low bonding strength. Formaldehyde undergoes condensation with resorcinol to give a three-dimensional crosslinked resin. Figure 11.19 shows the condensation mechanism. Bonding strength may also be enhanced by the ingredient penetration into the tissue and hydrophobicity of the resultant resin.

B. TOXICITY

Because of the formaldehyde component in GRF adhesive, its toxicity is of a major concern. Even if all the formaldehyde molecules applied are involved in the condensation reaction with gelatin and resorcinol, formaldehyde will be released from the cured adhesive when gelatin undergoes enzymatic hydrolysis. Therefore, the surgical application of GRF should be limited to special cases where high bonding strength is imperative. GRF is not commercially available in the U.S.

C. APPLICATIONS

Currently, GRF is largely used in Europe to treat acute aortic dissections because of its ability to reinforce the delicate structures of the acutely dissected aortic wall. Stassano et al. recently applied the GRF glue to two patients with aortic bioprosthetic endocarditis with annular abscesses.[39] The aortic valve was replaced with a bioprosthesis and the annular abscesses were debrided and closed with the aid of GRF. The glue completely sealed the abscess cavities. One year later the patients were asymptomatic and had no clinical or echocardiographic signs of aortic incompetence.

Bellotto et al. evaluated the ability of GRFG to seal incisional air leaks acutely in the lungs of rabbits under the condition of positive intratracheal pressure and persistent ventilation.[40] They established a technique for application of this adhesive and demonstrated its ability to consistently reduce the magnitude of air leaks, while generally providing complete pneumostasis in the presence of clinically relevant positive pressure ventilation. Their results are given in Figure 11.20. They concluded that this material can be prepared months in advance for occasional use as an effective means to deal with parenchymal air leaks encountered at surgery.

D. IMPROVEMENTS

Although refixation of dissected aortic layers with GRF adhesive represents a new option in the surgical treatment of aortic dissection, development of new tissue adhesive biomaterials is necessary because of the known mutagenicity of formaldehyde. Ennker et al. prepared a gelatin-dialdehyde glue by replacing formaldehyde with two less toxic aldehydes, glutaraldehyde and glyoxal.[41] They glued each pig's infrarenal aorta around an implanted prosthesis and found that the gelatin-dialdehyde glue was able to produce the same bonding effect in the area of the aortic wall as the substantially more toxic GRF glue. An observed tanning effect was attributed to the disintegration of the fiber texture, specifically collag-

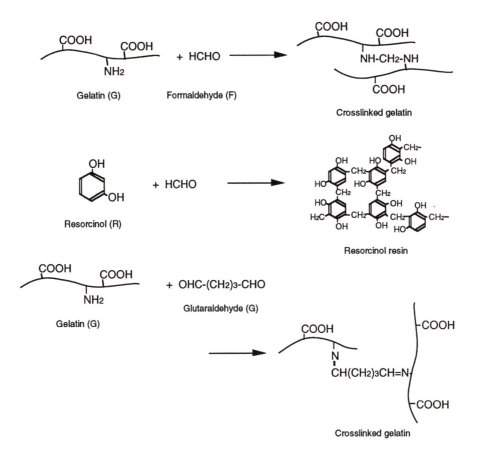

Figure 11.19 Plausible mechanisms of curing of the gelatin-resorcinol-formaldehyde-glutaraldehyde glue.

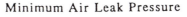

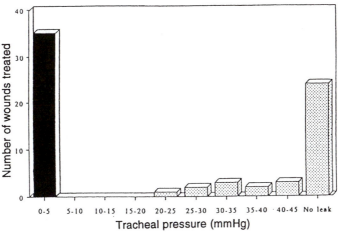

Figure 11.20 Number of wounds (glued vs. untreated) that leaked at any given intratracheal pressure (▨) glued; (■) untreated.

enous as well as smooth muscle fibers, and to the reciprocal alterations of the proteoglycan interstitial substances in the aortic wall.

Albes et al. studied the biophysical properties of GRFG by gluing aortic specimens from sheep with warm adhesive under wet and dry conditions and then submitting the specimens to compression.[42] GRFG

Table 11.8 Characteristics of Currently Available Tissue Adhesives

	Fibrin Glue	Cyanoacrylate	GRF
Handling	Excellent[a]	Poor[b]	Poor
Set time	Medium	Short	Medium
Tissue bonding	Poor	Good	Excellent
Pliability	Excellent	Poor	Poor
Toxicity	Low[c]	Medium[d]	High
Resorbability	Good	Poor	Poor
Cell infiltration	Excellent	Poor	Poor

[a] Spray type.
[b] Low viscous type.
[c] Not autologous.
[d] Long alkyl chains.

and cyanoacrylate glue showed similar results at 5 N and provided better adhesion when applied under dry conditions. Fibrin glue showed weak adhesion even under dry conditions, whereas GRFG exhibited good adhesive properties both for the wet and dry tissues.

V. NEW TISSUE ADHESIVE SYSTEMS

As described above, at least three kinds of tissue adhesives (fibrin glue, 2-cyanoacrylates, and GRF) are currently being used in surgery. However, all of them have several drawbacks, as summarized in Table 11.8. To overcome these problems, several attempts have been made to develop new tissue adhesives without using human blood-borne products (e.g., fibrinogen), cyanoacrylates, or formaldehyde. Four representative studies of new tissue adhesives were recently performed in Japan. They can be classified into two groups; gelatin-based and polyurethane-based adhesives.

A. GELATIN-BASED ADHESIVES

In this group, gelatin is the major component of tissue adhesives.

1. GTXIII®

A substitute of fibrin glue (GTXIII®), developed by Unitika Co., Osaka, Japan, mimics blood coagulation without using fibrinogen. GTXIII is now commercially available in Japan and is used mainly for hemostasis during surgery. GTXIII is composed of thrombin, coagulation factor XIII, and gelatin as carrier material. When GTXIII is injected into a bleeding site from a syringe, local hemostasis is accelerated because the added thrombin promotes fibrin formation. The risk of viral infection from GTXIII is much reduced, since fibrin is formed from fibrinogen present in a patient's own plasma. However, viral infection cannot be completely eliminated because the thrombin is obtained from multiple blood donors.

The hemostatic time of GTXIII was about 2 min when 166.7 units of thrombin, 5.2 units of factor XIII, and 150 mg of gelatin were applied to the liver of warfarinized rats after liver biopsy.[43] No adverse response was observed when 60 mg/kg of GTXIII with the above composition was injected into the ear vein of rabbit. It is reported that GTXIII was also able to accelerate wound healing.

2. Gelatin-poly(L-glutamic acid) Adhesive

It is known that carbodiimide is a coupling agent for amide bond formation between carboxyl and amino groups even in the presence of water.[44] An aqueous solution of gelatin sets to a gel when a water-soluble carbodiimide (WSC) is added to the solution due to the formation of intermolecular amide bonds in the gelatin molecules having both carboxyl and amino groups. An addition of poly(L-glutamic acid) (PLGA) to the gelatin solution shortens the incipient gelation time, as shown in Figure 11.21.[45] Since PLGA will be converted to acid anhydrides by an addition of WSC which functions also as an agent to produce acid anhydride from carboxyl groups, PLGA molecules with acid anhydrides will readily undergo crosslinking with gelatin molecules having amino groups to yield a hydrogel. This gelatin-PLGA hydrogel exhibited firm adhesion to the mouse skin and other soft tissues with a higher bonding strength than fibrin glue.[45] Table 11.9 shows a representative result of bonding strength of gelatin-PLGA hydrogel to various rabbit tissues when compared with fibrin glue. Bonding was performed using a mixture of

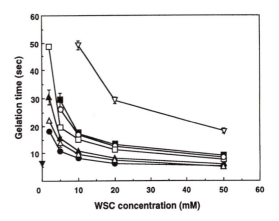

Figure 11.21 Effect of poly(L-glutamic acid) (PLGA) addition on the gelation time of gelatin aqueous solution with 1-ethyl-3-(3-dimethylaminopropyl) carbodiimide (the gelatin concentration is 100 mg/ml) (○) 1, (●) 5, (△) 10, (▲) 20, (□) 50, (■) 100 mg/ml of PLGA; (◁) gelation time of fibrin glue.

Table 11.9 Bonding Strength of Gelatin-PLGA Hydrogel and Fibrin Glue to Different Tissues of Rabbit

| | Bonding Strength (g/cm²) | | | | | |
| | Skin | Muscle | Peritoneum | | Small Intestine | |
			Inside	Outside	Inside	Outside
Gelatin-PLGA hydrogel	102.9 ± 11.3	90.5 ± 16.0	55.6 ± 10.6	76.2 ± 28.8	38.8 ± 10.2	42.1 ± 6.3
Fibrin glue	93.4 ± 14.0	86.0 ± 11.3	37.8 ± 4.4	59.9 ± 8.6	3.4 ± 0.0	17.7 ± 4.4

100 ml of aqueous solution containing 100 mg/ml gelatin, 100 mg/ml PLGA, and 35 ml of 9.6 mg/ml 1-ethyl-3-(3-dimethylamino-propyl) carbodiimide as WSC. The bonding strength of the gelatin-PLGA adhesive is higher than that of fibrin glue, irrespective of the tissue type. The difference in the bonding strength among the various soft tissues may be explained in terms of their surface properties. For example, the presence of hydrophobic fat in tissues will reduce the wettability of the fatty soft tissues by gelatin-PLGA solution or fibrin glue, resulting in a decrease in bonding strength. In addition, fat will reduce the anchoring effect of the crosslinked gelatin-PLGA adhesive on the soft tissues and hence the bonding strength. Contrary to fibrin glue, cohesive failure inside the crosslinked gel was observed when the gel-tissue bond was intentionally broken. The bonding strength of the gelatin-PLGA hydrogel became higher with an increase in PLGA concentration in the initial solution.

Histological sections of mouse subcutaneous tissues around the gelatin-PLGA hydrogel and fibrin glue are shown in Figure 11.22.[45] No severe inflammatory reaction is observed around both cured materials. The gelatin-PLGA hydrogel gradually disappeared through biodegradation in the body. The concentration of WSC required for hydrogel formation seems to be low enough not to cause an adverse reaction, but the toxicity of the remaining WSC, if any, should be checked carefully before clinical trial.

B. POLYURETHANE-BASED ADHESIVES

Polyurethane is synthesized by an addition polymerization between diisocyanate and oligomeric diol via the formation of urethane bond (–HNOCO–). If both ends of the formed prepolymer are capped with isocyanate, the resulting prepolymer will rapidly undergo gel formation upon contact with water. Therefore, the prepolymer with terminal isocyanate groups will be able to be used as a tissue adhesive if the gel itself and its biodegradation by-products are nontoxic.

1. Polyurethane from Fluorinated Hexamethylene Diisocyanate

Matsuda et al. synthesized a reactive hydrophilic urethane prepolymer in an attempt to develop a compliant tissue adhesive.[46] They used a random copolymer prepared from ethylene glycol (EG) and propylene glycol (PG) as the oligomeric diol and a fluorinated aliphatic diisocyanate like hexamethylene diisocyanate (FHMDI). The EG/PG ratio and average molecular weight of the copolymer were 2/1 and 4030, respectively. The addition polymerization between the EG-PG copolymer and an excess of FHMDI yielded a reactive urethane adhesive with terminal isocyanates. The chemical structure of the resultant

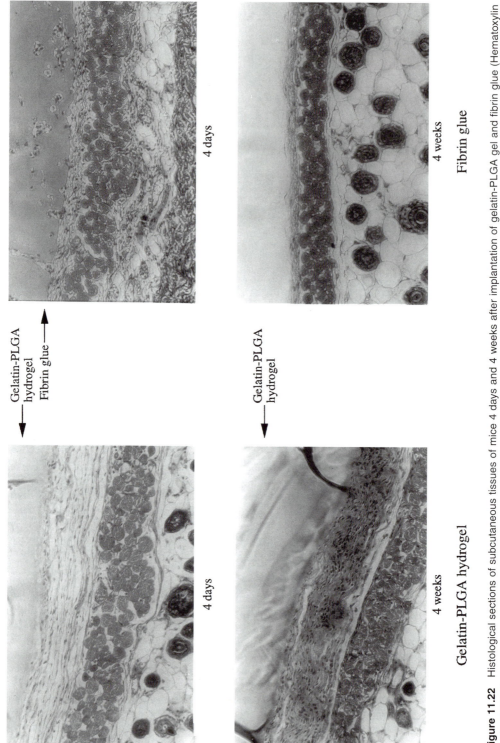

4 days

4 weeks

Fibrin glue

Gelatin-PLGA
hydrogel
Fibrin glue

Gelatin-PLGA
hydrogel

4 days

4 weeks

Gelatin-PLGA hydrogel

Figure 11.22 Histological sections of subcutaneous tissues of mice 4 days and 4 weeks after implantation of gelatin-PLGA gel and fibrin glue (Hematoxylin eosin staining).

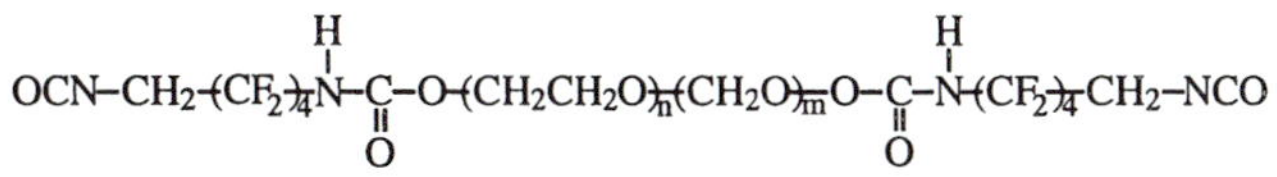

$$\underset{\text{O}}{\overset{\text{H}}{\text{OCN-CH}_2\text{-(CF}_2)_4\text{N-C-O-(CH}_2\text{CH}_2\text{O)}_n\text{(CH}_2\text{O)}_m\text{O-C-N-(CF}_2)_4\text{CH}_2\text{-NCO}}}$$

Figure 11.23 Chemical structure of urethane prepolymer synthesized using fluorinated hexamethylene diisocyanate.

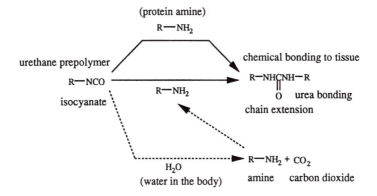

Figure 11.24 Reactions of the reactive urethane prepolymer with the tissue, moisture, and modified polyurethane.

adhesive is shown in Figure 11.23. This adhesive is in liquid form at room temperature and is cured when brought into contact with tissues. Figure 11.24 demonstrates plausible chemical reactions which will take place upon contact of the adhesive with the tissues and moisture. The isocyanate end groups of the prepolymer react with the amino groups of proteins of the tissue and water to produce an adhesive-tissue conjugate and the modified prepolymer having the terminal amino group, respectively. When the modified prepolymer reacts with the starting, reactive prepolymer, a gel is formed.

The EG-PG copolymer is not biodegradable, but the cured gel will undergo gradual degradation because of the introduction of biodegradable urethane bonds into the backbones of the gel. As a result of urethane hydrolysis, diamines will be released. Since aromatic amines are thought to be potentially carcinogenic, Matsuda et al. used aliphatic instead of aromatic diisocyanate like FHMDI. The resulting fluorinated aliphatic diamine is expected to be much less carcinogenic than aromatic diamines.

A histopathologic study conducted by implanting the adhesive in the subcutaneous and hepatic tissues for up to 20 months revealed that there were neither carcinogenic episodes nor tissue abnormalities. The cured polyurethane adhesive implanted subcutaneously was completely resorbed within 6 months. Although significant amounts of cured adhesive were biodegraded when applied to hepatic tissues, some remained even 20 months postimplantation. Based on the structure-carcinogenic potential relationship of diisocyanates, Matsuda et al. concluded that the FHMDI-based adhesive is noncarcinogenic, despite a high nucleophilic reactivity of FHMDI, and is one of the most reliable adhesives.[46]

The FHMDI-based adhesive was applied to tracheal anastomosis of dogs and the result was compared with that of conventional suture.[47] A half of the end-to-end anastomotic line was sutured by 3-0 absorbable polydioxanone or polyglactin, while the other half was adhered with the FHMDI adhesive. The result is summarized in Figure 11.25. One week after surgery, the cilia of the ciliated cells degenerated and disappeared from an extensive area of the sutured side, while the cilia were kept intact near the anastomotic line on the side where the adhesive was applied. Eight weeks after surgery, epithelialization was complete on both sides but regeneration of the cilia was still incomplete on the sutured side when compared with the side glued with the FHMDI adhesive. The infiltration of inflammatory cells was also less marked on the side treated with the adhesive. The polyurethane tissue adhesive was concluded to facilitate epithelialization and regeneration of cilia from the regenerated cells in tracheal anastomosis, due to a reduction in both foreign body reaction and mechanical damage.

2. Polyurethane from Biodegradable Polyester Diol

EG-PG copolymers are not readily biodegradable, but it is possible to synthesize biodegradable oligomeric diols which are a component of the polyurethane prepolymer. For this purpose, Kobayashi et al.

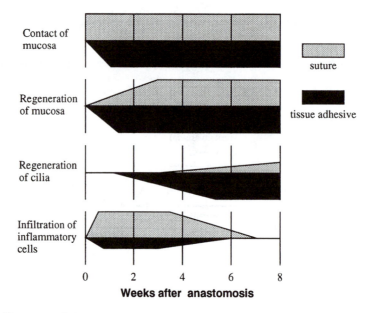

Figure 11.25 Ultrastructural changes at the site of tracheal anastomosis using either biodegradable suture or the reactive urethane prepolymer (PUP201).

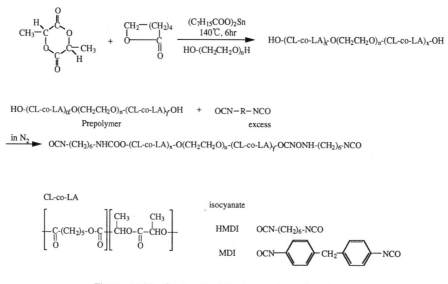

Figure 11.26 Synthesis of biodegradable polyurethane.

first synthesized D,L-lactide oligomer (PLA) or D,L-lactide-ε-caprolactone (50:50) copolymer [P(CL-co-LA)] using EG or poly(ethylene glycol) (PEG) as initiator to obtain hydroxy-terminated biodegradable polyesters.[48] Then, the polyesters were allowed to react with an excess of diisocyanate such as HMDI, toluene diisocyanate (TDI), and diphenylmethane diisocyanate (MDT) to introduce a reactive isocyanate group to both ends of the polyester. Figure 11.26 shows the synthetic route of these prepolymers. The isocyanate-capped prepolymers were curable in the presence of water.

The set time and mechanical appearance of the cured polymers are given in Table 11.10. The set time of the isocyanate-capped prepolymers is too long to be useful as a tissue adhesive, especially when

Table 11.10 Set Time and Mechanical Characteristics
of Cured Polymers

Prepolymer	Set Time	Property of Cured Polymer
EG-PLA500:HMDI	20–30 h	Brittle
EG-PLA500:TDI	2–3 h	Hard and brittle
EG-PLA500:MDI	2–3 h	Hard and brittle
EG-PLA1200:HMDI	20–30 h	Hard
PCL800:HMDI	12 h	Very soft
PCL800:TDI	2–4 h	Very soft
PCL1200:HMDI	12 h	Very soft
EG-P(CL-co-LA)1300:HMDI	25 h	Flexible
PEG400-P(CL-co-LA)2000		
HMDI	2 h	Soft
TDI	30–60 min	Flexible and strong
MDI	30–60 min	Flexible and strong
PEG1000-PLA2400		
TDI	20–30 min	Flexible
MDI	20–30 min	Flexible
PEG1000-P(CL-co-LA)2400:MDI	10–20 min	Flexible

Note: Curing condition: 2 g of prepolymer was mixed with 0.52 ml of water
and cured at 25°C under 60% relative humidity.

HMDI with low reactivity was used to introduce the terminal isocyanate group. However, the set time could be shortened when oligomeric diols, before capping, were mixed with diisocyanates *in situ*, as shown in Table 11.10.

The *in vitro* weight loss of the cured prepolymers as a function of hydrolysis time is given in Figure 11.27. The cured polymers having relatively high PEG contents became very brittle and were broken to small pieces after 3 weeks hydrolysis. Hydrolytic degradation of the cured polymers was accelerated as the PEG content increased. A study of the *in vivo* degradation of the cured PEG 400-P(CL-co-LA) 2000:MDI showed that the *in vivo* degradation rate was almost the same as, or slightly more enhanced than, the *in vitro* degradation. An acute inflammatory reaction was followed up to 2 weeks. Marked neovascularization was noticed around the implant at 1 week. After 4 weeks, the implant was encapsulated by tight collagen fibers and the inflammatory cells almost disappeared at 8 weeks. After 16 weeks, the implant was degraded to small pieces. When the degradation reaction proceeded to an appreciable extent, inflammatory cells appeared again and neovascularization was observed around the material pieces. After 12 months, the implanted materials could not be found anywhere in the tissue and no adverse tissue reactions, such as scar formation, were observed.

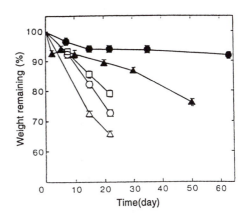

Figure 11.27 *In vivo* weight loss of various biodegradable polyurethanes as a function of hydrolysis time. (●) EG-P(CL-co-LA) 2400: MDI ([PEG] = 3 wt%); (▲) PEG400-P(CL-co-LA) 2000: MDI ([PEG] = 20 wt%); (□) PEG1000-P(CL-co-LA) 4000: MDI ([PEG] = 25 wt%); (○) PEG400-P(CL-co-LA) 1350: MDI ([PEG] = 30 wt%); (△) PEG1000-P(CL-co-LA) 2600: MDI ([PEG] = 38 wt%).

VI. SUMMARY

The currently available tissue adhesives have limited clinical applications because of the lack of favorable characteristics of an ideal tissue adhesive. An ideal tissue adhesive should cure rapidly *in situ*, generate strong bonding to a variety of tissues, and be gradually biodegradable in tissues without yielding toxic by-products. Synthetic cyanoacrylates have been used in surgery, although the cured polymers with short side chains release formaldehyde upon nonenzymatic hydrolysis in tissues, inciting acute inflammation. It is reported that butyl-2-cyanoacrylate appears to be safer when used for skin closure, although the polymer should not be allowed to infiltrate below the level of the skin, where it can contact vascularized tissues and incite a chronic foreign body giant cell reaction.[49] The cyanoacrylate tissue adhesive has also been tried in contaminated lacerations. On the other hand, fibrin glue has been more widely applied in surgery than cyanoacrylates, not only as tissue adhesive but also as hemostatic agent and sealant, although the bonding strength of fibrin glue is not sufficiently high for a secure closure. The hemostatic effect (in terms of blood loss) of fibrin glue is not significantly different between the areas treated with thrombin/fibrin glue and the areas treated with thrombin and placebo.[50]

The main reason for the slow progress in developing new tissue adhesives is the technical difficulty that tissue adhesives should be nontoxic and rapidly cured at 37°C in the presence of moisture under atmospheric pressure and, in addition, the cured adhesives should disappear from the tissues after wound healing without releasing any toxic biodegradation products. If the biodegradation of cured adhesives is too slow, they may act as a barrier to revascularization and tissue healing. Thus, since tissue adhesives must satisfy so many clinical requirements, their development is much more difficult than that of adhesives used for nonsurgical purposes. It seems likely that attempts to develop better tissue adhesives will be maintained despite these difficulties because of the continuing high demand from surgeons for good tissue adhesives.[1, 1a] Current rapid progress in biomedical engineering may introduce new tissue adhesives that incorporate novel growth factors to enhance healing in compromised wounds.

REFERENCES

1. Matsumoto, T., *Tissue Adhesives in Surgery*, Medical Examination Publishers, New York, 1972.
1a. Sierra, D. and Saltz, R., Eds., *Surgical Adhesives and Sealants,* Technomic Publishing Co., Inc., Lancaster-Basel, 1996.
2. Young, J.Z. and Medawar, P.B., Fibrin suture of peripheral nerves, *Lancet*, 2, 126, 1940.
3. Blombäck, B. and Blombäck, M., Purification of human and bovine fibrinogen, *Ark. Kemi*, 10, 415, 1956.
4. Matras, H., Dinges, H.P., Mamoli, B., and Lassman, H., Nonsutured nerve transplantation, *J. Maxillofac. Surg.*, 1, 37, 1973.
5. Kaetsu, H., Matsui, H., Tagawa, R., Shigaki, T., Goto, A., Iwanaga, N., Honda, M., Utsunomiya, F., Yamada, S., and Funatsu, A., Adhesive, hemostatic, and wound healing effect of Bolheal (HG-4), *Clin. Rep.*, 23, 3781, 1989 (in Japanese).
6. Matsui, H., Shigaki, T., Kaetsu, H., Utsunomiya, F., Iwanaga, N., Tagawa, R., Rikihisa, T., Nakagaki, T., Funatsu, A., and Yamada, S., Studies on absorption, distribution, and excretion of Bolheal (HG-4), *Clin. Rep.*, 23, 3775, 1989 (in Japanese).
7. Seifert, J., Klause, N., Stobbe, J., and Egbers, H.J., Antibodies formed against fibrin glue components and their circulatory relevance, *J. Invest. Surg.*, 7, 167, 1994.
8. Banninger, H., Hardegger, T., Tobler, A., Barth, A., Schupbach, P., Reinhart, W., Lammle, B., and Furlan, M., Fibrin glue in surgery: frequent development of inhibitors of bovine thrombin and human factor V, *Br. J. Haematol.*, 85, 528, 1993.
9. McKay, T.C., Albala, D.M., Gehrin, B.E., and Castelli, M., Laparoscopic ureteral reanastomosis using fibrin glue, *J. Urol.*, 152, 1637, 1994.
10. Seguin, J.R., Picard, E., Frapier, J.M., and Chaptal, P.A., Aortic valve repair with fibrin glue for type A acute aortic dissection, *Ann. Thorac. Surg.*, 58, 304, 1994.
11. Mester, U., Zuch, M., and Rauber, M., Astigmatism after phacoemulsification with posterior chamber lens implantation: small incision technique with fibrin adhesive for wound closure, *J. Cataract Refract. Surg.*, 19, 616, 1993.
12. Fasol, R., Schumacher, B., Schlaudraft, K., Hauenstein, K.H., and Seitelberger, R., Experimental use of a modified fibrin glue to induce site-directed angiogenesis from the aorta to the heart, *J. Thorac. Cardiovasc. Surg.*, 107, 1432, 1994.
13. Sheppard, B.B., De Virgilio, C., Bleiweis, Milliken, J.C., and Robertson, J.M., Inhibition of intra-abdominal adhesions: fibrin glue in a long term model, *Am. Surg.*, 59, 786, 1993.
14. Park, M.S. and Cha, C.I., Biochemical aspects of autologous fibrin glue derived from ammonium sulfate precipitation, *Laryngoscope*, 103, 193, 1993.
15. Tawes, R.L., Jr., Sydorak, G.R., and Du Vall, T.B., Autologous fibrin glue: the last step in operative hemostasis, *Am. J. Surg.*, 168, 120, 1994.

16. Wadstrom, J. and Wik, O., Fibrin glue (Tisseel) added with sodium hyaluronate in microvascular anastomosing, *Scand. J. Plast. Reconstr. Surg. Hand Surg.*, 27, 257, 1993.
17. Coover, H.W., Cyanoacrylate adhesives, a day of serendipity, a decade of hard work, *ACS Org. Coat. Appl. Polym. Sci. Proc.*, 48, 243, 1983.
18. Tseng, Y.C., Hyon, S.H., and Ikada, Y., Modification of synthesis and investigation of properties for 2-cyanoacrylates, *Biomaterials*, 11, 73, 1990.
19. Leonard, F., Kulkarni, R.K., Brandes, G., Nelson, J., and Cameron, J.J., Synthesis and degradation of poly(alkyl α-cyanoacrylates), *J. Appl. Polym. Sci.*, 10, 259, 1966.
20. Vezin, W.R. and Florence, A.T., In vitro heterogeneous degradation of poly(n-alkyl α-cyanoacrylates), *J. Biomed. Mater. Res.*, 14, 93, 1980.
21. Tseng, Y.C., Tabata, Y., Hyon, S.H., and Ikada, Y., In vitro toxicity test of 2-cyanoacrylate polymers by cell culture method, *J. Biomed. Mater. Res.*, 24, 1355, 1990.
22. Ciapetti, G., Stea, S., Cenni, E., Sudanese, A., Marraro, D., Toni, A., and Pizzoferrato, A., Cytotoxicity testing of cyanoacrylates using direct contact assay on cell cultures, *Biomaterials*, 15, 63, 1994.
23. Refojo, M. F., Dohlman, C. H., and Koliopoulos, J., Adhesives in ophthalmology: a review, *Surv. Ophthalmol.*, 15(4), 217, 1971.
24. Tseng, Y.C., Hyon, S.H., Ikada, Y., Shimizu, Y., Tamura, K., and Hitomi, S., In vivo evaluation of 2-cyanoacrylates as surgical adhesives, *J. Appl. Biomater.*, 1, 111, 1990.
25. Vanholder, R., Misstem, A., Roels, H., and Matton, G., Cyanoacrylate tissue adhesive for closing skin wounds: a double blind randomized comparison with suture, *Biomaterials*, 14, 737, 1993.
26. Caballero-Gómez, J.M. and Ortega-Moreno, J., Anastomosis of uterine serosa with cyanoacrylate versus suture in rats, *Acta Obstet. Gynecol. Scand.*, 72, 210, 1993.
27. Quillen, D.A. and Rosenwasser, G.O., Aerosol application of cyanoacrylate adhesive, *J. Refract. Corneal Surg.*, 10, 149, 1994.
28. Leahey, A.B., Gottsch, J.D., and Stark, W.J., Clinical experience with *N*-butyl cyanoacrylate (Nexacryl) tissue adhesive, *Ophthalmology*, 100, 173, 1993.
29. Sabanathan, S., Eng., J., and Richardson, J., The use of tissue adhesive in pulmonary resections, *Eur. J. Cardiothorac. Surg.*, 7, 657, 1993.
30. Eiferman, R.A. and Snyder, J.W., Antibacterial effect of cyanoacrylate glue, *Arch. Ophthalmol.*, 101, 958, 1983.
31. Noordzij, J.P., Foresman, P.A., Rodeheaver, G.T., Quinn, J.V., and Edlich, R.F., Tissue adhesive wound repair revisited, *J. Emerg. Med.*, 12(5), 645, 1994.
32. Howell, J.M., Bresnahan, K.A. et al., Comparison of effects of suture and cyanoacrylate tissue adhesive on bacterial counts in contaminated lacerations, *Antimicrob. Chemother.*, 39, 559, 1995.
33. Olson, M.E., Ruseska, I., and Costerton, J.W., Colonization of n-butyl-2-cyanoacrylate tissue adhesive by *Staphylococcus epidermidis*, *J. Biomed. Mater. Res.*, 22(6), 485, 1988.
34. Matthews, S.C., Tissue bonding: the bacteriological properties of a commercially-available cyanoacrylate adhesive, *Br. J. Biomed. Sci.*, 50, 17, 1993.
35. Tseng, Y.C., Hyon, S.H., and Ikada, Y., Physical modification of α-cyanoacrylate for application as surgical adhesives, in *Progress in Biomedical Polymers*, Gebelein, C.G. and Dunn, R.L., Eds., Plenum Press, New York, 1990, 53.
36. Tatooles, C.J. and Braunwald, N.S., The use of crosslinked gelatin as a tissue adhesive to control hemorrhage from liver and kidney, *Surgery*, 60, 857, 1966.
37. Braunwald, N.S., Gay, W., and Tatooles, C.J., Evaluation of crosslinked gelatin as a tissue adhesive and hemostatic agent: an experimental study, *Surgery*, 59, 1024, 1966.
38. Cooper, C.W. and Falb, R.D., Surgical adhesive, *Ann. NY Acad. Sci.*, 146, 224, 1968.
39. Stassano, P., Rispo, G., Losi, M., Caputo, M., and Spampinato, N., Annular abscesses and GRF glue, *J. Cardiovasc. Surg.*, 9, 357, 1994.
40. Bellotto, F., Johnson, R.G., Weintraub, R.M., Foley, J., and Thuser, R.L., Pneumostasis of injured lung in rabbits with gelatin-resorcinol formaldehyde-glutaraldehyde tissue adhesive, *Surg. Gynecol. Obstet.*, 174, 221, 1992.
41. Ennker, J., Ennker, I.C., Schoon, D., Schoon, H.A., Dorge, S., Meissler, J., Rimpler, M., and Helzer, R., The impact of gelatin-resorcinol glue on aortic tissue: a histomorphologic evaluation, *J. Vasc. Surg.*, 20, 34, 1994.
42. Albes, J.M., Krattek, C., Hausen, B., Rohde, R., Haverich, A., and Borst, H.G., Biophysical properties of the gelatin-resorcin-formaldehyde/glutaraldehyde adhesive, *Ann. Thorac. Surg.*, 46, 910, 1993.
43. Uemura, K., Miyagawa, T., and Sakamoto, I., Basic research for hemostatic agent, *J. Jpn. Soc. Biomater.*, 9, 56, 1991 (in Japanese).
44. Nakajima, N. and Ikada, Y., Mechanism of amide formation by carbodiimide for bioconjugation in aqueous media, *Bioconj. Chem.*, 6, 123, 1995.
45. Otani, Y., Tabata, Y., and Ikada, Y., A new biological glue from gelatin and poly(L-glutamic acid), *J. Biomed. Mater. Res.*, 31, 157, 1996.
46. Matsuda, T., Nakajima, N., Itoh, T., and Takakura, T., Development of a compliant surgical adhesive derived from novel fluorinated hexamethylene diisocyanate, *ASAIO Trans.*, 35, 381, 1989.
47. Fujino, S., Yamashita, N., Yamamoto, A., Asakura, S., Kato. H., and Mori, A., Tracheal anastomosis with a newly-developed tissue adhesive (PUP 201) in dogs: ultrastructural changes at the anastomotic site, *J. Clin. Electron Microscopy*, 24, 321, 1991.

48. Kobayashi, H., Hyon, S.H., and Ikada, Y., Water-curable and biodegradable prepolymers, *J. Biomed. Mater. Res.*, 25, 1481, 1991.

49. Toriumi, D.M., Raslan, W.F., Friedman, M., and Tardy, M.E., Variable histotoxicity of Histoacryl when used in a subcutaneous site: an experimental study, *Laryngoscope*, 101, 339, 1991.

50. Achauer, B.M., Miller, S.R., and Lee, T.E., The hemostatic effect of fibrin glue on graft donor sites, *J. Burn Case Rehabil.*, 15, 24, 1994.

Chapter 12

New Emerging and Experimental Materials for Wound Closure

C.C. Chu

CONTENTS

Recently, several polymeric and nonpolymeric materials have been tried as potential wound closure biomaterials, particularly as suture materials and tissue adhesives with a variety of objectives. These include (1) a strong need to curtail wound infection, particularly in contaminated cases (e.g., perforated appendicitis), (2) the ability to accelerate wound healing, particularly in healing-impaired clinic conditions, and (3) the desire for better mechanical properties and tissue biocompatibility. Although a few of these new materials have been tried and marketed outside the U.S., most of these biomaterials are still in their early development stage and their ultimate fate as wound closure biomaterials is still unknown. In this chapter, we summarize the current status of these emerging and/or experimental biomaterials for potential wound closure use.

I. ANTIMICROBIAL SUTURES

A. THE NEED TO CONTROL WOUND INFECTION

Wound infection is considered to be one of the oldest and most common complications in all injuries and every branch of surgery. The incidence of wound infection in this country ranges from 3% to 12%, with an average of 8%.[1] Despite many recent advances in surgical technique and medicine, such as new antibiotics and the alteration of the host immune system, the rate of wound infection has not changed significantly in recent years.[2] Wound infection often results in additional physiological, psychological, and economic burdens to patients as well as their families. Depending on the type of surgery and severity of infection, surgical infection has been reported to result in an average 7.4 additional d of hospitalization, with a range of up to 68 additional d.[3] Average additional expenses were $839, with a range of $0 to $7,900. When other factors, such as the patient's loss of productivity, compensation payments, the cost of implants, and current soaring health care expenses are taken into account, the total cost of wound infection is expected to be even higher.[4]

The development of wound infection depends on several factors, such as the degree of microbial contamination, host resistance, the nature of the wound, the type of surgery, and the presence of foreign materials. Foreign materials such as prosthetic devices have become increasingly important in wound infection because of their more frequent use in modern medicine.[5] The presence of foreign materials in a wound has been known to significantly enhance the propensity of surrounding tissues to infection. Suture materials are probably the most important biomaterials in wound infection because they are the most frequently used in surgery and because most wound infection begins along or near the suture lines. Thus, suture materials may contribute greatly to the genesis of surgical infections by lowering the clinical dose of a microorganism that is needed to cause wound infection. The role of suture materials in wound infection has already been discussed in Chapter 8 and will not be repeated here.

Although it is standard practice for surgeons not to use sutures to close wounds that are known to be heavily contaminated, most surgical wounds have some degree of microbial contamination which may or may not develop into clinically evident wound infection, depending on the degree of host resistance, the bacterial concentration, and its virulence.[6,7] The use of antimicrobial sutures could provide an extra degree of protection in clean or clean-contaminated wounds, particularly those associated with surgical implants. In addition, instead of healing by second intention, antimicrobial sutures may be useful for early secondary closure of incisional abscesses after adequate wound drainage to reduce healing time without complications.[8] Antimicrobial sutures may also be valuable in traumatic wounds like lacerations in automobile accidents, high-risk surgery like cardiovascular and orthopedic operations, frequently contaminated wound sites such as the colon, and in patients whose resistance has been compromised by diseases such as cancer, AIDS, diabetes, or hemorrhagic shock, or in elderly or newborn patients, organ transplantation, or chemotherapy.

B. CURRENT APPROACHES TO THE DEVELOPMENT OF ANTIMICROBIAL SUTURES

Basically, several approaches to the development of antimicrobial sutures have been reported in the literature. They are (1) the incorporation of silver metal on the surface of sutures or other biomaterials with or without electrically stimulated release of silver ions;[9–12] (2) the incorporation of conventional antibiotics, such as neomycin palmitate, penicillin, sulfonamide, quaternary ammonium complexes, chlorhexidine, and iodine, onto the surface of sutures;[6,13–20] (3) the incorporation of antibiotics into the interior (matrix type of drug delivery) of sutures through the mixing of antibiotics with suture polymers before spinning into suture fibers.[21,22] Each approach is described in the following sections.

1. Silver Metal-Coated Antimicrobial Suture (SAS)

A different approach to the control of wound infection around the vicinity of suture lines has been reported.[9,10] In these studies, Chu et al. examined the antimicrobial property of a new direct current-activated, silver metal-coated nylon 6,6 suture *in vitro*. It was found that a weak direct current (less than 400 μA) could significantly enhance the biocidal property of the new SAS against seven types of bacterial species.

The use of silver in both compound and elemental form for the treatment of wound infection has been known for centuries.[23] Recent typical examples are the use of silver sulfadiazine as a topical treatment for burns,[24–33] the silver-incorporated Gore-Tex® vascular graft for the control of prosthetic bacterial infection,[11,34] the silver anode treatment of chronic osteomyelitis,[12] and the silver-coated catheter tubes for reducing catheter-induced infections.[35–46]

The electrochemical features of direct current-activated silver and its results in animal trials and clinical cases were originally reported and recently reviewed by Spadaro.[47] Spadaro et al. have shown that silver is bacteriostatic when used as an anode with an extremely weak electric current.[48] Quantitative studies showed that most of this inhibition takes place in a few hours. Silver also exhibited fungicidal properties at concentrations as low as 1.9 μg/ml and its inhibitory and fungicidal concentrations are lower than those reported for other silver compounds.[49] Silver has also been incorporated in bone cement composites.[50] Even with the wide use of broad-spectrum antibiotics, effective control of osteomyelitis

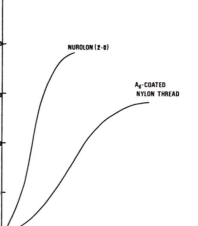

Figure 12.1 Stress and strain curves of both silver-coated antimicrobial nylon suture and commercial 2-0 Nurolon suture. (From Chu, C.C. et al., *J. Biomed. Mater. Res.*, 21, 1281, 1987. With permission.)

has not been consistent. However, Becker and Spadaro[51] and Webster et al.[12] used electrically generated silver ions to treat chronic osteomyelitis and controlled the infection in 80% (12 out of 15 patients)[51] and 64% (10 out of 15 patients).[12] Silver ions, because of their small size, are thought to be able to penetrate many tissues to some extent, particularly those that are poorly vascularized.

Several bacterial species, like *Escherichia coli*, *Staphylococcus aureus*, and *Pseudomonas aeruginosa* have been found to have minimum inhibitory and bactericidal concentrations for silver ions 10 to 100 times lower than antibiotics in current use[52] and bacterial resistance to the silver ion is rare.[53] Falcone and Spadaro have examined the inhibitory effect of an electrically activated, silver-coated fabric on six bacteria commonly found in cutaneous wounds.[54] Their results confirm previously reported effective diffusion of the silver ions and their local antibacterial action. Effectiveness of electrically activated silver in reducing bacterial colonization at a percutaneous implant in rats has also been examined.[55] A marked reduction or elimination of *S. aureus* was observed near the interface by intermittent electrical activation of the percutaneous silver implants.

The use of silver as a component of a suture for wound infection control was first reported by Chu et al.[9,10] They used silver metal-coated, multifilament nylon 6,6 yarns (obtained from Saquoit Industries, Inc., Scranton, PA) as antimicrobial sutures and examined their potential as antimicrobial wound closure biomaterials. The yarns were 129 denier and braided into size 2–0 sutures. The suture had a braid structure of 2/2, which indicated that each strand of yarn over- and under-passed two other strands. This braid structure is identical to commercially available nylon sutures (i.e., Nurolon® from Ethicon, Inc., Somerville, NJ). It was considered significant to develop an antimicrobial suture with a braid structure because braided sutures are more prone to wound infection than monofilament sutures. This 2–0 size synthetic absorbable suture (SAS) had a denier of 1278. (Denier is defined as the weight in grams per 9000 meters.) Its tensile strength (2.8 g per denier) was comparable to 2–0 size silk sutures, but is slightly lower than 2–0 size Nurolon suture (Figure 12.1). Characterization of this SAS by energy-dispersive spectrometer (EDS) X-ray elemental analysis indicated that metallic silver of 2 to 5 μm thickness was chemically bonded into the nylon substrate, and the characteristic Ag element peak at 3.0 KeV energy is evident. To identify further where the silver was located in the SAS, area maps of silver element distributions by EDS X-ray analysis along the longitudinal and cross-sectional directions of the SAS were studied (Figure 12.2). The metallic silver was found to be uniformly distributed on the surface of each nylon fiber within the SAS. The concentration of the metallic silver was about 320 μg Ag per centimeter length of the SAS. The 2–0 suture was electrically conductive with only 3 ohm resistance per 5 cm of SAS length.

The *in vitro* antibacterial properties of the SAS were evaluated qualitatively by the width and sterility of the clear zone in the bacterial culture plates,[9] and quantitatively by standard plate count methods.[10] Seven species of bacteria were tested: *Staphylococcus aureus*, *Escherichia coli*, *Pseudomonas aeruginosa*, *Klebsiella pneumonia*, *Shigella dysenteriae*, *Serratia marcescens*, and *Proteus mirabilis*. A weak direct current ranging from 0.4 to 400 μA was applied to the suture specimens to examine whether the

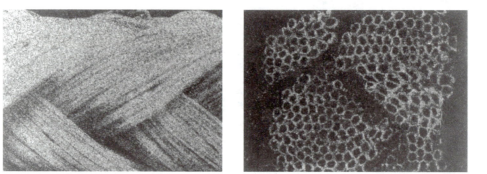

Figure 12.2 EDS area mapping of silver element for the silver metal-coated antimicrobial nylon suture. (Left) longitudinal view; (right) cross-sectional view.

biocidal property of the SAS could be enhanced by an anodic microcurrent. The commercial 2–0 Nurolon suture from Ethicon served as the control.

As summarized in Table 12.1, the SAS exhibited moderate to very good bactericidal activity toward these seven bacterial species. *P. aeruginosa* was the most sensitive, while *P. mirabilis* was the least sensitive. The observed width of the clear zone was further confirmed by the degree of sterility of the clear zone. In general, all stab tests in the clear region showed sterility when the width of a clear zone was greater than 2.0 mm. Application of direct current through the SAS specimens positively enhanced their antimicrobial properties, and the degree of enhancement depended on the direct current level, bacterial type, mode of current application, and the electrical polarity (anodic or cathodic polarization). pH measurement of the clear zone indicated that the observed clear zone in the bacterial culture plates was due solely to the antibacterial property of the SAS because of the observed constant pH (7.5). Figures 12.3 and 12.4 illustrate the observed clear zone in bacterial culture plates under various conditions.

An increasing current level was found to always increase the width of the clear zone, with *P. aeruginosa* the most sensitive. The ability to adjust the strength of the antimicrobial property would be very useful clinically because the SAS can be tailored to specific clinical conditions (heavily vs. lightly contaminated wounds) simply by either enlarging (increasing current level) or reducing (decreasing current level) its antimicrobial strength. It is interesting to note that SAS without any current application also exhibited some antimicrobial properties but at a significantly lower level.

The SAS also exhibited an antimicrobial activity toward well-established bacterial colonies, but the effect was less strong than when direct current was applied simultaneously with incubation. For example, the width of the clear zone at the anode site for *P. aeruginosa* was reduced from 7.5 mm to 2.5 mm when a direct current of 0.4 μA was applied 24 h after the bacterial colonies were established. These findings are believed to be clinically important because the risk of wound infection is directly proportional to the dose of contaminating bacteria and their virulence, but inversely proportional to the resistance of the host.[7] The observed antimicrobial property of the SAS toward well-established bacterial colonies may make SAS a useful tool to confine contaminated wounds.

Another interesting phenomenon associated with this observation was that the antimicrobial activity of the SAS toward 24 h well-established colonies was found at both anode and cathode sites instead of only at the anode site when direct current was applied simultaneously with incubation for 24 h. This finding suggests that elemental Ag itself has antimicrobial properties too, but its strength is weaker than Ag+ ions and is limited to the area immediately adjacent to the suture. Thus, only those bacteria adhered to the SAS would not survive.

As mentioned briefly before, the antimicrobial property of the SAS under the condition where direct current was applied simultaneously with incubation was observed only at the anode site (Figures 12.3 and 12.4). This unique finding suggests that the oxidation process of silver metal at the anode site under the influence of an electrical force must relate either directly or indirectly to the observed antimicrobial activity of the SAS. It is known that Ag+ ions would be released into the medium at the anode site (oxidation) and converted into Ag at the cathode site (reduction) as shown below:

$$Ag \rightarrow Ag^{+1} + e^{-1} \text{ (anode)}$$

$$Ag^{+1} + e^{-1} \rightarrow Ag \text{ (cathode)}$$

Table 12.1 Effects of the Mode of Direct Current Applied on the *In Vitro* Antibacterial Capability of Silver-Coated Nylon Braid Threads

Anti-Bacterial Performance	Width of Clear Zone in Culture Plate (mm, ± 0.5)								Sterility of Clear Zone in Culture Plate[a] (± 0.5)							
	Anode				Cathode				Anode				Cathode			
	24h		48h		24h		48h		24h		48h		24h		48h	
Bacterial Type and Current Level	X	Y	X	Y	X	Y	X	Y	X	Y	X	Y	X	Y	X	Y
Escherichia coli																
0.4 µA	3.2	2.0	4.0	2.0	0	1.6	0	2.0	IV	IV	IV	III	I	III	I	III
4.0 µA	3.5	2.0	5.0	2.0	0	2.0	0	2.2	IV	III	IV	III	I	III	I	IV
40 µA	4.1	2.4	6.0	2.0	0	1.0	0	1.6	IV	IV	IV	III	I	II	I	III
400 µA	5.0	2.5	6.2	2.8	0	0	0	2.4	IV	IV	IV	IV	I	I	I	IV
Pseudomonas aeruginosa																
0.4 µA	7.5	2.5	8.0	3.0	0	3.1	0	3.0	IV	IV	IV	IV	I	IV	I	IV
4.0 µA	8.1	2.0	9.5	3.0	0	2.8	0	2.5	IV	IV	IV	IV	I	IV	I	IV
40 µA	9.1	3.2	9.5	3.0	0	3.9	0	2.5	IV	IV	IV	IV	I	IV	I	IV
400 µA	10	4.1	9.5	4.7	0	4.1	0	4.1	IV	IV	IV	IV	I	IV	I	IV
Staphylococcus aureus																
0.4 µA	5.6	2.5	6.4	3.0	0	2.8	0	3.5	IV	IV	IV	IV	I	IV	I	IV
4.0 µA	7.0	2.7	7.0	3.0	0	2.3	0	2.8	IV	IV	IV	IV	I	IV	I	IV
40 µA	7.1	3.0	7.1	3.0	0	3.0	0	3.0	IV	IV	IV	IV	I	IV	I	IV
400 µA	8.0	3.1	8.0	3.1	0	3.0	0	3.0	IV	IV	IV	IV	I	IV	I	IV
Shigella dysenteriae																
0.4 µA	6.0	1.8	5.6	1.0	0	1.5	0	1.5	IV	IV	IV	II	I	III	I	III
4.0 µA	6.0	2.0	6.1	1.5	0	1.7	0	1.5	IV	IV	IV	III	I	III	I	III
40 µA	6.9	2.0	6.3	2.0	0	2.0	0	1.2	IV	IV	IV	IV	I	IV	I	II
400 µA	7.0	2.0	6.5	2.0	0	2.0	0	2.0	IV	IV	IV	IV	I	IV	I	IV
Serratia marcescens																
0.4 µA	4.5	1.1	4.0	2.1	0	1.9	0	1.4	IV	II	IV	IV	I	IV	I	III
4.0 µA	4.8	1.5	4.9	2.0	0	1.3	0	1.8	IV	III	IV	IV	I	II	I	IV
40 µA	5.0	1.8	5.3	2.0	0	1.9	0	2.1	IV	IV	IV	IV	I	IV	I	IV
400 µA	5.1	1.8	5.6	2.1	0	1.2	0	2.0	IV	IV	IV	IV	I	II	I	IV

[a] Determined by subculture tests. I, no antibacterial (all 3 stab tests nonsterile); II, slight antibacterial (1/3 of stab tests sterile); III, medium antibacterial (2/3 of stab tests sterile); IV, strong antibacterial (all 3 stab tests sterile). X, direct current applied simultaneously during incubation; Y, direct current applied after 24 h of incubation without current.

From Chu, C.C. et. al., *J. Biomed. Mater. Res.*, 21(11), 1281, 1987. With permission.

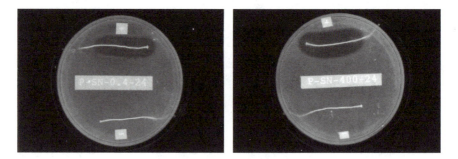

Figure 12.3 The effect of the magnitude of direct current on the antimicrobial activity of silver metal-coated antimicrobial nylon suture. The suture was impregnated with *P. aeruginosa*. (Left) 0.4 μA/24 h incubation. (Right) 400 μA/24 h incubation. (From Chu, C.C. et al., *J. Biomed. Mater. Res.*, 21, 1281, 1987. With permission.)

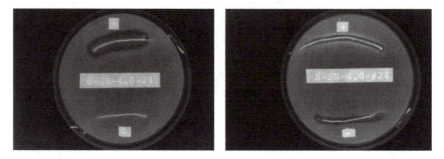

Figure 12.4 The effect of different modes of direct current application on the antimicrobial activity of silver-coated antimicrobial nylon suture. The suture was impregnated with *S. aureus*. (Left) 4.0 μA applied simultaneously with incubation for 24 h; (Right) 4.0 μA applied after the bacterial culture plate had been incubated for 24 h. (From Chu, C.C. et al., *J. Biomed. Mater. Res.*, 21, 1281, 1987. With permission.)

Because antimicrobial activity of the SAS was observed at the anode site when a direct current was applied, Ag⁺ ions generated at the anode site must be taken up by the surrounding bacteria and subsequently kill them. Thus, the anode-related antimicrobial activity of the SAS indirectly suggests that the uptake of Ag⁺ by bacteria must be the first step in the mechanism of the observed antimicrobial property of the SAS. Recent studies on the mechanism of bacterial sensitivity to silver indicated that the amount of silver uptake by bacteria is proportional to their sensitivity level toward silver.[56–61] For example, Kaur and Vadehra found that uptake of silver by a susceptible *K. pneumoniae* strain was three to four times higher than an experimentally derived silver-resistant *K. pneumoniae*.[56] Starodub and Trevors also reported that by energy dispersive X-ray analysis and transmission electromicroscopy, silver-sensitive *E. coli* contained dense silver particles inside their cells.[57] An Ag⁺-resistant strain, however, did not accumulate Ag ions.[57] Similar results have also been reported for other bacteria.[58–61]

The next questions to ask are how are Ag⁺ ions transported into the interior of cells, and how do the adsorbed Ag⁺ ions inside bacteria inhibit their metabolism? In order for cells to uptake any material from an environment, some type of specific transport system is required. Brierley et al. reported that accumulation of metals into bacterial cells usually occurs through a two-stage process.[62] The process involves (1) a rapid (in minutes), metabolic-independent surface binding to cells, followed by (2) a metabolic-dependent and gradual intracellular accumulation of the metal. Because Ag⁺ ions are not an essential nutrient, it is doubtful that their transport would go through a specific energy-dependent transport system; however, they could be carried into cells via a transport system for an essential metal. This hypothesized mechanism was supported by the study of silver resistance in *E. coli*.[57] It was reported that starved, washed resting cells of strain R1 *E. coli* were able to uptake Ag⁺ ions easily when assayed for Ag⁺ ions binding in a buffer lacking essential growth nutrients, but an actively growing *E. coli* of strain R1 (not washed, resting cells) could resist uptake of Ag⁺ ions. Ag⁺ ion uptake by bacteria could either interfere in their respiration or/and replication of DNA and hence exhibit antimicrobial activity.[63,64] In the former mechanism, AgNO₃ was

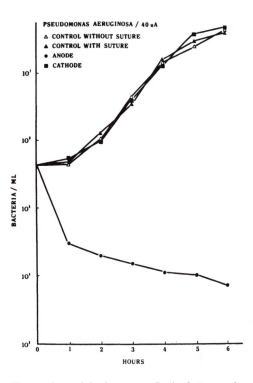

Figure 12.5 Standard plate counts of *P. aeruginosa* in the silver-coated antimicrobial nylon suture with a direct current of 40 μA. Two controls were without the suture and with the suture but with no direct current applied. (From Tsai, W.C. et al., *Surg. Gynecol. Obstet.*, 165, 207, 1987. With permission.)

found to inhibit an –SH-containing respiratory enzyme like succinate dehydrogenase. In the latter mechanism, Ag^+ ions were bound to bacterial DNA and interfered with its replication.

The qualitative antimicrobial properties of the SAS reported above was further confirmed in a later quantitative examination against *S. aureus, E. coli*, and *P. aeruginosa*, by Chu et al.[10] In that study, suture specimens of a fixed length were embedded in a custom-built plastic device filled with a fixed concentration of bacteria for predetermined periods of incubation. The bacterial suspension was then removed periodically for a standard plate count. The antibacterial property of the SAS was evident in the anode site of the suture fiber, and at a fixed current, the degree of bacteriostatic effect depended upon the bacterial species, as shown in Figures 12.5 and 12.6. For example, the *P. aeruginosa* was reduced to 7.5×10^4/ml, while the three controls (i.e., without suture, with a commercial nylon suture, Nurolon, and the cathode site of the SAS) all reached the same value of 4.5×10^7 over the same period. A reduction in the number of *P. aeruginosa* by a factor of 10^3 within a period of 6 h was observed. The data in Figure 12.5 also indicate that not only was growth of the initial *P. aeruginosa* inhibited, but also that the initial bacteria were killed over time. This excellent bactericidal property of the SAS toward *P. aeruginosa* is consistent with the previous qualitative antimicrobial data, and is clinically significant because this Gram-negative pathogen is frequently associated with wound infections resulting from severe skin damage, such as burns, and is resistant to many widely used antibiotics. Elimination of *S. aureus* and *E. coli* by SAS was not as dramatic as with *P. aeruginosa*. Bacteriostatic activity toward these two bacteria was not observed until about 3.5 h of direct current application (i.e., 40 μA).

The silver ion concentrations released from the SAS to the medium under various experimental conditions are shown in Figure 12.7. In general, the silver ion concentration increased with increasing current level or time, or both. The increase in Ag^+ ion concentration with time was much faster at a higher current level than at a lower current level. At the end of 6 h, the silver concentrations were 7.3 μg/ml at 0.4 μA and 305 μg/ml at 40.0 μA. It took 3 d for 0.4 μA to release an Ag^+ ion concentration that was achieved in only 3 h for 4.0 μA and less than 1 h for 40 μA.

A comparison between Figure 12.7 and Figures 12.5 and 12.6 indicates the different levels of bacterial sensitivity toward silver ion. As discussed before, Ag^+ ion uptake by bacteria was cell surface mediated.[61] The observed higher sensitivity of *S. aureus* toward Ag^+ ions than *E. coli* (as reflected in the lower Ag^+ ion concentration to achieve bacteriostatic effects in *S. aureus*) probably relates to the different cell surface structure and composition between *S. aureus* (Gram-positive) and *E. coli* (Gram-negative). Because Gram-positive bacteria do not have lipopolysaccharide-containing outer membranes, they are expected to be inherently more prone to the permeation and transport of Ag^+ ions released by SAS.

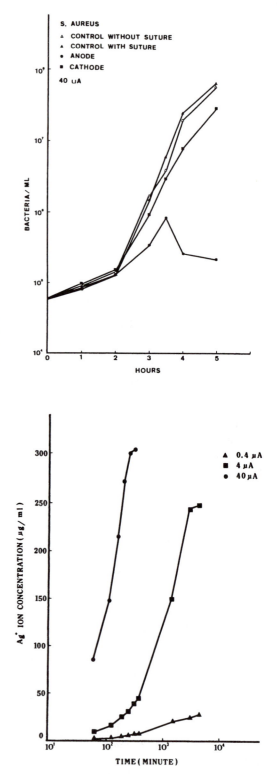

Figure 12.6 Standard plate counts of *S. aureus* in the silver-coated antimicrobial nylon suture with a direct current of 40 µA. Two controls were identical to those in Figure 12.5. (From Tsai, W.C. et al., *Surg. Gynecol. Obstet.*, 165, 207, 1987. With permission.)

Figure 12.7 The concentration of silver ions released from the SAS under a wide range of direct currents and times. (From Tsai, W.C. et al., *Surg. Gynecol. Obstet.*, 165, 207, 1987. With permission.)

A preliminary biocompatibility study of the SAS in rat gluteal muscle up to 60 d indicated that the total scores of histological evaluation of the SAS were always lower (less inflammatory response) than the control suture (Nurolon) up to 60 d postimplantation (Table 12.2).[9] Contrary to the findings in the control suture, the invasion of fibrous connective tissue into the interstitial space of the component yarns

Table 12.2 The Total Scores of Histologic Evaluation

Suture Material Implantation Period (d)	2/0 Nurolon (Control)	Ag-Coated Nylon Suture (Testing)
7	84	79.7 ± 1.2
14	—[a]	24.3 ± 3.1
30	36.3 ± 6.5	30.4 ± 2.5
60	32.7 ± 2.5	25.3 ± 0.6

[a] No score could be determined due to the difficulty of differentiating the cells in the slide.

From Chu, C.C. et al., *J. Biomed. Mater. Res.*, 21(11), 1281, 1987. With permission.

was not evident in the new SAS, even at the end of the study period (60 d). These results are parallel to the observed mild inflammatory reactions at silver implant sites in rats reported by Spadaro et al.[47,55]

In addition to the demonstrated antimicrobial property, the use of the electrically activated SAS in treating wound infection may also have one additional advantage — to improve the rate and quality of healing without infection. As reported by Becker,[65] a rapid and regenerative type of wound healing was found during the treatment of wound infection in humans by electrically activated silver. The production of many dedifferentiated (hence uncommitted) fibroblast cells in the wound under the influence of silver ions was suggested to be associated with the observed rapid healing rate. This preliminary finding is consistent with other studies which used endogenous and exogenous electric or magnetic fields to stimulate the healing rate of both soft and hard tissues, particularly the study reported by Dunn et al.[66] In that study, the effects of direct current on the healing of guinea pig dermal wounds were evaluated by using a collagen sponge model. Their preliminary data showed that fibroblast ingrowth and collagen fiber alignment were increased in the collagen sponge when it was stimulated with direct currents ranging from 20 to 100 µA through carbon electrodes. Similar results have also been found by Crisp and colleagues in their study of electrified metallic sutures in pigs.[67]

The data reported so far are from *in vitro* research. Does the SAS perform as well in animals and human beings as Chu et al. have demonstrated *in vitro*, and what are the mechanisms involved? To answer these questions and bring the concept of SAS closer to clinical reality, future animal implantation studies are essential to demonstrate the efficacy of the SAS *in vivo*. This may include the examination of other variables, such as (1) the performance of this SAS in deep intracorporeal sites, (2) the possibility of this SAS to directly improve the rate and quality of wound healing without infection, (3) the *in vivo* performance of this SAS in various types of knotted form, (4) the antimicrobial properties of the SAS in species whose immune response is compromised, and (5) a more thorough understanding of the underlying mechanism for the observed antimicrobial activity of the SAS.

It is desirable and beneficial to broaden the use of this SAS in intracorporeal sites, especially in sites having a history of above-average frequency of wound infection (e.g., intestine, wounds around surgical implants, deep-puncture wounds) to take full advantage of the antimicrobial property of the new SAS for wound infection control. The technical challenge of such a use will be the design of a noninvasive device to activate and enhance the antimicrobial capability of the new SAS in intracorporeal sites. As mentioned before, a rapid and regenerative type of wound healing was also reported by Becker during the treatment of wound infection in humans by electrically activated silver.[65] The increase in the rate of wound healing under the influence of silver compounds was also reported by Geronemus et al.[68] However, the role of silver and its compounds in the promotion of healing of cleaned wounds is not conclusive and controversy exists. For example, others reported that the presence of silver compounds as topical antimicrobial agents delayed wound healing.[69–71] Deitch et al. suggested that the toxicity of the topical antimicrobial agents of silver compounds (i.e., silver nitrate and silver sulfadiazine) is due to the anionic portion of the agent, like NO_3^-, not the silver ion.[72] Therefore, it will be beneficial to study the *in vivo* rate and quality of healing of the wounds treated with the new SAS.

In a quantitative biopsy culture assay of contaminated sutures in Swiss mice, Scher et al. reported that the number of *S. aureus* recovered from six throw-knotted sutures was higher than in unknotted ones.[73] This finding may suggest that tissues around a knotted suture could be more prone to wound infection than around an unknotted suture. Since all sutures are knotted in their clinical use, it is thus important to examine the *in vivo* antimicrobial performance of the new SAS in knotted form.

While it is known that the oxidation of metallic silver is an important part of the electrical silver activation mechanism, the activated surface under clinically appropriate conditions has not been characterized in detail. For example, serum proteins, which tend to decrease the persistence time of bacterial inhibitory effects, may bind to the surface and retard oxidation and precipitation of chlorides, or may affect subsequent dissolution rates and so influence effectiveness *in vivo*. Therefore, to characterize the sequence of surface morphological and chemical changes of the SAS as a function of current and time in various simulated physiological media, and to relate the microscopic surface characteristics of the SAS to bacterial inhibition observed *in vitro* and *in vivo* will provide investigators with a more complete understanding of the underlying antimicrobial mechanism of the SAS. Such an understanding is essential for possible future modification of the SAS, if needed, for specific clinical conditions.

In addition to reported use by Chu et al. of Ag-coated nylon sutures for wound infection control, Farrah and Erdos recently reported the use of silver salts-impregnated polyester suture (Ethibond®) to render it antimicrobial.[13] Ethibond sutures were modified by two different methods: adsorption of silver metals onto the suture surface pretreated either with manganese hydroxide [$Mn(NO_3)_2$ + NH_4OH] or sodium pyrophosphate [$Na_4P_2O_7$] to facilitate the precipitation of silver metal. Both precipitation methods resulted in polyester sutures having good antimicrobial properties toward *P. aeruginosa*, *E. coli*, and *S. aureus*. However, the manganese hydroxide pretreatment appeared to exhibit a better antimicrobial property toward *P. aeruginosa* than sodium pyrophosphate pretreatment, as evident in the larger zone of bacterial inhibition. For example, 2.4 ± 0.7 and 0.6 ± 0.5 mm zones of inhibition were found with manganese hydroxide and sodium pyrophosphate pretreatments, respectively. This tendency, however, was not found in *E. coli* and *S. aureus* in which both treatments showed a statistically insignificant difference in zone of inhibition, as shown in Table 12.3. Presoaking of the antimicrobial Ethibond suture in saline solution for 4 d before inhibition zone evaluation, however, reduced the antimicrobial capability of the treated suture, as indicated by the significant reduction in the size of the inhibition zone with both pretreatments.

2. IMPREGNATION OF NONMETALLIC-TYPE ANTIBIOTICS ONTO THE SUTURE SURFACE

The most frequent approach to achieving antimicrobial properties in sutures is to impregnate them with a variety of antimicrobial agents, such as neomycin palmitate, penicillin, sulfonamide, quaternary ammonium complexes, chlorhexidine, and iodine.[6,14–20,74] The main advantage of this approach is the ability to use far lower dosages of antibiotics than are needed with the oral or injected route because the drugs are in direct or close contact with the microorganisms in the wound and no loss of drugs occurs through the biotransformation found with systemic administration. This approach also helps reduce the possibility of bacteria seeding inside the crevices of braided sutures.

Based on the method of impregnation, there are two subgroups: (1) a simple dipping of sutures into antibiotic solutions without any pretreatment of the suture surface,[6,14–19] and (2) elaborate chemical modifications of the suture surface to provide better bonding sites for antibiotics.[20,74] The dipping method is the simplest and easiest. A variety of antimicrobial agents, such as neomycin palmitate, penicillin, sulfonamide, quaternary ammonium complexes, chlorhexidine, and iodine have been tried. Although these antibiotic- or antiseptic-impregnated sutures have achieved some degree of success in reducing wound infections in animals, their results are far from perfect for various reasons, such as the shortness of the effective domain and duration, and the narrowness of spectrum of the antibacterial effect. For example, the antibacterial activity of neomycin palmitate-impregnated silk and Dacron® sutures lasted from 4 to 8 h.[6] However, a recent study of iodine-impregnated nylon fibers reported antibacterial activity toward *E. coli*, *P. aeruginosa*, *S. aureus*, and *K. pneumoniae* even after 30 d iodine release in water.[19] It was suggested that triiodide ions (I_3^-) might be responsible for the observed antimicrobial capability. The benefits of using antiseptic agents to impregnate sutures have been questioned because they may be more tissue toxic than bactericidal.

Chemical modification of the suture surface to provide better bonding with antibiotics would solve some shortcomings of the simple dipping method. Tyagi et al.[74] used radiation grafting of 2-hydroxyethyl methacrylate (HEMA) onto polypropylene (PP) sutures to improve the hydrophilicity of PP sutures by introducing polar –OH functional groups from HEMA.[75] The poly(HEMA) modified PP sutures were subsequently immobilized with 8-hydroxy quinoline drug through the polar –OH group of the grafted PP suture to render it antimicrobial. The amount of the drug immobilized onto PP sutures depended on the amount of grafted poly(HEMA) and ranged from 2.5% (for 17% HEMA) to 7.5% (for 65% HEMA). Figure 12.8 illustrates the cumulative release of the drug with time. A sustained release of the drug for

Table 12.3 Inhibition of Bacterial Growth by Tubing, Sutures, and Gauze

Sample	Treatment	Zone of Inhibition (mm)[a]		
		P. aeruginosa	*E. coli*	*S. aureus*
Polyvinyl chloride tubing	None	0	0	0
	$Mn(NO_3)_2 + NH_4OH$	0	0	0
	$Na_4P_2O_7$	0	0	0
	$AgNO_3$	0	0	0
	$Mn(NO_3)_2 + NH_4OH + AgNO_3$	1.5 ± 0.5a	1.5 ± 0.5a	3.1 ± 1.2a
	$Na_4P_2O_7 + AgNO_3$	1.1 ± 0.2a	1.1 ± 0.2a	1.1 ± 0.3b
Silicone tubing	None	0	0	0
	$Mn(NO_3)_2 + NH_4OH$	0	0	0
	$Na_4P_2O_7$	0	0	0
	$AgNO_3$	0	0	0
	$Mn(NO_3)_2 + NH_4OH + AgNO_3$	2.4 ± 0.7a	2.5 ± 0.5a	1.1 ± 0.3a
	$Na_4P_2O_7 + AgNO_3$	1.5 ± 0.5b	3.0 ± 1.3a	1.1 ± 0.2a
Sutures	None	0	0	0
	$Mn(NO_3)_2 + NH_4OH$	0	0	0
	$Na_4P_2O_7$	0	0	0
	$AgNO_3$	0	0	0
	$Mn(NO_3)_2 + NH_4OH + AgNO_3$	2.4 ± 0.7a	1.4 ± 0.6b	1.3 ± 0.4a
	$Na_4P_2O_7 + AgNO_3$	0.6 ± 0.5b	2.4 ± 0.7a	1.5 ± 0.5a
Gauze	None	0	0	0
	$Mn(NO_3)_2 + NH_4OH$	0	0	0
	$Na_4P_2O_7$	0	0	0
	$AgNO_3$	0.6 ± 0.5c	0.6 ± 0.5c	0.1 ± 0.1c
	$Mn(NO_3)_2 + NH_4OH + AgNO_3$	1.7 ± 0.3b	2.0 ± 0.5b	2.4 ± 0.7a
	$Na_4P_2O_7 + AgNO_3$	2.4 ± 0.5a	4.0 ± 0.5a	1.3 ± 0.4b

[a] The inhibition zone was measured from four sides of the solids to the area of bacterial growth. The mean values and standard deviation for eight values from two solids are presented. Numbers followed by the same letter in each column for one material are not significantly different at the $P = 0.05$ level.

From Farrah, S.R. and Erdos, G.W., *Can. J. Microbiol.*, 37(6), 445, 1991. With permission.

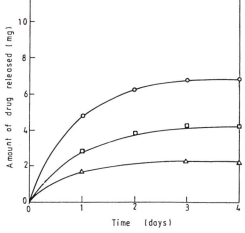

Figure 12.8 Cumulative release of drug from various poly(HEMA)-grafted polypropylene sutures. (△) 17% grafted poly(HEMA) with 2.5% 8-HQ drug; (□) 35% grafted poly(HEMA) with 4.6% 8-HQ drug; (○)65% grafted pol(HEMA) with 7.5% 8-HQ drug. (From Tyagi, P. K. et al., *J. Macromol. Sci. Pure Appl. Chem.*, A30(4), 303, 1993. With permission.)

a period of 4 to 5 d was observed with an accelerated release at the initial period. An *in vivo* study of this poly(HEMA) modified PP suture in the subcutis of female albino rats contaminated with 10^5 to 10^6 *S. aureus* indicated that the modified PP exhibited no clinical signs of wound infection, such as suppuration, 4 d postimplantation, while the control PP suture showed moderate suppuration. Another benefit of the poly(HEMA) grafting onto PP suture was the slight increase in tensile strength of the modified PP suture with less than 17% HEMA grafting. However, a higher level of HEMA grafting (>17%) was undesirable even though it would increase the incorporation of the drug because a deteriorated tensile strength was observed. For example, PP sutures grafted with 60% HEMA have only one third the tensile breaking strength of the ungrafted PP suture. The slight increase in strength with <17% HEMA grafting was attributed to the reinforcing effect of poly(HEMA). The grafted poly(HEMA) was expected to occur only in the amorphous domains without disrupting the crystallites of PP, as evident in a decrease in the overall level of crystallinity of poly(HEMA)-modified PP sutures due to the dilution of the crystalline regions by the incorporation of amorphous poly(HEMA) into the PP suture amorphous domains. Poly(HEMA) was dispersed in the amorphous domains of PP sutures and acted as a filler to improve the strength of the PP suture. The drastic reduction in tensile strength with >17% poly(HEMA)-modified PP sutures was thought to be due to the disruption of the microfibril structure and compactness of chains in the amorphous domains, since the excessive poly(HEMA) molecules could stretch or even break tie-chain segments located in the amorphous domains. The incorporation of poly(HEMA) molecules into the amorphous domains of PP sutures would also restrict the chain mobility in these domains, as evident in the continuous reduction in percent elongation at break with all levels of poly(HEMA) grafted PP sutures.

An unusual way to incorporate antibiotics onto the suture surface was recently reported by Guttmann and Guttmann.[20] Micropores were generated on the suture surface through a chemical reaction that generated gas.[76] These surface micropores were then filled with antibiotics through a coating process. The rate of drug release could be controlled by the size and amount of microporosity. Unfortunately, no clinical data were reported to reveal the antimicrobial properties of this type of antimicrobial suture.

The challenging issue of the proper retention of the impregnated or surface-bond antibiotics to sutures is further demonstrated by Knoop et al., who reported a study of bonding ofloxacin to Gore-Tex suture.[77] Although the bonding of ofloxacin to the suture was enhanced 22- and 75-fold in the presence of the cationic surfactant benzalkonium chloride or silver and organic solvents, respectively, the *in vitro* and *in vivo* retentions of the antibiotic were disappointing, 50% *in vitro* saline or serum and 8% *in vivo* for canine carotid arteries. This extreme low retention of ofloxacin *in vivo* was responsible for the failure of the ofloxacin-bonded Gore-Tex suture to ward off colonization by *S. aureus*.

II. BIOMATERIALS THAT COULD ACCELERATE WOUND HEALING: CHITIN

The best known nonsynthetic suture material that might possess some potential biological functions, such as the acceleration of wound healing, is the absorbable chitin. Chitin suture is a natural polysaccharide, poly-*N*-acetylglucosamine, with a (1-4) β-glycosidic linkage, which is found in the shells of crab, lobsters, shrimp, opossum shrimp, and insects. The chemical structure of chitin and its derivative chitosan are shown in Figure 12.9. Its chemical structure is similar to cellulose, except the –OH group at C_2 is replaced by an acetylated amino group. The chitin derivative, chitosan, is a deacetylation product of chitin. Chitin has three polymorphic forms α, β, and γ, which differ in their molecular chain arrangements.[78] Among these three forms, the α form is the most crystalline and exists as microfibrils in living systems. The chitin suture material was developed and, at this time, is used mainly in Japan.[79,80]

A. BIOLOGICAL FUNCTIONS OF *N*-ACETYLGLUCOSAMINE AND DERIVATIVES

Examination of the chemical structure of chitin, particularly the repeating unit *N*-acetylglucosamine, suggests that it may have some biochemical functions in addition to wound closure. These biochemical functions of chitin-based devices have recently been reviewed by Muzzarelli.[81] *N*-acetylglucosamine (NAGA) can be found in certain essential human glycoproteins in connective tissues like hyaluronic acid and keratin sulfate. The glycosamine moiety in chitin has been shown to exhibit a variety of biological functions, such as antiinflammatory, hepatoprotective, antireactive, and antihypoxic activities. Exogenous glucosamines could stimulate the synthesis of proteoglycans, an essential component of cell wall and matrix component in connective tissues. They also help to nurture cartilage and facilitate the formation of sulfate ester in chondroitin sulfate to counterbalance the degeneration of cartilage due to aging or disease. Recent discoveries of the immunomodulating capability of *N*-acetylglucosaminyl-*N*-acetylmuramyl-L-alanyl-D-isoglutamine (GMDP), whose structure is based on the chitin unit, to activate macrophage cytolytic activity toward tumor cells through the mechanisms of both stimulating superoxide radical production and suppressing of 5′-nucleotidase activity.[82] The antitumor effect of *N*-acetylglucosamine derivatives has also been confirmed in chitin and chitosan oligomers through the mechanism of enhancing the release of cytokines like interleukin-1 (IL-1) and tumor necrosis factor (TNF) from

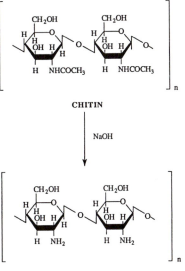

Figure 12.9 Chemical structure of chitin.

macrophage and polymorphonuclear leukocytes.[83–86] In addition to its potential antitumor effect, chitin and its derivatives have been reported as possible wound healing accelerators.[87] Chitosans have been reported to have antimicrobial activity against Gram-positive pathogens like *S. aureus, S. epidermidis,* and *S. haemolyticus*.[81] Electron microscopic data indicate that the bacterial cell wall in the presence of water-soluble chitosan became frayed and weakened and cell proliferation was depressed.

B. MANUFACTURING CHITIN SUTURES

There are several ways to obtain chitin suture fibers through wet spinning of chitin solutions. However, most of the resulting chitin fibers did not meet the requirement of sutures (i.e., 2 g/denier minimal tensile strength and 0.5 to 20 denier thickness). They were either too weak (if their diameter was small) or too thick (if their diameter was large enough to provide adequate strength).[88–90] A process for making chitin fibers disclosed in 1984 resulted in chitin fibers with adequate diameter and mechanical properties for suture use.[91] In principle, a dope solution of chitin solution with a concentration between 1% and 10% by weight in a chlorinated hydrocarbon like trichloroacetic acid is prepared; the dope solution is wet-spun by extruding the dope solution through a spinneret; the filament is coagulated in a coagulating solution of organic ketones or alcohol at 20 to 35°C (preferably anhydrous acetone, methanol, and ethanol); the filaments are further treated with a second coagulating solution consisting of an alcohol such as methanol, neutralized with aqueous caustic potash solution, washed, and dehydrated. Chitin sutures of USP size from 1/4 and 1/0 to 9/0 can be made by controlling the diameter of individual chitin filament, and the number of fibers per yarn for braiding. The resulting chitin sutures of 3/0 size have a dry tensile breaking strength ranging from 1.65 to 3.10 g/denier and an elongation of 8.7% to 20%. The corresponding knot strength ranged from 0.84 to 1.84 g/denier. The lower tensile strength, elongation, and knot strength values were those of chitin fibers under tension when passing through the second coagulation bath. This illustrates the importance that in the preparation of chitin fibers they should not be subject to tension during the second coagulation bath.

The other process reported for making chitin suture fibers meeting USP requirements is that of Nakajima et al.[79] In this process, amide-LiCl is used as the solvent for making chitin dope, which is wet-spun into a coagulation bath consisting of butyl alcohol. The dry tensile and knot strength of a 4/0 size chitin suture are 1.86 and 0.92 kg/mm^2, respectively.

C. *IN VITRO* AND *IN VIVO* PERFORMANCE OF CHITIN SUTURES

A comparison of the performance of chitin suture with other absorbable sutures like polyglycolide (PGA) and plain and chromic catgut *in vitro* and *in vivo* has been reported by Tachibana et al.[80] and Nakajima et al.[79] As shown in Figure 12.10, 3/0 size chitin suture had a straight and knot pull tensile strength between that of the same size PGA and chromic catgut sutures; however, chitin suture had the smallest elongation of the three absorbable sutures, particularly dry chitin suture. This low elongation was reflected

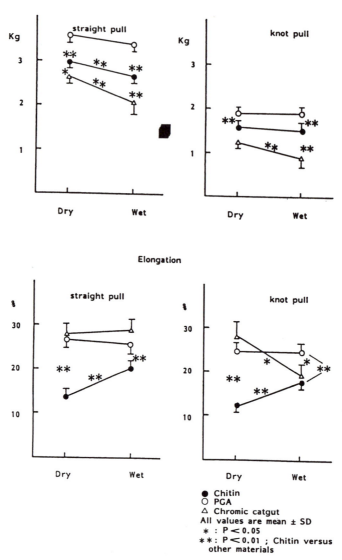

Figure 12.10 Mechanical properties of the strength and elongation of chitin. (●) Chitin; (○) PGA; (△) chromic catgut. (From Tachibana, M. et al., *Jpn. J. Surg.*, 218(5), 533, 1988. With permission.)

in the relatively poor handling property and knotting. Chitin suture has a lower straight pull strength when wet (90% of dry strength). Chitin sutures lose their strength in rabbit muscle at a rate similar to PGA sutures, as shown in Figure 12.11. For example, 3/0 chitin sutures retained 76% and 45% of their original tensile strength at 7 and 14 d postimplantation. However, chitin sutures had no measurable strength at 25 d postimplantation, while the same size PGA retained 7% of its original strength. The performance of chitin sutures under various media (artificial gastric juice, human bile, and pancreatic juices) was also examined. In artificial gastric juice (pH 1.2), chitin sutures lost strength faster than PGA sutures (35% retention in chitin vs. 60% retention in PGA at the end of 30 d) but slower than plain and chromic catguts, which showed no strength at the end of 3 d. In both human bile (pH 6.7) and pancreatic (pH 8.2) juices, chitin sutures exhibited virtually no loss of tensile strength over a period of 30 d. During the same period, PGA sutures lost 100% of their strength in human bile juice. No strength of PGA sutures could be measured at the end of 20 d in human pancreatic juice. Plain catgut exhibited no strength after 7 d in human bile juice, but chromic catgut retained about 60% of its original strength at the end of 30 d in human bile juice. No strength of plain and chromic catguts could be found after 7 and 30 d

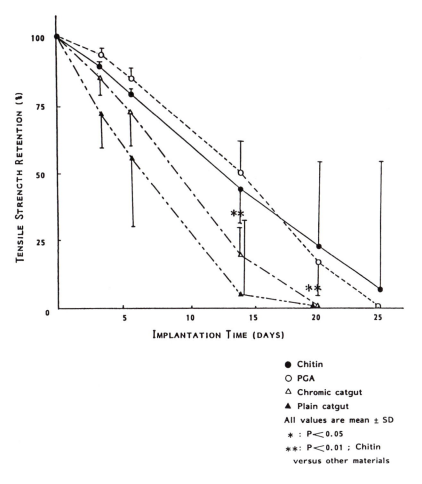

Figure 12.11 Tensile strength retention of chitin in muscle of mongrel dogs (*n*=5). (●) Chitin; (○) PGA; (△) chromic catgut; (▲) plain catgut. (From Tachibana, M. et al., *Japan J. Surg.*, 218(5), 533, 1988. With permission.)

in human pancreatic juice, respectively. Figure 12.12 illustrates these findings. As described later, the exceedingly high retention of chitin suture strength compared to PGA and catgut in digestive juices suggests that the degradation of chitin sutures must not be a pure water-induced hydrolytic mechanism like PGA and is probably closely related to certain enzymes (lysosomal enzymes) not found in these digestive juices. The findings also suggest that the degradation of chitin suture is affected more by acidic (lower pH) than alkaline media (higher pH). Similar findings were also reported by Nakajima et al.[79] Thus, it appears that chitin sutures are a better choice than PGA and catgut sutures in an alkaline environment as well as in the digestive tract and urological surgery.

Histopathologic data in mongrel dogs revealed no difference in tissue reactions between chitin and PGA sutures. Figure 12.13 illustrates the tissue response of chitin at 14 d and 6 months in dogs. However, there is a subtle difference between PGA and chitin in tissue response. At 14 d, phagocytic cells were rarely found around the chitin suture implantation site, while these cells could be found around PGA suture fibers. Chitin sutures showed accelerated collagen synthesis around the sutures. These sutures also required a considerably longer time to be absorbed (6 months) than PGA sutures (about 30 d in this case).

D. BIODEGRADATION MECHANISM OF CHITIN SUTURES

The degradation mechanism of chitin sutures *in vivo* is very different from PGA or catgut sutures and has been reported to have two pathways: (1) the degradation products of chitin are discharged as CO_2 through glycolysis of end product fructose, and (2) the degradation products are used to generate glycoproteins. The degradation of chitin sutures is controlled by lysozyme-catalyzed depolymerization.[92–97] Muzzarelli reported that lysozymes act as endohydrolases and catalyze the hydrolytic scission

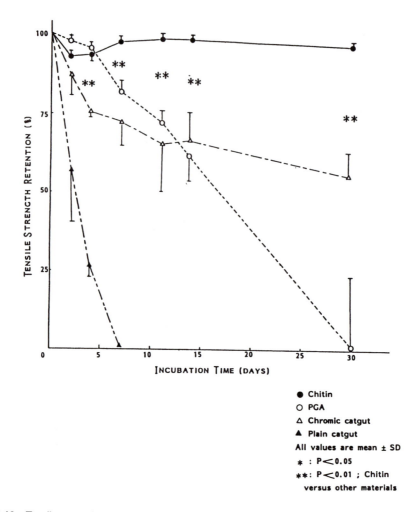

Figure 12.12 Tensile strength retention of chitin in human bile (pH 6.7, *n*=5). (●) Chitin; (○) PGA; (△) chromic catgut; (▲) plain catgut. (From Tachibana, M. et al., *Japan J. Surg.*, 218(5), 533, 1988. With permission.)

of the (1–4) β linkage in *N*-acetylglucosaminide. Other related lysozymes like N-acetylglucosaminidases may hydrolyze the terminal nonreducing *N*-acetylglucosamine unit of chitin. The different forms of chitins from different sources and/or processing conditions could also affect their susceptibility to lysozyme attack. For example, highly oriented and ordered chitins (having a more crystalline character-istic) and bleached chitins were found to have high resistance to lysozyme attack, while nascent or colloidal chitins are most readily degraded by lysozymes.[81]

Figure 12.14 illustrates the two metabolic pathways.[80] In the CO_2 pathway, chitin molecules are broken down into oligochitins by lysozymes which, in turn, are degraded into *N*-acetylglucosamine by β-*N*-acetylglucosaminidase. The resulting *N*-acetylglucosamine monomers are eventually converted into CO_2 through glycolysis via fructose. The most unique aspect of chitin biodegradation *in vivo* is the second pathway, which is the utilization of the degradation products, *N*-acetylglucosamine monomers, as a source for connective tissues through the synthesis of glycoproteins to facilitate wound repair. Figure 12.15 summarizes the degradation paths of chitin and chitosan. Their potential biological functions were described at the beginning of this section. Thus, lysozymes produced by macrophages hydrolyze chitin and chitosan into low-molecular-weight oligomers, which subsequently activate macrophages to produce cytokines like interferon, TNF, and IL-1 (one of the functions of IL-1 is to facilitate fibroblast proliferation). The activated macrophages also release *N*-acetyl-β-D-glucosaminidase, which catalyzes the breakdown of oligomers into D-glucosamine, *N*-acetylglucosamine, and substituted glucosamines. Proliferated fibroblasts under the action of IL-1 could use these amino sugars to make connective tissue components like hyaluronate and glycosaminoglycans.

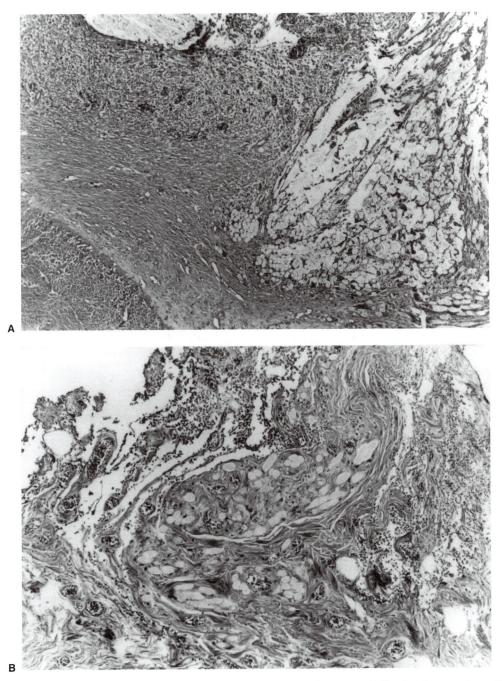

Figure 12.13   Tissue response to chitin. (A) 14 d (H & E, ×40). Inflammatory cell infiltration decreased, as with PGA, but phagocytosis was seldom seen. (B) 6 months (H & E, ×100). Chitin was almost absorbed and replaced by connective tissue. (From Tachibana, M. et al., *Japan J. Surg.*, 218(5), 533, 1988. With permission.)

III. BIOMATERIALS FOR BETTER MECHANICAL AND HANDLING PROPERTIES

In this category, there are several new materials: high-strength poly (vinyl alcohol), bioactive and more pliable PP-based monofilament suture, syndiotactic (instead of conventional isotactic) polypropylene monofilament for greater flexibility, elastomeric polyetherimide ester monofilament for better suture handling properties, composite sutures for reducing tissue ingrowth or better mechanical properties, creative copolymerization for improved biodegradation properties, polyvinylidene fluoride nonabsorbable suture for cardiovascular surgery, potentially biologically active synthetic absorbable sutures having the biological function similar to nitric oxide, and new tissue adhesives.

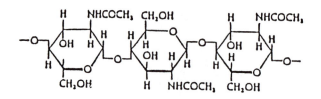

Chitin

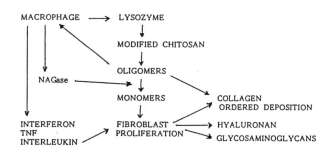

GNAc, N-Acetylglucosamine

GALAc, N-Acetylgalactosamine

Figure 12.14 *In vivo* two-pathway metabolism of chitin: one is that it is discharged as CO_2 through glycolysis after being resolved to *N*-acetylglucosamine; the other is that it is reused as glycoprotein. (From Tachibana, M. et al., *Japan J. Surg.*, 218(5), 533, 1988. With permission.)

```
MACROPHAGE  ———→  LYSOZYME
                       ↓
                  MODIFIED CHITOSAN
                       ↓
           NAGase ←  OLIGOMERS
                       ↓          → COLLAGEN
                  MONOMERS          ORDERED DEPOSITION
                       ↓
INTERFERON        FIBROBLAST  ——→ HYALURONAN
TNF               PROLIFERATION ——→ GLYCOSAMINOGLYCANS
INTERLEUKIN
```

Figure 12.15 *In vivo* lysozyme degradation of chitosan. Lysozyme, normally produced by macrophages, hydrolyzes susceptible modified chitosan to oligomers which activate macrophages to produce interferon, tumor necrosis factor, and interleukin-1. Activated macrophages also produce *N*-acetyl-β-D-glucosaminidase, which catalyzes production of D-glucosamine, *N*-acetylglucosamine, and substituted glucosamines from oligomers. These amino sugars are available to fibroblasts that proliferate under the action of interleukin-1, for incorporation into hyaluronate and lycosaminoglycans, thus guiding the ordered deposition of collagen, also influenced by oligomers. (From Muzzarelli, R., in *Polymeric Biomaterials*, Dumitriu, S., Ed., Marcel Dekker, New York, 1994, 179. With permission.)

A. HIGH-STRENGTH POLY(VINYL ALCOHOL) (HS-PVA)

Poly(vinyl alcohol) in hydrogel form or surface modified with RGD (Arg-Gly-Asp) has been reported to have some biomedical use, such as for synthetic vascular grafts and synthetic vitreous.[98-100] For suture use, PVA must be in fibrous form. HS-PVA fibers were developed initially by Hyon et al. in Japan.[101] This PVA fiber differs from conventional PVA fibers in that there was no formalization by formaldehyde.

Table 12.4 Mechanical Properties of Sutures
(USP-2 Standard)

Sutures	Tensile Strength (N)	One Knot Strength (N)	Knot Security
Silk	63.0 ± 0.7	39.2 ± 0.9	3
PET	118.0 ± 0.8	69.6 ± 3.4	3–4
E-PTFE(CV2)	49.4 ± 4.1	36.3 ± 3.1	—
UHMW-PE	421.1 ± 14.5	137.7 ± 7.1	6
HS-PVA	215 ± 8.7	84.7 ± 3.8	2
Stainless steel	163.2 ± 4.3	—	—

From Hyon, S.H. et al., in 32nd Int. Symp. Macromolecules, Kyoto, Japan, Aug. 1-6, 1988, pp. 798. With permission.

Thus, HS-PVA fibers are expected to be biocompatible with biological tissues. The two most distinctive characteristics of HS-PVA fibers that conventional suture fibers (except Gore-Tex) do not have are (1) a microporous surface structure for tissue ingrowth and (2) the surface of HS-PVA fibers can be easily modified chemically to facilitate a variety of biological functions.

Table 12.4 compares the tensile and knot properties of HS-PVA fibers with some common sutures like surgical silk, polyethylene terephthalate, PET (Ethibond), Gore-Tex (E-PTFE), and stainless steel. A 2/0 HS-PVA fiber is the strongest among these commercial sutures in terms of tensile breaking strength and knot strength (square knot). HS-PVA fibers also require fewer throws to secure a square knot than do silk and Ethibond sutures. Preliminary *in vivo* tissue biocompatibility studies in rat gluteal muscle indicate that HS-PVA was as biocompatible as Ethibond sutures.

B. POTENTIALLY BIOACTIVE AND MORE PLIABLE POLYPROPYLENE-BASED MONOFILAMENT SUTURE

Among the nonabsorbable monofilament sutures, polypropylene (PP) has been considered to be the most stable *in vivo*. However, existing PP sutures have two major drawbacks in their handling properties. They are pliability and knot security. Liu et al. reported the development of an innovative PP-based new monofilament suture which they claim to be more flexible, have better handling properties, and to have bioactive potential through chemical bonding of the surface active suture with antibiotic, growth factor, and anticlotting agents.[102,103]

This new PP-based suture is made by melt-blending of nonionic isotactic PP with an ionic copolymer of either ethylene or propylene and ethyleneically unsaturated carboxylic acids (e.g., acrylic or methacrylic acid) during the fiber melt-spinning process. The nonionic isotactic PP has a weight-average molecular weight M_w ranging from 200,000 to 350,000 and a number average molecular weight $\overline{M}_n$ of about 50,000 to 180,000 with a polydispersity of $\overline{M}_w/\overline{M}_n = 2.0$ to 4.0. The ionic copolymer was DuPont's Surlyn-8020 or 8920® which is an ethylene and methacrylic acid copolymer. Table 12.5 illustrates the mechanical properties of this new monofilament suture with various blend compositions of PP to ionic copolymer. When compared with 100% PP suture of identical size, the new PP/ionomer monofilament suture has slightly less unknotted tensile strength and elongation, but the new monofilament suture has a higher knot breaking strength.

Table 12.5 Physical Properties of PP/Ionomer Suture

Composition PP/Ionic (w/w %)	100/0	95/5	90/10
Diameter (mm)	0.238	0.245	0.245
Tensile strength (MPa)	396	348	335
Young's modulus (GPa)	2.59	0.53	0.48
Knot-pull (kg)	1.43	1.58	1.55
Straight-pull (kg)	1.76	1.64	1.58
Elongation at break (%)	40.2	39.5	38.1

From Liu, C.K. et al., Modified Polypropylene Suture with Ionomer, 20th Annu. Meet. Society for Biomaterials, April 5-9, 1994, Boston MA. With permission.

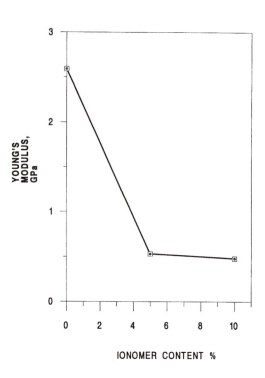

Figure 12.16 The effect of ionomer content (%) in polypropylene suture on its Young's modulus (GPa). (From Liu, C.K. et al., 20th Annual Meeting of the Society for Biomaterials, Boston, MA, 1994, 477. With permission.)

The most striking feature of this new monofilament suture is its relationship of Young's modulus, which indirectly relates to stiffness, to the ionic copolymer composition, as shown in Figure 12.16. There was a significant reduction in Young's modulus from 100% pure PP, as slight amounts (2% to 4%) of ionic copolymer were incorporated into 100% pure PP. A composition of only 5% ionic copolymer resulted in a Young's modulus only 19% of that of pure 100% PP suture, a reduction of 81%! A further increase in ionic copolymer content did not result in an appreciable reduction in Young's modulus. This relationship was responsible for the lower strain energy (toughness) of the new PP/ionomer monofilament suture compared to the conventional 100% pure PP suture. Liu et al. claimed that a reduction in toughness of a monofilament suture would facilitate the handling property of suture, particularly the straightening of kinked monofilament sutures from packaging before use. The new ionic copolymer modified monofilament PP suture has few voids and hence should be subject to a decreased incidence of premature breakage in use. Liu et al. also claimed that, due to the ionic nature of one of the constituents, the resulting new PP suture has the potential to chemically bond with cationic bioactive agents for a sustained release of such agents at wound sites. It is unclear, however, how a physically mixed blend of ionic copolymer and nonionic PP during melt-spinning would result in a preferential distribution of ionic copolymer onto the outermost layer of the resulting suture fibers. Such a preferential surface distribution is vital for facilitating chemical bonding of the new suture surface with bioactive agents. It is also unknown how such a chemically bonded bioactive agent would be released.

C. SYNDIOTACTIC POLYPROPYLENE SUTURES WITH GREATER FLEXIBILITY

All existing PP sutures are made mainly from isotactic PP in which all –CH$_3$ groups are located on one side of the backbone molecule. Syndiotactic PP has the 2 adjacent –CH$_3$ groups located alternatively along the backbone molecular plane. Because of this alternative arrangement of –CH$_3$ groups in syndiotactic PP, it is expected that PP with a syndiotactic structure would be expected to have a lower degree of crystallinity and hence a lower melting temperature, and be mechanically weaker than isotactic PP. Liu claimed syndiotactic PP sutures exhibited improved handling properties, such as greater flexibility, when compared with an isotactic PP suture.[104,105] Table 12.6 summarizes the mechanical and thermal properties of syndiotactic and isotactic PP sutures. The syndiotactic PP suture indeed has a lower tensile strength, Young's modulus, melting point, and level of crystallinity than the isotactic PP suture of equivalent size, as would be expected from polymer morphology. The considerably lower Young's modulus of syndiotactic PP should be expected to result in a filament that is less stiff than isotactic PP.

Table 12.6 Physical Properties of Monofilament Suture
from Syndiotactic and Isotactic Polypropylene Sutures

Physical Property	Syndio-PP	Isotactic-PP
Diameter (mm)	0.246	0.245
Tensile strength (MPa)	227	396
Young's modulus (GPa)	0.52	2.59
Elongation at break (%)	44	40

From Liu, C.K., 13th Southern Biomedical Engineering Conference,
Washington, D.C., 1994, 748. With permission.

Table 12.7 Physical and Mechanical Properties of Monofilament
Sutures

	Polyetherimide Ester	Polypropylene
Diameter (mm)	0.241	0.245
Tensile strength (MPa)	359	396
Young's modulus (GPa)	0.64	2.59
Elongation (%)	29	40

From Liu, C.K. et al., New Elastomeric Suture from Polyetherimide Ester, 20th Annu.
Meet. Society for Biomaterials, 1994, Boston, MA. With permission.

D. ELASTOMERIC POLYETHERIMIDE ESTER MONOFILAMENT SUTURE

It is always desirable to make monofilament sutures having the same handling properties as braided sutures of the same size. With this in mind, Liu et al. recently reported a new class of monofilament suture based on polyetherimide ester.[106,107] They claimed that this new suture has excellent mechanical and handling properties, such as resistance to creep, good knot security, and physical stability. The polyetherimide ester was prepared by polycondensation of a diol (1,4 butanediol), a dicarboxylic acid (dimethyl terephthalate), and a polyoxyalkylene diimide diacid. The resulting polymer has a melting point of 218°C.

Table 12.7 summarizes the essential mechanical properties of a 3/0 monofilament elastomeric polyetherimide ester suture with a PP suture as a control. The most significant characteristic of the new elastomeric polyetherimide ester suture is its Young's modulus (0.64 GPa), which was 25% of that of a PP suture. The elastomeric characteristic of this new suture is evident in its stress-strain curve. There was very little stress required to strain the suture to 10%; a very rapid increase in stress, however, was found after reaching about 10% strain and thereafter. This stress-strain behavior has been reported by Chu to be advantageous because the low stress exhibited at a small strain level of a suture (i.e., <10%) could allow wounds to swell easily during the first few days postoperation without cutting through the swollen wound by a suture.[108] Because of the lower modulus, elongation at break, and tensile strength, this new elastomeric polyetherimide ester suture has a lower toughness or strain energy (area under stress-strain curve) than a PP suture. Liu et al. claimed that sutures with lower toughness appear to have better flexibility. Another important mechanical property that this new elastomeric suture has is its low creep phenomenon. Creep is an increase in dimension of a material under a constant load, and creep is particularly important in surgical knots because suture fibers are under tension in a knot. A creep knot would elongate under tension, which may lead to wound dehiscence. Figure 12.17 provides a comparison of the creep property of three sutures (nylon, PP, and elastomeric polyetherimide ester).[107]

E. BICOMPONENT COMPOSITE SUTURE MATERIALS

The purpose of having composite sutures is to combine the merits of more than one component so that the resulting composite suture materials have advantages that neither of the constituents possess individually. The concept of composite sutures also permits the use of other polymers that currently cannot be used as sutures because of the lack of certain properties necessary for this application. This concept is not new and many research and development efforts have been reported in the patent literature. However, most of them have encountered a major technical problem in the manufacturing of composite suture materials: the lack of proper cohesion between the two constituent components. To solve this major technical difficulty, the approach of using constituents having functional groups that could chem-

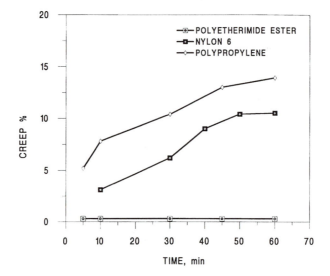

Figure 12.17 The % of creep of new polyetherimide ester suture vs. other synthetic sutures (From Liu, C.K., Brewer, J., and Kokish, M., 20th Annual Meeting of the Society for Biomaterials, Boston, MA, April 5-9, 1994, 243. With permission.)

Table 12.8 Possible Combination of Core-Sheath Composite Suture Materials

Composite	Matrix[c]	Extruding Polymer[c]
1	Polyethylene terephthalate	Isotactic Polypropylene
2	Kevlar[a]	Polypropylene
3	Kevlar[a]	Polyethylene
4	Kevlar[a]	Polyethylene terephthalate
5	Chain extended polyethylene[b]	Atatic polypropylene
6	Kevlar[a]	Polyglycolide
7	Nylon 6,6	Isotactic polypropylene
8	Nylon 6,6	Polyisobutylene
9	Polyethylene terephthalate	Nylon 11

[a] Aromatic polyamide product of DuPont Corporation.
[b] High strength polyolefin having straight pull tenacity of approximately 25 to 50 g/denier described in Keller, A. and Barham, P.J., *Plast. Rubber Int.*, 6(1), 1981.
[c] Matrix as the braided sheath; extruding polymer as the monofilament core.

From Kurtz, L.D., U.S. Patent 4,470,941 to Bioresearch Inc., Sept. 11, 1984.

ically bond together has been reported as the most frequent means. This approach has been considered to be costly, limiting the number and type of polymers that could be used, and has been largely unsuccessful. Kurtz and co-workers recently proposed an innovative approach to solve the adhesion problem between two constituents within bicomponent composite sutures.[109,110]

The principle behind Kurtz's approach is to use two constituents having vastly different melting temperatures. The component with a lower melting temperature will be used as a monofilament core material, while the constituent with a higher melting temperature will be braided over the monofilament core material. This core-sheath structure is then subject to heat and pressure such that the low-melting core component would melt and penetrate into and fill up the interstitial spaces of the braided suture. The resulting bicomponent composite suture will have a monofilament appearance but with a multifilament interior structure. Table 12.8 lists the types of combination of sheath and core materials that have been tried. The sheath materials ranged from polyethylene terephthalate (PET), Kevlar®, extended chain polyethylene to nylon 6,6, while the core materials include isotactic or atactic PP, PET, polybutylene, nylon 11, and absorbable polyglycolide.[109] Table 12.9 compares the knot-pull tensile strength, elongation,

Table 12.9 A Comparison of Mechanical Properties of Composite Sutures Made from Polyethylene Terephthalate Braided Sheath and Isotactic Polypropylene Monofilament Core with Some Commercial Sutures.

No.	Type of Suture	Knot-Pull Tensile Strength, F_{knot} (g)		Percent Elongation (%)	Knot Security		Gurley Stiffness G.S. (mg.)
		Required by USP	Measured		Ksec	$(n_{Ksec-1})/5$	
1	**CK suture 3/0**	1200	1456	15.0	2	—	8.2
2	Prolene 3/0 (from Ethicon)	1200	1504	58.3	3	$n_2/5=5$	19.8
3	PP yellow monofil 3/0	1200	1430	39.4	3	$n_2/5=5$	24.9
4	Nylon white monofil 3/0 (from Deknatel)	1200	1434	50.4	4	$n_3/5=5$	22.8
5	PET monofil 3/0	1200	2430	76.1	3	$n_2/5=5$	52.0
6	**CK suture 4/0**	750	930	12.8	2	—	5.9
7	Prolene 4/0 (from Ethicon)	750	946	56.7	3	$n_2/5=5$	9.9
8	PP blue monofil 4/0	750	841	29.1	3	$n_2/5=5$	14.4
9	Nylon white monofil 4/0 (from Deknatel)	750	950	47.8	4	$n_3/5=5$	12.6
10	PET green braid suture 4/0	750	1146	16.5	4	$n_3/5=5$	3.0
11	**CK suture 5/0**	500	649	14.2	2	—	2.2
12	Prolene 5/0 (from Ethicon)	500	646	44.9	3	$n_2/5=5$	3.1
13	PP blue monofil 5/0	500	532	31.5	3	$n_2/5=5$	5.9
14	Nylon white monofil 5/0 (from Deknatel)	500	577	51.0	4	$n_2/5=5$	5.4
15	PET green braid suture 5/0 (from Deknatel)	500	770	25.2	4	$n_3/5=1$	0.6
16	**CK suture 6/0**	250	318	11.0	2	—	0.4
17	Prolene 6/0 (from Ethicon)	250	270	50.0	3	$n_2/5=4$	0.6
18	PP blue monofil 6/0	250	192	29.9	3	$n_2/5=5$	1.1
19	PET monofil 6/0	250	485	37.0	3	$n_2/5=5$	3.3

CK - Composite suture

From Kurtz, L.D., U.S. Patent 4,470,941 to Bioresearch Inc., September 11, 1994.

and stiffness of four USP size (3/0, 4/0, 5/0, and 6/0) composite sutures consisting of a 40 denier PET braid sheath over a 265 denier isotactic PP core. All sutures tested including composite and noncomposite, showed better tensile knot breaking strength than USP specified. Noncomposite PET sutures always had the highest tensile knot breaking strength among all sutures tested for all four USP sizes. The composite sutures of size 3/0, 4/0, and 5/0 had tensile knot breaking strength similar to Prolene and nylon monofilament sutures of corresponding sizes. The composite sutures had the lowest Gurley stiffness values among all sutures tested for all four USP sizes, and the stiffness values were considerably lower than for the noncomposite sutures. Because of these very low stiffness values, the composite sutures had good knottability. All composite sutures required only a two-throw square knot to achieve knot security, while monofilament PP and PET sutures required a three-throw square knot, and nylon monofilament and PET braid sutures required four-throw square knots to achieve knot security. Scanning electron microscope (SEM) observation of this composite suture indicated infiltration of PP resin into the interstices of PET braids without any visible voids.

F. IMPROVED BIODEGRADATION OF ABSORBABLE SUTURES THROUGH COPOLYMERIZATION

The recent development of polydioxanone (PDS), Maxon®, Monocryl®, and Biosyn® sutures improves their mechanical properties and/or their tensile breaking strength retention both *in vitro* and *in vivo*. As described in Chapter 7, the biodegradation of all absorbable sutures could be described in terms of both strength loss and weight loss profiles. Due to the inherent structure-property relationship in fibers, an improvement in strength loss profile unfortunately also leads to a prolonged suture mass retention. Such a prolonged suture mass retention is undesirable because it elicits chronic inflammatory reaction and predisposes to infection, granuloma formation, etc., as described in detail in Chapter 8. Therefore, recent research efforts have been to develop new absorbable sutures with improved biodegradation properties from the random and segmented copolymerization of either existing absorbable suture components or new monomers chemically different from existing absorbable suture components, a concept similar to the composite sutures described above.

An example of such efforts is the copolymerization of PDS suture with glycolides, lactides, or morpholine-2,5-dione (MD).[111-114] A copolymer of PDS and PGA (20%) has an absorption profile similar to Dexon® and Vicryl® sutures, but it has a compliance similar to PDS. A copolymer of PDS and PLLA (15%) results in a more compliant suture than homopolymer PDS, but with a similar absorption profile to PDS. Copolymer sutures made from PDS and morpholine-2,5-dione (P-MD/PD) exhibit rather interesting biodegradation properties.[112] As shown in Figure 12.18, although P-MD/PD sutures were absorbed 10% to 25% earlier than PDS, the former retained a tensile strength profile similar to PDS with a slightly faster strength loss during the earlier stage, i.e., the first 14 d. This ability to break the inherent fiber structure-property relationship through copolymerization is a major improvement in the biodegradation properties of absorbable sutures. It is interesting to recognize that a small percent of MD (3%) in the copolymer suture P-MD/PD is sufficient to result in a faster mass loss profile without detriment to its tensile strength loss profile. The ability to achieve this ideal biodegradation property might be attributed to both an increasing hydrophilicity of the P-MD/PD copolymer and the disruption of crystalline domains due to the MD moiety. As described in Chapter 7, the loss of suture mass is mainly due to the destruction of crystalline domains, while the loss of tensile strength is chiefly due to the scission of tie-chain segments located in the amorphous domains. The question is why P-MD/PD copolymeric suture retains a similar strength loss to PDS. The possible explanation is that the amide functional groups in MD could form stronger intermolecular hydrogen bonds than ester functional groups. This stronger hydrogen bond contributes to the strength retention of P-MD/PD during *in vivo* biodegradation. Table 12.10 lists the essential mechanical properties of this unhydrolyzed P-MD/PD copolymeric suture along with others for comparison. The incorporation of the morpholine-2,5-dione moiety into PDS also lowers the unknotted and knotted strength of unhydrolyzed specimens, but increases elongation at break. This suggests that P-MD/PD copolymer should have a lower level of crystallinity than PDS, which is consistent with the observed faster mass loss of P-MD/PD *in vivo*.

Another possible chemical approach to the development of new absorbable polymers for wound closure use is based on modified monomers derived from glycolide or lactide. The advantage of this chemical approach is the well-known biocompatibility of glycolide and lactide. One example in this category of derivatives of poly(α-hydroxy acids) is the copolymer of L-lactide and 3-(S)[(alkyloxycarbonyl) methyl]-1,4-dioxane-2,5-dione, a cyclic diester.[115,116] The chemical structure of the resulting copolymer is shown in Figure 12.19. The most unique aspect of this new biodegradable polymer is the carboxyl acid pendant group which obviously would make the new polymer not only more hydrophilic

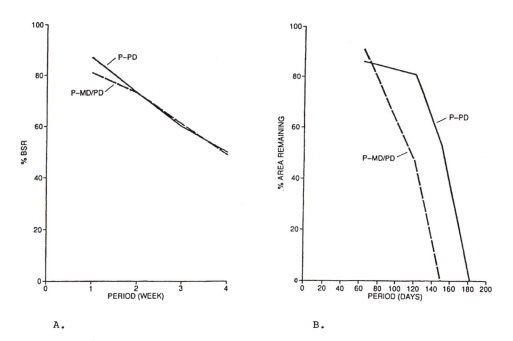

Figure 12.18 *In vivo* breaking strength (A) and cross-sectional area (B) remaining of copolymeric monofilament suture made of PDS and 3% morphine-2,5-dione (P-MD/PD) and homopolymer monofilament PDS (P-PD) as the control. (From Shalaby, S.W. and Koelmel, D.F., U.S. Patent 4,441,496 to Ethicon, 1984. With permission.)

Table 12.10 Comparative Physical Properties of 40/60 P-TMC/G (Maxon), P-PD (PDS), and 5/95 P-MD/PD Monofilament Sutures

	40/60 P-TMC/G	P-PD	5/95 P-MD/PD
Straight tensile strength (Kpsi)	88	87	62
Knot strength (Kpsi)	57	55	45
Elongation (%)	38	30	58
Young's modulus (Kpsi)	460	390	—

Note: TMC — Trimethylene carbonate; G — Glycolide; PD — p-dioxanone; MD — Morpholine-2,5-dione.

From Shalaby, S.W., in *Biomedical Polymers: Designed-to-Degrade Systems*, Shalaby, S.W., Ed., Hansere Publisher, New York, 1994, chap. 1. With permission.

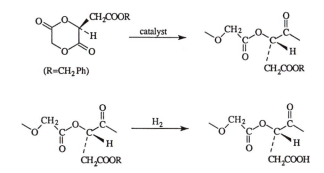

Figure 12.19 Schematic drawing of the synthesis of a biodegradable copolymer consisting of a carboxylic pendant group. (From Kimura, Y. et al., *Macromolecules*, 21, 3338, 1988. With permission.)

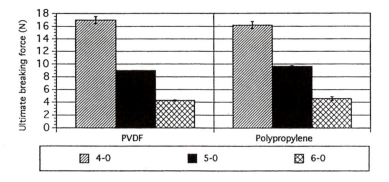

Figure 12.20 Ultimate breaking tensile force (Newton) of PVDF and Prolene sutures. (From Urban, E. et al., *Am. Soc. Artif. Intern. Org.*, 40(2), 145, 1994. With permission.)

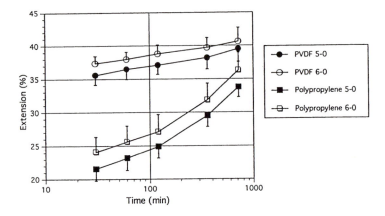

Figure 12.21 Creep properties of 5/0 and 6/0 PVDF and Prolene sutures. (From Urban, E. et al., *Am. Soc. Artif. Intern. Org.*, 40(2), 145, 1994. With permission.)

and hence subject to faster biodegradation, but also more reactive toward future chemical modification through the pendant carboxyl group. The availability of these carboxyl reactive pendant sites is very important and exciting because these sites could be used to chemically bond antimicrobial agents or other biochemicals, such as growth factors, producing future wound closure biomaterials having new and important biological functions. Unfortunately, there are no reported data to evaluate the performance of these new absorbable polymers for wound closure use, up to the present time.

G. POLYVINYLIDENE FLUORIDE NONABSORBABLE MONOFILAMENT SUTURE

The recent development of polyvinylidene fluoride (PVDF) nonabsorbable monofilament suture by Peters Laboratoire Pharmaceutique (Bobigny, France) was to provide a wound closure biomaterial in vascular surgery that would have very good antithrombogenicity with the same satisfactory handling characteristics as PP suture and yet be as durable as polyester sutures. The manufacturer hoped to replace PP with PVDF in vascular surgery for some of its unique properties not available with isotactic PP suture. The chemical, physical, mechanical, morphological, and biocompatible properties of 5/0 and 6/0 PVDF sutures (Teflene®) was recently reported by Urban et al.[117]

PVDF and PP sutures were found to be very similar in tensile breaking force and biocompatibility in blood vessels. The three properties that most differentiate PVDF from PP sutures are creep behavior, the extent of iatrogenic trauma by a needle holder, and sterilization by γ-irradiation. Figures 12.20 and 12.21 illustrate these differences. Over a period of 10^3 min, there was about 10% dimensional increase in PVDF sutures, while PP (Prolene) sutures had more than 50% dimensional increase. Thus, it appears that PVDF sutures have a better resistance to creep than PP sutures and hence are expected to be more dimensionally stable. However, PVDF exhibited more dimensional change than PP during the initial 30 min of creep testing.

PVDF sutures appeared to withstand the damage from needle holders better than PP suture, at least from the surface morphological point of view. PVDF sutures showed some flattening with a roughened surface, but they did not have the longitudinal cracks and fibrillar formation found with PP sutures. This morphological difference between PVDF and PP sutures, however, was not reflected to a marked degree in their tensile breaking force values. In other words, the iatrogenic trauma done by needle holders to PP and PVDF sutures did not reduce their tensile breaking force significantly.

PVDF and PP sutures have very similar melting temperatures (165 to 175°C), but distinctively different levels of crystallinity. PVDF has a level of crystallinity 59% ± 7%, while PP has 43% ± 3%. Because of the lack of an α-alkyl group, PVDF can be sterilized by the conventional γ-irradiation method, while PP requires the use of ethylene oxide gas. Thus, PVDF could take advantage of the efficiency and convenience of γ-irradiation sterilization. Like PP suture, PVDF sutures should not have any O_2 element in their chemical structure. However, the surface of PVDF and PP sutures showed oxidation products, as confirmed by electron spectroscopy for chemical analysis. The amounts of O_2 element on the surface of PVDF and PP sutures was 7.4% and 7.9%, respectively. However, bulk Fourier transform infrared (FTIR) data failed to reveal such oxidation products. This suggests that oxidation of PVDF and PP is introduced during melt-spinning of fibers and is mainly restricted to the surface of suture fibers.

PVDF sutures showed a similar histologic response as a PP suture. At the end of 6 months implantation in adult mongrel dogs, PVDF sutures were encapsulated by a thin layer of newly formed connective tissue with the absence of inflammatory cells. The explanted and cleaned PVDF sutures revealed no visible surface damage or degradation.

H. REINFORCED POLY(L-LACTIDE) ABSORBABLE SUTURE FOR LONGER RETENTION OF STRENGTH

The use of poly(L-lactide) (PLLA) as an absorbable suture material was tried by Cutright and Hunsuck in the early 1970s[118] and Jamshidi et al. in the 1980s.[119] Due to the presence of an α-methyl group, PLLA has been expected and indeed found to be hydrolyzed at a much slower rate than the unsubstituted polyglycolide (PGA). This very slow rate of biodegradation of PLLA makes it more like a nonabsorbable than an absorbable suture. The long retention of the mass of an absorbable implant after the loss of its function inside a living body has been a concern as a source of chronic inflammation, described in previous chapters (see Chapters 7 and 8). Besides this concern, which makes the use of PLLA suture less desirable than others, the considerably lower initial tensile strength of PLLA suture (0.7 GPa) than other synthetic absorbable sutures also makes the use of PLLA sutures less favorable, particularly in microsurgery. This relatively inferior mechanical property of PLLA suture fibers has been addressed in a study reported by Lam et al.,[120] which may revitalize the use of PLLA as the wound closure biomaterial for delayed wound healing.

Using unique dry-spinning and hot-drawing fiber processes, Lam et al. reported a newer generation of PLLA fibers for wound closure purposes. Due to the unique dry-spinning and hot-drawing processes, this new PLLA suture fiber exhibited a highly microfibrillar morphological structure which appears to reinforce the fiber. The fiber had a flat rather than round shape. This reinforced PLLA suture fiber has an initial tensile strength as high as 1.2 GPa right after manufacturing. The results from an *in vitro* degradation study of these new PLLA suture fibers indicate that the 8/0 reinforced PLLA suture fibers retained from about 70% to 100% of their original tensile strength over a period of 12 weeks, while a 7/0 PDS retained only about 8% at the end of the same period.

An *in vivo* implantation study in rat muscle indicated that this reinforced absorbable PLLA monofilament suture fiber induced an inflammatory reaction with an intensity similar to multifilament Vicryl sutures during an early stage postimplantation (<6 weeks). This early-stage inflammatory reaction toward PLLA suture fibers was characterized by several layers of macrophages surrounding the fibers. Lam et al. attributed the intensity of the observed inflammatory reaction of the PLLA suture fiber to morphological change in the fiber, which disintegrated into multi-microfilaments. The intensity of the inflammatory reaction decreased after 6 weeks and giant cells appeared around the PLLA suture fibers at week 12, and their inflammatory reaction remained the same between 12 and 52 weeks. The fragments of PLLA suture fibers started to appear within giant cells with an occasional macrophage and small fibrous encapsulation at week 80 postimplantation. After 80 weeks, PLLA suture fibers behaved like monofilament nylon suture (i.e., Ethilon) in terms of tissue reactions.

I. POTENTIALLY BIOLOGICALLY ACTIVE ABSORBABLE SUTURES

Chu, Lee, and Freed recently reported a new technology that permits the chemical bonding of nitric oxide derivatives to a series of synthetic absorbable polymers and fibers that may have a major impact on wound closure and cardiovascular biomaterials and devices.[121]

Nitric oxide (NO•) is a very small but highly reactive and unstable free radical biomolecule with expanding known biological functions. This small biomolecule and its biological functions have recently become one of the most studied and intriguing subjects, as recently reviewed by several investigators.[122-133] NO• is extremely labile and short-lived (about 6 to 10 seconds).

NO• and its radical derivatives have been known to play a very important role in a host of expanding biological functions, such as inflammation, neurotransmission, blood clotting, blood pressure, cardio- vascular disorders, rheumatic and autoimmune diseases, antitumor activity with a high therapeutic index, antimicrobial property, sensitization or protection of cells and tissues against irradiation, oxidative stress, respiratory distress syndrome, and cytoprotective property in reperfusion injury, to name a few.[122-144] NO• acts both as an essential regulatory agent to normal physiological activities and as cytotoxic species in diseases and their treatments. Nathan et al. reported that nitric oxide is a potent antiviral compound against two disfiguring poxvirus and herpes simplex virus type-1, which causes cold sores in humans.[126] Levi et al. also found that nitric oxide could protect the human heart against low oxygen supply, a condition known as myocardial ischemia, by widening blood vessels so that more oxygen-rich blood reaches the heart.[128] Elliott et al. reported that a new NO•-releasing, nonsteroidal anti-inflammatory drug has the benefits of accelerating gastric ulcer healing.[145,146] It is important to know, however, that excessive introduction of NO• into the body may have adverse effects, like microvascular leakage, tissue damage in cystic fibrosis, septic shock, B-cell destruction, and possible mutagenic risk, to name a few.[132,133,141,147-149]

NO• and NO•-derived radicals are not normal biological messengers whose trafficking depends on specific transporters or channels. Instead, nitric oxide radicals released by cells like macrophage and endothelial cells would diffuse randomly in all directions from the site of release. Because of this unusual property, the only way to control the biological functions of nitric oxide is to control its site of synthesis. This suggests that the only way to deliver the desirable biological functions of nitric oxide is through nature. Existing science and technology are not able to modulate the release of nitric oxide according to our wish for a variety of therapeutic purposes.

Although all existing synthetic absorbable and nonabsorbable polymeric biomaterials are different in their chemical constituents, they have one common characteristic: they do not have any inherent bio- logical functions to improve their role in human body repair. In other words, they are not biologically active and play only a passive instead of an active role in wound healing and tissue engineering. It would be ideal if these biomaterials could be made biologically "alive" and active by having some critical biological functions, such as the ability to modulate inflammatory reactions, to facilitate wound healing, or to mediate host defense system to combat diseases.

One approach to make biologically "alive" synthetic biomaterials is to find a suitable chemical means to incorporate nitroxyl radicals into biomaterials. Such an approach has become feasible due to a very recent invention by Chu and his associates.[121] They have been able to incorporate nitroxyl radicals into the carboxylic chain ends of synthetic absorbable biomaterials.[121] This new invention is based on the rationale that the –OH groups of the carboxylic acid chain ends of synthetic biomaterials could be replaced by an imidazole functional group, which subsequently would facilitate the nucleophilic substi- tution by nitroxyl radicals. The need to replace –OH by an imidazole is that –OH is known to be a difficult leave group for nitroxyl radical nucleophilic substitution reaction. If the –OH group of the carboxylic acid chain ends of biomaterial molecules could be replaced by an imidazole group, Chu et al. could transform carboxylic chain ends of biomaterials into imidazole chain ends. This transformation would dramatically facilitate the subsequent nucleophilic attack of nitroxyl radicals (e.g., 4-amino- 2,2,6,6-tetramethyl-piperidine-1-oxy) onto the carbonyl carbon of the biomaterials. An electron spin resonance study of these new biologically active biomaterials indicated that nitroxyl radicals indeed could be chemically bound to the carboxylic acid chain ends of synthetic biomaterials.[121]

The outcome of this novel discovery could form the foundation leading to the research and develop- ment of ideal "biologically alive" biomaterials for bioengineering of the next century. These new and biologically active biomaterials could permit scientists to actively reconstruct the injured, diseased, or aged human body. Some examples of the potential Chu et al.'s nitroxyl-radical-incorporated biomaterials are anticancer drugs, wound closure materials with improved healing and antimicrobial capability, vascular stents that could retard smooth muscle proliferation to eliminate restenosis, and synthetic vascular grafts that would not clot. In the anticancer drug area, the nitroxyl radical incorporated absorbable biomaterials could be used as the vehicles to precisely deliver the antitumor property of nitroxyl radicals to tumor sites via the biodegradation release of the incorporated nitroxyl radicals. The nitroxyl radical-incorporated biomaterials could also be used to improve the efficacy of radiation therapy in cancer because nitroxyl radicals are known to be able to considerably sensitize tumor cells toward radiation. The benefit will be a lower side effect of radiation therapy because a lower dosage of radiation could be used without compromising its therapeutic effect. In addition to the therapeutic effect and reconstruction of injured or diseased tissues, the nitroxyl radical-incorporated biomaterials may also be used as a useful tool for a fundamental study of a host of biochemical reactions involving free radicals and superoxide anions because these nitroxyl radical-labeled biomaterials could react with any reactive free radicals and neutralize them. These modified biomaterials could also be used to mimic the functions of superoxide dismutase (SOD), a naturally occurring enzyme, to neutralize superoxide anions and other reactive radicals. Thus, the modified biomaterials may be used to control local inflammatory reaction induced by wounds or/and surgical implants.

IV. NEW TISSUE ADHESIVES

As described in Chapter 11, all current commercial tissue adhesives are of either synthetic, e.g., α-cyanoacrylates, blood-based glue, e.g., fibrin, or proteins, e.g., GRF. These tissue adhesives have two major concerns: toxicity and viral contamination. To solve these problems, several new biodegradable tissue adhesives have very recently been introduced. They are: collagen-based tissue adhesives (Colcys®) by Imedex in France,[150-154] hydrogel-based FocalSeal®[156-161] and 3M Sealant,[162,163] and modified α-cyanoacrylates that can neutralize formaldehyde to reduce its toxicity.[155]

A. COLLAGEN-BASED TISSUE ADHESIVES

The first type of Colcys tissue adhesive is based upon a keratin-like protein (highly purified atelocollagen) that has been chemically modified so that aminothiols like cysteine or cysteamine are grafted onto the atelocollagen backbone molecule, shown in Figure 12.22A.[150] High adhesive strength with this tissue adhesive could be achieved through an *in situ* mild oxidation of the –SH groups, which leads to disulfide intermolecular crosslinkings and subsequent hydrogel formation. Iodine or H_2O_2 could serve as the oxidation agent. Based on *ex vivo* study, Constancis et al. reported that Colcys tissue adhesive achieved more rapid and stronger bonding than commercial fibrin glues (Tisseel® and Biocol®), as shown in Figure 12.23.[152] *In vivo* biocompatibility testing in rat skin indicated that Colcys showed the same classical tissue reactions as collagen biomaterials. The adhesive was slightly infiltrated by mononuclear cells and fibroblasts at the third day postimplantation and showed signs of degradation and more intense cell infiltration with sparse giant cells at day 7 and thereafter.

The second type of Colcys product is a collagen gel sealant which seals wounds with air and liquid tightness. It is known that adhesion due to wound healing of skin does not start until 24 h after the wound occurs, and reaches a peak at 15 d. In order to promote earlier adhesion of skin wounds, glues are needed to provide the required adhesion. Colcys gel sealant is based upon the same highly purified atelocollagen as Colcys tissue adhesive, but with a different chemical modification.[153,154] A controlled oxidation of carbohydrate and hydroxylysine residues of atelocollagen by periodic acid would create reactive aldehyde groups on collagen molecules. These newly created aldehyde groups could react with –NH$_2$ groups of both neighboring tissues and other collagen sealant molecules to form a crosslinking network that could seal wounds. Figure 12.22B illustrates the chemical sequences of this new type of gel sealant.[150] The crosslinking reaction between the aldehyde and amine groups could be initiated by adjusting the pH of the viscous solution toward the alkaline (e.g., phosphate/NaOH buffer) because the sealant before crosslinking reaction is stable in an acidic pH and low temperature (20°C). The shelf life of the collagen sealant is determined by the pH of the medium and temperature. With a combination of acidic pH and low temperature, e.g., 20°C, the sealant remains as a stable solid. During the application of the gel sealant, a higher temperature (37°C) is introduced so that the gel sealant can turn into a viscous fluid to be injected by an appropriate double syringe system. Colcys sealant appeared to provide a comparable adhesive force to Biocol fibrin glue but was stronger during the earlier period (<30 min) than Tisseel fibrin glue in an *ex vivo* study, as shown in Figure 12.23.[154] An *in vivo* histological study of the Colcys sealant in rats showed that the sealant was largely degraded by mononuclear and polynuclear cells at day 7 postimplantation, with residual inflammatory reactions at the injection site.[153]

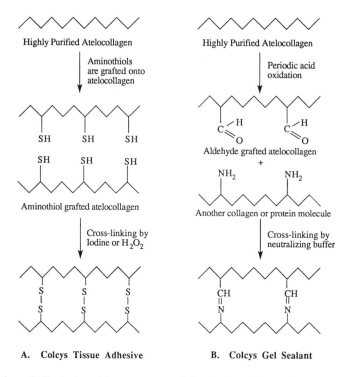

Figure 12.22 Schematic illustration of the sequences of chemical reactions of Colcys tissue adhesive (A) and sealant (B). (From Tiollier, J. et al., 21st Annual Meeting of the Society for Biomaterials and 27th Biomaterials Symposium, San Francisco, CA, 1995. With permission.)

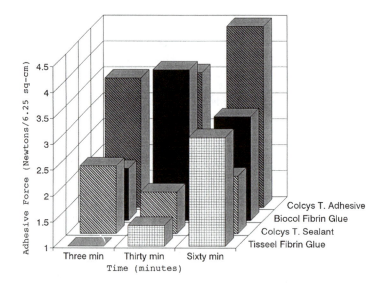

Figure 12.23 *Ex vivo* adhesive force in terms of tensile strength in N/6.25 cm² of Colcys tissue adhesive and sealant and Tisseel and Biocol fibrin glues in rabbit paravertebrate muscle. The Colcys tissue adhesive was from batch B, while the Colcys gel sealant was from sodium phosphate buffer neutralizing agent.

B. NEUTRALIZATION OF THE TOXICITY OF FORMALDEHYDE RELEASED FROM α-CYANOACRYLATE ADHESIVES

Because the toxicity of formaldehyde released from the α-cyanoacrylate tissue adhesives has been a major concern, any means to neutralize formaldehyde would be considerably interesting to biomaterials scientists and engineers for revitalizing the use of α-cyanoacrylates in wound closure. Leung et al.[155]

Poly(ethylene glycol)-co-Poly(d,l-lactide) Diacrylate Macromer*

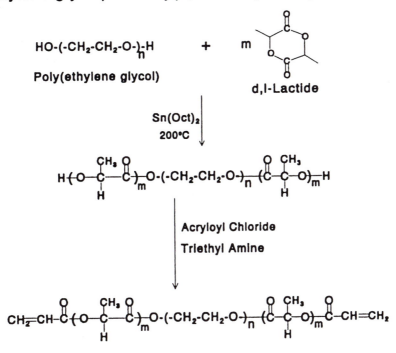

Figure 12.24 The chemical scheme for making poly(ethylene glycol)-co-poly(d,l-lactide) diacrylate macromer, the constituent of FocalSeal before photopolymerization. (From Sawhney, A.S., Pathak, C.P., and Hubbell, J.A., *Macromolecules*, 26, 581, 1993. With permission.)

very recently invented the use of formaldehyde scavenger-like alkali metal salts, e.g., sodium bisulfite, to neutralize formaldehyde released from α-cyanoacrylate tissue adhesives. In order to achieve a maximum neutralization effect of the released formaldehyde from α-cyanocrylate tissue adhesives, sodium bisulfite is microencapsulated by biodegradable polymers like the copolymers of glycolide and lactide. These microcapsules are then impregnated with α-cyanoacrylate monomers to make the final product. Depending on the type of biodegradable polymers, a wide range of the release rate of sodium bisulfite from the microcapsules could be achieved to match the release rate of formaldehyde to maximize the neutralization effect.

C. NEW HYDROGEL-BASED TISSUE ADHESIVES

Hydrogel-based tissue adhesives have several advantages over α-cyanoacrylates: better tissue biocompatibility, faster rate of biodegradation, better fluid mechanics for easy application to fill up small voids or cracks, and better viscoelasticity for a closer match to the biomechanics of the surrounding tissues. There are two types of hydrogel-based tissue sealants, FocalSeal and 3M Sealant. The former is a pure synthetic polymeric product, while the latter is semisynthetic.

FocalSeal is made from the macromer which consists of a copolymer of water-soluble polyethylene glycol (PEG) macromolecules with the two ends of each macromolecule capped with synthetic biodegradable oligomers like glycolide, lactide.[156-161] In order to be able to solidify or cure the sealant by a convenient means like light *in situ,* the two terminals of each of the FocalSeal macromer molecule are further capped by acrylates which provide the unsaturated hydrocarbon required for photoinitiated polymerization or curing by uv or visible light as shown in Figure 12.24. Depending on the type and molecular weight of capped biodegradable oligomers, the molecular weight of PEG, and degree of curing, the resulting sealant could have a wide range of biodegradation properties ranging from 1 day to 6 months, for example. The general concern of heat-related tissue necrosis due to *in situ* heat of polymerization has been minimized because the hydrogel-based sealant consists of a very high proportion (>80%) of water which would serve as a very good heat sinker.

PEG-derived crosslinker   Human serum albumin

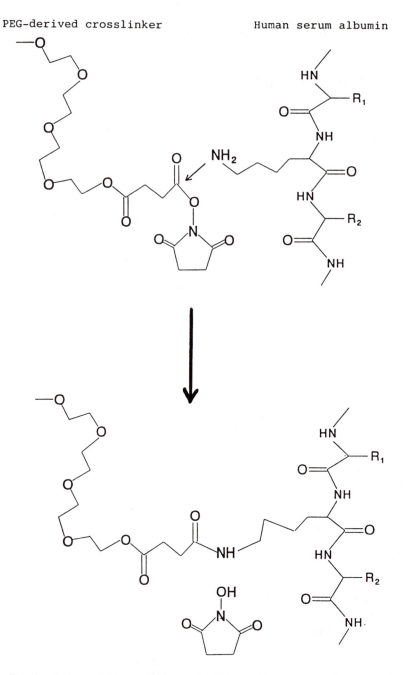

Figure 12.25 The chemical crosslinking or curing reaction between human serum albumin and poly(ethylene glycol) Disuccinimidylsuccinate crosslinker for 3M hydrogel-based tissue adhesives. (From Barrows, T.H., in *Medical Textiles and Biomedical Polymers and Materials,* 1996 Clemson University Conference, Sept. 11-12, 1996, Greenville, SC. With permission.)

The use of FocalSeal tissue sealant has been reported in a variety of clinical environments involving experimental animals, ranging from sealing of air leaks during lung surgery to use as a barrier for isolating a traumatized tissue from surrounding tissues/organs to prevent either tissue adhesion, particularly in abdominal surgery, or restenosis in transluminal balloon coronary angioplasty procedures.

3M tissue sealant is a hybrid of synthetic and natural products and has two basic components: a PEG-derived crosslinker, like PEG disuccinimidylsuccinate and FDA-approved clinical grade human serum albumin.[162,163] The formation of the hydrogel is achieved via the curing or crosslinking reaction between the terminal ester carbon of the PEG-derived crosslinker and the free amine end groups of albumin as shown in Figure 12.25. The biproduct, N-hydroxysuccinimide, is a stable product and appears to be biocompatible and nonmutagenic, nongenotoxic, and nonteratogenic.[163,164] Before curing or crosslinking with serum albumin, the PEG-derived crosslinker alone with molecular weight 3400, however, is cytotoxic in a standard L-929 mouse fibroblast agarose overlay diffusion assay.

This tissue sealant has the *in vitro* tissue bonding strength (measured by peel force) between α-cyanoacrylate and Beriplast® (fibrin glue) on guinea pig skin and the highest bonding strength on collagen among the three tissue adhesives. Preliminary *in vivo* study in dogs and pigs indicates that the 3M sealant appears to be able to stop air leaks in lungs. Such a capability is vital to the volume reduction thoracic surgery for those patients with chronic pulmonary emphysema to improve their quality of life.

REFERENCES

1. Coles, B., van Heerden, J.A., Keys, T.F., and Haldorson, A., Incidence of wound infection for common general surgical procedures, *Surg. Gynecol. Obstet.*, 154, 557, 1982.
2. Bergamini, T.M. and Polk, H.C., Jr., Pharmacodynamics of antibiotic penetration of tissue and surgical prophylaxis, *Surg. Gynecol. Obstet.*, 168, 283, 1989.
3. Brachman, P.S., Dan, B.B., Haley, R.W. et al., Nosocomial surgical infections: incidence and cost, *Surg. Clin. North Am.*, 60, 15, 1980.
4. Cruse, P.J. and Foord, R., The epidemiology of wound infection. A 10-year study of 62,939 wounds, *Surg. Clin. North Am.*, 60, 27, 1980.
5. Sugarman, B. and Young, E.J., *Infections Associated with Prosthetic Devices*, CRC Press, Boca Raton, FL, 1984.
6. Rodeheaver, G.T., Kurtz, L.D., Bellamy, W.T. et al., Biocidal braided sutures, *Arch. Surg.*, 118, 322, 1983.
7. Altemeier, W.A. and Culbertson, W.R., Surgical infection, in *Surgery, Principles and Practice*, 4th ed., Rhoads, J. and Moyer, C., Eds., J.B. Lippincott, Philadelphia, 1970, 48–74.
8. Hermann, G.G., Bagi, P., and Christofferson, I., Early secondary suture versus healing by second intention of incisional abscesses, *Surg. Gynecol. Obstet.*, 167, 16, 1988.
9. Chu, C.C., Tsai, W.C., Yao, J.Y., and Sindy B.L. Sheen, Newly-made antibacterial braided nylon sutures I. *In vitro* qualitative and *in vivo* preliminary biocompatibility study, *J. Biomed. Mater. Res.*, 21(11), 1281, 1987.
10. Tsai, W.C., Chu, C.C., Sindy B.L. Sheen, and Yao, J.Y., Newly-made antibacterial braided nylon sutures II. *In vitro* quantitative study, *Surg. Gynecol. Obstet.*, 165, 207, 1987.
11. Benvenisty, A.I., Tannenbaum, G., Ahlborn, T.N. et al., Control of prosthetic bacterial infection: evaluation of an easily incorporated, tightly bound, silver antibiotic PTFE graft, *J. Surg. Res.*, 44, 1, 1988.
12. Webster, D.A., Spadaro, J.A., Becker, R.O., and Kramer, S., Silver anode treatment of chronic osteomyelitis, *Clin. Orthop.*, 161, 105, 1981.
13. Farrah, S.R. and Erdos, G.W., The production of antibacterial tubing, sutures, and bandages by *in situ* precipitation of metallic salts, *Can. J. Microbiol.*, 37, 445, 1991.
14. Glassman, J.A., Fowler, E.F., and Novak, M.V., Experimental study of sulfonamide impregnated sutures, *Surg. Gynecol. Obstet.*, 78, 359, 1984.
15. Ludewig, R.M., Rudolf, L.E., and Wangensteen, S.U., Reduction of experimental wound infection with iodized gut sutures, *Surg. Gynecol. Obstet.*, 133, 946, 1971.
16. LeVeen, H.H., Falk, G., Mazzopira, F.A. et al., The suppression of experimental wound infections by biocidal sutures, *Surgery*, 64, 610, 1968.
17. Howell, J.J., Chlorhexidine and suture materials, *Br. Med. J.*, 5432, 449, 1965.
18. Echeverria, E. and Olivares, J., Clinical and experimental evaluation of suture material treated with antibiotics, *Am. J. Surg.*, 98, 695, 1959.
19. Singhal, J.P., Singh, J., Ray, A.R., and Singh, H., Antibacterial multifilament nylon sutures, *Biomater. Artif. Cell Immob. Biotech.*, 19, 631, 1991.
20. Guttman, B. and Guttmann, H., Sutures: properties, uses, and clinical investigation, in *Polymeric Biomaterials*, Dumitriu, S., Ed., Marcel Dekker, New York, 1994, chap. 10.
21. Dunn, R.L., Gibson, J.W., and Perkins, B.H., Fibrous delivery systems for antimicrobial agents, *ACS Polym. Mater. Sci. Eng.*, 51, 28, 1984.
22. Allard, S.J. and Song, J.H., Gradual release structures made from fibre spinning techniques, Eur. Patent 0,422,820, 1991.
23. Hill, W.R. and Pillsbury, D.M., *The Pharmacology of Silver*, Williams & Wilkins, Baltimore, 1939.
24. Fox, C.L., Jr., Topical therapy and the development of silver sulfadiazine, *Surg. Gynecol. Obstet.*, 157, 82, 1983.
25. Carr, H.S., Wlodkowski, T.J., and Rosenkranz, H.S., Silver sulfadiazine: In vitro antibacterial activity, *Antimicrob. Agents Chemother.*, 4, 585, 1973.
26. Adesunkanmi, K. and Oyelami, O.A., The pattern and outcome of burn injuries at Wesley Guild Hospital, *J. Tropic. Med. Hyg.*, 97, 108, 1994.

27. Fox, C.L., Jr., Rao, T.N.V., Azmeth, R., Gandhi, S.S., and Modak, S., Comparative evaluation of zinc sulfadiazine and silver sulfadiazine in burn wound infection, *J. Burn Care Rehabil.*, 11, 112, 1990.

28. Cruse, C.W. and Daniels, S., Minor burns treatment using a new drug delivery system with silver sulfadiazine, *South. Med. J.*, 82, 1135, 1989.

29. Dode, H., Hanslo, D., De-Wet, P.M., Millar, A.J.W., and Cywes, S., Efficacy of mupirocin in methicillin-resistant Staphylococcus aureus burn wound infection, *Antimicrob. Agents Chemother.*, 33, 1358, 1989.

30. Rakhry, S.M., Alexander, J., Smith, D., Meyer, A.A., and Peterson, H.D., Regional and institutional variation in burn care, *J. Burn Care Rehabil.*, 16, 86, 1995.

31. Edwards, J.V. and Foster, H.A., The effect of topical antimicrobial agents on the production of toxic shock syndrome toxin-1, *J. Med. Microbiol.*, 41, 408, 1994.

32. Russell, A.D. and Hugo, W.B., Antimicrobial activity and action of silver, *Prog. Med. Chem.* (Netherlands), 31, 351, 1994.

33. Hamilton-Miller, J.M.T., Shah, S., and Smith, C., Silver sulphadiazine: a comprehensive in vitro reassessment, *Chemotherapy*, 39, 405, 1993.

34. Shah, P.M., Modak, S., Fox, C.L., Babu, S.C., Sampath, L., Clauss, R.H., and Stahl, W.M., PTFE graft treated with silver Norfloxacin: drug retention and resistance to bacterial challenge, *J. Surg. Res.*, 42, 298, 1987.

35. Shafik, A., The electrified catheter. Role in sterilizing urine and decreasing bacteriuria, *World J. Urol.*, 11, 183, 1993.

36. Chole, R.A. and Hubbell, R.N., Antimicrobial activity of silastic tympanostomy tubes impregnated with silver oxide: a double-blind randomized multicenter trial, *Arch. Orolaryngol. Head Neck Surg.*, 121, 562, 1995.

37. Jansen, B., Rinck, M., Wolbring, P., Strohmeier, A., and Jahns, T., In vitro evaluation of the antimicrobial efficacy and biocompatibility of a silver-coated central venous catheter, *J. Biomater. Appl.*, 9, 55, 1994.

38. Sioshansi, P., New processes for surface treatment of catheters, *Artif. Organs*, 18, 266, 1994.

39. Gabriel, M.M., Swant, A.D., Simmons, R.B., and Ahearn, D.G., Effects of silver on adherence of bacteria to urinary catheters: in vitro studies, *Curr. Microbiol.*, 30, 17, 1995.

40. Goldschmidt, H., Hahn, U., Salwender, H., Jahns, T., Jansen, B., Wolbring, P., Rinck, M., and Hunstein, W., Prevention of catheter related infections by silver coated central venous catheters in oncological patients after chemotherapy, 34th Interscience Conference on Antimicrobial Agents and Chemotherapy, Orlando, FL, Oct. 4-7, 1994, 194.

41. Bodey, G.P., Zermeno, A., and Raad, I., Novel approach for the prevention of catheter infections: iontophoretic catheter using silver wire, 34th Interscience Conference on Antimicrobial Agents and Chemotherapy, Orlando, FL, Oct. 4-7, 1994.

42. Bach, A., Boehrer, H., Motsch, J., Martin, E., Geiss, H.K., and Sonntag, H.G., Prevention of bacterial colonization of intravenous catheters by antiseptic impregnation of polyurethane polymers, *J. Antimicrob. Chemother.*, 33, 969, 1994.

43. Bach, A., Geiss, M., Geiss, H.K., and Sonntag, H.G., Prevention of catheter-related colonization by silver-sulfadiazine-chlorhexidine (SSC) bonding: results of a pilot study in critical care patients, 33rd Interscience Conference on Antimicrobial Agents and Chemotherapy, New Orleans, LA, Oct. 17-20, 1993, 415.

44. Greenfeld, J., Sampath, L., Baradarian, R., Stylianos, S., and Modak, S., Intravascular placement of silver sulfadiazine-chlorhexidine impregnated catheters (SCC) in swine: evaluation of biofilm (BF) formation and bacterial adherence (BA), 33rd Interscience Conference on Antimicrobial Agents and Chemotherapy, New Orleans, LA, Oct. 17-20, 1993, 415.

45. McLean, R.J.C., Hussian, A.A., Sayer, M., Vincent, P.J., Hughes, D.J., and Smith, T.J.N., Antibacterial activity of multilayer silver-copper surface films on catheter material, *Can. J. Microbiol.*, 39, 895, 1993.

46. Mermel, L.A., Stolz, S.M., and Maki, D.G., Surface antimicrobial activity of heparin-bonded and antiseptic impregnated vascular catheters, *J. Infect. Dis.*, 167, 920, 1993.

47. Spadaro, J.A., *Modern Bioelectricity*, Marino, A.A., Ed., Marcel Dekker, New York, 1988, 629.

48. Spadaro, J.A., Berger, T.J., Barranco, S.D., Chapin, S.E., and Becker, R.O., Antibacterial effects of silver electrodes with weak direct current, *Antimicrob. Agents Chemother.*, 6, 637, 1974.

49. Berger, T.J., Spadaro, J.A., Bierman, R., Chapin, S.E., and Becker, R.O., Antifungal properties of electrically generated metallic ions, *Antimicrob. Agents Chemother.*, 10, 856, 1976.

50. Spadaro, J.A., Webster, D.A., and Becker, R.O., Silver polymethyl methacrylate antibacterial bone cement, *Clin. Orthop.*, 143, 266, 1979.

51. Becker, R.O. and Spadaro, J.A, Treatment of orthopaedic infections with electrically generated silver ions. A preliminary report, *J. Bone Joint Surg.*, 60, 871, 1978.

52. Berger, T.J., Spadaro, J.A., Chapin, S.E., and Becker, R.O., Electrically generated silver ions: quantitative effects on bacterial and mammalian cells, *Antimicrob. Agents Chemother.*, 9, 357, 1976.

53. Hendry, A.T. and Stewart, I.O., Silver-resistant Enterobacteriaceae from hospital patients, *Can. J. Microbiol.*, 25, 915, 1979.

54. Falcone, A.E. and Spadaro, J.A., Inhibitory effects of electrically activated silver material on cutaneous wound bacteria, *Plast. Reconstr. Surg.*, 77, 455, 1986.

55. Spadaro, J.A., Chase, S.E., and Webster, D.A., Bacterial inhibition by electrical activation of percutaneous silver implants, *J. Biomed. Mater. Res.*, 20, 565, 1986.

56. Kaur, P. and Vadehra, D.V., Mechanism of resistance to silver ions in Klebsiella pneumoniae, *Antimicrob. Agents Chemother.*, 29, 165, 1986.

57. Starodub, M.E. and Trevors, J.T., Silver resistance in Escherichia coli R1, *J. Med. Microbiol.*, 29, 101, 1989.

58. Trevors, J.T., Silver resistance and accumulation in bacteria, *Enzyme Microbial Technol.*, 9, 331, 1987.

59. Charley, R.C. and Bull, A.T., Bioaccumulation of silver by a multispecies community of bacteria, *Arch. Microbiol.*, 123, 239, 1979.

60. Pooley, F.D., Bacteria accumulate silver during leaching of sulfide ore minerals, *Nature*, 296, 642, 1982.

61. Silver, S., in *Molecular Biology, Pathogenicity, and Ecology of Bacterial Plasmids*, Levy, S.B. et al., Eds., Plenum Press, New York, 1981, 179.

62. Brierley, C.L., Kelly, D.P., Seal, K.J., and Best, D.J., in *Biotechnology Principles and Applications*, Higgins, J. et al., Eds., Blackwell Scientific, Oxford, 1985, 163.

63. Bragg, P.D. and Rainnie, D.J., The effect of silver ions on the respiratory chain of Escherichia coli, *Can. J. Microbiol.*, 20, 883, 1974.

64. Modak, S.M. and Fox, C.L., Jr., Binding of silver sulfadiazine to the cellular components of Pseudomonas aeruginosa, *Biochem. Pharmacol.*, 22, 2391, 1973.

65. Becker, R.O., *Proc. First Int. Conf. Gold and Silver in Medicine*, The Silver Institute, Washington, D.C., 1987, 227.

66. Dunn, M.G., Doillon, C.J., Berg, R.A., Olson, R.M., and Silver, F.H., Wound healing using a collagen matrix: effect of DC electrical stimulation, *J. Biomed. Mater. Res.*, 22, 191, 1988.

67. Crisp, W.E., Associated Gynecologist, Ltd., Phoenix, AZ, private communication, Dec. 15, 1989.

68. Geronemus, R.G., Merte, P.M. et al., Wound healing. The effects of topical antimicrobial agents, *Arch. Dermatol.*, 115, 1311, 1978.

69. Bellinger, C.G. and Conway, H., Effects of silver nitrate and sulfamylon on epithelial regeneration, *Plast. Reconstr. Surg.*, 45, 582, 1970.

70. McCauley, R.L., Linares, H.A., Pelligrin, V. et al., In vitro toxicity of topical antimicrobial agents to human fibroblasts, *J. Surg. Res.*, 46, 267, 1989.

71. McCauley, R.L., Li, Y.Y., Chopra, V., Herndon, D.N., and Robson, M.C., Cytoprotection of human dermal fibroblasts against silver sulfadiazine using recombinant growth factors, *J. Surg. Res.*, 56, 378, 1994.

72. Deitch, E.A., Marino, A.A., Gillespie, T.E., and Albright, J.A., Silver-nylon: a new antimicrobial agent, *Antimicrob. Agents Chemother.*, 23, 356, 1983.

73. Scher, K.S., Bernstein, J.M., and Jones, C.W., Infectivity of vascular sutures, *Am. Surg.*, 51, 577, 1985.

74. Tyagi, P.K., Gupta, B., and Singh, H., Radiation-induced grafting of 2-hydroxyethyl methacrylate onto polypropylene for biomedical applications. II. Evaluation as antimicrobial suture, *J. Macromol. Sci. Pure Appl. Chem.*, A30, 303, 1993.

75. Gupta, B.D., Tyagi, P.K., and Singh, H., Radiation-induced grafting of 2 hydroxyethylmethacrylate onto polypropylene for biomedical applications I. Effect of synthesis conditions, *J. Macromol. Sci. Chem. A*, 27, 831, 1990.

76. Lewin, M. and Guttmann, H., Method of improving the sorbtion capacity of polymers, U.S. Patent 4,066,387, 1978.

77. Knoop, F.C., Dworzack, D.L., Martig, R.J., Sterpetti, A.V., Bailey, R.T., and Schultz, R.D., Bonding of ofloxacin to polytetrafluoroethylene suture and colonization by *Staphylococcus aureus*, *Curr. Microbiol.*, 20, 27, 1990.

78. Singhal, J.P., Singh, H., and Ray, A.R., Absorbable suture materials: preparation and properties, *J. Macromol. Sci. Rev. Macromol. Chem. Phys.*, C28, 475, 1988.

79. Nakajima, M., Atsumi, K., and Kifune, K., Development of absorbable sutures from chitin, in *Chitin, Chitosan and Related Enzymes*, Zikakis, J.P., Ed., Academic Press, New York, 1984, 407–410.

80. Tachibana, M., Yaita, A., Taniura, H., Fukasawa, K., Nagasue, N., and Nakamura, T., The use of chitin as a new absorbable suture material — an experimental study, *Jpn. J. Surg.*, 218, 533, 1988.

81. Muzzarelli, R., *In vivo* biochemical significance of chitin-based medical items, in *Polymeric Biomaterials*, Dumitriu, S., Ed., Marcel Dekker, New York, 1994, 179.

82. Balitsky, K.L., Umansky, V.Y., Tarakhovsky, A.M., Andronova, T.M., and Ivanov, V.T., Glucosaminylmuramyl dipeptide-induced changes in murine macrophage metabolism, *Int. J. Immunopharmacol.*, 11, 429, 1989.

83. Suzuki, K., Mikami, T., Okawa, Y., Tokoro, A., Suzuki, S., and Suzuki, M., Antitumor effect of hexa-*N*-acetylchitohexaose and chitohexaose, *Carbohydr. Res.*, 151, 403, 1986.

84. Tokoro, A.N., Tatewaki, N., Suzuki, K., Mikami, T., Suzuki, S., and Suzuki, M., Growth-inhibitory effect of hexa-*N*-acetylchitohexaose and chitohexaose against Meth-A solid tumor, *Chem. Pharmacol.*, 36, 784, 1988.

85. Tsukada, K., Matsumoto, T., Aizawa, K., Tokoro, A., Naruse, R., Suzuki, S., and Suzuki, M., Antimetastatic and growth-inhibitory effects of *N*-acetylchitohexaose in mice bearing Lewis lung carcinoma, *Jpn. J. Cancer Res.*, 81, 259, 1990.

86. Suzuki, S., Suzuki, K., Tokoro, A., Okawa, Y., and Suzuki, M., Immunopotentiating effect of *N*-acetyl chitooligosaccharides, in *Chitin in Nature and Technology*, Muzzarelli, R.A.A., Jeuniaux, C., and Gooday, G.W., Eds., Plenum Press, New York, 1986, chapter 12.

87. Prudden, J.F., Migel, P., Hanson, P., Friedrich, L., and Balassa, L., The discovery of a potent pure chemical wound-healing accelerator, *Am. J. Surg.*, 119, 560, 1970.

88. Tokura, S., Nishi, N., and Noguchi, J., Studies on chitin. III. Preparation of chitin fibers, *Polym. J.*, 11, 781, 1979.

89. Austin, P.R. and Brine, C.J., Chitin films and fibers, U.S. Patent 4,029,727, 1977, June.

90. Capozza, R.C., Spinning and shaping poly-(N-acetyl-D-glucosamine), U.S. Patent 3,988,411, 1976, October.

91. Kifune, K., Inoue, K., and Mori, S., Process for the production of chitin fibers, U.S. Patent 4,431,601, 1984.

92. Sashiwa, H., Saimoto, H., Shigemasa, Y., Ogawa, R., and Tokura, S., Lysozyme susceptibility of partially deacetylated chitin, *Int. J. Biol. Macromol.*, 12, 295, 1990.

93. Fukamizo, T., Minematsu, T., Yanase, Y., Hayashi, K., and Goto, S., Substrate size dependence of lysozyme-catalysed reactions, *Arch. Biochem. Biophys.*, 250, 312, 1986.

94. Fukamizo, T. and Goto, S., Lysozyme-catalyzed reaction in continuous flow system, *J. Biochem.*, 109, 416, 1991.

95. Muzzarelli, R.A.A., *Chitin*, Pergamon Press, Oxford, 1977, 87–99.

96. Muzzarelli, R.A.A., Amphoteric derivatives of chitosan and their biological significance, in *Chitin and Chitosan*, Skjak-Braek, G., Anthonsen, T., and Sandford, P., Eds., Elsevier, Amsterdam, 1989.

97. Muzzarelli, R.A.A., Carboxymethylated chitins and chitosans, *Carbohydr. Polym.*, 8, 1, 1988.

98. Tamura, K., Hitomi, S., Natsume, T., Kobayashi, T., Kuwabara, O., Ohonishi, T., and Nakamura, K., Changes of elastic polyvinyl alcohol hydrogel after implantation, *Jpn. J. Artif. Organs,* 21, 176, 1992.

99. Iio, K., Minoura, N., Aiba, S., Nagura, M., and Kodama, M., Cell growth on poly(vinyl alcohol) hydrogel membranes containing biguanido groups, *J. Biomed. Mater. Res.*, 28, 459, 1994.

100. Tomita, N., Nagata, N., Ueda, Y., Tamai, S., Hyon, S.H., Ikeuchi, K., and Ikada, Y., Applications of high-strength poly(vinyl alcohol) fiber to biomaterials, in *Biomaterial-Tissue Interface*, Advances in Biomaterials, vol. 10, Doherty, P.J. et al., Eds., Elsevier Science, 1992, 483.

101. Hyon, S.H., Cha, W.I., and Ikada, Y., Preparation of high strength and modulus poly(vinyl alcohol) fibers, in *32nd International Symposium on Macromolecules*, Kyoto, Japan, Aug. 1-6, 1988, 798.

102. Liu, C.K., Brewer, J. and Kokish, M., Modified polypropylene suture with ionomer, *20th Annual Meeting of the Society for Biomaterials*, Boston, MA, April 5-9, 1994, 477.

103. Liu, C.K. and Brewer, J., Filament fabricated from a blend ofionomer resin and nonionic thermoplastic resin, U.S. Patent 5,284,489, US Surgical, 1994.

104. Liu, C.K., Suture fabricated from syndiotactic polypropylene, U.S. Patent 5,269,807, US Surgical, Dec. 14, 1993.

105. Liu, C.K., Medical fibers spun from polypropylene, *13th Southern Biomedical Engineering Conference*, Washington, D.C., April 16-17, 1994, 748.

106. Liu, C.K. and Brewer, J., Polyetherimide ester suture and its method of manufacture and method of use, U.S. Patent 5,225,485, US Surgical, July 6, 1993.

107. Liu, C.K., Brewer, J., and Kokish, M., New elastomeric suture from polyetherimide ester, *20th Annual Meeting of the Society for Biomaterials*, Boston, MA, April 5-9, 1994, 243.

108. Chu., C.C., Mechanical properties of suture materials: an important characterization, *Ann. Surg.*, 193, 365, 1981.

109. Kurtz, L.D., Preparation of composite surgical sutures, U.S Patent 4,470,941, Bioresearch Inc., Sept. 11, 1984.

110. Guttman, B., Lewin, M., and Kurtz, L., Composite surgical sutures with high knot security, *IUPAC International Symposium on Polymers for Advanced Technologies,* Jerusalem, 1987.

111. Shalaby, S.W., Synthetic absorbable polyesters, in *Biomedical Polymers: Designed-to-Degrade Systems*, Shalaby, S.W., Ed., Hanser Publisher, New York, 1994, chap. 1.

112. Shalaby, S.W. and Koelmel, D.F., U.S. Patent 4,441,496, Ethicon, 1984.

113. Bezwada, R.S., Shalaby, S.W., Newman, H.D., and Kafrauy, A., U.S. Patent 4,653,497, Ethicon, 1987.

114. Bezwada, R.S., Shalaby, S.W., Newman, H.D., and Kafrauy, A., U.S. Patent 4,643,191, Ethicon, 1987.

115. Kimura, Y., Shirotani, K., Yamane, H., and Kitao, T., Ring-opening polymerization of 3-(S)[(alkyloxycarbonyl) methyl]-1,4-dioxane-2,5-dione: a new route to a poly(α-hydroxy acid) with pendant carboxyl groups, *Macromolecules*, 21, 3338, 1988.

116. Kimura, Y., Biodegradable polymers, in *Biomedical Applications of Polymeric Materials*, Tsuruta, T., Hayashi, T., Kataoka, K., Ishihara, K., and Kimura, Y., Eds., CRC Press, Boca Raton, 1993, 163.

117. Urban, E., King, M.W., Guidoin, R., Laroche, G., Marois, Y., Martin, L., Cardou, A., and Douville, Y., Why make monofilament sutures out of polyvinylidene fluoride? *Am. Soc. Artif. Intern. Org.*, 40, 145, 1994.

118. Cutright, D.E. and Hunsuck, E.E., Tissue reaction to the biodegradable polylactic acid suture, *Oral Surg.*, 31, 134, 1971.

119. Jamshidi, K., Hyon, S.H., Nakamura, T., Ikada, Y., Shimizuand, Y., and Teramatsu, Y., *In vitro* degradation of poly-L-lactide fibers, in *Advances in Biomaterials, Biological and Biomechanical Performance of Biomaterials*, Christel, P., Meunier, A., and Lee, A.C.J., Eds., Elsevier, Amsterdam, 1986, 227.

120. Lam, K.H., Nijenhuis, A.J., Bartels, H., Postema, A.R., Jonkman, M.F., Pennings, A.J., and Nieuwenhuis, P., Reinforced poly(L-lactic acid) fibres as suture material, *J. Appl. Biomater.*, 6(3), 191, 1995.

121. Lee, K.H., Chu, C.C., and Freed, J., Aminoxyl-containing radical spin labeling in polymers and copolymers, U.S. Patent 5,516,881, May 14, 1996.

122. Zhdanov, R.I., *Bioactive Spin Labels,* Springer-Verlag, Berlin, 1992.

123. Snyder, S.H. and Bredt, D.S., Biological roles of nitric oxide, *Sci. Amer.*, 5, 68, 1992.

124. Moncada, S., Palmer, R.M.J., and Higgs, E.A., Nitric oxide: physiology, pathophysiology and pharmacology, in *Pharmacol. Rev.*, 43, 2, June 1991, 109-142.

125. Bredt, D.S., Hwang, P.M., Glatt, C.E., Lowenstein, C., Reed, R.R., and Snyder, S.H., Cloned and expressed nitric oxide synthase structurally resembles cytochrome P-450 reductase, *Nature,* 351(6329), 714, 1991.

126. Karupiah, G., Xie, Q.W., Buller, R.M.L., Nathan, C., Duarte, C., and Macmicking, J.D., Inhibition of viral replication by interferon-gamma-induced nitric oxide synthase, *Science,* 261(5127), 1445, 1993.

127. Esumi, H. and Tannenbaum, S.R., U.S.-Japan Cooperative Cancer Research Program: Seminar on nitric oxide synthase and carcinogenesis (Williamsburg, VA, January 19-20, 1993), *Cancer Res.,* 54(1), 297, 1994.

128. Park, K.H., Rubin, L.E., Gross, S.S., and Levy, R., Nitric oxide is a mediator of hypoxic coronary vasodilation relation to adenosine and cyclooxygenase-derived metabolites, *Circulation Res.,* 71(4), 992, 1992.

129. Darley-Usmar, V., Wiseman, H., and Halliwell, B., Nitric oxide and oxygen radicals: a question of balance, *FEBS Letters,* 369(2-3), 131,1995.

130. Sagar, S.M., Singh, G., Hodson, D.I., and Whitton, A.C., Nitric oxide and anti-cancer therapy, *Cancer Treatment Review,* 21(2), 159, 1995.

131. Morris, C.J., Trenam, C.W., and Earl, J.R., Reactive oxygen species in skin inflammation, in, *Handbook of Immunopharmacology: Immunopharmacology of Free Radical Species,* Academic Press, San Diego, 1995, 113-125.

132. Moilanen, E. and Vapaatalo, H., Nitric oxide in inflammation and immune response, *Ann. Med.,* 27(3), 359, 1995.

133. Liu, R.H. and Hotchkiss, J.H., Potential genotoxicity of chronically elevated nitric acid: A review, *Mutation Research,* 339(2), 73, 1995.

134. Pheng, L.H., Francoeur, C., and Denis, M., The involvement of nitric oxide in a mouse model of adult respiratory distress syndrome, *Inflammation,* 19(5), 599, 1995.

135. Amin, A.R., Vyas, P., Attur, M., Leszczynska-Piziak, J., and Patel, I.R., The mode of action of aspirin-like drugs: effect on inducible nitric oxide synthase, *Proceedings of Natl. Acad. Sci.,* 92(17), 7926, 1995.

136. Star, R.A., Rajora, N., Huang, J., Stock, R.C., Catania, A., and Lipton, J.M., Evidence of autocrine modulation of macrophage nitric oxide synthase by alpha melanocyte stimulating hormone, *Proceedings of Natl. Acad. Sci.,* 92(17), 8016, 1995.

137. Ikeda, M., Suzuki, M., Watarai, K., Sagai, M., and Tomita, T., Impairment of endothelium-dependent relaxation by diesel exhaust particles in rat thoracic aotra, *Japn. J. Pharmacol.,* 68(2), 183, 1995.

138. Barnes, P.J., Nitric oxide and airway disease, *Annals of Medicine,* 27(3), 389, 1005.

139. Ganz, M.B., Kasner, S.E., and Unwin, R.J., Nitric oxide alters cytosolic potassium in cultured glomerular mesangial cells, *Am. J. Physiol.,* 268(6 Part 2), F1081, 1995.

140. Lovchik, J.A., Lyons, C.R., and Lypscomb, M.F., A role for gamma interferon-induced nitric oxide in pulmonary clearance of cryptococcus neoformans, *Am. J. Respir. Cell & Mole. Biol.,* 13(1), 116, 1995.

141. Dusting, G.J., Nitric oxide in cardiovascular disorders, *J. Vasc. Res.,* 32(3), 143, 1995.

142. Halliwell, B., Oxygen radicals, nitric oxide and human inflammatory joint disease, *Ann. Rheum. Dis.,* 54(6), 505, 1995.

143. Wink, D.A., Cook, J.A., Krishna, M.C., Hanbauer, I., Degraff, W., Gamson, J., and Mitchell, J.B., Nitric oxide protects agains alkyl peroxide-mediated cytotoxicity: Further insights into the role nitric oxide plays in oxidative stress, *Arch. Biochem. Biophys.,* 319(2), 402, 1995.

144. Sotomayor, E.M., Dinapoli, M.R., Calderon, C., Colsky, A., Fu, Y.X., and Lopez, D.M., Decreased macrophage-mediated cytotoxicity in mammary-tumor-bearing mice is related to alteration of nitric-oxide production and-or release, *Int. J. Cancer,* 60(5), 660, 1995.

145. Elliott, S.N., McKnight, W., Cirino, G., and Wallace, J.L., A nitric oxide-releasing nonsteroidal anti-inflammatory drug accelerates gastric ulcer healing in rats, *Gastroenterology,* 109(2), 524, 1995

146. Wallace, J.L., Cirino, G., McKnight, G.W., and Elliott, S.N., Reduction of gastrointestinal injury in acute endotoxic shock by flurbiprofen nitroxybutylester, *Europ. J. Pharmacol.,* 280(1), 63, 1995.

147. Schmidt, H.H. and Walter, U., NO at work, *Cell,* 78, 919, 1994.

148. Nussler, A.K., Billiar, T.R., and Simmons, R.L., Inducible nitric oxide synthase: Its role in inflammation, sepsis, and shock, in, *Modulation of the Inflammatory Response in Severe Sepsis,* J.M. Telladoo et al., Eds., Progress in Surgery, Vol.20, S. Karger AG, Basel, A.K., Switzerland, 1995,

149. Francoeur, C. and Denis, M., Nitric oxide and interleukin-8 as inflammatory components of cystic fibrosis, *Inflammation,* 19(5), 587, 1995.

150. Tiollier, J., Constancis, A., Gagnieu, C. et al., Novel developments of collagen/gelatin surgical adhesives for surgical soft tissue application, 21st Ann. Meet. Society for Biomaterials and 27th Biomaterials Symposium, San Francisco, CA., March 18-22, 1995.

151. Tiollier, J., DuPont, D., Rossin, D., Lathuilliere, S., and Constancis, A., Colcys as surgical adhesives: in vivo characterization and biocompatibility, 21st Ann. Meet. Society for Biomaterials and 27th Biomaterials Symposium, San Francisco, CA., March 18-22, 1995.

152. Constancis, A., Barc, G., and Tiollier, J., Colcys as surgical adhesives: ex vivo characterization of mechanical and adhesive, 21st Ann. Meet. Society for Biomaterials and 27th Biomaterials Symposium, San Francisco, CA., March 18-22, 1995.

153. DuPont, D., Rossin, D., Lathuilliere, S., Tardy, M., Gravagna, P., and Tiollier, J., New surgical sealant (Glue) based on controlled oxidized collagen: ex vivo and in vivo characterization, 21st Ann. Meet. Society for Biomaterials and 27th Biomaterials Symposium, San Francisco, CA., March 18-22, 1995.

154. Tardy, M., Gravagna, P., Revet, L., Uhlrich, S., Tiollier, J., and Tayot, J.L., New surgical sealant (Glue) based on controlled oxidized collagen: design and physico-chemical characterization, 21st Ann. Meet. Society for Biomaterials and 27th Biomaterials Symposium, San Francisco, CA., March 18-22, 1995.

155. Leung, J.C. and Clark, J.G., Biocompatible monomer and polymer compositions, U.S. Patent 5,328,687, July 12, 1994.

156. Sawhney, A.S., Pathak, C.P., and Hubbell, J.A., Bioerodible hydrogels based on photopolymerized poly(ethylene glycol)-co-poly(α-hydroxy acid) diacrylate macromers, *Macromolecules,* 26, 581, 1993.

157. Sawhney, A.S., Pathak, C.P., van Rensburg, J.J., Dunn, R.C., and Hubbell, J.A., Optimization of photopolymerized bioerodible hydrogel properties for adhesion prevention, *J. Biomed. Mater. Res.,* 28, 831, 1994.

158. Hill-West, J.L., Chowdhury, S.M., Slepian, M.J., and Hubbell, J.A., Inhibition of thrombosis and intimal thickening by *in situ* photopolymerization of thin hydrogel barriers, *Proc. Natl. Acad. Sci., USA,* 91, 5967, 1994.

159. Hill-West, J.L., Chowdhury, S.M., Sawhney, A.S., Pathak, C.P., Dunn, R.C., and Hubbell, J.A., Prevention of postoperative adhesions in the rat by *in situ* photopolymerization of bioresorbable hydrogel barriers, *Obstet. Gynecol.,* 83, 59, 1994.

160. Lyman, M.L. and Sawhney, A.S., Design of a synthetic pneumosealant, 5th World Biomaterials Congress, Toronto, Canada, May 29-June 2, 1996, 212.

161. Lyman, M.L., Pichon, D., Jarrett, P.K., Rudowsky, R., and Sawhney, A.S., Use of a synthetic photopolymerized biodegradable hydrogel as a pneumosealant, 5th World Biomaterials Congress, Toronto, Canada, May 29-June 2, 1996, 313.

162. Barrows, T.H., Truong, M.T., Lewis, T.W., Grussing, D.M., Kato, K.H., Gysbers, J.E., and Lamprecht, E.G., Evaluation of a new tissue sealant materials: Serum albumin crosslinked *in vivo* with polyethylene glycol, 5th World Biomaterials Congress, Toronto, Canada, May 29-June 2, 1996, 8.

163. Truong, M.T., Barrows, T.H., and Wilson, T.J., In vitro analysis of mechanical properties of a new tissue sealant material: Polyethylene glycol crosslinked serum albumin, 5th World Biomaterials Congress, Toronto, Canada, May 29-June 2, 1996, 73.

164. Dannenberg, N-hydroxy-scuuinimid. Eine nicht krebserzeugende N-hydroxy-Verbindung (N-hydroxysuccinimide, a non-carcinogenic N-hydroxy compound), *Z. Krebsforsch,* 76, 216, 1971.

Index